Accession no.
36059302

WITHDRAWN £32.99

29/2/8
9

FACULTY OF HEALTH + SOCIAL CARE
Library
3 1 AUG 2010
Wirral Campus
Clatterbridge
UNIVERSITY OF CHESTER

KU-508-382

WIRRAL EDUCATION CENTRE
LIBRARY
0151 604 72

URINARY & FECAL INCONTINENCE

CURRENT MANAGEMENT CONCEPTS

URINARY
&
FECAL
INCONTINENCE
CURRENT MANAGEMENT CONCEPTS

DOROTHY B. DOUGHTY, MN, RN, FAAN, CWOCN

Director, Wound Ostomy Continence Nursing Education Center
Emory University
Atlanta, Georgia

THIRD EDITION

LIBRARY

ACC. No | DEPT.

CLASS No.
616.62 Dou

UNIVERSITY
OF CHESTER

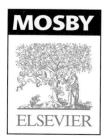

MOSBY

ELSEVIER

MOSBY
ELSEVIER

11830 Westline Industrial Drive
St. Louis, Missouri 63146

URINARY & FECAL INCONTINENCE, CURRENT
MANAGEMENT CONCEPTS
Copyright © 2006, Elsevier, Inc. All rights reserved.

ISBN-13: 978-0-323-03135-6
ISBN-10: 0-323-03135-8

No part of this publication may be reproduced or transmitted in any form or by any means, electronic or mechanical, including photocopying, recording, or any information storage and retrieval system, without permission in writing from the publisher. Permissions may be sought directly from Elsevier's Rights Department: phone: (+1) 215 239 3804 (US) or (+44) 1865 843830 (UK); fax: (+44) 1865 853333; e-mail: healthpermissions@ elsevier.com. You may also complete your request on-line via the Elsevier website at http://www.elsevier.com/ permissions.

Notice

Nursing is an ever-changing field. Standard safety precautions must be followed, but as new research and clinical experience broaden our knowledge, changes in treatment and drug therapy may become necessary or appropriate. Readers are advised to check the most current product information provided by the manufacturer of each drug to be administered to verify the recommended dose, the method and duration of administration, and contraindications. It is the responsibility of the licensed prescriber, relying on experience and knowledge of the patient, to determine dosages and the best treatment for each individual patient. Neither the publisher nor the author assumes any liability for any injury and/or damage to persons or property arising from this publication.

The Publisher

Previous editions copyrighted 1991, 2000

ISBN-13: 978-0-323-03135-6
ISBN-10: 0-323-03135-8

Executive Publisher: Darlene Como
Developmental Editor: Barbara Watts
Publishing Services Manager: Jeffrey Patterson
Project Manager: Jeanne Genz
Designer: Andrea Lutes

Working together to grow
libraries in developing countries

www.elsevier.com | www.bookaid.org | www.sabre.org

ELSEVIER   BOOK AID International   Sabre Foundation

Printed in the United States of America

Last digit is the print number: 9 8 7 6 5 4 3 2

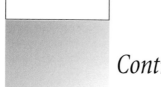

Contributors

DONNA ZIMMARO BLISS, PhD, RN, FAAN
Professor
University of Minnesota School of Nursing
Minneapolis, Minnesota

LEA R. CRESTODINA, MSN, RN, GNP, CWOCN, CDE
Assistant Director, Wound Ostomy Continence Nursing
  Education Center
Emory University
Atlanta, GA

JOANN ERMER-SELTUN, MSN, RN CWOCN, ARNP
Family Nurse Practitioner
Mercy Medical Center North Iowa
Women's Health Center Continence Clinic
Mason City, Iowa

MIKEL L. GRAY, PhD, FNP, PNP, CUNP, CCCN, FAAN
Professor and Nurse Practitioner
University of Virginia
Department of Urology and School of Nursing
Charlottesville, Virginia

MARGARET McLEAN HEITKEMPER, PhD, RN, FAAN
Professor and Chairwoman
Department of Biobehavioral Nursing and Health Systems
University of Washington
Seattle, Washington

LINDA L. JENSEN, BS, RN, BCIAPC
Clinical Research Nurse
Colon and Rectal Surgery Associates
Minneapolis, Minnesota

ANNE K. JINBO, MSN, MPH, CWOCN, CPNP
Wound, Ostomy, Continence Coordinator
Kapiolani Medical Center for Women and Children
and
Kapiolani Medical Center at Pali Momi
Honolulu, Hawaii

MARTA KRISSOVICH, MS, RN, CNS, NP, CCCN
Continence Consultant
New Assurance Continence Consultants
Heber City, Utah

DEBORAH LEKAN-RUTLEDGE, MSN, RNC, CCCN
Duke University School of Nursing
Durham, North Carolina

KATHERINE N. MOORE, PhD, RN, CCCN
Associate Professor
Faculty of Nursing University of Alberta Edmonton
Alberta, Canada

JOANNE P. ROBINSON, PhD, APRN, BC
Associate Professor
Rutgers, The State University of New Jersey
College of Nursing
Newark, New Jersey

JOANN MERCER SMITH, BSN, RN, CWOCN, CRNI
Clinical Specialist
Medical Services and Support
C.R. Bard, Inc.
Covington, Georgia

MARIALIANA STARK, DrPH, APRN, PNP
Assistant Professor
University of Hawaii at Manoa
School of Nursing and Dental Hygiene
Honolulu, Hawaii

DONNA L. THOMPSON, MSN, CRNP, CCCN
Assistant Professor of Nursing
Neumann College
Aston, Pennsylvania
and
Continence Specialist
Fair Acres Geriatric Center
Lima, Pennsylvania

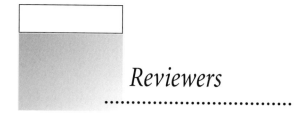

Reviewers

JUDY A. DUTCHER, MSN, APRN-BC, CWOCN
Director of Clinical Services
Connecticut Support Services, LLC
Plainville, Connecticut

DIANA PARKER, BSN, MS, CWOCN
Wound, Ostomy, and Continence Nurse Specialist
St. Joseph Hospital
Bellingham, Washington

NANCY S. WALSH, BS, RN, CWOCN
Wound, Ostomy, and Continence Nurse
Greenwich Hospital
Greenwich, Connecticut

Preface

··

When the first edition of this text was published in 1991, incontinence was beginning to gain recognition as a very prevalent condition and one that significantly affected the quality of life. Current studies indicate that it remains very common and that it affects individuals across their life span. Although it is most frequent in women and the elderly, enuresis is a common problem for children, and stress incontinence is reported among nulliparous female athletes. Fortunately, the increasing awareness of incontinence as a significant health care problem has stimulated research into its causes, presentation, and management; as a result, we have clearer insights into the mechanisms of incontinence and, even more importantly, into options for correction or management. These insights and options are reflected throughout the pages of this text.

The emphasis in this text is on principle-based nursing management. It is clear that optimal continence care is multidisciplinary in focus, because many individuals will require physician evaluation and some will require pharmacologic or surgical intervention. However, most of the preventive strategies and behavioral interventions fall within the domain of nursing. The nurse is frequently the first to detect the patient's problem with bladder or bowel function, and nurses have traditionally been charged with providing for containment and skin care, that is, *in*continence management. The nurse who has a firm grasp of the physiologic and pathologic mechanisms affecting controlled elimination is prepared to provide much more than just containment or skin care; she or he is prepared to provide continence care, that is, care directed toward restoration of continence. Effective continence care is dependent on thorough assessment, accurate identification of the causative and contributing factors, and implementation of a comprehensive management plan (which may include referrals to other health care providers). This text provides an in-depth review of the physiology of continence, the pathologic mechanisms producing incontinence, and current treatment options for the various types of incontinence, with an emphasis on behavioral therapy. Chapter 1 also provides a profile of the qualifications and competencies that define a continence care nurse.

The organization of the text is designed to support the clinician in acquiring and accessing the information needed to provide comprehensive continence care across the life span. The text includes a thorough review of normal voiding physiology and normal bowel function as a basis for understanding the various disorders. Because effective management of any individual with urinary incontinence begins with determination of the "type" of incontinence and with correction of reversible factors, Chapter 12 provides in-depth guidelines for comprehensive assessment of the individual with urinary incontinence or voiding dysfunction, and Chapter 3 addresses transient incontinence and reversible factors. Many of the chapters on urinary incontinence are devoted to a particular type of incontinence; this organizational approach is based on the fact that the pathology, presentation, and treatment options differ according to the specific type of incontinence or voiding dysfunction. However, there are some universal challenges in management of the individual with lower urinary tract dysfunction, and these are addressed in chapters on containment devices, absorptive products, and catheter management.

The chapters on bowel dysfunction address the most common issues and problems faced in the management of these individuals: the pathology and management of diarrhea, constipation, irritable bowel syndrome, and fecal incontinence. The focus throughout these chapters is on accurate assessment and individualized management, with the primary goal being restoration of normal bowel function and the secondary goal being effective management of any residual dysfunction.

Because the pediatric population presents unique problems and challenges in terms of bowel and bladder dysfunction, Chapter 16 provides a comprehensive review of bowel and bladder management in this population.

As in the previous editions, each chapter is preceded by behavioral objectives and is followed by review questions and answers. These features are provided to assist the clinician to assess her or his level of comprehension and may be used either as a "pretest" or as a "posttest."

It is exciting to see the many advances and changes in continence care. I am grateful to all of the authors for taking the time and expending the effort to share their knowledge of current concepts in continence care, and I am grateful to you, the reader, for your own commitment to continence!

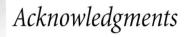

Acknowledgments

I extend sincere appreciation to the following people; without their help this book would not have been possible:

My husband, Mac, who has provided nonstop computer assistance and moral support, stepped over the paper stacks, met many of my home obligations, and tolerated my frequent nonavailability

My parents, Warren and Vicky Beckley, who taught me the importance of lifelong learning and accomplishment

Barbara Watts, my Mosby editor, for her guidance, support, and *patience*

Dorothy B. Doughty

Contents

·····························

CHAPTER 1

Introductory Concepts

DOROTHY B. DOUGHTY & LEA R. CRESTODINA

OBJECTIVES

1. Identify factors that contribute to the lack of accurate data regarding prevalence and incidence of urinary and fecal incontinence.
2. Describe current data regarding prevalence of urinary and fecal incontinence among the following populations: children, community-dwelling adults, institutionalized elders.
3. Describe the physical, psychosocial, and financial effects of incontinence.
4. Define the following terms: stress incontinence, overactive bladder/urge incontinence, acute and chronic retention, neurogenic lower tract dysfunction, enuresis, functional incontinence.
5. Describe current trends in assessment and management of the incontinent individual.
6. Describe the role of the continence care nurse.

Incontinence is not a newly discovered clinical problem—its occurrence and impact have been documented for decades. However, until recently it was generally "accepted" as an inevitable consequence of childbearing or aging, and there was little attention or research devoted to understanding either its causes or its potential cures; containment and skin protection were identified as the goals of care. The geriatrician Bernard Isaacs characterized incontinence as one of the "giants" dominating the care of geriatric patients and suggested that until recently incontinence could be used as an example of the "inverse care law, which states that the more common a condition is, the less attention is devoted to it."[1] Fortunately, these attitudes are changing, and incontinence is now recognized as being both significant and frequently reversible. This change is reflected in the growing number of texts, articles, and research reports devoted to the assessment and management of the incontinent individual. The inclusion of urinary incontinence (UI) in the first group of clinical conditions to be addressed by the AHCPR (Agency for Health Care Policy and Research) Guidelines is potent testimony to the prevalence and cost of incontinence in the United States and to the confusion among health care practitioners as to its management.

Although incontinence is frequently associated with physical complications such as skin breakdown and falls, its greatest impact is usually on the individual's or caregiver's quality of life. Because it is more likely to affect *quality* of life than *length* of life, its effect is frequently minimized. In addition, continence care is typically provided in the home, outpatient, or long-term care setting as opposed to the acute care setting, and effective management frequently involves behavioral therapy as opposed to surgery or medications. All these factors contribute to the perception that incontinence is not a significant medical problem. The fact that most physicians lack interest in incontinence creates a tremendous opportunity for the continence care nurse; she or he can play a major role in community education and casefinding as well as in individual patient assessment and management. Effective intervention for the incontinent individual involves assessment and management of psychosocial factors as well as correction or management of the physical factors causing or contributing to the incontinence. This chapter addresses the prevalence and impact of incontinence, currently accepted terminology and classification systems for the various "types" of incontinence, barriers to continence care, and current guidelines for management of incontinence, including the role of the continence care nurse. Subsequent chapters address the physiology of normal voiding and defecation, assessment of the incontinent individual, and the pathology, presentation, and management of each type of incontinence.

DEFINITIONS

A single episode of incontinence is fairly easy to define: the involuntary and uncontrolled passage of urine or stool or both. However, it is more difficult to define the *condition* of incontinence, because most incontinent individuals experience some combination of controlled and uncontrolled elimination of urine and stool. Multiple definitions have been used in the study of UI; the two most commonly cited are the definitions proposed by the International Continence Society (ICS) and by the Urinary Incontinence Guidelines Panel. The ICS defines UI as "the complaint of any involuntary leakage of urine,"[2] and the Urinary Incontinence Guidelines Panel defines UI as "the involuntary loss of urine which is sufficient to be a problem."[3] Both of these definitions are primarily subjective. Although subjective definitions can be problematic when used as the basis for prevalence studies, they capture the essence of the incontinence problem—it *is* intensely subjective, in that the volume and frequency of leakage perceived as very problematic by one individual may be a minor nuisance to another. (Incontinence is much like pain; it is a problem if the patient or caregiver perceives it as such.) The ICS states that incontinence always requires further definition/description to include factors such as type, frequency, and severity of the leakage, the effect on quality of life, and whether or not the individual wishes to seek treatment.[2] Some authors suggest the use of a validated tool to "quantify" the severity or impact of the incontinence; these severity indices are typically based on the frequency of the incontinence and the quantity of urine lost or the interference with the individual's quality of life.[4] The Second International WHO (World Health Organization) Consultation on Incontinence recommends the severity index developed by Sandvik and colleagues;[5] this tool utilizes frequency and volume of leakage to classify the incontinence as slight, moderate, or severe (Box 1-1). This index has been validated

BOX 1-1   Severity Index

Questions Used to Assess the Degree of Urinary Incontinence in Women
How often do you experience leakage?
1. Less than once a month
2. A few times a month
3. A few times a week
4. Every day and/or night
How much urine do you leak each time?
1. Drops
2. Small splashes
3. More
The severity index is created by multiplying the results of these two questions.
In the three-level severity index, responses to the second question are aggregated into drops (1) and more (2) and are then multiplied times the frequency, resulting in the following index values (1-8):
   1-2 = Slight
   3-4 = Moderate
   6-8 = Severe
The four-level severity index is based on the following index values (1-12):
   1-2 = Slight
   3-6 = Moderate
   8-9 = Severe
   12 = Very severe

Reprinted with permission from Dr. Hogne Sandvik.

against pad weight tests and used in a number of studies;[6,7] the results indicate a positive and significant correlation between the severity index and the patient's subjective rating of "bother" associated with the UI.

The condition of fecal incontinence also lacks a "consensus" definition. *Fecal incontinence* is usually defined as the involuntary passage of liquid or solid stool (or as loss of voluntary control of stool elimination), whereas the term *anal incontinence* includes the inability to control the elimination of flatus.[8,9] Many authors include some measure of social impact in their definition; for example, the WHO defines anal incontinence as "the involuntary loss of flatus, liquid, or solid stool that is a social or hygienic problem."[10] Fecal incontinence may be further defined in terms of sensory and cognitive awareness (recognized, or "urge" incontinence, versus unrecognized, or "passive" incontinence) and in terms of etiology (functional versus organic).[9,11]

PREVALENCE AND INCIDENCE
General Concepts

Prevalence and incidence rates provide us with insight into the scope and magnitude of the problem of incontinence. Prevalence refers to the total number of individuals with incontinence (as compared with the total population being studied) at a specific point in time; prevalence data provide a static view of incontinence. Incidence is defined as the number (or percentage) of individuals who develop incontinence over a specific period of time; incidence data provide a dynamic view of the problem of incontinence.

Incontinence is generally studied within a specific population group; for this reason, overall prevalence rates (that is, prevalence across the life span) are not available for UI. The prevalence data that are available are difficult to summarize and impossible to generalize to the general population because of extremely wide variations (that is, 2% to 55%).[12] These variations in prevalence rates can be attributed to a lack of conformity among prevalence studies in the following areas: definition of UI, demographics of the study population, survey method, and study design.[6,13] The definition of UI obviously significantly affects prevalence outcomes; some researchers classified respondents as incontinent if they had ever experienced an episode of uncontrolled or unexpected urinary loss, whereas others used definitions that addressed the frequency or severity of urine loss.[6,13-15] Study methodology also significantly affects prevalence rates; in most studies of UI, the type or severity of incontinence was elicited through a written questionnaire or interview without validation by objective measures such as physical exam, pad tests, or urodynamic testing. Analysis indicates that prevalence studies based on broad definitions of UI and studies using subjective reports without objective validation yielded higher prevalence rates than studies in which strict definitions were used and incontinence was validated.[6,16] The method in which the data are collected, such as

a mailed questionnaire, phone survey, or personal interview, also affects the prevalence rates, with higher rates reported for interviews versus mailed surveys.[12,14] (Interestingly, some studies suggest that anonymous questionnaires provide the most accurate data for conditions associated with social stigma.[8]) A final factor affecting prevalence rates is the study population; studies involving the "general population" yield prevalence rates different from those of studies focused on the institutionalized elderly or on individuals visiting urology or gastroenterology clinics.

It is evident that studies reporting prevalence rates suffer from inconsistencies in definitions, demographics, and methodology. Use of standardized definitions and validated measures to define urinary and fecal incontinence would increase the accuracy of data regarding prevalence and incidence and the ability to compare and compile data across studies.

Incidence Data

Data regarding incidence are limited because of the difficulty in following a population over a period of time. Study groups must be large enough to account for participants who are lost to follow-up, move out of the geographic study area, or die. Some researchers have tracked the "natural history" of UI for specific populations by gathering data regarding the development of "new-onset" incontinence, risk factors for incontinence development, and remission rates. The studies done to date, although limited, suggest that urinary continence and UI are highly dynamic conditions, with "new-onset" incontinence being partially offset by individuals who regain continence. For example, Nygaard and Lemke tracked development and remission rates of UI in older rural women (more than 65 years of age). Within the first 3 years of this study, 20.4% of the women who were continent at baseline had developed urge incontinence, and 24% had developed stress incontinence; during years 3 to 6, 28.5% of the women who were continent at the 3-year study point had developed urge incontinence, and 20.7% had developed stress incontinence. However, these researchers also found impressive remission rates; 31.7% of the women with urge incontinence and 28.6% of the women with stress incontinence at baseline experienced remission within the first 3 years of the study, and remission rates during years 3 to 6 were 22.1% for women with urge incontinence and 25.1% for women with stress incontinence.[17] Hampel and associates assessed the development of UI in pregnant women 16 to 45 years of age and reported a 49% incidence rate; 86.2% of these cases resolved spontaneously after delivery.[16] Incidence rates of 30% and 21% occurred after hysterectomy and in women with uterine prolapse who did not undergo surgery.[16] In a small study of UI among Swedish women aged 20 to 59 years, Samuelsson and colleagues found a baseline prevalence of 23.6%, an annual incidence rate of 2.9%, and an annual spontaneous remission rate of 5.9%. The incidence rate for UI occurring at least weekly was much lower than the incidence rate for any episodes of urinary leakage (0.5% as compared with 2.9%).[18] Moller and colleagues studied the incidence and remission rates for lower urinary tract symptoms (including UI) over the course of a year among 2284 Danish women aged 40 to 60 years. Baseline prevalence was 28.5%; during the following year, 10% of the women who were asymptomatic at baseline developed lower urinary tract symptoms, and 27.8% of the women who were symptomatic at baseline experienced spontaneous remission.[19] A recent study in the United Kingdom addressed storage symptoms among 23,182 community-dwelling men and women more than 40 years of age and generated the following data: prevalence of 28.5%, 1-year incidence rate of 14.1%, and 1-year remission rate of 26%.[20] Although incidence and remission data are limited, the studies that have been done consistently demonstrate that continence and incontinence are not "steady-state" conditions; they also all demonstrate a steady increase in overall prevalence with aging. (Although remission rates exceed incidence rates, the overall prevalence of incontinence continues to rise, because remission rates affect the *minority* of patients who are incontinent, whereas incidence rates affect the *majority* of individuals who are continent.) The hope is that additional studies focused on factors associated with incidence and with remission will enable clinicians to develop programs that reduce incidence and promote remission.

Prevalence According to Age

UI has long been associated with aging, and many prevalence studies have focused on the geriatric population. Although the elderly are at increased risk for incontinence, the problem of incontinence is certainly not unique to the elderly population; it is a problem for people of all ages, including children and female athletes. For example, nocturnal enuresis affects approximately 10% of 7-year-old children,[21] and as many as 28% of elite female athletes (average age 19.9 years) experience incontinence while participating in their sport.[22] Incontinence is particularly common among women participating in gymnastics (67%), basketball (66%), tennis (50%), and field hockey (42%).[22] However, incontinence is much more common among middle-aged and elderly adults; current prevalence data suggest a marked increase in prevalence of UI during middle age (from 10% to 20% among young adults to 20% to 30% among middle-aged adults), and a steady increase in prevalence with advancing age (up to 30% to 50% among elderly adults).[23]

Community-Dwelling Adults. The prevalence of UI among community-dwelling adults ranges from less than 5% to more than 58%, depending on sample population, survey methodology, and definition of incontinence.[24-27] Minassian and colleagues compiled the results of 35 studies conducted in multiple countries and involving more than 230,000 community-dwelling adults, with a median response rate of 80%. The compiled "median prevalence rate" across all studies was 27.6% for women and 10.5% for men. The major difficulty in compiling results from the various studies was a wide range in the definition used for incontinence (from "any urinary incontinence, past or present" to "2 or more episodes of urinary incontinence within a week").[27] These findings are consistent with those of the EPINCONT study, in which 25% of the participating women ($n = 27,936$ women) reported urinary leakage. However, the EPINCONT study also addressed severity, and only 7% of the women reported incontinence that was moderate to severe and "bothersome."[26] These data again point out the need for standardized definitions that include a severity factor. The WHO's Committee on Epidemiology suggested the following as key elements of a "minimum data set" for future prevalence studies: screening question for any incontinence; frequency measure; quantity of urine lost during a typical incontinence episode; type of incontinence; duration of incontinence; and severity measure, preferably via a validated index.[5]

Institutionalized Elderly. As stated previously, most prevalence studies have targeted the elderly both in the community and in long-term care institutions. Elderly persons are at increased risk for incontinence because of factors such as dementia, urinary tract infection (UTI), pharmaceuticals, restricted mobility, and constipation. The profound effect of incontinence among this population is reflected in the fact that incontinence is a common impetus for institutionalization.[13] This fact helps to explain the high prevalence of incontinence among the institutionalized elderly; the data of Hampel and colleagues indicate a prevalence of 22% to 90%, with a mean of 55.7%.[14] The mean prevalence rate reported by Hampel and colleagues is consistent with the 50% prevalence reported by multiple other investigators.[28-35] It is interesting to compare the prevalence rates for UI in the nursing home population in the United States with prevalence rates for the same patient population in other countries. One study of seven industrialized countries indicated prevalence rates for UI ranging from a low of 42.9% in Japan to a high of 61.6% in Sweden; the prevalence rate for the United States in this study was 46.4%.[36] (More recent data for institutionalized elderly in the United States suggest prevalence rates ranging from 50% to 65%.)[37] When one considers the high prevalence rates among the elderly and the increasing age of our population, it is clear that we need to conduct incidence studies to determine the factors that produce and prevent incontinence in this population.

Prevalence of Urinary Incontinence According to Ethnicity

There are very limited data relating prevalence to ethnic background; however, the data that are available provide interesting insights. For example, some data suggest a higher prevalence of incontinence (especially stress incontinence) among white women than among black women or Hispanic women, and investigators have theorized that these differences could result from differences in urethral pressures, urethral length, pelvic muscle strength, or the birth process.[5,38,39] However, the limited data available make it difficult to draw any firm conclusions, and some investigators have found only minor differences in prevalence among the various ethnic groups.[40] In addition, some data suggest ethnic differences in *type* of incontinence; for example, some studies suggest that black women are more likely to develop overactive bladder, whereas other investigators report comparable rates of overactive bladder/urge incontinence among white, black, and Hispanic women..[41,42] It is clear that we need many more studies involving ethnically diverse populations before we can provide any definitive answers to questions regarding incontinence and ethnicity.

One ethnic study that may provide clues to etiologic factors for incontinence involved Pakistani women; this study documented a significantly higher prevalence of incontinence among Pakistani women who used a commode than among Pakistani women who voided in the squatting position (28.5% as opposed to 12.3%).[14]

Prevalence of Urinary Incontinence by Type of Incontinence

There have been few studies designed to measure the prevalence of specific types of UI, despite the importance of such data in developing prevention and management programs. Sandvik and colleagues[43] conducted an epidemiologic survey for prevalence and type of incontinence that was corrected for validity. They did this by initially classifying a group of women with known incontinence as having "stress," "urge," or "mixed" incontinence based on their responses to an epidemiologic survey. These women were then evaluated by means of urodynamics and a gynecologic evaluation, and the gynecologist's final classification was compared with the initial classification derived from the epidemiologic survey. An epidemiologic survey using a questionnaire was then completed, and the results were "corrected for validity" based on the correction formulas derived from the original study. Interestingly, the percentage of women with stress incontinence increased from 51% to 77%, the percentage with pure urge incontinence increased from 10% to 12%, and the percentage of mixed incontinence decreased from 39% to 11%.[43] (These data point out the difficulty in accurately identifying the type of incontinence; although questionnaires are thought to be less accurate than objective studies such as urodynamics, we need further data to ascertain clearly the optimal use of patient report versus urodynamic findings for accurate classification.)[17,38] The EPINCONT study indicated that 50% of women reporting incontinence reported "stress-type" incontinence, 11% reported symptoms of "overactive bladder/urge" incontinence, and 36% reported mixed symptoms.[26] (These classifications were based only on patient reports and were not validated by objective diagnostic studies.) Thom's data also revealed a higher prevalence of stress incontinence in younger women; however, he found urge incontinence and mixed incontinence to be predominant among older women.[12] Such apparently contradictory data indicate the need for additional studies.

Prevalence of Fecal Incontinence

The data regarding prevalence of fecal incontinence are even more limited than the data for UI; in addition, the data available are considered to be compromised by a significant reluctance on the part of patients to report any problem with bowel control, as a result of the social stigma. Reported rates among adults are quite variable, depending on the population sampled, method of data collection, and definition of incontinence.[44] For example, Johanson and Lafferty conducted a survey of patients visiting either their primary care physician or a gastroenterologist and found a prevalence of 18.4%; the prevalence rate was higher in men and increased progressively with age.[45] In contrast, Locke reported prevalence rates of 2.2% to 7.4% based on general population surveys; risk factors in his study included female gender, advancing age, and general debilitation.[46] The higher prevalence rates reported by Johanson and Lafferty are thought to result from sample bias (use of gastroenterology and general practice patients); most studies indicate that the prevalence among the community-dwelling population as a whole is about 2% to 5%, which is consistent with Locke's findings.[44] In contrast, the prevalence among institutionalized adults is reported to approach 50%.[37,47]

The populations at greatest risk for fecal incontinence include women who sustain sphincteric injuries during vaginal delivery, individuals who have undergone anorectal surgery, and the institutionalized elderly. However, fecal incontinence also occurs in children, most commonly as a result of anorectal anomalies or chronic constipation; the overall prevalence of fecal incontinence in children more than 4 years of age is 1% to 4%,[11] and the rates among otherwise healthy school-aged children are even lower (1% to 2%).[48]

Risk factors for fecal incontinence following *vaginal delivery* include forceps delivery, an infant greater than 4 kg, prolonged second stage of labor, and abnormal presentation, especially occipitoposterior presentation; transient fecal incontinence occurs in up to 20% of women who have delivered vaginally, although most of these women experience rapid and spontaneous remission.[44] Reported prevalence rates for incontinence following common *anorectal surgical procedures* average 1% to 5%;[44] Nyam and Pemberton reported high initial prevalence (45%) among patients undergoing lateral sphincterotomy for anal fissure, but only a 1% prevalence at 5 years following the procedure.[49] By far the highest risk population is the *institutionalized elderly*; reported prevalence rates range from 20% to 46%, with major risk factors including UI, neurologic disease, cognitive impairment, compromised mobility, and age greater than 70 years.[37,44,50]

When one considers the high prevalence rates for incontinence (both urinary and fecal) among the elderly and the "graying of America," it is clear that we need to conduct additional studies to determine the factors that produce and prevent incontinence in this population.

IMPACT OF INCONTINENCE

It is apparent that incontinence is a prevalent health condition that affects people regardless of age, sex, or ethnic background. Consideration of the physical, psychosocial, and economic impact of incontinence further substantiates the significance of the problem. Accurate data regarding the magnitude of urinary and fecal incontinence provide critical guidance to payers, policy makers, and health care providers in appropriately allocating resources and in establishing appropriate programs for the prevention and management of incontinence.

Physical Consequences

The major physical consequences occurring as a result of incontinence are skin lesions and skin breakdown, UTIs, and falls; each of these contributes to the adverse economic effect of incontinence as well as its profound physical effect. Incontinence-related skin damage includes maceration, friction, and dermatitis; typically, these conditions require use of skin care products in addition to nursing care. One survey found that 35% of the patients in a long-term care setting had skin damage, and 12% of these patients required pharmaceutical treatment.[51] Incontinence is also a risk factor for pressure ulcers; however, the causative factor is more likely to be the associated reduction in mobility and activity, as opposed to a direct effect of the incontinence.

Falls represent a major health problem for the elderly and are influenced by multiple risk factors, such as medications, cognitive impairment, restricted mobility, or environmental obstacles that may be overlooked because of visual deficits. Nocturia, a symptom that occurs in up to 80% of ambulatory elderly persons, can predispose these individuals to falls as they maneuver to the bathroom in minimal light or in complete darkness.[52] Approximately 20% to 30% of individuals more than 65 years of age get up two or three times a night to void, and this has been demonstrated to increase the risk for falls (from 10% in patients without nocturia to 21% in patients with nocturia three or more times a night).[52]

UTIs and urosepsis are also more common in the incontinent population.[53] A major cause of UTI is the use of indwelling catheters for the management of incontinence; however, the use of absorptive products is also a risk factor for UTI (because the increased microbial counts on the skin increase the risk of ascending bacteriuria).[54] UTI may also occur as a result of urinary retention, which produces urinary stasis and bacterial overgrowth.[55,56]

The postmenopausal woman is at increased risk for both incontinence and UTI, partly because of the effects of estrogen deficiency. Estrogen promotes the growth of lactobacilli in the vagina; these "good" bacteria are a major portion of the normal vaginal flora. Lactobacilli produce lactic acid from glycogen, which reduces the intravaginal pH; the low pH, in turn, inhibits the growth of uropathogens. Decreased estrogen levels reduce the levels of lactobacilli; this contributes to a higher intravaginal pH and to colonization by uropathogens, specifically *Escherichia coli*.[55] Most studies of systemic estrogen therapy have shown no reduction in incidence of UI or UTIs, and some studies indicate that the incidence of UI may actually be *increased* by systemic therapy. However, topical estrogen replacement *has* been associated with a reduction in UTIs among women with atrophic vaginitis and urethritis, and it may also reduce the incidence of UI.[57] This is another area in which additional data are desperately needed. An additional consideration related to UTIs is the direct and indirect cost of antibiotic therapy; in addition to the primary cost associated with the antibiotic itself, there is the potential for a secondary vaginal yeast infection (which increases the patient's discomfort and adds the cost of another pharmaceutical agent).

Patients with significant fecal incontinence are also at risk for nutritional compromise, which develops as a result of deliberate fasting to reduce the risk of embarrassing fecal accidents. Patients often realize that food intake triggers incontinent episodes, and they may then severely limit food intake whenever they need to travel away from home.[9]

Economic Consequences

Few studies have calculated the financial burden associated with UI; however, direct and indirect costs related to UI in the United States have been estimated at $16.3 billion annually.[58] Direct economic expenditures for UI include costs incurred in routine care, costs of diagnostic evaluation and treatment of incontinence, and costs related to the consequences of incontinence.[9,51,59,60] Indirect costs are associated with lost productivity resulting from incontinence (such as loss of income attributable to the individual's or caregiver's inability to work or forced early retirement).[60,61] See Box 1-2.

Interestingly, most of the "direct costs" associated with incontinence are related to containment, management of complications, and nursing home admissions; only 10% to 11% of the costs are related to diagnosis and treatment.[5,58] Absorptive products, containment products, and laundry costs are estimated to account for 50% to 75% of the annual expenditures for incontinence management.[5,58] Reusable products and some containment devices have an associated laundering or cleaning cost just as soiled clothing and bed linens do. When laundering costs are being considered, depreciation of equipment, supplies for washing, and electricity must also be factored into the total cost. These costs are incurred whether the patient is in the community or is institutionalized.

Time spent on incontinence-related care by nurses, nursing assistants, laundry personnel, and housekeepers should be included when the economic effect is calculated. In Baker and Bice's study on publicly financed home care services for low-income elderly persons, the overall cost of care was significantly greater for patients with urinary or fecal incontinence; the major areas of increased cost were for paraprofessional services (such as home health aides and homemakers), day care, medical equipment and supplies, and transportation.[62] The excess costs associated with management of the incontinence were estimated as $860 to $950 over 18 months.[62] Frenchman studied the cost

BOX 1-2 Economic Costs of Incontinence

Direct Costs

Routine Care

Labor
Nursing, housekeeping, laundry personnel
Supplies
Disposable absorptive products (linen savers, pads, briefs)
Reusable absorptive products (bed pads, briefs, bed linens)
Containment
Indwelling catheters, intermittent catheters, external catheters, bedside commodes, urinals, bedpans
Equipment
Depreciation of laundry equipment, laundering supplies, water and electricity

Diagnostic and management therapies

Labor
Physician, nursing, and technician costs for diagnostic procedures, patient education and management, follow-up and monitoring, housekeeping and laundry personnel
Supplies
Educational materials, biofeedback and electrical stimulation equipment, vaginal cones, pessaries, penile clamps, procedural supplies, skin care supplies

Medications

Procedure Costs
Lab tests, urodynamic tests, anorectal manometry, surgical procedures, charges for biofeedback and electrical stimulation
Other
Equipment depreciation, room charges for procedures, travel costs

Complications Related to Incontinence

Skin damage/breakdown
Topical therapy (creams, ointments, dressings)
Urinary tract infection
Lab tests, antibiotic therapy
Longer hospitalization
Supplies, labor, room charge, etc.
Injury from falls
Potential hospitalization, rehabilitation, home care services, supplies
Institutionalization

Indirect Costs

Loss of wages because of time away from work
Decreased work productivity
Pain and suffering
Loss of earnings for caregiver

of care for individuals with UI in two long-term care facilities in New Jersey and found the average cost to be $17.21/resident/day.[63]

Direct costs also encompass the resources utilized in the evaluation and management of incontinence. Labor expenses include physician, nurse, and technician charges for performance and interpretation of laboratory results. The average cost of diagnostic evaluation was estimated to be $603 in 1995 for the patient with UI;[60] although no data are available regarding the average cost of diagnostic evaluation for the patient with fecal incontinence, the cost of anorectal manometry is typically less than the cost of urodynamic studies.[9] Treatment costs can be broken down into behavioral, medical or pharmacologic, and surgical therapy. The cost of behavioral therapy may comprise equipment charges such as electrical stimulation units or biofeedback equipment, in addition to follow-up clinic or office visits. Pharmaceutical costs are quite variable, depending on the agent prescribed and the dose. Medical costs may also include special devices used to support continence such as pessaries, urethral inserts, penile clamps, intermittent catheters, or indwelling catheters. Surgical treatment may initially appear to be the most costly treatment modality; however, long-term behavioral or pharmacologic treatment may surpass the cost of a one-time surgery charge.[60] When calculating the cost of care, it is critical to consider both the cost of treatment and the benefit derived. For example, three to four biofeedback sessions that result in resolution of the incontinence comprise a very cost-effective treatment approach; in contrast, ongoing use of a pharmaceutical that provides only partial improvement is generally *not* cost-effective. (Cost-effectiveness analysis requires comparative assessment of the cost of treatment and the benefit of treatment as opposed to basing decisions only on cost data.[5])

The physical complications of incontinence (skin damage, UTIs, and falls) are associated with significant additional costs, which affect both the individual and society. Management of incontinence-induced problems may require additional diagnostic studies, product utilization, and possibly hospitalization. All of these interventions represent additional costs.[64] For example, a patient who is injured in an incontinence-related fall may require surgery, rehabilitative care, and home care; some may even require institutionalization. Wagner and Hu estimated the cost associated with adverse consequences of UI to be $13.1 billion; 80% of these dollars are spent on additional hospital days and on treatment of UTIs.[60]

Indirect costs are usually represented as loss of actual or potential earnings by the patient or the caregiver, and disability payments related to the inability to work. Indirect costs are much more difficult to calculate but are estimated to be hundreds of millions of dollars per year.[9] For the patient, this would include time missed from work because of frequent toileting, illness related to the incontinence, or treatment (surgery, clinic visits, etc.). The inability to work because of incontinence is much more common among patients with fecal incontinence or large-volume UI; one survey in the United States found that 13.2% of individuals with *any* degree of fecal incontinence and 29.4% of those with large-volume fecal leakage reported that they were unable to go to work or school.[65] When calculating indirect costs, one must also consider the impact on the caregiver's ability to work; these individuals may also miss work because of the demands of caring for the individual or of obtaining treatment for the incontinence and related conditions.[9] The cost of emotional pain and suffering related to incontinence is usually not included in the cost of care because it is difficult to attach a price to this aspect of incontinence. However, if the patient is so distressed that psychotropic medications and psychologic counseling are necessary, these costs could appropriately be incorporated into the total "cost picture" for the incontinence.

It is difficult to accurately determine the true costs associated with incontinence for several reasons: variable prevalence rates, probable underreporting of incontinence with "self-managed" care, and variable pricing. However, the data that *are* available regarding indirect and direct costs reflect a significant economic loss. As the actual costs of incontinence rise, reimbursement for continence care is shrinking. The implications for research are clear: data are urgently needed that define the cost and the outcomes of prevention and management programs for specific patient populations. (Up to now, many of the studies have focused only on the elderly patient population.)

Psychosocial Consequences

Incontinence is unfortunately viewed by many as a "societal norm" for the elderly and for childbearing women; despite this, it has a substantial negative psychosocial effect on these individuals and an even greater effect on individuals for whom incontinence is viewed as "abnormal." Children with enuresis may feel shame at not being fully "potty trained" and fear ostracism by their peers. For working adults, incontinence can influence career and relationships, specifically sexual relationships. For the elderly, there is the fear of loss of independence and institutionalization. People with incontinence engage in numerous activities to conceal their secret, such as dark clothing, frequent toileting, fluid restriction, use of absorptive products, and potent fragrances to conceal odor.[66] A common response to clinically significant incontinence is social withdrawal, caused by the fear of accidents and embarrassment associated with the incontinence; this is particularly true of individuals with fecal incontinence and large-volume UI, who may consider themselves "tethered" to the toilet.[9,67] This social isolation, whether self-imposed or initiated by others, contributes to loss of self-esteem, loneliness, and alienation. Incontinence that is perceived as "severe" by the individual is also frequently associated with anxiety and depression; the relationship between severe UI and depression and anxiety is well documented among both men and women.[68-70] Anger and hostility are also common among individuals with significant incontinence, and they may be directed either at the event that led to their incontinence or at the health care team who fails to provide either significant improvement or compassionate and sensitive management.[9]

The effect of incontinence on quality of life has been emphasized in an effort to raise awareness and support for a health condition that has minimal influence on mortality but may cause significant psychosocial disability.[71] Multiple quality of life instruments and illness-impact tools have been used to assess the psychosocial effect of incontinence.

Some tools are general illness-effect scales, whereas others have been specifically targeted to the condition of incontinence.[72-76] These tools are discussed in greater depth in Chapter 12.

One factor affecting the degree of psychosocial effect is the type of incontinence. Current data indicate that fecal incontinence has a greater effect than UI and that UI caused by detrusor instability, that is, urge incontinence, has a greater effect than stress incontinence in terms of mental or emotional distress, practical inconvenience (measures to hide the incontinence), social limitations, and sleep disturbance.[9,72,73,77,-80] In one contradictory study, patients with stress incontinence perceived their incontinence to be worse than those with urge incontinence; no explanation was offered for this finding.[73] Physical activity did not appear to be so highly affected in patients with urge incontinence, possibly because urge incontinence is not consistently correlated to activity, as is stress incontinence. However, travel to locations more than 30 minutes from home or to places where the person is unfamiliar with the bathroom facilities is an activity associated with much anxiety and much "negative psychosocial effect" for the individual with urge incontinence.[75,80] Urge incontinence is usually associated with larger volumes of urine leakage at unpredictable times; as a result, individuals with this type of incontinence frequently live in fear of a socially disastrous "accident." Additionally, there are multiple precipitating factors for urge incontinence, and these factors reduce the individual's sense of control over bladder function and urinary leakage. Sleep disturbance related to frequency and nocturia, which are common with urge incontinence, may further exacerbate psychosocial problems; these issues are an important component of management for the patient with urge incontinence.[73,77,78]

Other factors that may influence the psychosocial effect of UI are severity of the incontinence, duration of the problem, and age of the individual. Severity or perceived severity of incontinence positively correlated with a decreased quality of life and increased distress.[76,79,81] Severity of incontinence is difficult to measure, and until recently there were no widely accepted guidelines for severity classification;

as a result, some researchers utilized "self-report of symptoms" to determine severity, whereas others established specific criteria. However, as noted earlier in this chapter, Sandvik and colleagues developed and validated a simple severity index that correlates positively to patients' perceptions of UI severity; the tool utilizes frequency of incontinent episodes and volume of leakage to classify the UI as slight, moderate, or severe.[6,7] There are no widely accepted tools to measure the severity of fecal incontinence, although some clinicians are using a scale similar to that developed by Sandvik. Obviously, as the severity of incontinence increases, so do the behaviors to conceal it and the associated emotional distress. There are very limited data regarding the relationship between duration of the incontinence and psychosocial disturbance; the few studies that have addressed this issue have generated conflicting results, possibly because of the influence of uncaptured variables.[79]

Age is another factor shown to influence psychosocial distress. One particular study of urge and stress incontinence in women 40 years of age and older demonstrated a positive correlation between age and degree of emotional disturbance. In this study, elderly subjects (women 70 years of age or older) with stress incontinence reported less effect on physical recreation, community activities, and outside entertainment than their younger counterparts (women 40 to 60 years of age); the younger women perceived a severe impact on quality of life.[72] With *urge* incontinence, however, there was no significant difference in impact scores for elderly women as compared with younger women.[72] In contrast, Wyman and colleagues did not find a notable correlation between psychosocial effect and age; however, this may be because the study participants were all more than 55 years of age.[80]

A particular concern for the elderly is the threat of institutionalization. Incontinence is a major driving force for admission into a long-term care facility because primary caregivers or family members may be unable to manage or deal with the incontinence.[9,37] UI has been found to substantially increase the risk of nursing home admission; in women the risk is doubled, and in men it is more than tripled.[64] There also exists an increased tendency

to institutionalize incontinent individuals in rural, less densely populated regions than in small or medium-sized metropolitan areas.[82] This predisposition may be attributable in part to a lack of resources or support for incontinent individuals in this setting.

It is apparent that incontinence affects people of all ages and affects them physically, socially, and emotionally. More comparative studies using standard quality of life impact tools would be valuable in further clarifying the scope and magnitude of the psychosocial issues. Increased awareness of the psychosocial, economic, and physical consequences of incontinence may help to change attitudes regarding this very common problem. Increased knowledge and acceptance may positively influence care-seeking behaviors and support for prevention and management programs.

RISK FACTORS

Identification of risk factors related to urinary or fecal incontinence may help avert some cases of incontinence through early interventions to counteract or minimize the effect of identified risk factors. In cases of existing UI or fecal incontinence, a management plan that addresses related risk factors can reverse or minimize the problem of incontinence. Current data suggest that risk factors vary based on the type of incontinence. For example, vaginal delivery, multiparity, and hysterectomy are consistently identified as risk factors for stress incontinence in women; some data suggest that obesity, chronic cough, depression, and genetic differences in collagen are risk factors as well.[5,27] In contrast, diabetes (especially poorly controlled diabetes), a history of stroke, and advanced age seem to be risk factors for overactive bladder/urge incontinence, and family history appears to be the most significant risk factor for nocturnal enuresis among children.[5,27] General debilitation and dementia appear to be the primary risk factors for both functional UI and fecal incontinence in the institutionalized elderly.[37] More research into the risk factors for specific types of incontinence is clearly needed, along with data regarding strategies to correct the risk factors or to minimize their negative impact.

CARE-SEEKING BEHAVIORS

In contrast to the prevalent nature of incontinence, care-seeking behavior is quite limited, and this holds true across multiple studies, countries, and cultures; even among individuals with severe incontinence, fewer than 50% report seeking help from a health care professional.[27] The factors limiting care-seeking behavior include acceptance of the incontinence as normal, embarrassment, concerns regarding the cost of treatment, the belief that nothing can be done, failure of health care providers to provide effective treatment when incontinence *is* reported, and the individual's perception that his or her incontinence is too limited in severity to necessitate treatment. Factors that promote care-seeking behavior include the belief that incontinence is a common and treatable condition affecting their friends as well as themselves, appropriate and effective treatment when incontinence is reported, and incontinence of greater severity.[14,32]

IMPLICATIONS OF PREVALENCE, EFFECT, AND CARE-SEEKING DATA

The data clearly indicate that incontinence is a common problem with a significant effect on the individual, family, and society. It is also clear that the degree of effect is determined partly by the severity and nature of the incontinence; that is, fecal incontinence typically has a greater effect than UI, and urge UI frequently has a greater effect than stress UI.[78] Although these are very treatable conditions, many individuals live out their lives without obtaining treatment because of their perception of incontinence as "normal," the embarrassment associated with the condition, or the failure of clinicians to provide effective treatment or appropriate referrals. The implications for continence clinicians are clear: (1) we need to provide more preventive care, such as pelvic muscle training for adolescent girls and young women, (2) we need to provide community education to change the perception that incontinence is "inevitable" and "not treatable," and (3) we need to provide professional education so that clinicians are equipped either to manage incontinence effectively or to refer patients appropriately.

CLASSIFICATION AND TERMINOLOGY ISSUES

Standard terminology is important in the study and management of any condition, because it permits comparison and compilation of research data and supports information sharing. The development of standard classification and terminology in the field of continence care has been complicated by the fact that continence does not "belong" to any one specialty and by the natural tendency of each involved specialty (such as urology, neurourology, and gynecology) to use its own "system" and vocabulary. For example, several classification systems that focused only on neurogenic forms of incontinence were developed,[83] and gynecologists developed terminology related specifically to stress incontinence in women.

International Continence Society Classification System

It is the ICS that has led the way in the development of a "cross-specialty" vocabulary and classification system. The ICS established a committee to develop standard terminology related to lower urinary tract function in 1973; the committee's first report was approved and published in 1975. This original set of recommendations clarified the use of the term "incontinence" as a symptom, as a sign, and as a condition and defined the "condition" of incontinence as "a social or hygienic problem that is objectively demonstrable."[84] The report further identified and defined the following specific "types" of incontinence: stress incontinence, urge incontinence, reflex incontinence, and overflow incontinence. Subsequent reports by the standardization committee provided additional recommendations for standardization of terminology, and in 1988 a major summary report that provided comprehensive guidelines for the assessment and classification of lower urinary tract dysfunction was published.[85] This report introduced a conceptual classification system for lower urinary tract dysfunction based on the underlying functional abnormality; this broad classification system was not designed to replace the previously established definitions and descriptions of the specific "types" of incontinence, but rather to provide an overarching framework that was physiologically based. The ICS system, with some modifications, is the system most widely used by clinicians. For example, the North American Nursing Diagnosis Association (NANDA) patterned its classification of UI after the ICS system, and the current ICS system is the basis for the classification system used by the AHCPR Guidelines Panel as well.[3,86]

Overview. The "functional" classification system developed by the ICS was based on the two major components of lower urinary tract function, that is, urinary storage and urinary elimination, and on the critical roles of the bladder and sphincter. Any problem with continence or voiding dysfunction was therefore conceptualized as either a problem with storage or a problem with urine elimination (voiding). Problems were further classified as being caused by bladder dysfunction or sphincter dysfunction. This broad classification provided a simple and easily understood four-point grid: problems with storage caused by bladder dysfunction, problems with storage caused by sphincter dysfunction, problems with elimination caused by bladder dysfunction, and problems with elimination caused by sphincter dysfunction.[85] Specific types of incontinence were defined within the context of "storage problem" or "emptying problem" and the area of dysfunction. (For example, urge incontinence was classified as a problem with storage, caused by bladder dysfunction.) Advantages of this system include the physiologic framework and the focus on the underlying dysfunction, which directs assessment and management. A significant limitation is the failure to address incontinence caused by conditions outside of the urinary tract, such as cognitive dysfunction or immobility.

Types of Incontinence. The original classification system proposed by the ICS identified four major types of incontinence: stress incontinence, urge incontinence, reflex incontinence, and overflow incontinence.[54] (See Appendix B.) This original system provides the basis for the system most commonly used in clinical practice today. Subsequent reports have added types and terms to the original system and revised many of the original definitions.

Current definitions for the various types of incontinence are outlined as follows:

- *Stress incontinence* is defined subjectively as "the *complaint* of involuntary leakage on effort or exertion, or on sneezing or coughing" and objectively as "the *observation* of involuntary leakage from the urethra, synchronous with exertion/ effort, or sneezing or coughing"; stress incontinence is thought to be caused by increased abdominal pressure. *Urodynamic stress incontinence* is defined as "the involuntary leakage of urine during increased abdominal pressure, in the absence of a detrusor contraction"; the ICS recommends use of this term as opposed to "genuine stress urinary incontinence."[2] Urodynamically demonstrated stress incontinence is further classified as either "incompetent urethral closure mechanism" (leakage occurring in the absence of a detrusor contraction) or "urethral relaxation incontinence" (leakage occurring in the absence of either a detrusor contraction *or* increased abdominal pressure, the syndrome clinically designated as "intrinsic sphincteric deficiency.")[2]

- *Urge UI* is defined subjectively as "the complaint of involuntary leakage accompanied by or immediately preceded by urgency"; *urgency* is defined as "the complaint of a sudden compelling desire to pass urine which is difficult to defer." (The terms "motor urgency" and "sensory urgency," previously used to differentiate between leakage associated with urgency and sudden leakage with no accompanying urgency, are no longer recommended.)[2] *Overactive bladder syndrome,* also known as "urge syndrome" or "urgency-frequency syndrome," is described as "urgency, with or without urge incontinence, and usually with frequency and nocturia." Increased daytime frequency is defined as "the complaint by the patient who considers that he/she voids too often by day" (also known as pollakiuria), and nocturia is "the complaint that the individual has to wake at night one or more times to void." These symptoms suggest detrusor overactivity, but detrusor overactivity can only be *confirmed* by urodynamic studies demonstrating involuntary detrusor contractions during bladder filling.[2] *Detrusor overactivity incontinence* (urodynamically demonstrated "overactive bladder/urge incontinence") is "incontinence due to an involuntary detrusor contraction."[2]

- *Mixed UI* (also known as mixed stress-urge incontinence) is defined as "the complaint of urinary leakage associated with urgency and also with exertion, effort, sneezing, or coughing".[2]

- The term *reflex incontinence* is no longer recommended, although it is still commonly used in clinical practice to indicate loss of volitional control of voiding caused by a neurologic lesion between the sacral cord and the pons.[2] The currently recommended term for lower urinary tract dysfunction and incontinence caused by a disturbance in the neurologic structures and processes that control voiding is *neurogenic lower urinary tract dysfunction.*[87] By definition, this type of dysfunction occurs only in patients with neurologic disorders. *Detrusor-sphincter dyssynergia* is commonly associated with this type of dysfunction and is defined as "a detrusor contraction that occurs concurrently with an involuntary contraction of the urethral and/or periurethral striated muscle."

- *Overflow incontinence* was previously defined as "any involuntary loss of urine associated with over-distention of the bladder"; however, the ICS no longer recommends use of this term unless it is clearly defined in terms of pathophysiology (such as bladder outlet obstruction or detrusor underactivity).[2,85] Problems with bladder emptying should now be classified as acute or chronic urinary retention, which are defined as follows: *acute retention of urine* is "a painful, palpable, or percussible bladder, when the patient is unable to pass any urine," and *chronic retention of urine* is "a non-painful bladder, which remains palpable or percussible after the patient has passed urine." The ICS notes that the patient with chronic retention of urine may be incontinent (the condition formerly known as "overflow incontinence").[2] Terms and definitions for etiologic factors contributing to impaired bladder emptying include the following: "detrusor underactivity" is "a contraction of reduced strength and/or duration, resulting in prolonged bladder emptying and/or a failure to achieve complete bladder emptying within a normal time span"; "acontractile detrusor"

is "detrusor that cannot be demonstrated to contract during urodynamic studies"; and "bladder outlet obstruction" is a "generic term for obstruction during voiding, and is characterized by increased detrusor pressures and reduced urinary flow rates."[2]

- *Enuresis* is a synonym for incontinence and is defined as "any involuntary loss of urine"; *nocturnal enuresis* is the term that should be used to denote "loss of urine occurring during sleep."[2]

- *Extraurethral incontinence* is defined as the "observation of urine leakage through channels other than the urethra";[2] this type of incontinence is typically the result of an ectopic ureter or a fistula.

- *Uncategorized incontinence* is a new "general use term" and is defined as the observation of involuntary leakage that cannot be classified into one of the foregoing categories on the basis of signs and symptoms."[2]

Additional Categories and Terminology Relevant to Clinical Practice

UI caused by factors outside the urinary tract, such as immobility or cognitive impairment, is currently labeled "functional incontinence." The AHCPR Guidelines define functional incontinence as urinary leakage associated with "chronic impairments of physical and/or cognitive functioning."[3]

A specific term sometimes used in relation to urge incontinence and overflow incontinence is "detrusor hyperactivity with impaired contractility"; this is a "combination term" used to denote unstable contractions occurring during the filling phase in conjunction with impaired contractility and ineffective emptying. This condition is sometimes encountered in older adults.[3,88]

Fig. 1-1 provides a correlation between the broad conceptual classification developed by the ICS (that is, problems with storage versus problems with emptying) and the "type" classification system commonly used in clinical practice.

Classification Based on Duration, Reversibility, and Management

In addition to the disorder-based ICS classification system, there are classification systems based on the duration, reversibility, and management of the

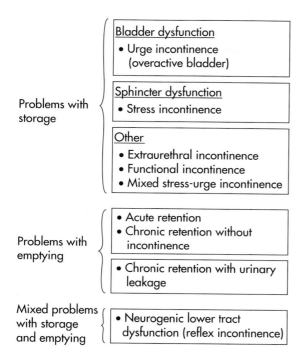

Problems with storage
- **Bladder dysfunction**
  - Urge incontinence (overactive bladder)
- **Sphincter dysfunction**
  - Stress incontinence
- **Other**
  - Extraurethral incontinence
  - Functional incontinence
  - Mixed stress-urge incontinence

Problems with emptying
- Acute retention
- Chronic retention without incontinence
- Chronic retention with urinary leakage

Mixed problems with storage and emptying
- Neurogenic lower tract dysfunction (reflex incontinence)

Fig. 1-1 Types of incontinence.

incontinence. Each of these systems provides a unique perspective for the continence clinician; they are, in general, complementary rather than competitive.

One classification that directs clinical management is the differentiation between incontinence that is transient and incontinence that is established. Transient incontinence is caused by reversible factors; the most common of these are captured in the mnemonic DIAPPERS (delirium, infection or inflammation, atrophic vaginitis and urethritis, pharmaceuticals, psychologic conditions, conditions resulting in excess urine production, restricted mobility, and stool impaction).[89] Established incontinence, in contrast, cannot be easily reversed; established incontinence is usually caused by a pathologic condition within the urinary tract or neurologic system or by irreversible cognitive impairment.[28] The relevance to clinical practice is clear; the clinician begins by addressing all reversible factors and then addresses any residual "established" incontinence.

A second "management-based" system has been incorporated into the updated version of the AHCPR Guidelines. The guidelines address the issue of "chronic intractable incontinence," that is, incontinence in individuals with cognitive or physical deficits that render them unable to participate in behavioral interventions and who are not candidates for surgical or pharmacologic correction of their incontinence. Individuals with intractable incontinence can be further classified according to an Australian model that categorizes continence as independent, dependent, or social. Within this system, "independent continence" indicates that the individual is able to maintain continence without assistance, whereas "dependent continence" indicates that the individual is kept clean and dry through the efforts of caregivers. "Social continence" is the category used for individuals who utilize continence aids such as absorbent products or external collection devices to manage their incontinence.[3]

MANAGEMENT TRENDS AND ISSUES

Incontinence is now recognized as a very treatable condition; the primary options for treatment are behavioral interventions, pharmacologic agents, and surgical procedures. The specific management plan for any patient must be based on the specific type of incontinence, the causative and contributing factors, and the patient's candidacy and interest in the various treatment options.

Effective treatment is always dependent on a thorough and accurate assessment, which is designed to identify reversible factors contributing to the incontinence and the type or pattern of any established incontinence as well as the environmental and psychosocial factors affecting management. The key components of assessment include the patient-and-caregiver interview, a focused physical assessment, evaluation of a bladder chart, and simple laboratory studies to rule out infection and retention. More complex evaluation may be required for patients with complex clinical presentations or comorbidities, patients who present with unexplained hematuria, patients in whom primary management fails, and patients who elect surgical intervention.[3]

One of the most important advances in the area of continence care is the development of inexpensive, noninvasive, and effective interventions labeled collectively as "behavioral therapy." This category includes strategies such as dietary and fluid management, toileting programs, bladder and bowel retraining programs, and pelvic muscle reeducation (with or without biofeedback). In general, these strategies should be utilized as first-line therapy for patients with amenable conditions (such as patients with urge incontinence, stress incontinence, or functional incontinence). Pharmacologic agents may be used as adjunct therapy. Surgical procedures are usually reserved for patients who "fail" primary therapy or who present with specific problems not amenable to behavioral therapies (such as the patient with stress incontinence and comorbid pelvic organ prolapse). In establishing a management plan, the clinician must always be cognizant of the need to protect the upper urinary tract from hostile conditions such as reflux and retention; this is of particular concern in management of the patient with a neurologic lesion producing neurogenic lower urinary tract dysfunction (reflex incontinence).

Nurses are well equipped to provide primary continence care and to work collaboratively with other providers to provide complex continence care. Box 1-3 outlines the critical competencies and qualifications of the continence care nurse at both the primary and the advanced levels.[90]

BOX 1-3   Abstract of Position Statement Re: Continence Care Nurse

Continence care nursing is the identification, assessment, and management of urinary, fecal, and double incontinence. Nursing involves the examination of health care problems from a holistic perspective, including management of both urinary and fecal loss, causative factors, and complications. Continence care nursing practice should include prevention, risk assessment, and management of secondary complications, including changes in perineal skin integrity.

Primary continence management is based on an understanding of normal voiding and defecation physiology and common alterations in bowel and bladder function. Specific competencies of the primary continence nurse include the following:

- Identification of risk factors for urinary and fecal incontinence
- Assessment of urinary and fecal incontinence to include relevant history; focused physical examination; record of bladder and bowel elimination and incontinent episodes; simple bedside cystometry; identification of complicating factors such as infection, retention of urine, fecal impaction, perineal skin damage, and neurologic disorders
- Establishment of an appropriate management program to include dietary and fluid management; bowel training or stimulated defecation program; bladder retraining, prompted voiding, or scheduled voiding program; pelvic muscle reeducation without biofeedback; indwelling catheter management; intermittent catheterization program management; recommendations regarding containment and absorptive devices and skin care; education and counseling for patient and caregivers
- Identification of patients requiring referral for assessment and management of complex urinary or fecal incontinence

Advanced continence nursing is based on a more in-depth understanding of the pathophysiology associated with various types of incontinence. In addition to the competencies possessed by the primary continence care nurse, the advanced level practitioner possesses some or all of the following competencies:

- Assessment: Detailed physical examination to include evaluation of prolapse and urethral hypermobility; performance of complex multichannel urodynamic studies with or without fluoroscopic imaging; performance of anorectal manometry studies
- Management and interventions: Pelvic floor rehabilitation and reeducation by means of electrical muscle stimulation and biofeedback; fitting and placement of vaginal pessaries

From the Wound, Ostomy and Continence Nurses Society, Mt. Laurel, NJ, 1996.

REGULATORY ISSUES

The advances in continence knowledge and continence management are reflected in new regulatory guidelines; the Centers for Medicare and Medicaid Services (CMS) have recently released guidelines for the longterm care setting related to continence care and use of indwelling catheters. These guidelines, known as F315, became effective on June 27, 2005, and they provide clear guidance for the development of programs to optimize bladder function and continence and to minimize complications such as urinary tract infections. Key elements of this guidance document include the following:[91]

- Use of indwelling catheters is limited to individuals who have medical conditions that require catheterization and that cannot be effectively managed by other interventions, such as significant urinary retention in a patient who cannot tolerate intermittent catheterization, Stage 3 or 4 pressure ulcers complicated by urine contamination that is impeding healing, or terminal illness or severe pain. The document provides specific guidance regarding assessment of any individual admitted with an indwelling catheter as well as guidelines for discontinuation of the catheter as soon as medically feasible.
- Each resident is assessed for bowel and bladder function and for factors known to impact on continence (such as comorbidities, mobility status, cognition, and medications); following assessment, an individualized plan is implemented to optimize the resident's functional status and level of continence, through a combination of behavioral strategies, medications, and devices such as pessaries (when indicated). Bladder retraining programs and pelvic muscle reeducation programs are recommended only for individuals with intact cognition who are motivated to improve their bladder function and control. In contrast, prompted voiding and habit training/scheduled voiding programs may be used for individuals with cognitive impairment who retain the ability to ambulate with assistance and to say their name or reliably point to one of two objects.
- Treatment of urinary tract infections is limited to individuals with symptomatic urinary tract infections (fever, flank pain or suprapubic pain or tenderness, change in character of urine, and/or worsening of mental or functional status). Very specific guidance is provided for diagnosis of urinary tract infection in patients with and without an indwelling catheter.

SUMMARY

The cost-effectiveness of care is a critical issue in today's health care environment; as the United States health care dollar continues to shrink, the demand for interventions that produce the best outcome for the least cost continues to escalate. To meet the needs of the incontinent individual today and in the future, we must provide evidence-based care, document our costs and our outcomes, collaborate with legislators, regulators, and other professionals to assure appropriate coverage for care, and contribute to research. Because none of us can do all of this independently, we must build strong collaborative relationships with other providers and with our consumers. It is a tremendous challenge with equally tremendous rewards, both for ourselves as professionals and, most importantly, for our patients.

The Wound, Ostomy and Continence Nurses Society has published a position paper[90] on the role of the continence care nurse that clearly delineates the competencies and qualifications of the continence care nurse at both the primary and the advanced level. The relevant portions of that position statement are outlined in Box 1-3.

SELF-ASSESSMENT EXERCISE

1. Explain why prevalence rates vary so widely from study to study and the implications for future studies.

2. Identify groups at high risk for incontinence based on prevalence data currently available.

3. List the three major types of physical complications associated with UI and explain the relationship.

4. Rate the following statement as true or false: UI is primarily a social and hygienic problem and is a relatively low—cost health care problem because most of the cost is managed by the individual.

5. Identify the types of incontinence associated with the greatest effect on quality of life and explain your answer.

6. Briefly define each of the following "types" of incontinence and explain whether it represents a problem with storage, a problem with emptying, or both.
   a. Stress incontinence
   b. Overactive bladder/Urge incontinence
   c. Neurogenic lower tract dysfunction/Reflex incontinence
   d. Chronic retention with urinary leakage
   e. Functional incontinence
   f. Extraurethral incontinence
   g. Nocturnal enuresis

7. Describe current trends in assessment and management of incontinence.

8. Outline key responsibilities and competencies of the primary continence nurse.

REFERENCES

1. Isaacs B: Incontinence. In *The challenge of geriatric medicine,* Oxford, 1992, Oxford University Press, pp 101-122.
2. Abrams P, Cardozo L, Fall M, et al: The standardisation of terminology in lower urinary tract function: report from the standardisation sub-committee of the International Continence Society, *Urology* 61(1):37-49, 2003.
3. Urinary Incontinence Guidelines Panel: *UI in adults: clinical practice guideline update,* AHCPR Pub. No. 96-0686, Rockville, Md, 1996, Agency for Health Care Policy and Research, Public Health Service, US DHHS.
4. Castleden CM: The Marjory Warren lecture: incontinence—still a geriatric giant? *Age Ageing* 26(suppl 4):47-52, 1997.
5. Brown J, Nyberg L, Kusek J, et al: Proceedings of the National Institute of Diabetes and Digestive and Kidney Diseases international symposium on epidemiologic issues in urinary incontinence in women, *Am J Obstet Gynecol* 188(6):S77-S88, 2003.
6. Nihira M, Henderson N: Epidemiology of urinary incontinence in women, *Curr Womens Health Rep* 3:340-347, 2003.
7. Sandvik H, Seim A, Vanvik A, Hunskaar S: A severity index for epidemiological surveys of female urinary incontinence: comparison with 48-hour pad weighing tests, *Neurourol Urodyn* 19(2):137-145, 2000.
8. Macmillan A, Merrie A, Marshall R, Parry B: The prevalence of fecal incontinence in community-dwelling adults: a systematic review of the literature, *Dis Colon Rectum* 47:1341-1349, 2004.
9. Miner P: Economic and personal impact of fecal and urinary incontinence, *Gastroenterology* 126:S8-S13, 2004.
10. Norton C: The development of bowel control. In Norton C, Chelvanayagam S, editors: *Bowel continence nursing,* Beaconsfield Publishers, 2004, Beaconsfield, UK: 1-7.
11. Whitehead W, Wald A, Diamant N, et al: Functional disorders of the anus and rectum. *Gut* 45:1155-1159, 1999.
12. Thom D: Variation in estimates of urinary incontinence prevalence in the community: effects of differences in definition, population characteristics, and study type, *J Am Geriatr Soc* 46:473-480, 1998.
13. Teunissen T, Lagro-Janssen A, van den Bosch W, van den Hoogen H: Prevalence of urinary, fecal and double incontinence in the elderly living at home, *Int Urogynecol J* 15:10-13, 2004.
14. Hampel C, Wienhold D, Benken N, et al: Definition of overactive bladder and epidemiology of urinary incontinence, *Urology* 50(suppl 6A):4-14, 1997.
15. Roberts RO, Jacobsen SJ, Rhodes T, et al: Urinary incontinence in a community-based cohort: prevalence and healthcare-seeking, *J Am Geriatr Soc* 46:467-472, 1998.
16. Hampel C, Wienhold D, Benken N, et al: Prevalence and natural history of female incontinence, *Eur Urol* 32(suppl 2):3-12, 1997.
17. Nygaard I, Lemke J: Urinary incontinence in rural older women: prevalence, incidence, and remission, *J Am Geriatr Soc* 44(9):1049-1054, 1996.
18. Samuelsson E, Mansson L, Milson I: Incontinence aids in Sweden: users and costs, *BJU Int* 88:893-898, 2001.
19. Moller L, Lose G, Jorgensen T: Incidence and remission rates of lower urinary tract symptoms at one year in women aged 40-60: longitudinal study, *BMJ* 320(7247): 1429-1432, 2000.
20. McGrother C, Donaldson M, Shaw C, et al: Storage symptoms of the bladder: prevalence, incidence, and need for services in the UK, *BJU Int* 93(6):763-769, 2004.
21. Haggloff B, Andren O, Bergstrom E, et al: Self-esteem before and after treatment in children with nocturnal enuresis and urinary incontinence, *Scand J Urol Nephrol* 183:79-82, 1997.
22. Nygaard IE, Thompson FL, Svengalis SL, Albright JP: Urinary incontinence in elite nulliparous athletes, *Obstet Gynecol* 84:183-187, 1994.
23. Hunskaar S, Arnold E, Burgio K, et al: Epidemiology and natural history of urinary incontinence, *Int Urogynecol J* 11:301-319, 2000.
24. Temml C, Haidinger G, Schmidbauer J, et al: Urinary incontinence in both sexes: prevalence rates and impact on quality of life and sexual life, *Neurourol Urodyn* 19:259-271, 2000.
25. Roberts R, Jacobsen S, Reilly W, et al: Prevalence of combined fecal and urinary incontinence: a community-based study, *J Am Geriatr Soc* 47(7):837-841, 1999.
26. Hannestad Y, Rortveit G, Sandvik H, Hunskaar S: A community-based epidemiological survey of female urinary incontinence, *J Clin Epidemiol* 53(11):1150-1157, 2000.
27. Minassian V, Drutz H, Al-Badr A: Urinary incontinence as a worldwide problem, *Int J Gynecol Obstet* 82(3): 327-338, 2003.

28. Brandeis GH, Baumann MM, Hossain M, et al: The prevalence of potentially remediable urinary incontinence in frail older people: a study using the Minimum Data Set, *J Am Geriatr Soc* 45:179-184, 1997.

29. Cummings V, Holt R, van der Sloot C, et al: Cost and management of urinary incontinence in long term care, *J Wound Ostomy Continence Nurs* 22(4):193-198, 1995.

30. Diokno AC: Epidemiologic and psychosocial aspects of incontinence, *Urol Clin North Am* 22(3):481-485, 1995.

31. Fultz NH, Herzog AR: Epidemiology of urinary symptoms in the geriatric population, *Urol Clin North Am* 23(1):1-10, 1996.

32. Johnson V, Gary MA: Urinary incontinence: a review, *J Wound Ostomy Continence Nurs* 22:8-16, 1995.

33. Pinkowski P: Prompted voiding in the long term care facility, *J Wound Ostomy Continence Nurs* 23:110-114, 1996.

34. Prosser S, Dobbs F: Casefinding incontinence in the over 75, *Br J Gen Pract* 47:498-500, 1997.

35. Weksler M: Urinary incontinence: taking action against this silent epidemic, *Geriatrics* 51(4):47-51, 1996.

36. Sgadari A, Topinkova E, Bjornson J, Bernabei R: Urinary incontinence in nursing home residents: a cross-national comparison, *Age Ageing* 26(suppl 2):49-54, 1997.

37. Schnelle J, Leung F: Urinary and fecal incontinence in nursing homes, *Gastroenterology* 126:S41-S47, 2004.

38. Hunskaar S, Burgio K, Diokno A, et al: Epidemiology and natural history of urinary incontinence in women, *Urology* 62(4, suppl 1):16-23, 2003.

39. Espino D, Palmer R, Miles T, et al: Prevalence and severity of urinary incontinence in elderly Mexican-American women, *J Am Geriatr Soc* 51(11):1580-1586, 2003.

40. Novielli K, Simpson Z, Hua G, et al: Urinary incontinence in primary care: a comparison of older African-American and Caucasian women, *Int Urol Nephrol* 35:423-428, 2003.

41. Duong T, Korn A: A comparison of urinary incontinence among African American, Asian, Hispanic, and white women, *Am J Obstet Gynecol* 184:1083-1086, 2001.

42. Sze E, Jones W, Ferguson J, et al: Prevalence of urinary incontinence symptoms among black, white, and Hispanic women, *Obstet Gynecol* 99(4):572-575, 2002.

43. Sandvik H, Hunskaar S, Vanvik A, et al: Diagnostic classification of female urinary incontinence: an epidemiological study corrected for validity, *J Clin Epidemiol* 48(3):339-343, 1995.

44. Kenefick N: The epidemiology of faecal incontinence. In Norton C, Chelvanayagam S, editors: *Bowel continence nursing*, Beaconsfield Publishers, 2004, Beaconsfield, UK, pp 14-22.

45. Johanson J, Lafferty J: Epidemiology of fecal incontinence: the silent affliction, *Am J Gastroenterol* 91(1):33-36, 1996.

46. Locke GR, III: The epidemiology of functional gastrointestinal disorders in North America, *Gastroenterol Clin North Am* 25(1):1-12, 1996.

47. Nelson R: Epidemiology of fecal incontinence, *Gastroenterology* 126:S3-S7, 2004.

48. DiLorenzo C, Benninga M: Pathophysiology of pediatric fecal incontinence, *Gastroenterology* 126:S33-S40, 2004.

49. Nyam D, Pemberton J: Long-term results of lateral internal sphincterotomy for chronic anal fissure with particular reference to incidence of fecal incontinence, *Dis Colon Rectum* 42(10):1306-1310, 1999.

50. Chassagne P, Landrin I, Neveu C, et al: Fecal incontinence in the institutionalized elderly: incidence, risk factors, and prognosis, *Am J Med* 106(2):185-190, 1999.

51. Wyman JF: The costs of urinary incontinence, *Eur Urol* 32(suppl 2):13-19, 1997.

52. Stewart RB, Moore MT, May FE, et al: Nocturia: a risk factor for falls in the elderly, *J Am Geriatr Soc* 40:1217-1220, 1992.

53. Diokno AC, Brock BM, Herzog AR, Bromberg J: Medical correlates of urinary incontinence in the elderly, *Urology* 36:129-138, 1990.

54. Brown DS: Diapers and underpads, part 1: skin integrity outcomes, *Ostomy/Wound Manage* 40(9):20-32, 1994.

55. Bjornsdottir LT, Geirsson RT, Jonsson PV: Urinary incontinence and urinary tract infections in octogenarian women, *Acta Obstet Gynecol Scand* 77(1):105-109, 1998.

56. Raz R, Stamm W: A controlled trial of intravaginal estriol in postmenopausal women with recurrent urinary tract infections, *N Engl J Med* 329(11):753-756, 1993.

57. Eriksen B: A randomized, open, parallel-group study on the preventive effect of an estradiol-releasing vaginal ring (Estring) on recurrent urinary tract infections in postmenopausal women, *Am J Obstet Gynecol* 180(5):1072-1079, 1999.

58. Wilson L, Brown J, Park G, et al: Annual costs of urinary incontinence, *Obstet Gynecol* 98:398-406, 2001.

59. Kobelt G: Economic considerations and outcome measurements in urge incontinence, *Urology* 50(suppl 6A):100-107, 1997.

60. Wagner T, Hu TW: Economic costs of urinary incontinence in 1995, *Urology* 51(3):355-361, 1998.

61. Resnick N: Urinary incontinence, *Lancet* 346:94-99, 1995.

62. Baker D, Bice T: The influence of urinary incontinence on publicly financed home care services to low income elderly people, *Gerontologist* 35(3):360-389, 1995.

63. Frenchman I: Cost of urinary incontinence in two skilled nursing facilities: a prospective study, Available at: http://www.mmhc.com/cg/archives/01jan.shtml, 2003.

64. Thom D, Haan M, Eeden SK: Medically recognized urinary incontinence and risk of hospitalization, nursing home admission, and mortality, *Age Ageing* 26:367-374, 1997.

65. Drossman D, Li Z, Andruzzi E, et al: US householder survey of functional gastrointestinal disorders: prevalence, sociodemography, and health impact, *Dig Dis Sci* 38:1569-1580, 1993.

66. Umlauf MG, Goode PS, Burgio KL: Psychosocial issues in geriatric urology, *Geriatr Urol* 23(1):127-136, 1996.

67. Chelvanayagam S, Wilson S: Psychosocial aspects of patients with faecal incontinence. In Norton C, Chelvanayagam S, editors: *Bowel continence nursing*, Beaconsfield Publishers, 2004, Beaconsfield, UK, pp 33-44.

68. Nygaard I, Turvey C, Burns T, et al: Urinary incontinence and depression in middle-aged US women, *Obstet Gynecol* 101:149-156, 2003.

69. Stewart W, Van Rooyen J, Cundiff G, et al: Prevalence and burden of overactive bladder in the US, *World J Urol* 20:327-336, 2003.

70. Melville J, Walker E, Katon W, et al: Prevalence of comorbid psychiatric illness and its impact on symptom perception, quality of life, and functional status in women with urinary incontinence, *Am J Obstet Gynecol* 187:80-87, 2002.

71. Herzog AR, Diokno AC, Brown MB, et al: Urinary incontinence as a risk factor for mortality, *J Am Geriatr Soc* 42:264-268, 1994.

72. Hunskaar S, Vinsnes A: The quality of life in women with urinary incontinence measured by the sickness impact profile, *J Am Geriatr Soc* 39(4):378-382, 1991.

73. Kelleher CJ, Cardozo LD, Khullar V, Salvatore S: A new questionnaire to assess the quality of life of urinary incontinent women, *Br J Obstet Gynaecol* 104:1374-1379, 1997.

74. Lee PS, Reid DW, Saltmarche A, Linton L: Measuring the psychosocial impact of urinary incontinence: the York Incontinence Perceptions Scale (YIPS), *J Am Geriatr Soc* 43:1275-1278, 1995.

75. Valerius AJ: Quality of life tools for assessment of urinary incontinence, *Urol Nurs* 17(3):104-105, 1997.

76. Wagner TH, Patrick DL, Bavendam TG, et al: Quality of life of persons with urinary incontinence: development of a new measure, *Urology* 47(1):67-72, 1996.

77. Grimby A, Milsom I, Molander U, et al: The influence of urinary incontinence on the quality of life of elderly women, *Age Ageing* 22:82-89, 1993.

78. Payne C: Epidemiology, pathophysiology, and evaluation of urinary incontinence and overactive bladder, *Urology* 51(suppl 2A):3-10, 1998.

79. Seim A, Hermstad R, Hunskaar S: Management in general practice significantly reduced psychosocial consequences of female urinary incontinence, *Qual Life Res* 6:257-264, 1997.

80. Wyman JF, Harkins SW, Choi SC, et al: Psychosocial impact of urinary incontinence in women, *Obstet Gynecol* 70(3):378-381, 1987.

81. Robinson D, Pearce KF, Preisser JS, et al: Relationship between patient reports of urinary incontinence symptoms and quality of life measures, *Obstet Gynecol* 91(2):224-228, 1998.

82. Coward RT, Horne C, Peek CW: Predicting nursing home admissions among incontinent older adults: a comparison of residential differences across six years, *Gerontologist* 35(6):732-743, 1995.

83. Wein A: Classification of neurogenic voiding dysfunction, *J Urol* 125:605-609, 1981.

84. Bates P, Bradley W, et al: First report on the standardisation of terminology of lower urinary tract function, *Br J Urol* 48:39-42, 1976.

85. Abrams P, Blaivas JG, Stanton SL, Andersen JT: The standardisation of terminology of lower urinary tract function, *Scand J Urol Nephrol* 114(suppl): 5-19, 1988.

86. NANDA-approved nursing diagnoses and definitions. In *Mosby's medical, nursing, and allied health dictionary,* ed 5, St. Louis, 1999, Mosby.

87. Stohrer M, Goepel M, Kondo A, et al: The standardization of terminology in neurogenic lower urinary tract dysfunction with suggestions for diagnostic procedures, *Neurourol Urodyn* 18:139-158, 1999.

88. Ouslander J, Schnelle J: Incontinence in the nursing home, *Ann Intern Med* 122:438-449, 1995.

89. Resnick N: Geriatric incontinence, *Urol Clin North Am* 23(1):55-71, 1996.

90. Wound, Ostomy and Continence Nurses (WOCN) Society: *Position statement: role of wound, ostomy, and continence (ET) nurses in continence management,* Mt. Laurel, NJ, 1996, WOCN Society.

91. Department of Health and Human Services, Centers for Medicare and Medicaid Services. Surveyor Guidance for Incontinence and Catheters (S&C-05-23). Baltimore, MD, 2005.

CHAPTER

2

Physiology of Voiding

MIKEL L. GRAY

OBJECTIVES

1. List three goals for management of the individual with urinary incontinence.
2. Explain why conditions associated with high intravesical pressures place the individual at risk for upper urinary tract damage.
3. Identify the primary mechanism for control of smooth muscle contractility in the upper tracts (pelves and ureters) and in the bladder.
4. Identify key structures and functions of the "pelvic floor" (to include the role of the levator ani).
5. Compare the role of neural regulation in control of smooth muscle contractility in: (a) the upper urinary tracts, and (b) the bladder and urethra.
6. List three major factors affecting lower urinary tract function and urinary continence.
7. Describe the detrusor reflex.
8. Describe the role of each of the following structures in modulating detrusor contractility and the detrusor reflex: cerebral cortex, extrapyramidal nervous system, pontine micturition center, parasympathetic nerve pathways, and sympathetic nerve pathways.
9. Explain the role of the following neurotransmitters in the control of bladder and urethral function and the implications for pharmacologic management of patients with voiding dysfunction or incontinence: acetylcholine, norepinephrine, and adenosine triphosphate (ATP).
10. Explain the significance of urethral softness, urethral mucus production, and the submucosal vascular cushion in maintenance of urinary continence.
11. Explain the composition (in terms of slow-twitch, or Type 1, versus fast-twitch, or Type 2,

muscle fibers) and the roles of the rhabdosphincter, periurethral striated muscle, and the levator ani in the maintenance of continence.
12. Explain why continence is partially dependent on maintenance of an intraabdominal position for the bladder base and the proximal portion of the urethra.
13. Identify assessment parameters that could be used to determine a child's readiness for toilet training.
14. Identify the pathologic changes in bladder wall histologic characteristics and innervation that may result in impaired detrusor contractility in the older adult.
15. Explain how each of the following may affect bladder function and continence: cerebrovascular accident (CVA), Parkinson's disease, Alzheimer's disease, impaired perfusion of the frontal cortex, benign prostatic hypertrophy, and estrogen deficiency.

The normal lower urinary tract performs two primary functions: it stores urine to maintain continence and it evacuates urine via micturition. **Continence** is the act of storing urine in the bladder until a "socially appropriate" opportunity for bladder evacuation occurs; the term continence also implies absence of any urine loss between episodes of micturition, even during periods of physical activity or in the presence of a strong desire to urinate. Micturition is a coordinated act of bladder elimination. It requires relaxation of the pelvic floor muscles, opening of the urethral sphincter, contraction of the detrusor, and complete or nearly complete evacuation of urine from the bladder. Although continence is a complex phenomenon influenced by psychosocial, physiologic, and mechanical factors, it is frequently viewed from a single (behavioral, physiologic, or mechanical) perspective that fails to account for the complex interrelationship among all three factors.[1] For example, many lay persons (including many educators and employers) view continence as a "learned behavior" that is mastered during childhood and is expected to persist throughout adulthood.[2,3] Taken from this perspective, toilet access becomes a privilege that is regulated, and incontinence is implicitly defined as misbehavior or immature behavior. Similarly, clinicians with a strong physiologic perspective sometimes view continence exclusively as a series of neuromuscular events; these individuals may prescribe the correct drug for an incontinent patient but typically fail to address the behavioral changes needed to achieve optimal results with pharmacologic therapy. When the patient fails to respond as well as these clinicians expect, they express frustration. During the early 1970s, urodynamicists learned the peril of viewing continence from an exclusively mechanical perspective; they attempted to define lower urinary tract function via a series of equations describing relationships between detrusor pressure and urethral flow but found that these equations failed to explain continence or incontinence adequately in the clinical setting.

Nevertheless, research over the past several decades has considerably increased our understanding of lower urinary tract function and its role in maintaining urinary continence.[4,5] We now enjoy a much better understanding of many of the physiologic aspects that control lower urinary tract function and the mechanical factors that influence the delicate balance between pressure and urinary flow rates. However, many other factors affecting urinary continence remain poorly understood or unknown, and further research into lower urinary tract function and dysfunction is urgently needed.

Effective nursing management of the individual with urinary incontinence requires both careful assessment of all factors affecting continence and development of a comprehensive, rational, and individualized plan of care designed to meet the following goals: reduction or elimination of urinary leakage, protection of the upper urinary tracts against the complications of voiding dysfunction, maintenance of perineal skin integrity, and preservation of dignity. To assess and manage the patient with voiding dysfunction or urinary incontinence appropriately, the nurse must possess a thorough understanding of normal urinary tract function, the relationship between voiding dysfunction and upper urinary tract damage, and the factors affecting urinary continence. This chapter is designed to provide the nurse with an overview of upper urinary tract function and the potential effect of voiding dysfunction on the upper tracts and with a clear understanding of the three key components of urinary continence: (1) anatomic integrity of the lower urinary tract, (2) neurologic control of the detrusor (bladder) muscle, and (3) competence of the urethral sphincter mechanism. A brief review of the anatomy of the upper and lower urinary tracts and pelvic floor is provided, followed by a detailed discussion of the physiology of urinary continence and urine elimination and of changes across the life span.

UPPER URINARY TRACTS

The urinary system is commonly divided into the paired upper urinary tracts (comprising the kidneys, renal pelves, and ureters), and the lower urinary tract, which consists of the urinary bladder, urethra, and adjacent pelvic floor structures (Fig. 2-1). The kidneys are a pair of bean-shaped, symmetric organs located in the retroperitoneal space, parallel to vertebral levels T12 to L3. The lateral aspects of the kidneys assume a rounded, convex shape, and the medial aspects are marked by the smooth, concave surface known as the "hilum." The hilum is the point of entry and exit for the renal artery, renal veins, lymphatics, and nerves; the hilum also serves as the point of origin for the renal pelvis and urinary transport system. If the kidney is viewed in cross section, the renal cortex and renal medulla can be appreciated. The renal cortex is the outer section; it bounds the inner medulla and has a granular appearance when viewed by the naked eye.

The renal pyramids and adjacent cortex contain the functional unit of the kidney, the nephron.

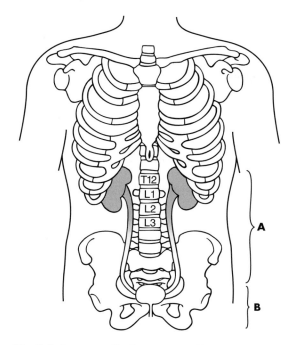

Fig. 2-1 Anatomy of urinary system. Upper urinary tracts, *A,* comprise the paired kidneys, renal pelves, and ureters; lower urinary tract, *B,* comprises the bladder and urethra.

Each nephron consists of a glomerulus and a tubular system, which are jointly responsible for urine production. The glomerulus is a capillary network that is supplied by the afferent arteriole and is surrounded by the collecting structure known as "Bowman's capsule"; as blood is forced through this capillary network under pressure, a large volume of dilute filtrate is produced. This filtrate is collected in Bowman's capsule and transported through the tubular system, whereas the remaining blood leaves the glomerulus through the efferent arteriole and subsequently passes through the peritubular capillary network. Most of the filtered water and electrolytes are reabsorbed (from the filtrate into the bloodstream) in the proximal tubule. Additional sodium and water exchange occurs in the loop of Henle according to a complex homeostatic system, and further exchange of water and specific ions takes place in the distal tubule and collecting

duct, partly under the influence of antidiuretic hormone. Collectively, these systems function to maintain internal homeostasis through the following processes: excretion of metabolic waste products and solutes, excretion or conservation of hydrogen ions and excretion or production of bicarbonate ions (to provide long-term preservation of pH balance), and regulation of blood pressure and hydration through the renin-angiotensin system and the selective excretion of water. The final product of the processes of filtration and reabsorption is urine, and the remainder of the urinary system is responsible for the transport, storage, and elimination of urine.

Urine transportation occurs in the renal pelves and ureters. The renal pelvis is a funnel-shaped structure that stores approximately 15 to 30 mL of urine. From its origin at the renal hilum, the paired renal pelves narrow until they join the ureters at the level of the ureteropelvic junction. The ureters are long, tubular structures that describe an inverted-S course as they travel from the renal pelvis to the base of the bladder. The ureters enter the bladder through the ureterovesical junction. This junction consists of three components: the intravesical ureter, the trigone, and the adjacent bladder wall. These components act together to permit urinary efflux (passage of urine from upper to lower urinary tract) and to prevent urinary reflux (retrograde movement of urine from lower to upper urinary tract). Any condition that causes loss of this one-way flow pattern and permits reflux of urine into the upper urinary tracts places the individual at risk for recurrent episodes of pyelonephritis and possible renal damage.

The renal pelves and ureters transport urine from the kidneys to the lower urinary tract by means of peristalsis. As the renal pelvis fills, pacemaker cells located in the calyces propagate a peristaltic contraction that transports a bolus of urine from the upper urinary tract through the ureter to the bladder. This peristaltic wave transports 5 to 15 mL of urine at relatively low pressures, varying from 20 to 60 cm H_2O. Because the system transporting urine from the upper tracts to the lower tract is a low-pressure system, conditions causing elevated intravesical pressures (such as conditions associated with low bladder wall compliance or bladder outlet obstruction) increase the risk of upper urinary tract distress; this condition is characterized by recurrent febrile urinary tract infections, hydroureteronephrosis, vesicoureteral reflux, and possibly compromised renal function.[6]

LOWER URINARY TRACT

The urinary bladder is a hollow, muscular organ that lies within the lower abdomen of the infant and within the true pelvis of the adult (the section of pelvis below an oblique plane extending from the symphysis pubis through the sacrum).[7] It is anatomically divided into two segments, the body and the base. The base of the bladder, sometimes called the "lissosphincter," is a triangular, fixed, and nondistensible structure located in the true pelvis[7,8] (Fig. 2-2). In the male, the bladder base is superior to the seminal vesicles and prostate gland and adjacent to the rectum. It is usually visualized as lying just above the superior margin of the symphysis pubis on cystography. In the female, the base of the bladder lies in proximity to the anterior vaginal wall, and it is seen just above the inferior margin of the symphysis pubis. The bladder base is characterized by two inlets and a single outlet. The inlets are the ureteral orifices that lie at the termination of the ureterovesical junctions; the outlet is the urethral orifice, commonly referred to as the "bladder neck." The triangular area formed by the two ureteral and one urethral orifice is known as the "trigone"; the ureteral orifices lay mediolaterally to the trigone.

The body of the bladder is anatomically continuous with the bladder base, although each structure has a unique embryonic origin. The dome of the bladder is attached to the anterior abdominal wall by the urachus. The body of the bladder is commonly referred to as the "detrusor," which is the primary smooth muscle of the bladder wall; the detrusor plays an essential role in bladder filling, urine storage, and urine expulsion. In contrast to the base, the body of the normal bladder is easily distensible. In the empty bladder, the body collapses onto the fixed base, assuming a roughly tetrahedron shape. As it fills with urine, the bladder assumes a roughly spherical shape; the adult bladder is normally able to accommodate approximately 300 to 600 mL of urine.

The urethra is a collapsible tube that extends from the bladder neck to an external meatus located just above the vaginal introitus in the female and in the glans penis of the male. The female urethra is approximately 3.5 to 5.5 cm in

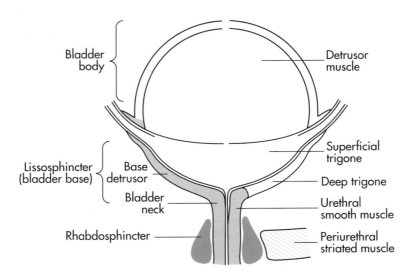

Fig. 2-2 The bladder can be divided into two regions: the fixed base, sometimes called the lissosphincter, and the flexible bladder body containing the detrusor muscle.

length; it exits the body at an approximate 16-degree angle with respect to the fixed bladder base. The distal two-thirds of the female urethra is fused to the anterior vaginal wall; these structures share vascular elements as well as muscular and endopelvic fascial support. Almost the entire female urethra functions as a sphincter mechanism with epithelial, vascular, and muscular components (Fig. 2-3).

The male urethra is approximately 23 cm long and is divided into two functional segments[9] (Fig. 2-4). The proximal portion of the urethra traverses the prostate gland and the pelvic muscles to form the sphincter mechanism; it is also known as the "posterior urethra" because of its anatomic position. The distal urethra provides little contribution to sphincter function; instead, it serves as a conduit for the expulsion of urine during micturition or semen during ejaculation. The posterior (proximal) urethra can be subdivided into three segments: the bladder neck (also called the "preprostatic urethra"), the prostatic urethra, and the membranous urethra.

The bladder neck is less than 1 cm in length and ends as the urethra intersects with the base of the prostate. The prostatic urethra is approximately 3 cm long; it courses through the prostate gland near its anterior aspect, traveling from its base (located just below the bladder base) to its apex (located just above the membranous urethra and adjacent pelvic floor muscle). The membranous urethra is approximately 2.5 cm long; it is bounded by pelvic floor muscles and contains specialized, striated muscle fibers within the urethral wall. The membranous urethra is the least distensible portion of the urethra and is often called the external sphincter. However, the entire proximal urethra contains compressive and muscular elements that form a sphincter mechanism functionally comparable to the female urethra.

The distal, or conduit, urethra in the male begins with a bulbous dilatation at the base of the erectile bodies of the penis (the corpora cavernosa). From this point, it courses through the posterior aspect of the flaccid penis to its termination at the

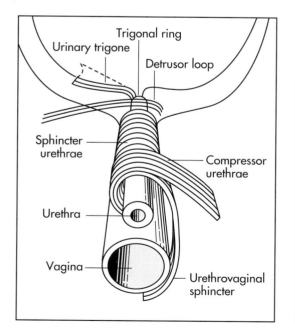
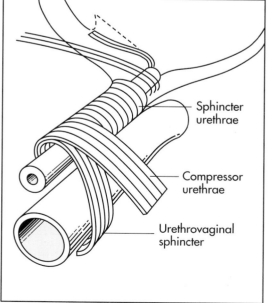

Fig. 2-3 The female urethra and muscular components of the female rhabdosphincter: sphincter urethrae, urethrovaginal sphincter, and compressor urethrae.

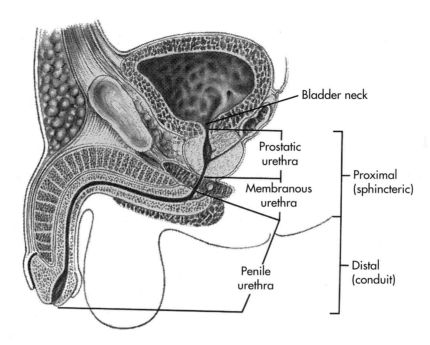

Fig. 2-4 The male urethra is divided into two functional units: the proximal (sphincteric) urethra and the distal (conduit) urethra. (From Thompson JM, McFarland GK, Hirsch JE, Tucker SM: *Mosby's clinical nursing,* ed 4, St. Louis, 1997, Mosby.)

glans penis. The penile urethra is surrounded by the corpus spongiosum, a rich, vascular structure that lies between the inferior aspects of the two erectile bodies.

CELLULAR ANATOMY OF THE URINARY TRACT

The walls of the urinary tract distal to the nephron consist of four distinctive histologic layers that contribute to urinary transport, storage, and evacuation: the urothelium, lamina propria, smooth muscle (muscular tunic), and serosa.[10,11]

The urothelium of the urinary bladder is primarily composed of transitional epithelium that can be roughly subdivided into three layers: (1) smaller cells at the base of the urothelium (closest to the underlying submucosa) that reproduce rapidly to replace cells lost from the superficial layer that is exposed to urine, (2) a middle layer of medium-sized cells, and (3) a superficial layer of very large cells (the largest epithelial cells in the human body) that line the vesicle of the bladder and are called umbrella cells. Immediately beneath the urothelium is the lamina propria (sometimes called the submucosa), which contains blood vessels, lymphatics, nerves, and extracellular matrix (connective tissues and proteins critical to the structural integrity of organs and tissues within the body).

Beneath the lamina propria is a tunic of smooth muscle. Smooth muscle cells differ from skeletal muscle cells in several important aspects that are relevant to bladder function.[5,10] Smooth muscle cells tend to be smaller than skeletal muscle cells, and they are arranged in bundles, in contrast to the striated fibers that characterize skeletal muscle. Smooth muscle cells develop a contraction relatively slowly; however, they are generally able to sustain the contraction much longer than a skeletal muscle.

Both smooth and skeletal muscles contain actin and myosin protein filaments, and the interaction between these filaments creates the mechanical shortening (contraction) that allows movement. However, unlike striated muscle, the actin and myosin in smooth muscle cells are arranged in a variable configuration that links individual cells to neighboring cells. Because of this characteristic, smooth muscle is more adaptable than skeletal muscle; it can adjust its length over a much wider range than skeletal muscle, which is essential because the urinary bladder fills to accommodate widely varying volumes of urine.

Although the precise mechanisms that regulate smooth muscle contraction and relaxation are not fully understood, it is known that depolarization (contraction) relies on release of intracellular calcium ions, which bind to the protein calmodulin. Calmodulin activates an enzyme called kinase that promotes the transfer of phosphate from adenosine triphosphate (ATP), resulting in interactions between actin and myosin and contraction of the muscle cell. Relaxation of smooth muscle cells requires a reduction in intracellular calcium ions that is modulated by the opening of potassium ion channels. All smooth muscles of the urinary tract are likely to develop phasic contractions when subjected to unopposed stretch. Contraction of smooth muscle cells within the bladder is primarily provoked by autonomic stimulation, which causes release of neurotransmitters at the abundant neuromuscular junctions within the detrusor and urethra. However, smooth muscle cells also maintain a steady level of tension that is modulated by hormones and local factors such as nitric oxide (NO), as well as neurotransmitters released by autonomic nerves throughout the urinary tract and particularly in the bladder and urethra.

The smooth muscle bundles of the renal pelves and ureters are loosely organized into an outer longitudinal layer and an inner circular layer. The smooth muscle bundles of the upper urinary tracts have particularly tight connections, including gap junctions; this construction allows for rapid spread of an electrical stimulus, which results in synchronized muscle contraction. Thus, a contractile wave can rapidly propel urine from the renal pelvis

through the ureter and into the bladder; this peristaltic contraction typically occurs in response to stretch as the renal pelvis fills with urine and is independent of neural stimulation.[12] The contractile wave is initiated in pacemaker cells believed to be located near the ureterocalyceal border, and the resulting contraction is rapidly propagated throughout the length of the ureter.

Because of the close connections between the smooth muscle cells of the upper urinary tracts, neuromuscular junctions are relatively uncommon in the renal pelvis and ureter. Nonetheless, the nervous system exerts an indirect modulatory influence on the smooth muscle of the renal pelvis and ureter. Although the mechanisms of this modulation remain unclear, it is believed that stimulation of the parasympathetic nervous system (PSNS) increases the frequency and amplitude of ureteral peristalsis and that sympathetic nervous stimulation (SNS) inhibits this activity. Specific drugs are also known to affect ureteral peristalsis. Antihistamines and morphine have been shown to enhance ureteral peristalsis, whereas calcium-channel blockers, anticholinergics, and ampicillin have been shown to inhibit ureteral contractility.

The smooth muscle of the bladder is noticeably different from that found in the renal pelves and ureters.[13] Smooth muscle bundles in the detrusor are arranged in a complex meshwork so that no distinctive layers can be identified. The detrusor muscle also lacks the gap junctions characteristic of the smooth muscle in the renal pelves and ureters, and detrusor muscle bundles exhibit comparatively poor electrical coupling when compared with smooth muscle within the renal pelvis, ureter, or bowel.[14,15] This characteristic promotes continence by rendering the detrusor muscle resistant to spontaneous, stretch-induced mass contractions during bladder filling and storage. In contrast to the upper tracts, neuromuscular junctions are found throughout the detrusor muscle in a ratio of nearly 1:1, indicating that neural control plays a very significant role in detrusor contraction.

In addition to the smooth muscle bundles and neuromuscular junctions of the detrusor, the bladder wall contains an extensive extracellular matrix composed chiefly of collagen and elastin, with collagen the predominant of the two. Sheaths of collagen invaginate the smooth muscle of the detrusor or form bundles that penetrate the mucosa. Collagen bundles are relatively noncompliant (that is, poorly distensible), and an overabundance of collagen produces the visible trabeculation commonly seen in neuropathic or obstructed bladders. Elastin fibers are comparatively sparse throughout the bladder wall and detrusor muscle. They are arranged in a spiral, springlike configuration and are more distensible than collagen.

The urethra is distinguished from the upper urinary tract and bladder in that it contains both smooth muscle and a specialized form of striated muscle. The smooth muscle bundles of the male bladder neck form a circular ring; this does not occur in the female bladder neck. However, in both sexes, longitudinally arranged smooth muscle bundles extend into the proximal portion of the urethra; these bundles may represent an extension of the detrusor or trigonal smooth muscle. In addition to this smooth muscle, specialized striated (skeletal) muscle is found in the membranous urethra of the male and throughout almost the entire length of the female urethra. These skeletal muscles are "specialized" in that they are designed to maintain tone over long periods of time.

PELVIC FLOOR

The term "pelvic floor" typically refers to the bony structures, endopelvic fascia, and muscles that support the pelvic organs and contribute to the sphincter mechanism for both the urinary and intestinal tracts. Because the pelvic floor is difficult to visualize, its components bear multiple names, and one segment of a muscle or fascial sheet may be distinctly labeled as if it were a separate structure. For the purposes of this discussion, the bony pelvis, endopelvic fascia, and pelvic muscles are described as functional units, and the individual structures frequently named and described in surgical texts are described separately only if they directly contribute to our current understanding of continence or serve as a surgical landmark or point of attachment for the various surgical procedures used to manage urinary incontinence.

Female Pelvic Floor

The bony pelvis of the female is a ring of bones that can be described according to their relative positions on the face of a clock[16] (Fig. 2-5, *A*). The 6 o'clock position is occupied by the symphysis pubis, and the pubic bones occupy the regions between 3 and 5 o'clock and between 7 and 9 o'clock. The 12 o'clock position is occupied by the sacral bone, and the areas between 9 and 11 o'clock and

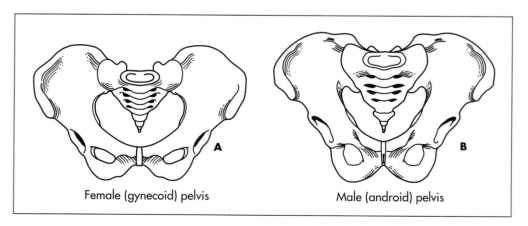

Female (gynecoid) pelvis   Male (android) pelvis

Fig. 2-5 The bony pelvis of the female, *A*, and the male, *B*.

between 1 and 3 o'clock are occupied by the pelvic side walls. (The pelvic side walls include the ischial spine, the sciatic foramen, and the sacral attachments.) All the muscles and endopelvic fascia of the female are anchored to the bony structures of the pelvis.

The endopelvic fascia of the female is continuous with the retroperitoneal fascia; it consists of fibromuscular tissue that contributes to the support of the pelvic organs, including the bladder base and the urethra.[16,17] The endopelvic fascia can be subdivided into the endopelvic and levator portions,[18] but for the purposes of this discussion the pelvic floor fascia is considered a single functional unit. In addition to connective tissue, the endopelvic fascia also contains varying portions of smooth muscle and vascular elements; the specific "mix" of tissue types is dependent on the location and functional role of the specific structure. Condensations of the endopelvic fascia are referred to as ligaments, although it is important to remember that these ligaments typically constitute only one aspect of a larger fascial plane. Collectively, the endopelvic fascia invaginates the pelvic viscera and provides a secondary source of support for these organs; the *primary* support structure for the pelvic organs is the levator ani muscle.

The upper vagina, cervix, and uterus are attached to the pelvic side walls by a relatively large sheet of endopelvic fascia,[16] which originates at the greater sciatic foramen of the bony pelvis and inserts into the lateral walls of the cervix and the proximal third of the vagina (Fig. 2-6). Condensations of this fascia are separately labeled as the cardinal and uterosacral ligaments, although these two structures are anatomically contiguous. Downward reflections of this fascial sheet support the middle portion of the vagina and attach to the pelvic side walls.

The endopelvic fascia also forms a hammock that stretches and supports the vagina between the side walls of the pelvis; this hammock helps to prevent the bladder from prolapsing into the potential space of the vaginal vault. Posterior fascial structures extend this support and form a horizontal sheet that supports the rectum and prevents it from prolapsing forward into the potential space of the vagina. These sheets of connective tissue are often labeled the "pubocervical" and "rectovaginal" fascia. Again, it is important to remember that they represent individual aspects of a larger, functionally continuous fascial sheet that provides support to the cervix, vagina, and upper uterus and indirect support to the bladder and rectum.

Specific fascial ligaments or condensations of larger fascial tissue planes are significant to any discussion of continence because they are used to create compensatory support during surgical correction of urethral hypermobility and pelvic organ prolapse associated with stress urinary incontinence.[16,18] Table 2-1 summarizes specific areas of the endopelvic fascia that form important surgical landmarks and their functional significance to continence management.

The primary supportive muscle of the female pelvic floor is the levator ani.[16,18] In the standing woman, the levator ani provides a horizontal plane of support for the bladder base, vagina, and adjacent pelvic organs. The levator also contributes to urethral sphincter function, particularly during periods of physical exertion. As is true of the endopelvic fascia, various descriptions of the levator

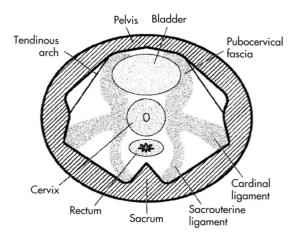

Fig. 2-6 Schema of endopelvic fascial structures in the female. (Modified from Wahle GR, Young GPH, Raz S: Anatomy and physiology of pelvic support. In Raz S, editor: *Female urology*, ed 2, Philadelphia, 1996, WB Saunders.)

TABLE 2-1 Condensations of the Female Endopelvic Fascia

LIGAMENT	DESCRIPTION
Pubourethral ligaments	Condensations of endopelvic fascia that bridge lower, inner surface of symphysis pubis and middle of urethra
Urethropelvic ligaments	Endopelvic fascia providing support for bladder neck and proximal urethra
Vesicopelvic ligaments	Fascial condensations that attach to pelvic side walls providing lateral support to bladder base and pelvic side wall; loss of this fascial support creates a paravaginal wall defect
Cooper's ligament	Condensation of connective tissue at the top of the crural arch from the inferior iliac to the pubic bone; provides support and structure for the floor of the inguinal canal
Broad ligament	Triangular fold of the peritoneum; supports uterus and fallopian tube
Round ligament	Passes from superior lateral angle of the uterus to the internal inguinal ring and supports uterus and fallopian tube
Uterosacral ligament (sacrouterine ligament, or cardinal-uterosacral complex)	Two short cords that pass from cervix toward sacrum; holds the cervix upward and backward and provides forward slant of uterus
Mackenrodt's ligament (cardinal ligament)	Condensation of uterosacral fascial complex; contributes to support of upper vagina, cervix, and uterus
Sacrospinous ligaments	Attaches ischial spine to lateral aspect of sacrum and coccyx; used for repair of severe uterine prolapse
Arcus tendineus fasciae pelvis/"white line"	Linear condensation extending from the pubic bone to the ischial spine; acts as important surgical landmark

ani have led to confusion concerning its anatomic description; a review of 265 studies of the levator muscle in humans consistently revealed five pairs of origin and insertion points carrying as many as 16 labels in women alone.[19] Despite the variety of labels, the levator ani in female humans can be described according to these five pairs of origins and insertions, most commonly described as: (1) puboperineal, (2) pubovaginal, (3) pubococcygeal (frequently called pubovisceral and puboanal), (4) puborectal, and (5) iliococcygeal. Two portions are thought to play the most direct role in maintaining urinary continence, the pubococcygeal (pubovisceral or puboanal) and the iliococcygeus (Color Plate 1). The first portion consists of U-shaped muscle fibers that arise from the pubic bones, attach to the lateral walls of the vagina and rectum, and extend around the posterior portion of the rectum. This portion of the levator ani is called the "pubococcygeus," or the "pubovisceral" muscle. The second portion of the levator ani is the relatively thin ileococcygeus muscle that originates from the pelvic side walls and inserts into the bony pelvis behind the rectum. Although five origin and insertion pairs for the levator ani have been identified (and assigned a wide variety of names), the continence nurse should remember that it comprises a single functional unit, particularly when viewed from the perspective of pelvic muscle rehabilitation.

Male Pelvic Floor

The pelvic floor in the male, as in the female, is composed of the bony pelvis, endopelvic fascia, and pelvic muscles. The bony pelvis of the male is comparable to the female pelvis in many aspects. The anterior portion of the male pelvis is formed by the symphysis pubis and pubic bones, the side walls are comparable, and the posterior surface comprises the coccyx and sacrum and their bony attachments. However, the pelvic side walls of the male have a steeper angle than the female's, and the pelvic inlet is narrower than that of the female and is shaped more like a heart rather than the circular shape of the female inlet (Fig. 2-5, *B*).

The pelvic fascia in the male is analogous to the pelvic fascia of the female in several ways: it is continuous with the retroperitoneal fascia, it can be divided into the endopelvic (abdominal) fascia and the levator ani fascia, and individual segments have been given specific names.[17,20] However, it functions as a single unit, and for the purpose of this discussion, the term "pelvic fascia" is used to describe those elements that serve as a secondary supportive structure for the pelvic viscera in the male. The puboprostatic fascia is the section that extends from the inner aspects of the symphysis pubis and pubic bones to the junction of the prostatic and membranous urethra; condensations of this fascia are known as the "puboprostatic ligaments." The puboprostatic fascia provides lateral support for the bladder base and urethra and inserts into the ischial spines of the male's pelvic side walls. The pelvic fascia is located posteriorly to the ischial spines in the male; this segment extends from the rectum to the pelvic side walls, thus providing posterior support and separating the urethra, bladder base, seminal vesicles, and prostate gland from the rectum. The anterior rectal wall, prostate gland, and seminal vesicles are separated by a thin layer of pelvic connective tissue called "Denonvilliers' fascia"; this fascial sheet covers the posterior aspect of the prostate gland and then extends above the prostatic base to partially enfold the posterior aspect of the seminal vesicles. Denonvilliers' fascia is densest at the base of the prostate and the seminal vesicles but thins significantly as it approaches the membranous urethra (Table 2-2).

As in the female, primary support for the bladder base and urethra is provided by the levator ani muscle. Similar to the female, two portions of the levator ani are considered most important to a discussion of continence, the U-shaped pubococcygeus (pubovisceral) and the ileococcygeus.[20] In contrast to the female, the levator ani in the male is generally thicker and narrower, and it lacks a vaginal opening.

TABLE 2-2 Condensations of the Male Endopelvic Fascia

LIGAMENT	FUNCTIONAL SIGNIFICANCE
Puboprostatic ligament	Attached to back of pelvic bone and to visceral layer of pelvic fascia on prostate, providing support for the prostate gland and bladder base
Denonvilliers's fascia	Covers and fuses with pelvic endopelvic fascia covering the prostate; actually a reflection of peritoneal connective tissue
Arcus tendineus/ "white line"	Linear condensation extending from the pubic bone to the ischial spine; indicates the origin of the levator ani

Microscopic Anatomy of the Pelvic Floor

The endopelvic fascia is primarily composed of the connective tissues collagen and elastin.[16,17] However, it may also contain vascular elements, neural elements, and smooth muscle, depending on its location in the pelvis and its functional role. For example, the cardinal ligaments contain vascular elements as well as connective tissue, whereas the perirectal fascia contains few vascular elements and more collagen. Similarly, the pubovesical fascia contains smooth muscle, which is postulated to interact with muscular elements of the urethra to promote urethral closure during bladder filling and urethral funneling during micturition. Thus, the endopelvic fascia provides a dynamic rather than a static source of support for the bladder base and urethra. This flexibility is an essential element of support for the varied functions of the pelvic floor, which include storage and elimination of urine and stool as well as labor and delivery in the female.

The microscopic anatomy of the levator ani muscle also provides important clues to its function. The levator ani muscle consists of skeletal muscle fibers that are innervated by branches of the pudendal nerve.[7] As in all skeletal muscles, the functional element of the levator ani is the motor unit.[21] A motor unit consists of an anterior horn cell (neuron), its axon, a neuromuscular junction, and the muscle fibers; the neuromuscular junction provides "connection" and "communication" between the nervous system and the muscle fibers. Skeletal muscles can be divided into slow-twitch and fast-twitch fibers.[21] Type 1 (slow-twitch) fibers are adapted to maintain muscle tone over prolonged periods of time, whereas Type 2 (fast-twitch) fibers are physiologically designed to provide the rapid contraction required for sudden physical exertion. The levator ani is composed of approximately 70% Type 1 fibers and 30% Type 2 fibers. The preponderance of slow-twitch fibers allows the muscle to provide sustained support for an individual in the upright (standing) position, whereas the fast-twitch fibers provide rapid contraction of the periurethral and perianal fibers whenever there is a need to increase sphincter tone to offset a sudden increase in abdominal force (as when a person coughs, sneezes, or lifts a heavy object).

FACTORS AFFECTING CONTINENCE
Anatomic Integrity of the Urinary System

The urinary tract can be conceptualized as a single tube that extends from the glomerulus to the urethral meatus. Effective transport, storage, and elimination of urine and maintenance of continence are dependent partially on the anatomic integrity of this contiguous tube. Two conditions may interrupt the anatomic continuity of the urinary tract and allow urine to bypass the urethral sphincter mechanism.[6] The first is ectopia of the ureter or bladder. Ectopia of the ureter occurs when a duplicated ureter bypasses the urethral sphincter mechanism and opens into a structure other than the bladder. For example, some women have an ectopic ureteral orifice that empties into the vagina; this results in continuous urinary leakage that is typically superimposed on an otherwise normal voiding pattern. Ectopia, or "exstrophy," of the bladder is a relatively uncommon defect characterized by externalization of the entire bladder as well as pelvic diastasis (widening of the pelvis and separation of the

symphysis pubis) and splaying of the urethra to the level of the bladder neck. The second condition that may interrupt the anatomic integrity of the urinary tract and produce urinary leakage is a fistula. A fistula is an acquired condition characterized by an abnormal passage or epithelialized tube that connects the urethra or bladder with the skin or vagina; it causes extraurethral urine loss that varies from a continuous dribble to a constant leakage that replaces any identifiable voiding pattern.

Control of the Detrusor Muscle

The concept of detrusor control is based on clinical observations that spontaneous contraction of the detrusor muscle, before a person desires to urinate, is a common (but not universal) characteristic of urge urinary incontinence and overactive bladder dysfunction.[22,23] Based on the relationship between overactive detrusor contractions and urge urinary incontinence, it has been traditionally presumed that the detrusor muscle remains relaxed until the person voluntarily (albeit indirectly) initiates a detrusor contraction via the act of micturition.[24] However, the concept of a "stable" detrusor, defined as one that remains entirely relaxed throughout bladder filling and storage and contracts only during micturition, has been challenged by multiple researchers; these investigators used urodynamic techniques to demonstrate the presence of low-pressure contractions during bladder filling that do not produce urine loss or an immediate and strong desire to urinate.[25-28] These observations have led some researchers to advocate the following terminology (labels) for bladder contractions that occur during the filling phase: (1) "phasic"[28] or "filling"[25] contractions, that is, contractions not associated with bothersome urgency or with urine loss; and (2) "overactive" contractions, that is, contractions associated with overactive bladder symptoms (urgency and frequency) and/or urge urinary incontinence.

A more recent study using an animal model has significantly increased our understanding of the detrusor response to bladder filling. Gillespie and colleagues[29] differentiated two types of detrusor activity: (1) phasic activity characterized by activation of small regions of the bladder wall in response to localized stretch, and (2) global contractions involving most of the bladder wall. These experiments were able to demonstrate clinically relevant differences in phasic versus global contractions based on response to antimuscarinic agonists, nicotinic agonists, and nerve stimulation. Although it is tempting to apply results of this experiment to the clinical setting and to conclude that the phasic or filling contractions observed during urodynamic testing in normal human subjects corresponds to the two types of detrusor activity seen in the animal model, there are insufficient data to determine whether localized phasic detrusor contractions do occur in humans and whether these can be observed via urodynamic testing. However, if phasic and global contractions can be demonstrated in the human detrusor, we will gain important answers to persistent questions about the absence of overactive detrusor contractions in many patients with overactive bladder dysfunction, and the presence of measurable contractions in normal subjects.

Whether or not phasic detrusor activity occurs in humans, it is known that proprioceptive stretch receptors are stimulated by distension of the bladder wall and that activation of these receptors produces an awareness of bladder filling that is perceived as the "desire to urinate." As the intravesical volume increases, the magnitude of this desire increases, and this prompts the individual to find a socially appropriate time and place to relieve this desire via micturition. Thus, continence demands control of the detrusor during both phases of bladder function, filling/storage and micturition. As noted previously, this control is primarily neurologic and originates in modulatory centers found within the central nervous system.

Neurologic control of the detrusor is only partly understood. Although we have identified most of the major structures in the brain involved in lower urinary tract function, little is known about the complex cross-talk that exists among these centers and about the roles of the surprisingly large variety of neurotransmitters within the central nervous system that regulate lower urinary tract function[30] (Fig. 2-7). This discussion of detrusor control is divided into two sections, efferent and afferent pathways. "Efferent pathway" is a broad term used

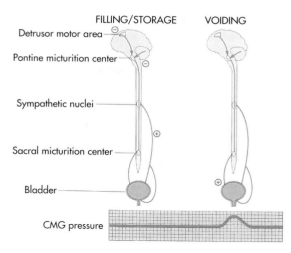

Fig. 2-7 Schema of neurologic control of detrusor during bladder filling and storage and during micturition. (From Gray M: *Genitourinary disorders,* Mosby's clinical nursing series, St. Louis, 1992, Mosby.)

to describe motor control of the detrusor muscle via peripheral nerves acting under the influence of the central nervous system. The term "afferent pathways" is used to describe neurologic mechanisms that alert the individual to bladder distension, the desire to urinate, and bothersome lower urinary tract symptoms such as urgency and pain.

Efferent Pathways in the Brain. Sophisticated brain imaging has significantly improved our understanding of the principal modulatory areas in the brain that are responsible for continence. For example, a "detrusor motor area" (paired collection of nuclei in the prefrontal cortex) has long been associated with lower urinary tract function[31]; however, functional imaging studies (positron emission tomography and related techniques) have more recently demonstrated that the anterior cingulate gyrus and frontal cortex exert considerable control over both bladder filling and micturition and that nuclei within the right hemisphere of the brain predominate.[32-36] Further evidence of this influence on lower urinary tract function is provided by research into the associations among detrusor overactivity, urge urinary incontinence, and dysfunction of the frontal lobe and anterior cingulate gyrus. For example, it is well known that the blood supply of these areas is derived from branches of the middle and anterior cerebral arteries, and these arteries are the most common locations of CVAs in the United States.[37,38] Data indicate that lesions involving the frontal lobe are associated with detrusor overactivity and urge urinary incontinence, whereas those affecting the occipital lobe are not.[39] Similarly, detrusor overactivity resulting in urinary incontinence in frail elders is associated with poor perfusion of the cerebral cortex, a condition not seen in age-matched controls who remain continent.[40]

The thalamus is a relay center connecting the cerebral cortex with lower centers of the brain. Activation of the thalamus occurs during bladder distension, but not when the bladder is provoked by iced saline cystometry (bladder filling using saline that is chilled to 0° Celsius).[35,36] Although the relationships between the thalamus and frontal cortex or cingulate gyrus remain unclear, these observations provide further support that the thalamus promotes bladder filling and storage and acts in conjunction with multiple other modulatory areas in the brain.

The extrapyramidal nervous system consists of the basal ganglia, caudate nuclei, red nuclei, substantia nigra, putamen, and globus pallidus. Collectively, these nuclei interact with the cerebellum and the corticospinal tracts (pyramidal system) to coordinate motor movements and to maintain the body's position in space. Two areas, the basal ganglia and cerebellum, are hypothesized to influence lower urinary tract function and to promote bladder filling and storage.

The association between the basal ganglia and lower urinary tract function is principally derived from strong clinical correlations between basal ganglia dysfunction (Parkinson's disease) and overactive detrusor contractions leading to urgency and urge urinary incontinence.[41-43] In addition, stimulation of the subthalamic nucleus in patients with parkinsonism has been found to increase both bladder capacity and the cystometric volume required to stimulate an overactive detrusor contraction.[44] These observations have led clinicians to hypothesize that the basal ganglia contribute to inhibition of detrusor contractions, thus promoting bladder filling and storage, and that this is compromised when dopamine levels are diminished by parkinsonism.

The cerebellum is located within the posterior fossa of the cranium. It helps to coordinate voluntary movements and the ability to maintain an upright (standing) position without support. Although neurologic communication between the detrusor and the cerebellum has not been clearly delineated, cerebellar dysfunction is associated with detrusor overactivity in humans,[45,46] and cerebellar lesions in multiple sclerosis are associated with bladder dysfunction and urinary incontinence.

Imaging studies and research using animal models have identified multiple other areas in the brain that are activated during bladder filling/storage or during micturition. They include the midbrain (mesencephalon), additional areas in the gyrus, hypothalamus, globus pallidus, and the vermis.[32,36,47] However, there is insufficient evidence to define their role in lower urinary tract function.

Research in both animals and humans clearly demonstrates that the brainstem exerts a significant effect on continence.[33,34,35,48] Three areas in the brainstem play an important role in control of the detrusor. One collection of nuclei in the pons promotes bladder filling and storage (L region), and another set of nuclei coordinates bladder contraction and sphincter relaxation (M region). The coordination of detrusor and sphincter response is essential for effective evacuation of urine during micturition. A third center, the periaqueductal gray, receives communication from nuclei in the pons and is thought to act as an integration center, primarily promoting bladder filling and storage.[49-52] These brainstem centers do not receive direct input from the sacral spinal cord; instead, they receive input from various regions of the brain.[5,53] Although the mechanisms by which modulatory areas in the brainstem control the detrusor reflex remain unclear, these pathways for neural communication add weight to the theory that multiple areas of the brain work together to control detrusor function.[54]

Efferent Pathways in the Spinal Cord and Peripheral Nerves. The spinal cord also plays a critical role in control of lower urinary tract function,[6] in that the spinal cord provides the pathways that permit communication between the central nervous system and the bladder and sphincter. Detrusor control is modulated by fibers of the autonomic nervous system.[55] SNS efferents originate from spinal nuclei typically located between the tenth thoracic and the second lumbar segments. Stimulation of the sympathetic nerve roots innervating the bladder and proximal portion of the urethra promotes detrusor muscle relaxation and contraction of the proximal urethral musculature, thus promoting bladder filling and urine storage.[56] Efferent pathways from the PSNS originate from spinal nuclei located in sacral segments 2 to 4. Stimulation of the parasympathetic nerve roots innervating the bladder causes contraction of the detrusor muscle (by direct stimulation) and urethral opening (primarily via indirect, inhibitory mechanisms). Two efferent peripheral nerve pathways carry the sympathetic and parasympathetic signals from the spinal cord to the urinary bladder. The inferior hypogastric nerve plexus is postulated to provide the primary sympathetic input to the detrusor muscle, whereas parasympathetic input is provided primarily by the pelvic plexus (see Fig. 2-7).

Neural stimulation produces muscle contraction or relaxation through the release of chemical messengers known as "neurotransmitters."[57] Neurotransmitters are released from the neuromuscular junction in response to neural stimulation and then bind to receptors on the target muscle cells, producing a physiologic response. Table 2-3 provides a description of the specific neurotransmitters significant to detrusor function.

Neurotransmitters in the Bladder. Neurotransmitters are substances that act as messengers within the nervous system or between the nervous system and target organs such as a muscle. Within the lower urinary tract, neurotransmitters act on efferent pathways to stimulate or inhibit muscular activity. To qualify as a neurotransmitter, a substance must have the following characteristics: (1) it must be found within a neuron, (2) it must be synthesized within the neuron, (3) it must be released when the neuron is stimulated, (4) it must act on receptors in another neuron or muscle cell to create a biologic effect (such as contraction of a muscle), and (5) it must be inactivated following its release (via reuptake or by a deactivating enzyme). Our understanding of neurotransmitters and the receptors that they act on has grown dramatically (within the past several

decades in particular), as has our appreciation for the remarkable complexity with which multiple neurotransmitters interact to accomplish a single physiologic function such as micturition (Table 2-3). This chapter reviews some of the best-known physiologic responses directly attributable to the action of neurotransmitters acting on the lower urinary tract; however, all these responses are continuously modulated and altered by the action of other neurotransmitters acting within the central nervous system and the lower urinary tract, and each of these substances is subject to "cross-talk." The concept of cross-talk is clinically relevant because it provides a more accurate understanding of the complexity of the neuromuscular regulation of the lower urinary tract and the remarkably variable responses among different patients when given a single pharmacologic agent.

Acetylcholine. Detrusor contraction is primarily mediated by stimulation of cholinergic receptors, which release acetylcholine in response to parasympathetic stimulation.[5] Cholinergic receptors and the neurotransmitter acetylcholine are found throughout the central and peripheral nervous systems as well as within the bladder wall; the response of a specific organ is determined by the type of receptors within the synapse or neuromuscular junction. For example, preganglionic nerve synapses within the PSNS contain nicotinic receptors, which are inhibited by curare. In contrast, the postganglionic receptors (including those found in the neuromuscular junctions of the detrusor muscle) are muscarinic; these receptors are inhibited by anticholinergics such as atropine. Recent research has led to additional subdivision of the muscarinic cholinergic receptors based on their pharmacologic affinity for specific cholinergic radioligands.[58,59] Although at least five muscarinic receptor subtypes have been identified, receptors within the detrusor muscle are limited to the M_2 and M_3 subtypes. Familiarity with muscarinic receptors, and their distribution throughout the body, is significant because they are the primary targets for pharmacologic agents developed for treatment of overactive bladder (Fig. 2-8). For example, some of the widely available "anticholinergic" medications (such as oxybutynin) act at the

TABLE 2-3   **Principal Receptors within the Lower Urinary Tract and their Pharmacologic Significance**

NEUROTRANSMITTER/ PHYSIOLOGIC ACTION	ASSOCIATED RECEPTORS	PHARMACOLOGIC SIGNIFICANCE
Acetylcholine	**Smooth muscle** Muscarinic	Cholinergic agents used to stimulate bladder muscle contraction (bethanechol chloride).
Stimulates contraction of smooth and striated muscle	Muscarinic subtypes: M_1 to M_5, M2 and M3 predominate in lower urinary tract Striated muscle nicotinic	Antimuscarinic agents: inhibit overactive detrusor contractions Oxybutynin (nonspecific, readily penetrates CNS) Tolterodine (evidence of organ but not receptor specificity, less likely to penetrate CNS) Trospium (poor penetrance into CNS) Solefenacin* (receptor specificity, higher affinity for M_3 receptors) Darifenacin* (receptor specificity, higher affinity for M_3 receptors)
Norepinephrine Stimulates smooth muscle contraction (via alpha- adrenergic receptors) or smooth muscle relaxation (via beta-2 or beta-3 receptors)	**Smooth muscle** Beta-3 adrenergic receptors in the bladder body Beta-2 adrenergic receptors in bladder neck Alpha-1a adrenergic receptors in urethral (and prostatic) smooth muscle	Nonspecific beta-adrenergic agents not found effective in the treatment of overactive bladder dysfunction (primarily because of intolerable cardiovascular or pulmonary side effects) but beta-3 specific agonists currently under investigation may overcome these limitations. Nonspecific alpha-adrenergic agonists increase bladder outlet resistance Ephedrine Pseudoephedrine Imipramine Alpha-adrenergic antagonists reduce bladder outlet resistance in bladder neck and urethra resulting from benign prostatic hypertrophy Terazosin (long-acting alpha-1 antagonist) Doxazosin (long-acting alpha-1 antagonist) Tamsulosin (greater receptor specificity to alpha-1a adrenergic subtypes reduces associated hypotension) Alfuzosin (greater receptor specificity to alpha-1a adrenergic subtypes reduces associated hypotension, reduced risk for retrograde ejaculation when compared with tamsulosin, doxazosin, or terazosin)

CNS, central nervous system.
* Investigational agent.

level of the muscarinic receptors to cause inhibition of detrusor muscle contractions; however, these agents also bind to muscarinic receptors in other organs. (This explains the constipation, blurred vision, dry mouth, and heat intolerance that constitute the common side effects of these drugs.)

Newer antimuscarinic drugs are designed to be either "organ-specific" or "receptor-specific."[60] To illustrate, tolterodine is an organ-specific agent; although it demonstrates comparable affinity for all muscarinic receptor subtypes, it does show greater affinity for receptors in the bladder wall as

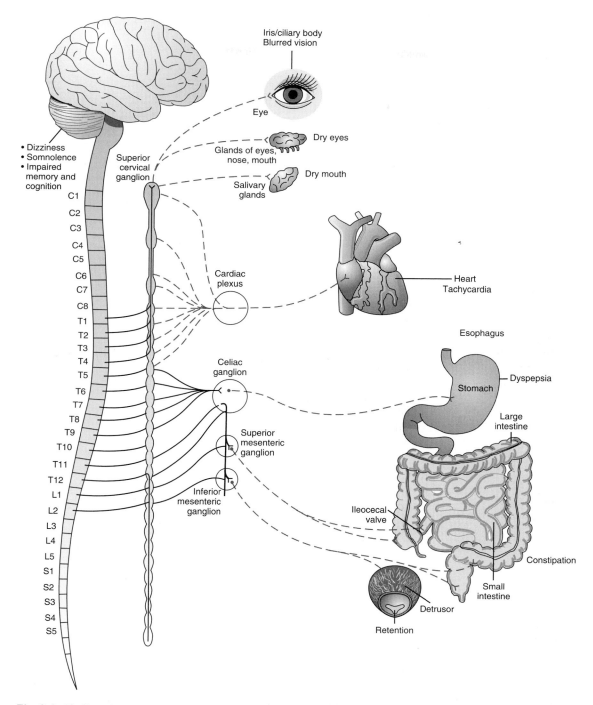

Fig. 2-8 Cholinergic receptors are located throughout the body, and administration of an antimuscarinic agent may produce multiple unintended side effects including those illustrated here. (Modified from Copstead LC, Banasik JL: *Pathophysiology,* 3e, St. Louis, Saunders, 2005.)

compared with those in the parotid glands (in both animal models and in humans).[61-63] In contrast, two agents currently undergoing clinical trials (that is, solifenacin and darifenacin) demonstrate *receptor* specificity; these agents exhibit higher affinity for the M_2 or M_3 receptor subtypes than either tolterodine or oxybutynin.[64,65] Although academic arguments can be made for either approach (that is, organ-specific versus receptor-specific agents), it is important to remember that clinical effectiveness represents a combination of efficacy and tolerability that must be demonstrated in the clinical research and practice settings as opposed to the laboratory.

Norepinephrine. Norepinephrine (sometimes called noradrenaline) is released from adrenergic receptors found in the bladder body (detrusor muscle) and the bladder base (lissosphincter). As is true of muscarinic subtypes, multiple beta-adrenergic receptor subtypes have been identified. Beta-1 adrenergic receptors are predominant in the heart muscle, and beta-2 receptors are present in the lungs. Both beta-2 and beta-3 adrenergic receptors have been identified in the lower urinary tract, including the detrusor muscle.[66] As anticipated, stimulation of these receptors occurs under SNS control and promotes detrusor relaxation.[66] At least one substance has been identified that acts as a beta-3 receptor agonist; these receptors are now undergoing investigation as potentially new targets in the pharmacologic management of overactive bladder dysfunction.[67]

Adenosine triphosphate. ATP is released from nonadrenergic, noncholinergic (NANC) receptors located throughout the detrusor.[68] Stimulation of these purinergic (P2X or P2Y) receptors causes detrusor contraction. The relationship between cholinergic and purinergic detrusor contractions remains unclear. Some researchers believe that ATP may act to initiate a detrusor contraction, and acetylcholine may then act to provide the sustained contraction needed for bladder evacuation.[58] Although ATP appears to play a secondary, or supportive, role in mediation of detrusor contractions in the normal bladder, it may play a more significant role in the unstable detrusor or in the patient with interstitial cystitis.[5]

Nitric oxide. NO is a gaseous substance that is neither produced nor stored in vesicles like other neurotransmitters. Instead, it is produced as needed by hydroxylation of L-arginine to citrulline. NO has a short half-life and three endogenous forms: (1) endothelial NO, (2) neuronal NO, and (3) macrophage-inducible NO. Among other biologic effects, NO acts as a potent vasodilator. Based on this knowledge, several NO-potentiating agents have been developed for treatment of erectile dysfunction (such as sildenafil, vardenafil, and tadalafil). Although existing evidence has not demonstrated that NO is produced by smooth muscle cells in the bladder wall, it is present in the urinary tract, and it may play an as yet undefined role in detrusor muscle relaxation.[69]

Central Nervous System Neurotransmitters. Central nervous system neurotransmitters also affect detrusor control.[5] Serotonin (5-HT), norepinephrine, and gamma-aminobutyric acid (GABA) are found in the brain and brainstem, and they are believed to promote bladder filling and storage. Oxytocin and NO are also present in the brain and brainstem, and they are believed to promote micturition. Although comparatively little is known about how these neurotransmitters affect continence or about the magnitude of their effects, clinical and basic science research is beginning to elucidate some of these previously unknown mechanisms of detrusor control. For example, clinical studies have identified a relationship between depression (a condition that is characterized by a deficit of serotonin in the brain) and detrusor overactivity.[70,71] In addition, research using an animal model[72] demonstrated that altered serotonin levels seen with depression resulted in cystometric changes consistent with overactive bladder dysfunction in female (but not male) rats. The results of these studies challenge existing notions that urinary incontinence causes depression and suggest instead that depression may predispose individuals to detrusor overactivity and urge or mixed urinary incontinence. In addition to multiple ongoing investigations into the mechanisms by which central nervous system neurotransmitters affect continence, researchers are also exploring whether pharmacologic agents that target dopamine or GABA receptors may play a role in the management of overactive bladder dysfunction.[67]

Endocrine and Paracrine Substances. Detrusor function in the human may also be affected by endocrine and paracrine substances.[5] Endocrine substances are those manufactured and secreted by specific glands located throughout the body and then carried through the bloodstream to act on distant organs or tissues. For example, estrogen receptors have been found in the urinary bladder,[73] and estrogen is thought to exert an indirect influence on detrusor muscle function by altering the production of prostaglandins.[5] In support of this hypothesis, women frequently relate changes in urinary urgency and the severity of urge urinary incontinence to their menstrual cycle. Whether these changes can be entirely attributed to the influence of estrogen or whether progestins also affect detrusor function is not known. Oxytocin receptors may also exist in the human bladder, although the influence of this hormone on the detrusor is unknown.[74,75]

Corticotropin-releasing factor (CRF) is another endocrine substance with potential impact on bladder function; it is a neuropeptide that is released from the pituitary and acts on the pituitary gland to promote the release of the hormone corticotropin. Excessive CRF release is associated with panic, anxiety, and depressive disorders, and with post-traumatic stress responses. Immunohistochemical studies have shown that CRF may affect bladder function,[72] and a clinical study revealed that patients with urge and mixed urinary incontinence have an unexpectedly high prevalence of panic and anxiety disorders.[76] Initial research in an animal model showed that infusion of CRF into awake rats lowered functional bladder capacity and promoted detrusor overactivity, and administration of a CRF antagonist (astressin) partially blocked this effect.[77] Although these data do not provide conclusive evidence that CRF causes detrusor overactivity, they do raise the possibility that this hormone may influence lower urinary tract function, and they may provide greater understanding of the physiologic mechanisms that underlie the often quoted adage "I was so frightened I wet my pants."

Paracrine substances are manufactured locally, and their action is limited to adjacent organs or tissues.[57] For example, the prostaglandins PGE_2, PGE_{2a}, and PGI_2 are paracrine substances that are manufactured in the lower urinary tract and the reproductive systems. They may influence detrusor function directly, by exciting the detrusor muscle, or indirectly, by promoting relaxation of the urethral smooth muscle.[5]

Afferent pathways. We have comparatively little knowledge about the afferent pathways of the lower urinary tract and how they regulate the two principal sensory disorders affecting the lower urinary tract: urgency and pain.[10] Several classes of afferent sensory receptors, including neurokinin (NK1, NK2 and NK3), vanilloid (VR1), and purinergic receptors are located in the smooth muscle, lamina propria, and urothelium of the bladder and urethra. They communicate with the central nervous system via finely myelinated A-delta fibers and unmyelinated C fibers. A-delta fibers sense bladder filling and tension within the bladder wall, whereas C fibers transmit discomfort or pain in response to excessive stretching of the bladder wall. These axons travel within the pelvic, hypogastric, and pudendal nerves, and they transmit information from the lower urinary tract to the central nervous system via the lumbosacral spinal cord.[78]

Multiple neurotransmitters are involved in transmission of sensation from the bladder wall, including substance P, neurokinin A, calcitonin gene-related peptide (CGRP), vasoactive intestinal polypeptide (VIP, so named because it was first discovered in the gastrointestinal tract), pituitary adenylate cyclase-activating peptide (PACAP), ATP, and various enkephalins. Intensive research into these substances is ongoing, with significant clinical implications, because many of these neurotransmitters are released in large quantities in response to inflammation. Further research may yield important clues regarding the pathophysiology and treatment of bladder pain syndrome (interstitial cystitis).

Research into possible causes of interstitial cystitis (bladder pain syndrome) have also focused on the role of the mucoid lining of the urothelium, that is, whether defects in this layer may create bladder pain by exposing the underlying epithelium to irritating chemical substances within the urine.[79,80] The mucoid layer is principally composed of glycosaminoglycans (GAG; unchained polysaccharide molecules) that are hypothesized to account for the urothelium's barrier property. However, other researchers remain unconvinced that this mucoid layer serves as a barrier; they have pointed out that the GAG layer fails to prevent specific substances such as nystatin or amiloride from reaching urothelial cells.[10]

Although our knowledge of the afferent mechanisms that determine perceptions of lower urinary tract filling (and micturition) remains incomplete, research to date clearly indicates that afferent receptors exist within the urothelium, lamina propria, and smooth muscle cells of the bladder and urethra. These receptors respond to factors other than the stretch caused by bladder filling; they also respond to a variety of chemical characteristics, including pH and possibly osmolarity. Acting on as yet unclear physiologic triggers, they may initiate a short-term or prolonged response leading to inflammation, pain, or bothersome urgency; these symptoms may persist long after the initial insult and may contribute to the syndromes we call interstitial cystitis and overactive bladder.

Sphincter Mechanism Competence

Traditionally, a sphincter is defined as an annular, or circular, muscle designed to occlude an opening of the body.[81] Two urethral sphincters have been described as acting together and in concert with the periurethral muscles of the levator ani to maintain closure of the urethra during bladder filling and storage: an internal sphincter, composed of the smooth muscle of the bladder neck, and an external sphincter, composed of the intrinsic striated muscle fibers of the urethra. However, advances in our understanding of lower urinary tract physiology have led to a more accurate and complete description of the urethral sphincter mechanism as a mixture of compressive, tension, and supportive elements.[82] During bladder filling and storage, these elements form a watertight urethral seal to prevent urinary leakage, even in the presence of sudden or strenuous physical exertion or precipitous rises in abdominal and intravesical pressure caused by coughing or sneezing. In addition, this remarkable mechanism accommodates bladder evacuation by providing a low-resistance conduit for urinary outflow during micturition.

Elements of Compression. The compressive elements of the urethral sphincter mechanism are necessary to provide a watertight seal against the passage of urine from the bladder into the urethra during bladder filling and storage. The primary compressive elements include inner urethral softness, the mucoid lining of the urethral epithelium, and the submucosal vascular cushion.

Urethral softness. Inner urethral softness is the first essential compressive component of the urethral sphincter.[83] In the physiologically normal individual, the urethral epithelium rapidly alters its shape to maintain a watertight seal during storage and to allow an unobstructed flow of urine during micturition. This ability to deform itself to create a watertight seal can be observed when one is passing a stiff catheter into the bladder. Even though the catheter is smaller than the potential diameter of the urethra, urine exits exclusively through the lumen of the catheter rather than around the tube. This occurs because the inner lining of the urethra deforms to the shape of the catheter and forms a watertight seal around the catheter. Unfortunately, prolonged catheterization may cause erosion of the urethral lining; in this case, leakage of urine around the tube occurs passively or with minimal exertion, even if a relatively large-diameter (French size) catheter is placed. Leakage around an indwelling catheter may also occur as a result of bladder spasms, which act to force urine out around the catheter; this phenomenon can occur whenever the bladder is abnormally irritable, as in the setting of bladder infection, constipation, or use of an overly large catheter or balloon.

Surface tension. The second element of compression is the mucoid-like GAG layer within the urethra.[84] GAG molecules alter the surface tension of the urethral epithelium, thus promoting coaptation and closure of the urethral walls.[85] The combined effects of urethral softness and GAG molecules within the urethral wall can be conceptualized by the example of a soft condom. If a condom is unrolled and held by its distal end, the walls of this tubular structure will fall together, reflecting their softness. If the condom is shaken briskly, its walls easily fall apart, indicating low surface tension (that is, a low propensity of the walls to cling together). However, if the walls of the condom are coated with a water-soluble lubricant (such as K-Y Jelly), they will tend to "coapt," or adhere to one another, even if the condom is again shaken briskly; this is the result of the higher surface tension produced by the addition of the lubricant. The GAG lining of the urethral epithelium increases surface tension in a comparable manner.

Vascular cushion. The vascular cushion located immediately beneath the urethral epithelium is the third element contributing to urethral compression.[85,86] This rich network of arteries, veins, and arteriovenous communications contributes to the compressive effects of the muscular elements of the sphincter; that is, the cushion acts as an incompressible sponge, thus transmitting the compressive forces to the urethral epithelium. The volume of blood contained within the vascular cushion of the urethra is evidenced by the surprisingly high volume of blood loss that occurs after transurethral surgery or traumatic catheterization (Fig. 2-9).

The effect of deficiencies in the compressive elements of the urethra can be illustrated by the occurrence of stress urinary incontinence and obstructed voiding in a male patient after radical prostatectomy (Fig. 2-10). In this case, the softness of the urethral epithelium has been disrupted by scarring at the anastomotic site. As a result, the urethral walls are unable to coapt (close) effectively, and this results in stress pattern incontinence; in addition, the loss of urethral softness prevents "funneling" of the urethra and therefore causes obstructed voiding (bladder outlet obstruction). In women, estrogen is known to promote cellular reproduction in the urethral epithelium, to stimulate mucus production in both the vagina and the urethra, and to sustain the submucosal vascular cushion.[87,88] These estrogenic effects may partly explain the association between estrogen deficiency and stress pattern incontinence and the complementary role of estrogens in the management of stress incontinence in women.[89]

Elements of tension. The smooth and striated muscles of the proximal portion of the urethra in the male, the muscular elements of the entire female urethra, and the periurethral striated muscle comprise the tension elements of the urethral sphincter mechanism (Fig. 2-11).

Smooth muscle. Circular bundles of smooth muscle are found at the bladder neck of males[6]; their importance to continence remains somewhat controversial. Contraction of the smooth muscle of the bladder neck is known to support antegrade ejaculation of semen,[90] and surgical preservation of the bladder neck during radical prostatectomy has been found to promote early recovery of continence.[91,92] In addition, dyssynergic contraction of the smooth muscle of the bladder neck during voiding causes significant obstruction.[93] All these findings support a significant role for this component of urethral smooth muscle, but the exact importance remains unclear.[94] Longitudinal smooth muscle bundles are also found within the urethral wall;[7,95] contraction of these bundles may shorten and widen (funnel) the urethra during micturition or may promote urethral closure during bladder filling and storage. Of important note, smooth muscle bundles are also found within the prostate gland, and their tone affects the prostatic urethra. An increase in resting tone is seen with aging and benign prostatic hyperplasia (BPH). Excessive tone within the prostatic smooth muscle interferes with funneling of the prostatic urethra and may contribute to the obstruction associated with BPH.

In the female, smooth muscle bundles extend nearly the entire length of the urethra, but they thin significantly as they approach the meatus.[68] The easily identifiable circular layer of smooth muscle present within the bladder neck of the male is not found in the bladder neck of the female. Instead, smooth muscle bundles run obliquely or longitudinally along almost the entire urethral course. Similar to the controversy noted in males, some investigators hypothesize that smooth muscle bundles contract during micturition to shorten and widen the urethra, whereas other investigators postulate that these bundles contribute to urethral narrowing and sphincter closure during bladder filling and storage.[95]

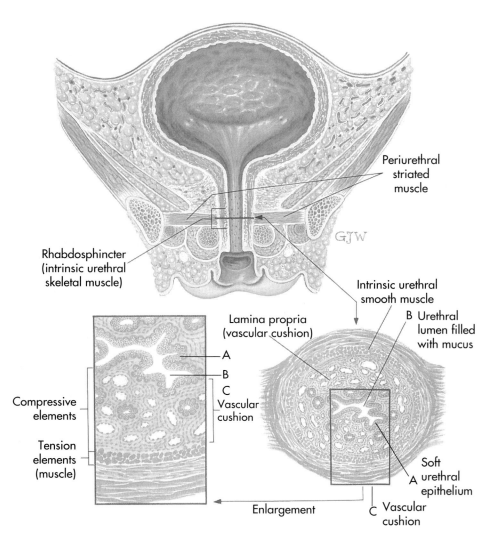

Fig. 2-9 Compressive elements of urethral sphincter mechanism. *A,* Urethra is lined by soft epithelial tissue that deforms to create a watertight seal; *B,* mucosal secretions produced by epithelium fill the microscopic holes left as epithelium seals shut; *C,* vascular cushion transmits intraabdominal pressure to seal epithelium in response to muscular tone. (From Gray M: *Genitourinary disorders,* Mosby's clinical nursing series, St. Louis, 1992, Mosby.)

Rhabdosphincter. The intrinsic striated muscle of the urethral sphincter is called the rhabdosphincter.[8,96] It is located in the membranous urethra, just below the apex of the prostate gland in the male and the middle third of the urethra in the female. In both genders it consists of unique omega-shaped fibers, and it thins as it joins connective tissue in the posterior urethra.[16,96] Most of these fibers (65% to 100%) are Type 1, or slow-twitch fibers, which are ideally suited to maintaining tone over prolonged periods of time between voiding. *The rhabdosphincter is thought to be the most important element of tension in the competent urethral sphincter mechanism.*

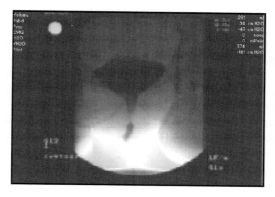

Fig. 2-10 Scarring of the urethra after radical prostatectomy causes loss of compression, obstruction, and stress urinary incontinence.

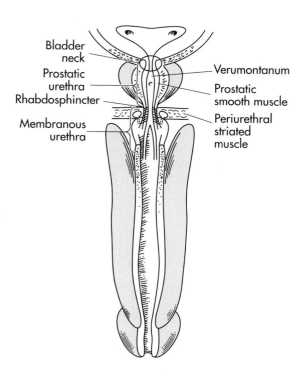

Bladder neck
Prostatic urethra
Rhabdosphincter
Membranous urethra
Verumontanum
Prostatic smooth muscle
Periurethral striated muscle

Fig. 2-11 Muscular components of the male urethral sphincter mechanism: smooth muscle of bladder neck, smooth muscle of the preprostatic and prostatic urethra, rhabdosphincter located at membranous urethra, and periurethral striated muscle.

Periurethral striated muscle. The periurethral striated sphincter of the female is divided into three distinctive portions: the sphincter urethrae, compressor urethrae, and urethral vaginal sphincter (see Fig. 2-3). These muscles contain both fast- and slow-twitch striated muscle fibers that increase urethral closure pressure during brief periods of physical exertion or in response to voluntary commands. In the male, the periurethral striated muscle is located adjacent to the membranous urethra. Similar to the female, it contains a mixture of slow- and fast-twitch skeletal muscle fibers, providing for rapid contraction in response to sudden rises in abdominal pressure and for maintenance of tone for prolonged periods, which is needed to ensure continence during routine physical activity. The rhabdosphincter, periurethral muscles, and pelvic floor muscles also contribute to the individual's ability to delay voiding; this is because sustained contraction of the pelvic muscles stimulates a spinal reflex that inhibits detrusor contraction.[97,98] This has clinical significance, in that patients with urge pattern incontinence can be taught (usually with biofeedback) to voluntarily contract the pelvic muscles in order to inhibit bladder contraction and delay voiding.

Elements of support. The pelvic floor provides support for the bladder and urethra, which is essential to competence of the urethral sphincter.[6] The pelvic floor contributes to continence by maintaining the bladder base in an intraabdominal position. This position promotes transmission of abdominal pressure to *both* the bladder and the urethra, which is thought to assist with maintenance of urethral closure during activities that cause a sudden increase in abdominal pressure (such as coughing or sneezing). The primary support structure is the levator ani muscle.[16] The levator ani contains an abundance of slow-twitch muscle fibers, which maintain tone throughout the hours that a person remains in the upright position; it also contains fast-twitch fibers that are able to respond rapidly to precipitous rises in abdominal pressure. The endopelvic fascia provides supplemental support, as described earlier in this chapter. It is important to remember that these structures are designed to provide dynamic support for the pelvic viscera. This flexibility is necessary for the passage of urine and stool and for the extraordinary demands created by vaginal delivery.

Several characteristics of the levator ani contribute to the confusion and contradictions that pervade our understanding of this remarkable muscle. Unlike the muscles of the arms, legs, or chest, the levator ani is rarely viewed in its entirety, and hypertrophy of this muscle is not readily apparent to the unaided eye. As a result, it is often difficult for men and women to distinguish contraction of the levator ani muscle from contraction of the abdominal, thigh, or gluteal muscles. In addition, exhaustion of the levator ani is not easily recognized, because repeated, purposive contraction does not produce the panting or muscle aches typically associated with muscle fatigue. This may result in subconscious substitution of the abdominal or gluteal muscles when the levator becomes fatigued. Finally, the levator muscle, unlike the large muscles of the extremities, is primarily composed of slow-twitch fibers, and our understanding of effective techniques for exercising these muscle fibers is limited.[38,96,99] Because of the unique characteristics of this muscle, effective rehabilitation typically requires biofeedback and repeated monitoring by a qualified health care professional.

Neurologic Modulation of the Sphincter Mechanism

The smooth muscle of the urethral sphincter mechanism contains both cholinergic and adrenergic receptors; adrenergic receptors promote urethral closure during bladder filling and storage, and cholinergic receptors promote urethral relaxation and funneling during micturition (see Table 2-3). During voiding, cholinergic (muscarinic) receptors within the urethra are thought to mediate contraction that reduces urethral length and increases urethral diameter; muscarinic receptors may also indirectly facilitate micturition by inhibiting norepinephrine release. During storage, adrenergic receptors mediate increased urethral smooth muscle tone, which is responsible for as much as 50% of urethral closure pressure. Specifically, urethral closure is promoted by the action of the neurotransmitter norepinephrine which acts on alpha-1a

adrenergic receptors, found throughout the urethral (and prostatic) smooth muscle.[100] Knowledge of specific receptor subtypes is clinically relevant because this knowledge has led to the development of pharmacologic agents that selectively antagonize alpha-1a receptors; these agents produce urethral sphincter relaxation in men with obstruction resulting from BPH *without* significantly lowering blood pressure. (The risk for hypotension or dizziness in men being managed by most alpha-adrenergic blocking agents is significant, because both the prostatic and arteriolar smooth muscles contain rich supplies of alpha-1 receptors; however, those in the prostate are predominantly alpha-1a subtypes, whereas those in the arteriolar smooth muscle are predominantly alpha-1b receptor subtypes.) The bladder neck and urethral smooth muscle also contains beta-adrenergic receptors,[100] but this knowledge has not yet led to any effective pharmacologic agents for the management of stress urinary incontinence or BPH, probably because beta-2 receptors are also abundant in the lungs.

The potential role of NO in urethral smooth muscle relaxation has gained increased recognition, due in part to increasing clinical experience with phosphodiesterase-5 (PDE-5) inhibitors such as sildenafil or vardenafil. The manufacture and release of NO are related to activation of cyclic guanosine monophosphate, which ultimately leads to relaxation of urethral smooth muscle. With the development of long acting PDE-5 inhibitors such as tadalafil, it is feasible that an existing or yet to be developed drug within this class may play a role in the management of BPH or bladder neck dyssynergia. Other neurotransmitters that have been linked to urethral smooth muscle relaxation include vasoactive intestinal polypeptide and ATP.

Cholinergic receptors are also abundant in both the periurethral and pelvic floor striated muscles. However, the receptors for these striated muscles are primarily *nicotinic* rather than muscarinic, and they respond to different pharmacologic agonists or antagonists than does the smooth muscle of the lower urinary tract. The type and physiologic role of receptors within the rhabdosphincter remain controversial. As is true of the pelvic floor and

LIBRARY, UNIVERSITY OF CHESTER

periurethral striated muscles, nicotinic receptors predominate within the striated fibers of the rhabdosphincter; however, there is some evidence that the rhabdosphincter may also be innervated by autonomic fibers, specifically by adrenergic nerve fibers.[101]

It is particularly important to understand central nervous system modulation of the smooth and striated muscle of the sphincter mechanism and pelvic floor muscles because this is the basis for pharmacologic intervention in the management of stress urinary incontinence. The smooth muscle of the urethra is innervated by branches of the autonomic nervous system; parasympathetic (cholinergic) nerves synapse with neurons at sacral segments 2 to 4, whereas adrenergic (sympathetic) nerves synapse with neurons in the spinal cord segments T10 to L2. Innervation of the *striated* muscle of the urethra arises from branches of the pudendal (and not the pelvic) nerve, which synapse with neurons at Onuf's nucleus (a collection of motor neurons located at the lateral border of the ventral horn of sacral segments 2 to 4).[10] During bladder filling and storage, activation of afferent pathways in the bladder provokes sphincter closure, primarily under the influence of reflex mechanisms within the spinal cord.[10] Specifically, neurons within Onuf's nucleus mediate contraction of the rhabdosphincter via the neurotransmitter glutamine. This neurotransmitter may be thought of as activating an "on/off" mechanism that promotes sphincter closure during bladder filling (the "on" position) and inhibits contraction to allow urethral opening for micturition (the "off" switch). As noted previously, these actions are coordinated by the pontine micturition center. As long as glutamine is physiologically active, the tone of the rhabdosphincter can be further modulated by two additional neurotransmitters produced by neurons in Onuf's nucleus: norepinephrine and serotonin. However, when glutamine is transiently eliminated in preparation for micturition, the activity of these complementary neurotransmitters is also eliminated, thus ensuring that micturition occurs without resistance from a partially contracted rhabdosphincter.

The clinical significance of these pathways and neurotransmitters is reflected in recent development of an investigational drug for the treatment of stress incontinence. This agent, duloxetine,[102] acts on neurons within the spinal cord to increase urethral resistance by increasing the availability of the neurotransmitters serotonin and norepinephrine. These neurotransmitters help to modulate striated muscle tone during bladder filling, as explained above.

BLADDER FUNCTION ACROSS THE LIFE SPAN

Infancy

During infancy, micturition occurs by means of a classic reflex mechanism.[103] The bladder fills until proprioceptive stretch receptors stimulate the brain center or spinal reflex mechanisms to provoke a detrusor contraction. For the majority of infants (about two-thirds), this triggers coordinated voiding under the influence of the pontine micturition center. However, about 33% of full-term neonates demonstrate an interrupted voiding pattern and vesicosphincter dyssynergia (uncoordinated contraction of urethral and pelvic floor muscle), leading to interrupted voiding and functional obstruction.[104] Fortunately, this pattern of vesicosphincter dyssynergia usually resolves within the first year of life, resulting in more efficient bladder emptying and fewer voids during a 24-hour period. The developmental processes that account for this resolution are not known, but maturation of the pontine micturition center remains a strong possibility. During the first 6 months of life, the bladder capacity is small in relation to hourly urine production, and voiding occurs about 20 times daily. At about 6 months of age, the frequency of voiding begins to diminish. This change in the pattern of urine elimination may occur as a result of increased ability to inhibit micturition unconsciously as the brain matures or because of changes in the functional capacity of the bladder in relation to the volume of urine produced by the kidneys.[103,105,106]

Mastering Continence

Between 1 and 2 years of age, the neurologically normal child develops a conscious awareness of bladder filling.[103] This event probably marks the first major milestone toward the mastery of continence.

Initially, this perception of urinary urgency occurs immediately before voiding. The child is also learning to identify, contract, and relax the pelvic muscles, including the periurethral striated muscles. Mastery of these skills allows the child to temporarily postpone micturition and to briefly interrupt the urinary stream during micturition, and this ability marks the second milestone toward continence. Nonetheless, a third developmental milestone must be reached before the child can be described as "ready" for toilet training. Direct control over the detrusor is thought to occur when modulatory centers in the frontal cortex, thalamus, hypothalamus, and basal ganglia establish inhibitory control over the micturition centers in the pons and spinal cord. The processes by which these milestones are reached are unknown.

The neurologically normal child reaches a stage of readiness for toilet training between 1 and 4 years of age. Although it is not currently possible to determine the precise point at which the developing child gains control over detrusor contractions, several signs indicate a readiness to achieve urinary continence.[107] Nighttime bowel control is typically mastered first, followed by diurnal fecal continence. However, unlike fecal continence, daytime urinary continence typically precedes nocturnal control over micturition. Successful toilet training is feasible when a child has gained fecal continence, is able to verbalize the perception of urinary urgency, is able to postpone urination briefly, and is able to interrupt the urinary stream voluntarily. Attempts to toilet train a child before mastery of these skills are likely to fail or to produce a child who experiences urinary frequency and frequent episodes of urinary leakage when she or he is unable to reach the toilet after the onset of an unstable detrusor contraction.

Although most children master an adult voiding pattern by 4 years of age, as many as 10% to 15% experience persistent voiding problems.[103] The most common voiding problem is so-called "nocturnal enuresis," a condition characterized by episodes of urinary leakage during sleep. A smaller percentage of children will experience episodes of urge urinary incontinence associated with unstable detrusor contractions that occur during waking hours.[108]

Further growth and maturation typically resolve these conditions, although a few of these individuals experience urinary frequency or occasional episodes of enuresis that persist into adulthood.

Aging and Continence

Although it is known that aging by itself does not cause urinary incontinence, there are many age-related changes in the central nervous system, urinary bladder, and adjacent organs that increase the risk of incontinence in the elderly.[13,109,110] Specifically, elderly individuals tend to urinate smaller volumes more frequently during waking hours and are more likely to experience nocturia. In addition, elderly persons are more prone to urinary incontinence and urinary retention when compared with younger adults. Unfortunately, although a great deal of research has focused on voiding dysfunction in the elderly, less work has been done on physiologic changes of the lower urinary tract directly associated with aging. Nonetheless, valuable research has been completed in this area, and some age-associated changes in the lower urinary tract have been described.

Changes in Microscopic Anatomy. Changes in the microscopic architecture of the bladder wall can be observed with aging. Susset and colleagues reported an increase in the collagen content of the bladder wall in women older than 50 years of age, although these changes have not been observed by others.[111,112] However, further studies *have* demonstrated that collagen fibers in the aging bladder cross-link and stiffen, even if there is no increase in volume.[113] In addition, a growing body of evidence suggests that the number of cholinergic receptors tends to diminish with aging, whereas the number of purinergic and adrenergic receptors increases.[100,114,115] The implications of these observations are not totally clear; however, they may provide partial explanations for detrusor hyperactivity with insufficient contractility, a voiding disorder characterized by both urge incontinence and incomplete bladder emptying. This change in receptor distribution also may account for the often disappointing clinical response of elders to antimuscarinic medications. In addition, because circulating catecholamines reach a peak during the morning, an enhanced adrenergic response may account for the relatively common complaint among men of a poor urinary stream during the morning hours, followed by improved voiding efficiency as the day progresses.

Elbadawi and colleagues[116-118] correlated histologic changes in the detrusor (as evidenced by biopsy studies), urodynamic findings, and clinical signs and symptoms related to bladder function for a group of elderly patients. They were able to identify three distinctive types of histologic characteristics that correlated with the following three "clinical-urodynamic" categories among elderly individuals: those with normal voiding function, those with detrusor instability, and those with a combination of detrusor instability and impaired contractility. It is not known whether these changes represent primary *causes* of voiding dysfunction in the elderly or a secondary *effect* of changes originating in the nervous system.

Changes in the Central Nervous System.

Alterations in central nervous system function also affect continence in the elderly person.[119] CVAs affect approximately 1% of the population,[37] and epidemiologic studies have demonstrated that age is the most powerful predictor of the risk for stroke; the risk is estimated at 5% among Americans 55 to 59 years of age, but it increases to 25% among persons 80 to 84 years of age.[120]

The occurrence of a stroke places the elderly person at risk for urinary incontinence for several reasons. First, the neurologic damage caused by the infarction itself and by the edema and ischemia in surrounding tissues may damage the detrusor motor center or other modulatory areas essential to detrusor muscle control, resulting in detrusor instability and urge incontinence.[121] In addition, a significant stroke acutely impairs the functional status of the elderly person. Alterations in mobility, cognition, speech, and dexterity limit the individual's ability to recognize the cues of bladder filling and to act on these cues by moving to the toilet or by alerting caregivers of the need to toilet.[122] The influence of functional impairment on continence is demonstrated by studies regarding the prevalence of urinary incontinence after a stroke. In one study,[123] 47% of a group of 935 patients admitted to the hospital for acute CVA experienced urinary

incontinence. However, the prevalence of urinary incontinence fell to 19% 6 months after the stroke, at which point functional status had improved as a result of recovery and rehabilitation.

Parkinsonism, also called Parkinson's disease, is a progressive neurodegenerative disease that affects the neurons of the basal ganglia. Although parkinsonism is clearly not a normal part of aging, age *is* the primary risk factor for development of this disorder[124]; the prevalence of parkinsonism is approximately 0.2% in the general population but rises to approximately 3% among persons 79 years of age and older. Because the basal ganglia are known to contribute to detrusor control, parkinsonism is associated with detrusor hyperreflexia and urge urinary incontinence.[41,43] However, the likelihood of urinary incontinence associated with parkinsonism is influenced by the individual's functional status and by the urodynamic characteristics of the lower urinary tract. In advanced cases, the bradykinesia, resting tremors, and postural reflex disorders associated with parkinsonism impair balance, mobility, and dexterity, and the ability to toilet.

Parkinsonism is sometimes confused with a condition called "multiple system atrophy" (MSA), or the Shy-Drager syndrome.[125,126] MSA is an autonomic disorder affecting the intracerebral and spinal cord tracts; as a result of these mixed effects, detrusor instability typically coexists with intrinsic sphincter deficiency. This disease affects approximately twice as many men as women, and aging is a risk factor. Differentiation between MSA and parkinsonism is particularly important among men when prostatic resection is being considered. Although men with parkinsonism may benefit from prostatectomy, those with MSA are likely to develop significant stress urinary incontinence when the prostate is removed.

Dementia or senile dementia is defined as the diffuse deterioration of mental function, causing changes in memory, behavior, and emotional stability.[37] Alzheimer's disease is the primary cause of dementia, accounting for more than 50% of all cases of senile dementia in the elderly.[127] Alzheimer's disease is a neurohistopathologic diagnosis based on identification of senile plaques and neurofibrillary tangles in the brain.[37] However, in the clinical setting, the diagnosis of Alzheimer's disease is typically based on its clinical features and on the exclusion of related disorders causing senile dementia (such as hydrocephalus, cerebrovascular disorders, intracranial tumors, metabolic disorders, or Pick's disease). Alzheimer's disease affects approximately 3 to 4 million Americans, and its incidence rises steadily with aging. However, unlike the pattern with CVA or parkinsonism, urinary incontinence does not commonly occur during the early stages of the disease. Instead, urinary incontinence typically occurs during the advanced stages of the disease, and the functional decline associated with Alzheimer's probably plays an important role in the loss of bladder control.

Although Alzheimer's disease is not known to cause unstable detrusor contractions, Griffiths and colleagues[40,128, 129] identified evidence of a cerebral component in the development of urge incontinence in many older persons. They correlated single-photon emission computerized tomography scans, clinical signs and symptoms, and urodynamic findings and suggested that impaired perfusion of specific areas in the frontal lobes of the cerebral cortex may cause detrusor instability in many elderly persons. This detrusor instability was distinctive from that seen among younger persons because it was associated with impaired sensation of bladder filling. Unlike the younger person with urge incontinence, who experiences urinary urgency at low volumes, their elderly subjects experienced no sense of urinary urgency before the onset of an unstable detrusor contraction resulting in urinary leakage. In addition, this form of urge incontinence was associated with impaired cognitive function, especially with orientation to time.

Sphincter Mechanism Function. The function of the urethral sphincter mechanism is affected by alterations in nervous system function and also by changes in the urethra itself. The maximum urethral closing pressure is lower in elderly women than in younger women.[130] Multiple factors may contribute to this alteration in sphincter function, and estrogens clearly play a central role. Estrogens are known to increase smooth muscle sensitivity to alpha-adrenergic stimulation, and this increase may partly account for the lower maximum urethral

closure pressure noted in older, postmenopausal women. However, estrogen treatment of postmenopausal women with atrophic vaginal changes and stress urinary incontinence rarely resolves the stress-related urine loss.[131] Rather, exogenous estrogens are more effective for the treatment of irritative voiding symptoms and urge incontinence than for the treatment of stress incontinence. In addition, the proportion of elderly women who experience stress urinary incontinence is relatively stable, particularly when compared with the increasing prevalence of urge incontinence within this group,[132] a finding that reflects the increasing significance of detrusor instability as a cause of urinary leakage in the elderly.

Clearly, the greatest change in sphincter mechanism function in the male occurs as a result of prostatic enlargement.[133] BPH is the gradual enlargement of the glandular elements of the prostate gland. Aging, in combination with functioning testes, is the primary risk factor for BPH, and its prevalence rises steadily with age. Although as many as 10% of men demonstrate some evidence of glandular hyperplasia as early as 30 years of age, clinical symptoms of BPH seldom occur before the fifth decade of life. Among men more than 60 years of age, the prevalence of BPH rises to approximately 50%, and it reaches 90% among men 85 years of age.

BPH is rarely a direct cause of mortality; rather, it typically is a quality-of-life disorder because of the associated voiding symptoms.[134] The enlarging prostate produces bladder outlet obstruction by encroaching on the lumen of the prostatic urethra and by increasing the smooth muscle tone in the bladder neck and prostatic urethra. In some cases, the bladder outlet obstruction remains mild, and the detrusor muscle is able to compensate for the increased outlet resistance by increasing the power of its contraction. In other cases, more significant obstruction causes decompensation of the detrusor muscle and bothersome voiding symptoms including diminished urinary stream, intermittency of the stream, frequent urination, and incomplete bladder emptying. In particularly severe cases, episodes of acute urinary retention occur.

The effects of bladder outlet obstruction involve more than just the sphincter mechanism. Studies of animals and humans have demonstrated that bladder outlet obstruction also produces unstable detrusor contractions, which contribute to or cause the irritative voiding symptoms frequently associated with BPH.[9,135] Although this instability is associated with morphologic changes in the bladder wall,[111] it has also been shown that obstruction causes changes in spinal pathways in the rat;[136] a positive response to iced saline cystometry in humans further supports involvement of the central nervous system.[137] These relationships are particularly significant when one is considering treatment for the elderly male with BPH and symptoms of urgency. Although the obstructive prostate may cause detrusor instability, it also provides a "protective" mechanism, and the presence of prostate enlargement has been associated with preservation of *continence,* whereas prostate surgery that removes this protective mechanism has been associated with the presence of urinary *incontinence.*[134,138]

Changes in Renal and Metabolic Function.

Changes in renal and metabolic functions may also affect voiding function in the elderly. Unlike younger persons, who produce the bulk of their urine during waking hours, older adults produce roughly equal volumes of urine during the day and night.[109] As a result, more than half of adults older than 70 years of age experience two episodes of nocturia on a regular basis.[139,140] Kikuchi[141] studied human atrial natriuretic peptide and vasopressin, also called the "antidiuretic hormone," in a group of "younger" versus "older" elderly men. They found that the "older" subjects experienced changes in the circadian rhythm of these hormones as well as higher urinary output at night as compared with the "younger" subjects enrolled in the study. Specific diseases associated with aging also predispose the elderly person to nocturia. Chronic venous insufficiency, edema of the lower extremities, congestive heart failure, and diabetes predispose to increased urine production during nighttime hours. Although the elderly person who is relatively mobile and alert can manage this increase in nighttime urine production by getting up to void during the night, the person with immobility or altered cognition may be unable to recognize the urge to urinate or to move to the toilet; immobility and altered cognition are common among elderly individuals who are acutely ill or hospitalized or who have been given sleeping aids.

Functional Aspects of Continence.

In addition to factors that directly affect lower urinary tract function, any discussion of the physiology of the aging bladder must involve consideration of the functional aspects of aging and its effect on continence. Although most elderly persons remain alert and mobile, many disorders associated with aging reduce mobility, dexterity, and the ability to maintain continence. Elderly persons are at risk for arthritis, osteoporosis, hip fractures, peripheral vascular disease, and other disorders that affect balance, mobility, and dexterity. In some cases, these disorders may cause urinary incontinence in a person with an otherwise healthy lower urinary tract. In other cases, these conditions push an elderly person from a condition of mild voiding dysfunction to clinically significant urinary leakage.

Drugs also affect the functional status of the elderly individual. Sedative hypnotic medications and narcotic analgesics impair alertness and mobility and may lead to urinary incontinence. Diuretics cause polyuria and may lead to urinary incontinence, particularly in the individual with preexisting detrusor instability. Antidepressants, anticholinergic or antispasmodic agents, decongestants, antiparkinsonian drugs, or calcium-channel blockers can predispose elderly individuals to urinary retention, particularly those who have preexisting impairment of detrusor contractility or bladder outlet obstruction.

Despite all the previously mentioned challenges to urinary continence associated with aging, it is important to remember that most elderly persons living in the community and nearly half of those confined to their homes or a long-term care facility retain continence.[142]

SUMMARY

Urinary continence is a complex set of behaviors that requires physiologic modulation of the lower urinary tract and adherence to a set of learned, culturally prescribed behaviors. Because of an increased awareness of the problem of urinary incontinence, our knowledge of the physiologic mechanisms that govern continence has grown significantly. Nonetheless, our understanding of urinary continence will remain incomplete until we learn to integrate the physiologic, mechanical, and psychosocial aspects of urinary continence into a holistic approach to lower urinary tract and voiding function.

SELF-ASSESSMENT EXERCISE

1. Identify four goals to be addressed in a comprehensive management program for the individual with urinary incontinence.
2. Which of the following individuals is at greatest risk for upper tract damage and why?
   a. Individual with vesicovaginal fistula and constant urinary leakage
   b. Individual with detrusor instability and normal detrusor contractility resulting in urge urinary incontinence and low residual urine volumes
   c. Individual with bladder outlet obstruction resulting in high intravesical pressures and incomplete bladder emptying with high residual urine volumes
3. Explain why anticholinergic medications have a much greater influence on bladder contractility than on ureteral peristalsis.
4. Explain the role of the "pelvic floor" in maintenance of normal bladder and urethral function and in preservation of continence.
5. Identify the importance of each of the following in preservation of continence:
   a. Anatomic integrity of the lower urinary tract
   b. Neurologic control of the detrusor (bladder)
   c. Competence of the urethral sphincter mechanism
6. Rate the following statement as true or false and explain your answer. "Voiding in the neurologically intact and continent adult is controlled by the sacral micturition center by means of the 'detrusor reflex'."
7. Compare the role of the cerebral cortex and the role of the pons in the regulation of voiding.

8. Medications that mimic the SNS (that is, alpha-adrenergic agonists) would be helpful in which of the following situations? Why?
   a. Patient with impaired detrusor contractility
   b. Patient with excessive urethral resistance
   c. Patient with inadequate urethral resistance
   d. Patient with detrusor instability and impaired contractility
9. Explain why women are at greater risk for urinary leakage after menopause.
10. Explain the role of fast-twitch fibers and the role of slow-twitch fibers in the maintenance of urinary continence and the implications for pelvic muscle reeducation.
11. Your friend asks you when she should start trying to toilet train her child. How would you respond to her?
12. Explain the following statement: "The elderly individual is at increased risk for urinary incontinence, although incontinence in the elderly always represents an abnormal (pathologic) condition."

REFERENCES

1. Moore KN, Paul P: A historical review of selected nursing and medical literature on urinary incontinence between 1850 and 1976, *J Wound Ostomy Continence Nurs* 24:106-122, 1997.
2. Cooper CS, Abousally CT, Austin JC, et al: Do public schools teach voiding dysfunction? Results of an elementary school teacher survey, *J Urol* 170(3):956-958, 2003.
3. Fitzgerald ST, Palmer MH, Kirkland VL, Robinson L: The impact of urinary incontinence in working women: a study in a production facility, *Womens Health* 35(1):1-16, 2002.
4. Steers WD: Physiology of the urinary bladder. In Walsh PC, Retik AB, Vaughan ED, Wein AJ, editors: *Campbell's urology,* ed 6, Philadelphia, 1992, WB Saunders.
5. Steers WD: Physiology and pharmacology of the bladder and urethra. In Walsh PC, Retik AB, Vaughan ED, Wein EJ, editors: *Campbell's urology,* ed 7, Philadelphia, 1998, WB Saunders.
6. Gray ML: *Genitourinary disorders,* St. Louis, 1992, Mosby.
7. Dixon J, Gosling J: Structure and innervation in the human. In Torrens M, Morrison JFB, editors: *Physiology of the lower urinary tract,* London, 1987, Springer-Verlag.

8. Elbadawi A: Anatomy and innervation of the vesi-courethral muscular unit of micturition. In Krane RJ, Siroky MB, editors: *Clinical neuro-urology,* Boston, 1991, Little, Brown.

9. Rosier PFWM: *Bladder function in elderly male patients.* Thesis presented to the Department of Urology, School of Medicine, University of Nijmegen, Nijmegen, The Netherlands, 1996.

10. de Groat WC, Fraser MO, Yoshiyama M, et al: Neural control of the urethra, *Scand J Urol Nephrol Suppl* 207:35-43, 2001.

11. Zderic SA, Chacko S, DiSanto ME, Wein AJ: Voiding function: relevant anatomy, physiology, pharmacology and molecular aspects. In: Gillenwater JY, Grayhack JT, Howards SS, Mitchell ME, editors: *Adult and pediatric urology,* ed 4, Philadelphia, 2002, Williams & Wilkins, pp 1061-1113.

12. Weiss RM: Physiology and pharmacology of the renal pelvis and ureter. In Walsh PC, Retik AB, Vaughan ED, Wein AJ, editors: *Campbell's urology,* ed 7, Philadelphia, 1998, WB Saunders.

13. Baker JC, Mitteness LS: Nocturia in the elderly, *Gerontologist* 28:99-104, 1988.

14. Brading AF, Mostwin JL: Electrical and mechanical responses of guinea-pig bladder muscle to nerve stimulation, *Br J Pharmacol* 98(4):1083-1090, 1989.

15. Parekh AB, Brading AF, Tomita T: Studies of longitudinal tissue impedance in various smooth muscles, *Prog Clin Biol Res* 327:375-378, 1990.

16. DeLancey JO: Functional anatomy of the female pelvis. In Kursh ED, McGuire EJ, editors: *Female urology,* Philadelphia, 1994, JB Lippincott.

17. Brooks JD: Anatomy of the lower urinary tract and male genitalia. In Walsh PC, Retik AB, Vaughan ED, Wein AJ, editors: *Campbell's urology,* ed 7, Philadelphia, 1998, WB Saunders.

18. Wahle GR, Young GPH, Raz S: Anatomy and physiology of pelvic support. In Raz S, editor: *Female urology,* Philadelphia, 1996, WB Saunders.

19. Kearney R, Sawhney R, DeLancey JO: Levator ani muscle anatomy evaluated by origin-insertion pairs, *Obstet Gynecol* 104(1):168-173, 2004.

20. Redman JF: Anatomy of the genitourinary system. In Gillenwater JY, Grayhack JT, Howards SS, Dukett JW, editors: *Adult and pediatric urology,* St. Louis, 1996, Mosby.

21. Siroky MB: Electromyography of the perineal striated muscles. In Krane RJ, Siroky MB, editors: *Clinical neurourology,* Boston, 1991, Little, Brown.

22. Couillard DR, Webster GD: Detrusor instability, *Urol Clin North Am* 22(3):593-612, 1995.

23. Wein AJ, Rovner ES. Definition and epidemiology of overactive bladder, *Urology* 60(5 suppl 1):7-12, 2002.

24. Abrams RM, Stanley H, Carter R, Notelovitz M: Effect of conjugated estrogen on vaginal blood flow in surgically menopausal women, *Am J Obstet Gynecol* 143:375,1982.

25. Gray M: Urodynamic evaluation of detrusor instability. Doctoral dissertation, University of Florida, Gainesville, Fla, 1990.

26. Thuroff JW, Jonas U, Frohneberg D, et al: Telemetric urodynamic investigations in normal males, *Urol Int* 35(6):427-434, 1980.

27. van Waalwijk van Doorn ES, Remmers A, Janknegt RA: Conventional and extramural ambulatory urodynamic testing of the lower urinary tract in female volunteers, *J Urol* 147(5):1319-1326, 1992.

28. Zinner NR: Clinical aspects of detrusor instability and the value of urodynamics, *Eur Urol* 34(suppl 1):16-19, 1998.

29. Gillespie JI, Harvey IJ, Drake MJ: Agonist- and nerve-induced phasic activity in the isolated whole bladder of the guinea pig: evidence for two types of bladder activity, *Exp Physiol* 88(3):343-357, 2003.

30. Klausner AP, Steers WD: Research frontiers in the treatment of urinary incontinence, *Clin Obstet Gynecol* 47(1):104-113, 2004.

31. Andrew J, Nathan PW, Spanos NC: Cerebral cortex and micturition, *Proc R Soc Med* 58:533, 1964.

32. Athwal BS, Berkley KJ, Hussain I, et al: Brain responses to changes in bladder volume and urge to void in healthy men, *Brain* 124(2):369-377, 2001.

33. Blok BF, Sturms LM, Holstege G: Brain activation during micturition in women, *Brain* 121(11):2033-2042, 1998.

34. Blok BF, Willemsen AT, Holstege G: A PET study on brain control of micturition in humans, *Brain* 120(1):111-112, 1997.

35. Matsuura S, Kakizaki H, Mitsui T, et al: Human brain region response to distention or cold stimulation of the bladder: a positron emission tomography study, *J Urol* 168(5):2035-2039, 2002.

36. Nour S, Svarer C, Kristensen JK, et al: Cerebral activation during micturition in normal men, *Brain* 123(4):781-789, 2000.

37. Bannister R: *Brain and Bannister's clinical neurology,* ed 7, Oxford, 1992, Oxford University Press.

38. Kandel ER, Schwarz JH: *Principles of neural science,* New York, 1981, Elsevier/North Holland, pp 672-679.

39. Sakakibara R, Hattori T, Yasuda K, Yamanishi T: Micturitional disturbance after acute hemispheric stroke: analysis of the lesion site by CT and MRI, *J Neurol Sci* 137(1):47-56, 1996.

40. Griffiths DJ, McCracken PN, Harrison GM, Gormley EA: Cerebral etiology of geriatric urge urinary incontinence, *Age Ageing* 23:246-250, 1994.

41. Aranda B, Cramer P: Effects of apomorphine and L-dopa on the parkinsonian bladder, *Neurourol Urodyn* 12:203-209, 1993.

42. Fitzmaurice H, Fowler CJ, Richards D, et al: Micturition disturbance in Parkinson's disease, *Br J Urol* 57:652-656, 1985.

43. Khan Z, Starer P, Bohla A: Urinary incontinence in female Parkinson disease patients: pitfalls of diagnosis, *Urology* 33:486-489, 1989.

44. Finazzi-Agro E, Peppe A, D'Amico A, et al: Effects of subthalamic nucleus stimulation on urodynamic findings in patients with Parkinson's disease, *J Urol* 169(4):1388-1391, 2003.

45. Berciano J: Olivopontocerebellar atrophy: a review of 117 cases, *J Neurol Sci* 53(2):253-272, 1982.
46. Chami I, Miladi N, Ben Hamida M, Zmerli S: Continence disorders in hereditary spinocerebellar degeneration: comparison of clinical and urodynamic findings in 55 cases, *Acta Neurol Belg* 84(4):194-203, 1984.
47. Marson L: Identification of central nervous system neurons that innervate the bladder body, bladder base, or external urethral sphincter of female rats: a transneuronal tracing study using pseudorabies virus, *J Comp Neurol* 389(4):584-602, 1997.
48. Griffiths DJ, Holstege G, Dalm E, de Wall H: Control and coordination of bladder and urethral function in the brainstem of the cat, *Neurourol Urodynam* 9:63-92, 1990.
49. Matsuura S, Allen GV, Downie JW: Volume-evoked micturition reflex is mediated by the ventrolateral periaqueductal gray in anesthetized rats, *Am J Physiol* 275(6):R2049-2055, 1998.
50. Matsumoto S, Levendusky MC, Longhurst PA, et al: Activation of mu opioid receptors in the ventrolateral periaqueductal gray inhibits reflex micturition in anesthetized rats, *Neurosci Lett* 363(2):116-119, 2004.
51. Snowball RK, Dampney RA, Lumb BM: Responses of neurones in the medullary raphe nuclei to inputs from visceral nociceptors and the ventrolateral periaqueductal grey in the rat, *Exp Physiol* 82(3):485-500, 1997.
52. Taniguchi N, Miyata M, Yachiku S, et al: A study of micturition inducing sites in the periaqueductal gray of the mesencephalon, *J Urol* 168(4):1626-1631, 2002.
53. de Groat WC, Steers WD: Autonomic regulation of the urinary bladder and sexual organs. In Lowey AD, Spyer KM, editors: *Central regulation of the autonomic functions,* Oxford, 1990, Oxford University Press.
54. Leach GE: Urodynamic manifestations of cerebellar ataxia, *J Urol* 128:348-350, 1982.
55. Ghoneim G, Hassouno M: Options for the pharmacologic management of stress and urge urinary incontinence in the elderly, *J Wound Ostomy Continence Nurs* 24:311-318, 1997.
56. McGuire EJ, Herlihy E: Bladder and urethral responses to sympathetic stimulation, *Invest Urol* 17:9-15, 1979.
57. Seeley RR, Stephens TD, Tate P: *Anatomy and physiology,* St. Louis, 1989, Mosby.
58. Levin RM, Staskin DR, Wein AJ: The muscarinic cholinergic binding kinetics of the human urinary bladder, *Neurourol Urodyn* 1:221, 1982.
59. Wang P, Luthin GR, Ruggieri MR: Muscarinic acetylcholine receptor subtypes mediating urinary bladder contractility and coupling to GTP binding proteins, *J Pharmacol Exp Ther* 273:959-966, 1995.
60. Wein AJ: Pharmacological agents for the treatment of urinary incontinence due to overactive bladder, *Expert Opin Investigat Drugs* 10(1):65-83, 2001.
61. Brynne N, Stahl MM, Hallen B, et al: Pharmacokinetics and pharmacodynamics of tolterodine in man: a new drug for the treatment of urinary bladder overactivity, *Int J Clin Pharmacol Ther* 35(7):295, 1997.
62. Nilvebrant L, Andersson KE, Gillberg PG, et al: Tolterodine: a new bladder-selective antimuscarinic agent, *Eur J Pharmacol* 327(2-3):195-207, 1997.
63. Nilvebrant L, Hallen B, Larsson G: Tolterodine: a new bladder selective muscarinic receptor antagonist: preclinical pharmacological and clinical data, *Life Sci* 60(13-14):1129-1136, 1997.
64. Ikeda K, Kobayashi S, Suzuki M, et al: M(3) receptor antagonism by the novel antimuscarinic agent solifenacin in the urinary bladder and salivary gland, *Naunyn Schmiedebergs Arch Pharmacol* 366(2):97-103, 2002.
65. Miyamae K, Yoshida M, Murakami S, et al: Pharmacological effects of darifenacin on human isolated urinary bladder, *Pharmacology* 69(4):205-211, 2003.
66. Morita T, Iizuka H, Iwata T, Kondo S: Function and distribution of beta3-adrenoceptors in rat, rabbit and human urinary bladder and external urethral sphincter, *J Smooth Muscle Res* 36(1):21-32, 2000.
67. Andersson KE: Treatment of overactive bladder: other drug mechanisms, *Urology* 55(5A suppl):51-59, 2000.
68. Burnstock G: The changing face of autonomic neurotransmission, *Acta Physiol Scand* 126:67-91, 1986.
69. Ehren I, Adolfsson J, Wiklund NP: Nitric oxide synthase activity in the human urogenital tract, *Urol Res* 22:287-290, 1994.
70. Meade-D'Alisera P, Merriweather T, Wentland M, et al: Depressive symptoms in women with urinary incontinence: a prospective study, *Urol Nurs* 21(6):397-399, 2001.
71. Zorn BH, Montgomery H, Pieper K, et al: Urinary incontinence and depression, *J Urol* 162(1):82-84, 1999.
72. Lee KS, Na YG, Dean-McKinney T, et al: Alterations in voiding frequency and cystometry in the clomipramine induced model of endogenous depression and reversal with fluoxetine, *J Urol* 170(5):2067-2071, 2003.
73. Bussolati G, Tizzani A, Casetta G, et al: Detection of estrogen receptors in the trigone and urinary bladder with an immunohistochemical technique, *Gynecol Endocrinol* 4:205-213, 1990.
74. Fahrenholz F, Eggena P, Kojro E, et al: Synthesis and biological activities of a photoaffinity probe for vasotocin and oxytocin receptors, *Int J Pept Prot Res* 30:577-582, 1987.
75. Roy C, Bockaert J, Rajerison R, Jard S: Oxytocin receptor in frog bladder epithelial cells: relationship of (^{3}H)oxytocin binding to adenylate cyclase activation, *FEBS Lett* 30:329-334, 1973.
76. Melville JL, Walker E, Katon W, et al: Prevalence of comorbid psychiatric illness and its impact on symptom perception, quality of life, and functional status in women with urinary incontinence, *Am J Obstet Gynecol* 187(1):80-87, 2002.
77. Klausner AP, Yong-Gil N, Kyu-Sung L, et al: The role of corticotropin releasing factor and its antagonist, astressin on micturition in the awake rat. Chicago, 2003, American Urological Association; abstract published in *J Urol* 169(4):43-44 (abstract 167), 2003.

78. Yoshimura N, de Groat WC: Neural control of the lower urinary tract, *Int J Urol* 4(2):111-125, 1997.

79. Nickel JC, Downey J, Morales A, et al: Relative efficacy of various exogenous glycosaminoglycans in providing a bladder surface permeability barrier, *J Urol* 160(2):612-614, 1998.

80. Parsons CL, Boychuk D, Jones S, et al: Bladder surface glycosaminoglycans: an epithelial permeability barrier, *J Urol* 143(1):139-142, 1990.

81. *Webster's new collegiate dictionary,* Springfield, Mass, 1979, G & C Merriam, p 1111.

82. Gray ML, Rayome RG, Moore KN: The urethra! sphincter: an update, *Urol Nurs* 15:40-55, 1995.

83. Zinner NR, Sterling AM, Ritter R: Role of inner urethral softness in urinary incontinence, *Urology* 16:115-117, 1980.

84. da Silva EA, Sampaio FJ, Ortiz V, Cardoso LE: Regional differences in the extracellular matrix of the human spongy urethra as evidenced by the composition of glycosaminoglycans, *J Urol* 167(5):2183-2187, 2002.

85. Staskin DR, Zimmern PE, Hadley HR, Raz S: Pathophysiology of stress incontinence, *Clin Obstet Gynecol* 12:357-368, 1985.

86. Raz S, Caine M, Zeigler M: The vascular component in the production of urethral pressure, *J Urol* 108:93-96, 1972.

87. Abrams RM, Stanley H, Carter R, Notelovitz M: Effect of conjugated estrogen on vaginal blood flow in surgically menopausal women, *Am J Obstet Gynecol* 143:375, 1982.

88. Bergman A, Karram MM, Bhatia NN: Changes in urethral cytology following estrogen administration, *Gynecol Obstet Invest* 29:211, 1990.

89. Elia G, Bergman A: Estrogen effects on the urethra and beneficial effects in women with genuine stress urinary incontinence, *Obstet Gynecol Surv* 48:509-517, 1993.

90. Aust TR, Lewis-Jones DI : Retrograde ejaculation and male infertility, *Hosp Med (Lond)* 65(6):361-364, 2004.

91. Selli C, De Antoni P, Moro U, et al: Role of bladder neck preservation in urinary continence following radical retropubic prostatectomy, *Scand J Urol Nephrol* 38(1):32-37, 2004.

92. Lowe BA: Comparison of bladder neck preservation to bladder neck resection in maintaining postprostatectomy urinary continence, *Urology* 48(6):889-893, 1996.

93. Noble JG, Bruce-Jones ADA, Mathias CJ, Milroy EJG: Autonomic and pharmacologic dysfunction in bladder neck dyssynergia, *Neurourol Urodyn* 11:400-401, 1992.

94. Moore KN: Electrical stimulation for the treatment of urinary incontinence: do we know enough to accept it as part of your practice? *J Adv Nurs* 20:1018-1022, 1994.

95. Brading AF, Teramoto N, Dass N, McCoy R: Morphological and physiological characteristics of urethral circular and longitudinal smooth muscle, *Scand J Urol Nephrol Suppl* 207:12-18, 2001.

96. Gosling J, Dixon J: Pelvic floor. In Mundy AR, Stephenson TP, Wein AJ, editors: *Urodynamics: principles, practice and application,* London, 1994, Churchill Livingstone.

97. Elbadawi A: Comparative neuromorphology in animals. In Torrens M, Morrison JFB, editors: *The physiology of the lower urinary tract,* London, 1987, Springer-Verlag.

98. Torrens M: Human physiology. In Torrens M, Morrison JFB, editors: *Physiology of the lower urinary tract,* London, 1985, Springer-Verlag.

99. Johnson VY: *Effects of a submaximal exercise protocol to recondition the circumvaginal musculature in women with genuine stress urinary incontinence.* Unpublished dissertation, University of Texas at San Antonio, 1997.

100. Andersson KE, Hedlund P: Pharmacologic perspective on the physiology of the lower urinary tract, *Urology* 60(5 suppl 1):13-21, 2002.

101. Yalla SV, Rossier AB, Fam BA, et al: Functional contribution of autonomic innervation to urethral striated sphincter: studies with parasympathomimetics, parasympatholytics and alpha adrenergic blocking agents in spinal cord injured and control male subjects, *J Urol* 117:494, 1977.

102. Van Kerrebroeck P: Duloxetine: an innovative approach for treating stress urinary incontinence, *BJU Int* 94 (suppl 1):31-37, 2004.

103. Rushton HG: Enuresis. In Kelalis PP, King LR, Belman AB: *Clinical pediatric urology,* ed 3, Philadelphia, 1992, WB Saunders.

104. Sillen U: Bladder function in healthy neonates and its development during infancy, *J Urol* 166(6):2376-2381, 2001.

105. Goellner MH, Ziegler EE, Forman SG: Urination during the first three years of life, *Nephron* 28:174-177, 1981.

106. Gray ML: Genitourinary embryology, anatomy and physiology. In Karlowicz K, editor: *Urologic nursing: principles and practice,* Philadelphia, 1996, WB Saunders.

107. Brazelton TB: A child-oriented approach to toilet training, *Pediatrics* 21:121-123, 1962.

108. Gray M: Incontinence in the school-aged child, *Progressions* 5:16-23, 1993.

109. Brockelhurst JC: Aging, bladder function and incontinence. In Brockelhurst JC, editor: *Urology in the elderly,* London, 1994, Churchill Livingstone.

110. Broderick GA, Wein AJ: Pharmacologic therapy for incontinence. In O'Donnell PD, editor: *Geriatric urology,* Boston, 1994, Little, Brown.

111. Elbadawi A: Pathology and pathophysiology of detrusor in incontinence, *Urol Clin North Am* 22:499-512, 1995.

112. Susset JG, Servot-Viguier D, Lamy F, et al: Collagen in 155 human bladders, *Invest Urol* 16:204-206, 1978.

113. Monnier VM, Kohn RR, Cerami A: Accelerated age related browning of human collagen in diabetes mellitus, *Proc Natl Acad Sci USA* 81:583, 1984.

114. Gilpin SA, Gilpin JC, Dixon JS, et al: The effect of age on the autonomic innervation of the urinary bladder, *Br J Urol* 58:378-381, 1986.

115. Hampel C, Gillitzer R, Pahernik S, et al: Changes in the receptor profile of the aging bladder, *Urology* 43(5):535-541, 2004.

116. Elbadawi A, Yalla SV, Resnick NM: Structural basis of geriatric voiding dysfunction. II. Aging detrusor: normal vs. impaired contractility, *J Urol* 150:1657-1667, 1993.

117. Elbadawi A, Yalla SV, Resnick NM: Structural basis of geriatric voiding dysfunction. III. Detrusor overactivity, *J Urol* 150:1668-1680, 1993.

118. Elbadawi A, Yalla SV, Resnick NM: Structural basis of geriatric voiding dysfunction. IV. Bladder outlet obstruction, *J Urol* 150:1681, 1993.

119. Steers WD, Barrett DM, Wein AJ: Voiding function and dysfunction. In Gillenwater JY, Grayhack JT, Howards SS, Duckett J, editors: *Adult and pediatric urology,* St. Louis, 1996, Mosby, pp 1159-1219.

120. Thompson DW, Furlan AJ: Clinical epidemiology of stroke, *Neurol Clin* 14:309-315, 1996.

121. Badlani GH: Incontinence associated with cerebrovascular accidents. In O'Donnell PD, editor: *Geriatric urology,* Boston, 1994, Little, Brown.

122. Ween JE, Alexander MP, D'Esposito M, Roberts M: Incontinence after stroke in a rehabilitation setting: outcome associations and predictive factors, *Neurology* 47:659-663, 1996.

123. Nakayama H, Jørgensen HS, Pedersen PM, et al: Prevalence and risk factors of incontinence after stroke, *Stroke* 28:58-62, 1997.

124. Tanner CM, Goldman SM: Epidemiology of Parkinson's disease, *Urol Clin* 14:317-335, 1996.

125. Kirby RS: Nontraumatic neurogenic bladder dysfunction. In Mundy AR, Stephenson TP, Wein AJ, editors: *Urodynamics: principles, practice, and application,* London, 1994, Churchill Livingstone, pp 365-373.

126. Staskin DR: Intracranial lesions that affect lower urinary tract function. In Krane RJ, Siroky MB, editors: *Clinical neurourology,* Boston, 1991, Little, Brown.

127. Keefover RW: The clinical epidemiology of Alzheimer's disease, *Neurol Clin* 14:337-351, 1996.

128. Griffiths DJ, McCracken PN, Harrison GM, Moore KN: Urge incontinence in elderly people: factors predicting the severity of urine loss before and after pharmacologic treatment, *Neurourol Urodyn* 15:53-57, 1995.

129. Griffiths DJ, McCracken PN, Harrison GM, Moore KN: Urinary incontinence in the elderly: the brain factor, *Scand J Urol Nephrol Suppl* 157:83-88, 1994.

130. Ouslander JG: Lower urinary tract disorders in the elderly female. In Raz S, editor: *Female urology,* Philadelphia, 1994, WB Saunders.

131. Fantl JA, Bump RC, McClish DK, Wyman JF: Efficacy of estrogen supplementation in treatment of urinary incontinence, *Obstet Gynecol* 88:745-749, 1996.

132. Nygaard IE, Lemke JH: Urinary incontinence in rural older women: prevalence, incidence and remission, *J Am Geriatr Soc* 44:1049-1054, 1996.

133. BPH Clinical Guideline Panel: *Benign prostatic hyperplasia: diagnosis and treatment,* Rockville, Md, 1994, Department of Health and Human Services, Agency for Health Care Policy and Research.

134. Steers WD, Zorn B: Benign prostatic hyperplasia, *Dis Mon* 41:437-500, 1995.

135. O'Connor LT, Vaughan ED Jr, Felsen D: In vivo cystometric evaluation of progressive bladder outlet obstruction in rats, *J Urol* 158:631-635, 1997.

136. Steers WD, deGroat WC: Effect of bladder outlet obstruction on micturition pathways in the rat, *J Urol* 140:864, 1988.

137. Chai TC, Gray M, Steers WD: Incidence of a positive iced water test in bladder outlet obstructed patients: evidence for bladder neuroplasticity, *J Urol* 160:34-38, 1998.

138. Umlauf MG, Sherman SM: Symptoms of urinary incontinence among older community-dwelling men, *J Wound Ostomy Continence Nurs* 23:314-321, 1996.

139. Homma Y, Imajo C, Takahashi S, et al: Urinary symptoms and urodynamics in a normal elderly population, *Scand J Urol Nephrol Suppl* 157:27-30, 1994.

140. Matthiessen TB, Rittig S, Norgaard JP, et al: Nocturnal polyuria in male patients with lower urinary tract symptoms, *J Urol* 156:1292-1299, 1996.

141. Kikuchi Y: Participation of atrial natriuretic peptide (hANP) levels and arginine vasopressin (AVP) in aged persons with nocturia, *Jpn J Urol* 86:1651-1659, 1995.

142. Agency for Health Care Policy and Research Clinical Guideline Panel for Urinary Incontinence: *Acute and chronic urinary incontinence in adults,* Rockville, Md, 1996, Department of Health and Human Services.

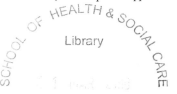
SCHOOL OF HEALTH & SOCIAL CARE
Library

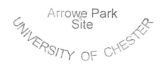
Arrowe Park Site
UNIVERSITY OF CHESTER

Assessment and Management of Acute or Transient Urinary Incontinence

JOANN ERMER-SELTUN

OBJECTIVES

1. Define the following terms: acute incontinence, chronic incontinence, and transient incontinence.
2. Explain why screening for reversible factors is the first step in assessment and management of any patient with urinary incontinence (UI).
3. Use the acronym DIAPPERS to identify common reversible factors contributing to UI.
4. Identify specific data to be gathered during the patient interview, focused physical examination, and initial laboratory tests to screen for transient factors.
5. Explain why elderly persons are at particular risk for acute onset of incontinence caused by transient factors.
6. Explain the potential effects of each of the following types of medications on bladder function and continence: alpha-adrenergic receptor antagonists and agonists; angiotensin-converting enzyme (ACE) inhibitors; calcium-channel blockers; tranquilizers, sedatives, alcohol, nicotine, and narcotic analgesics; skeletal muscle relaxants; anticholinergics; imipramine.
7. Describe the two types of voiding symptoms that may occur with bladder outlet obstruction and the pathologic mechanisms of each.
8. Explain the effect of reduced compliance on upper tract function and the implications for management.
9. Identify factors that increase risk for incontinence among patients who have undergone major surgery.
10. Discuss the guidelines for assessment and management of a patient with acute onset of UI.

Incontinent states are sometimes subdivided into acute and chronic, based on duration. The term "acute" is used to designate incontinence of recent and abrupt onset; the patient may report new onset of urinary leakage or may report sudden worsening of preexisting minor incontinence, such as a sudden and significant increase in the volume of urine loss. New-onset incontinence is frequently caused by reversible, or transient factors, and acute incontinence is sometimes known as "transient incontinence." However, the continence nurse should be aware that the terms "acute incontinence" and "transient incontinence" are not synonymous; in some patients, the acute onset of incontinence is attributable to an illness or injury that ultimately results in chronic incontinence. For instance, acute UI caused by a stroke may persist and become chronic UI if the patient does not regain the ability to delay voiding. The continence nurse should also be aware that "transient" or "reversible" factors frequently play a contributing role in conditions of established incontinence. For example, a woman who has experienced occasional leakage during activity for many years may have an acute exacerbation when she is prescribed an ACE inhibitor for blood pressure control, as a result of the chronic cough commonly caused by this medication. Therefore, screening for and correction of reversible factors are of primary importance in the management of any patient with UI.

UI is quite common; the prevalence among the community-dwelling elderly population is as high as 33%, and the prevalence among institutionalized elderly individuals is as high as 50%.[1] In a survey of 45,000 US households, the prevalence of UI within the preceding 30 days was found to be 37%[2];

the sample demographics matched the demographics of the US census. Interestingly, a report by the International Continence Society confirmed a prevalence rate of UI in Europe similar to that of the United States.[3]

One type of voiding dysfunction that imposes astonishing social, economic and psychologic burdens is overactive bladder (OAB). OAB is a constellation of bladder symptoms that include urgency and urinary frequency with or without UI; it is estimated to affect more than 33 million Americans.[4] It affects both men and women equally, but "wet" OAB (OAB with UI) affects more women, whereas "dry" OAB (OAB without UI) is more prevalent in men.[5]

The sudden onset of UI is very distressing to persons who have never experienced it before; patients may experience alarm, anxiety, and fear over the loss of bladder control and independence. Also, because of embarrassment related to the UI, the patient may reduce or even eliminate social contacts and sexual relationships. These factors contribute to an increased risk for depression.[6-8] Several studies have confirmed the negative impact of UI on quality of life, social activities, and psychologic status; in addition, UI creates an astronomical financial burden for patients and caregivers.[2] Furthermore, the onset of incontinence is known to be a common reason for admission of the elderly to long-term care settings.[9,10] Thus, aggressive assessment and management of voiding dysfunction and UI disorders are indicated to correct the problem whenever possible.

The geriatric population is at particularly high risk for transient episodes of incontinence because of age-related changes in the anatomy and physiology of the lower urinary tract (Box 3-1). These changes include a reduction in sensory awareness of bladder filling, reduced ability to empty the bladder effectively, increased rate of urine production at night, reduced bladder capacity, and reduced ability to delay voiding, as well as gender-specific changes.[7,11] In addition to changes in the function of the lower urinary tract, continence in the elderly is also affected by altered mobility and dexterity and by alterations in cognitive status. Any alteration in the fine balance among lower urinary tract function,

> **BOX 3-1** **Age-Related Changes in the Lower Genitourinary Tract**
>
> 1. Increased nocturnal urinary output related to change in levels of arginine vasopressin and atrial natriuretic hormone
> 2. Reduction in urethral closing pressure and urethral length resulting from estrogen loss
> 3. Reduced ability to delay voiding
> 4. Reduced bladder capacity
> 5. Reduced sensory awareness of filling
> 6. Reduced urinary flow rates
> 7. Elevated postvoid residual
> 8. Elevated risk for bladder outlet obstruction secondary to prostatic hypertrophy
> 9. Increased frequency of sensory and motor urgency
>
> Data from Miller M: Nocturnal polyuria in older people, *J Am Geriatr Soc* 48:1321-1329, 2000; Naeem M, Naeem L, Morley JE: Aging urinary bladder. In Morley JE, Armbrecvht HJ, Coe RM, Vellas B, editors: *Science of geriatrics*, vol II, New York, 2000, Springer-Verlag, pp 659-667; and Wagg A, Malone-Lee J: The management of urinary incontinence in the elderly, *Br J Urol* 82(suppl 1):11-17, 1998.

mobility/dexterity, and cognition can abruptly change continence status.[12] Thus, the continent elderly person is frequently borderline in terms of bladder function and continence; in this situation the addition of a "reversible" factor that negatively affects the function of the urinary tract, such as a bladder infection, can precipitate incontinence. This is in contrast to the younger person with stable bladder and sphincter function; in this individual, a bladder infection is manifest as frequency, urgency, and dysuria, but continence is maintained. In fact, acute onset of incontinence in the younger patient population is more likely to be induced by illness, injury, or surgery, and it may or may not be reversible.

This chapter provides a review of the known causes of acute and transient UI in adults and addresses interventions to restore continence. In many cases, multiple etiologic factors exist simultaneously; in these situations, management strategies must be aimed at correcting as many of the reversible factors as possible, within the limitations posed by the individual patient's overall clinical status and management plan.

ETIOLOGIC FACTORS FOR ACUTE-ONSET INCONTINENCE

As noted earlier, multiple factors can contribute to the sudden onset or worsening of urinary leakage. One approach to "classifying and remembering" the most common reversible factors is the acronym DIAPPERS (Box 3-2); although this acronym was originally designed as a guide for assessment of the elderly patient, many of the factors are relevant to the assessment of any individual with urinary leakage. Another way to classify the causes of acute UI is by the causative factor's relationship to the urinary tract, that is, factors within the urinary tract and factors outside the urinary tract. In this chapter, factors outside the urinary tract are discussed first, and then factors within the urinary tract are reviewed.

Factors Outside the Urinary Tract

It is frequently factors outside the urinary tract that produce acute or transient UI. The most common of these factors are discussed; they include delirium, dehydration, dietary bladder irritants, pharmaceuticals, psychological problems, conditions resulting in excessive urine production or in retention, conditions causing restricted mobility or dexterity, and stool impaction. The health care provider should take a proactive approach by screening for these factors when assessing the patient with new onset of incontinence and should then intervene to reduce or eliminate any factors contributing to the incontinence. Successful intervention frequently requires creativity and an ability to tactfully suggest life-style changes that may seem easy and simple, almost too simple for the patient to believe they are the solution to the UI. Patients are frequently accustomed to extensive testing and medical-surgical interventions for correction of health care problems. Thus, simple measures such as environmental alterations or dietary changes may not seem aggressive enough to make a difference and may not feel like "treatment." Success in helping the patient to value these treatment measures requires clear explanations of the pathologic processes resulting in UI (in lay terms), along with a discussion regarding the impact of behavioral therapies on the UI. Continence nurses must recognize the importance of patient education as well as documentation and follow-up programs to reinforce and to monitor the effectiveness of these measures.

Delirium. Delirium is defined as an acute confusional state characterized by cognitive deficits and behavior disturbances. It is often a causative factor in transient UI; the alteration in cognitive function compromises the individual's ability to recognize and respond appropriately to the sensation of a full bladder. Many clinical conditions may result in acute confusion, including systemic illnesses, central nervous system diseases, medications, dehydration, alcohol use, sleep deprivation, a reaction to anesthesia, or metabolic conditions such as renal or hepatic failure. The cause of delirium is often multifactorial, with a complex interplay of predisposing and precipitating factors. The most commonly cited "causative" factors in the elderly are polypharmacy and sepsis; fluid and electrolyte imbalances may also contribute to alterations in mental status.[13] Almost every drug class can alter cognition in the elderly because of age-related alterations in drug metabolism, renal function, and brain perfusion.[14] A simple mnemonic can be used to identify classes of drugs that are most likely to cause changes in mental status in the elderly (Box 3-3).[15] In the elderly, acute confusion may also be precipitated by a urinary tract or respiratory infection, and altered

---

BOX 3-2   **Reversible (Transient) Causes of Urinary Incontinence**

D	Delirium, Dehydration, Dietary irritants
I	Infection of urinary tract, symptomatic
A	Atrophic urethritis and vaginitis; acute urogenital prolapse
P	Pharmaceuticals
P	Psychological, especially depression
E	Excess urine output (endocrine disorders, congestive heart failure, overhydration, sleep apnea)
R	Restricted mobility, Retention
S	Stool impaction

Adapted from Resnick NM: Geriatric incontinence, *Urol Clin North Am* 23:55-74, 1996.

BOX 3-3 Drugs Causing Acute Change in Mental Status in Elderly Persons

Initial	Drug Class
A	Antiparkinsonian drugs
C	Corticosteroids
U	Urinary incontinence drugs
T	Theophylline
E	Emptying drugs*
C	Cardiovascular drugs
H	H2-blockers
A	Antimicrobials
N	Nonsteroidal antiinflammatory drugs
G	Geropsychiatric drugs†
E	ENT drugs‡
I	Insomnia drugs
N	Narcotics
M	Muscle relaxants
S	Seizure drugs

Adapted from Flaherty JH: Commonly prescribed and over the counter medications: causes of confusion, *Clin Geriatr Med* 14:101-127, 1998.

*Emptying drugs: a class of medications that enhances activity of the upper gastrointestinal tract (e.g., metoclopramide).

†Geropsychiatric drugs: includes any medication that crosses the brain-blood barrier and possibly impairs cognition (e.g., tricyclic antidepressants, selective serotonin reuptake inhibitors, benzodiazepines, antipsychotics, anticholinergics).

‡ENT drugs: ear, nose, and throat; drugs taken for problems of the respiratory system and sinuses (e.g., decongestants, antihistamines, expectorants, antitussives).

mental status may be the only clinical indicator of that infection. The elderly may also experience acute confusion in response to illness and hospitalization. When the nurse is dealing with incontinence related to delirium, the focus is on correction of the confusional state; once this is resolved, the incontinence typically resolves as well. (The patient is again able to recognize and respond to the sensation of a full bladder.)

It is obviously important to differentiate between delirium, which is reversible, and dementia, which is not. When assessment reveals an irreversible alteration in mental status, the nurse must focus on strategies for managing (rather than correcting) the chronic incontinence; this may involve an individualized or routine scheduled toileting program, prompted voiding, and/or use of collection devices or absorbent pads. These options are discussed further in Chapters 6 and 11.

Dehydration. Inadequate fluid intake has been related to the onset of OAB symptoms (urgency and frequency), and it may even lead to urge incontinence. It is not uncommon for a patient experiencing these symptoms to reduce fluid intake in a futile attempt to reduce the number of trips to the bathroom and the episodes of leakage. In actuality, the concentrated urine produced by fluid restriction may actually irritate the bladder lining, thus worsening OAB symptoms and UI. Inadequate fluid intake also contributes to constipation and difficult elimination of stool (this is discussed further under the section on stool impaction). It is therefore important to spend time educating patients regarding the importance and benefits of adequate fluid intake and emphasizing the detrimental effects of limited fluid consumption. Many persons find it difficult to remember to drink adequate amounts of fluids because of lack of thirst, aversion to the taste of water, or just poor intake habits. However, when patients become aware of the relationship between their fluid intake and their OAB symptoms and UI, they are frequently more motivated to make this change in daily behavior. In helping patients to change their behavior, it may be helpful to set "progressive" goals, that is, to gradually increase the volume of fluid intake over a period of days to weeks as opposed to imposing an immediate expectation of an intake of eight glasses of water-based fluid per day. Some "fluid for thought" could be to increase their daily fluid intake by one glass of fluid each week until the fluid goal is achieved. Patients should be encouraged to drink small amounts of fluids regularly throughout the day, as opposed to consuming large amounts at one sitting; this is generally easier for the individual and is also less likely to result in sudden production of large volumes of urine.

Dietary Irritants. Numerous studies have suggested that bladder irritants may play a causal or contributing role in UI; however, the specific role played by these substances remains unclear, with a limited evidence base.[16] The substance with the strongest evidence base is caffeine, which is thought to contribute to both stress UI and urge UI.

Caffeine administration has been shown to increase bladder pressure during urodynamic tests,[17] and it has also been shown to increase urgency and frequency (as a result of its diuretic and irritant effects). Some investigators have found dietary caffeine to be a statistically significant risk factor for detrusor instability, even after controlling for variables such as age and smoking.[18,19] Caffeine is found in coffee, tea, many types of soft drinks (especially colas), chocolate, and nonprescription medications such as Anacin, Excedrin, and Midol. Other types of foods and beverages that have been associated with altered bladder control include carbonated beverages, milk or milk products, artificial sweeteners such as Nutrasweet, sugar, honey, corn syrup, citrus fruits and juices, highly spiced foods, and even decaffeinated sodas, coffee, and tea. It is important to note that these are "potential" irritants, and they do not affect all patients equally; a substance that causes increased frequency and urgency for one individual may have no impact on another. Therefore, patients should be counseled to "experiment" by eliminating potential irritants from their diet one at a time for a week to determine the impact on their own symptoms.

Alcoholic beverages affect bladder control because they increase urinary volume, alter mentation, and produce sedation. Alcohol is discussed in depth under pharmaceuticals.

Pharmaceuticals. Medications can actually cause incontinence, and they are a common contributing factor to incontinence; therefore, the assessment of any incontinent individual must include a complete listing of all medications, including prescription, over-the-counter, and herbal agents. Many patients are unable initially to provide a complete listing of all medications they are currently taking; they may be able to report only that they take "a dozen" pills every day and that they cost a fortune. However, it is important to persevere to obtain this information; most patients are able to compile a list or to bring all their medications to the clinic once they are convinced of the importance and relevance of the data. If the patient is not able to provide the information, it may be helpful to inquire about the types of medical specialists they have seen and any recent visits and recommendations. The patient's

pharmacy may be another resource; often the pharmacist can provide a complete listing of the medications routinely taken by the patient. Any medication that alters the normal levels of neurotransmitters in the lower urinary tract can contribute to UI or voiding dysfunction; Table 2-3 (see Chapter 2) provides a review of the relevant neurotransmitters and their effects on voiding physiology, which clarifies the effects of various pharmaceuticals.

Alpha-adrenergic receptor antagonists such as prazosin or terazosin are typically prescribed for hypertension. These drugs, also known as alphablockers, are also known to cause or worsen UI; this is because they produce relaxation of the smooth muscle in the bladder neck and urethra, which may cause or worsen stress incontinence in the female. A woman who already has some degree of stress incontinence is likely to experience an increase in the frequency and severity of leakage, and the woman with no prior history of leakage may experience new onset of stress incontinence depending on the degree of urethral relaxation.

Unlike the alpha-adrenergic "antagonist" medications, the alpha-adrenergic "agonist" medications promote increased smooth muscle tone in the proximal urethra and bladder neck. Commonly used medications in this group include those used for cold and allergy symptoms, such as pseudoephedrine and ephedrine. These medications enhance urethral resistance, and therefore they may be used to treat stress UI. However, these drugs may contribute to emptying problems or even overflow incontinence in an individual with bladder outlet obstruction, such as an older man with an enlarged prostate gland or the individual with a urethral stricture. Because these medications are available over the counter, the continence specialist must query any patient who presents with symptoms of urinary retention regarding recent ingestion of cold remedy type drugs.

ACE inhibitors, such as enalapril or catapril, are another type of antihypertensive medication that may contribute to stress incontinence. This is caused primarily by the dry cough that is a common side effect of these drugs; the cough can aggravate stress incontinence in women who have weak pelvic support and in men who have had a prostatectomy.[20]

When the patient's antihypertensive drug appears to be causing or contributing to his or her incontinence, the continence care nurse should consult the primary care provider regarding a possible change in medication (that is, another type of antihypertensive).

Some cardiac drugs can also affect continence. One of the most common "offenders" is the dihydropyridine class of calcium-channel blockers (nifedipine, nicardipine, israpidine, felodipine, and nimodipine). These drugs have a relaxing effect on the detrusor muscle, which may precipitate urinary retention.[20] In addition, this class of calcium-channel blockers causes increased urine production at night, and this may result in nocturia or enuresis. Finally, calcium-channel blockers may cause constipation, which can result in outflow obstruction or increased bladder contractility and urge pattern incontinence.

Diuretics are another type of medication commonly prescribed for cardiac conditions that are likely to precipitate or worsen UI. Although these drugs are clearly necessary for the management of congestive heart failure and hypertension, the sudden increase in urine production may cause leakage; this is particularly common in the elderly patient with detrusor overactivity, who may be unable to make it to the bathroom "in time." The timing of diuretic administration can be adjusted to allow the patient to accommodate the sudden increase in urine volume. For example, if the diuretic is taken at night, the patient will experience nocturia, urgency, urge incontinence, and enuresis; in contrast, a late afternoon or early evening dosage schedule accompanied by 1 to 2 hours of rest with leg elevation can promote evening diuresis and a subsequent reduction in nocturia. The continence nurse can also assist the patient to maintain continence during periods of increased urine output by teaching the patient urge-inhibition strategies such as relaxation, distraction, and "quick flick" pelvic floor muscle contractions.

Although the mechanisms are not well understood, smoking is strongly associated with altered bladder control.[21] Nicotine has been shown to cause detrusor instability and the resulting symptoms of urgency, frequency, and even urge UI. In addition, the classic "smoker's cough" can cause new onset of stress UI or an exacerbation of stress UI among individuals with pelvic floor weakness. The chronic repetitive cough may also, in itself, cause or contribute to pelvic floor weakness and loss of vaginal and urethral support.[21] In fact, the risk for stress UI increases by a factor of 2.5 in women who smoke, and studies indicate that smoking is an "independent" risk factor.[21] Moreover, smoking has been linked to an increased risk for bladder cancer.[22] Continence nurses have an opportunity, along with primary care providers, to provide anticipatory guidance regarding the health benefits of a smoking cessation program; such a program may prevent nicotine-related bladder disorders.[22]

Sedatives and tranquilizers can adversely affect continence in several ways. Perhaps the most common is a direct consequence of the drug's desired effect; that is, the patient who normally wakes readily to the sensation of a full bladder and typically gets up twice during the night to void may fail to wake to the sensation of a full bladder, thus resulting in nocturnal enuresis. Elderly patients who experience detrusor hyperactivity with impaired contractility (DHIC) may be particularly vulnerable to this effect, because their bladders are both "overactive" and "poorly contractile." These drugs may also cause reduced sensory awareness of bladder filling and temporary confusion (delirium) in the elderly and may exacerbate any preexisting impairment in mobility; these conditions, in turn, contribute to incontinence.

Alcohol is another contributing factor to incontinence because of its sedative and diuretic effects. The potential effects of moderate alcohol intake on continence include polyuria, frequency, and urgency; excessive alcohol ingestion may also produce delirium, sedation, and transient immobility. Patients who experience occasional problems with incontinence at night may find that elimination of alcohol intake during the evening eliminates the problem; many patients make this association on their own in the course of keeping a bladder diary.

Narcotic analgesics prescribed for control of postoperative or chronic pain may produce effects similar to those associated with tranquilizers and alcohol, such as transient delirium, sedation, and immobility. In addition, narcotic analgesics commonly produce constipation or urinary retention, or both; therefore, patients who require narcotic analgesics for more than a few days should be prescribed a bowel regimen that includes daily fiber therapy and stool softeners as needed to prevent constipation and impaction, and they should be monitored for evidence of urinary retention.

Anticholinergic drugs are an important category of medications in terms of impact on continence, and many prescription drugs have anticholinergic effects. Among the most common of the "anticholinergic component" drugs are those used to treat psychosis, depression, gastrointestinal problems, and Parkinson's disease. The drug classification for many anticholinergic agents begins with the prefix "anti": these include antidepressants, antipsychotics, antiparkinsonian drugs, antispasmodics, and some antihypertensives.[23] All anticholinergic drugs have the potential to produce urinary retention, as evidenced by the fact that drugs with significant anticholinergic effects are frequently prescribed for the treatment of urgency, frequency, and urge incontinence. When used to treat these urinary symptoms, the desired effects of anticholinergics are reduction of "unstable" bladder contractions and reduced sensory urgency in response to bladder filling. However, when anticholinergic medications are prescribed for other medical problems in the patient with "normal" bladder function, urinary retention with incomplete bladder emptying or overflow incontinence may result. Anticholinergic medications may also produce sedation, delirium, immobility, and constipation, all of which are associated with incontinence. In addition, a common side effect of anticholinergic drugs is "dry mouth" (xerostomia); patients commonly increase their fluid intake to counteract this effect, and this may increase their episodes of UI, although in actuality increased fluid intake is more likely to reduce incontinent episodes than to increase them.

In addition to the many drugs with anticholinergic components, some pure anticholinergic drugs are prescribed for a variety of medical conditions, such as irritable bowel syndrome. These drugs may also result in some degree of urinary retention; examples include hyoscyamine (Levsin or Levbid).

Dicyclomine (Bentyl) is an antispasmodic that is also used for irritable bowel; it can induce similar adverse urinary effects, specifically bladder relaxation and incomplete emptying. Skeletal muscle relaxants, commonly prescribed for patients with multiple sclerosis or spinal cord injury, may also cause problems with retention and incomplete emptying; common examples include diazepam (Valium), baclofen (Lioresal), and dantrolene sodium (Dantrium).

As noted earlier, anticholinergic drugs can contribute to urinary retention and voiding dysfunction; however, these agents may also be used to treat specific urinary symptoms, such as urgency, frequency, and nocturia. Drugs commonly used in this manner include oxybutynin (Ditropan), tolterodine (Detrol), trospium (Sanctura), solifenacin succinate (Vesicare), and darifenacin (Enablex). Flavoxate HCl (Urispas) and hyoscyamine (Cystospaz) were used for these symptoms in the past, but they have fallen out of favor as a result of their limited uroselectivity and increased incidence of side effects. The newer generation of anticholinergic drugs for OAB and urge UI (tolterodine, trospium, solifenacin succinate, and darifenacin) produce fewer systemic side effects because they demonstrate much greater uroselectivity; that is, they have greater affinity for the cholinergic receptor sites in the bladder than those elsewhere in the body. (The cholinergic receptors in the bladder wall are primarily M2 and M3, and the newer drugs, the antimuscarinics, bind selectively to these receptor sites.[24]) Some of the newer agents also have less ability to cross the blood-brain barrier (as a result of reduced lipophilicity); this may reduce the incidence of confusion, which is a potential side effect of many anticholinergics, especially in the elderly population.[24]

Patients receiving anticholinergic drugs for treatment of their urinary symptoms must be carefully monitored for incomplete emptying, retention, and overflow incontinence. It is important to realize that the clinical presentation of overflow incontinence is very similar to that of "urge" incontinence, that is, frequency, urgency, small voided volumes, and leakage on the way to the bathroom; therefore, it is necessary to question the patient regarding feelings of incomplete emptying, to palpate the bladder, and to perform a postvoid residual check when there is any question regarding incomplete emptying. In some situations, patients with overflow incontinence have had their anticholinergic dose inappropriately increased in an effort to control their increasing urgency, frequency, and incontinence, when in fact they needed a reduction in dose or complete elimination of the drug. (When evaluating the patient's drug profile for evidence of anticholinergic agents, the clinician must remember that many over-the-counter medications, such as cold preparations, contain anticholinergics that may precipitate or contribute to retention.)

Imipramine is another drug that is sometimes prescribed for patients who suffer from OAB and urge UI as well as stress UI. Although it is classified as a tricyclic antidepressant, imipramine also has systemic anticholinergic effects, a strong direct inhibitory effect on the detrusor muscle,[25] and alpha-adrenergic effects at the level of the bladder neck and urethra. The anticholinergic and direct inhibitory effects reduce detrusor irritability, whereas the adrenergic effects increase urethral and bladder neck resistance; thus, this drug is beneficial for both OAB and stress UI. The recommended dose of imipramine for management of incontinence is 10 to 25 mg; much higher doses (75 mg or more) are required for the treatment of depression. Therefore, patients who are receiving imipramine for depression need to be carefully monitored for retention and overflow incontinence.

A final factor to consider when medications are being evaluated is the potential for synergistic effects if a patient is taking more than one medication with a potentially adverse effect on continence. For example, a hypertensive patient who is taking an alpha-adrenergic antagonist (which relaxes the bladder neck) or an ACE inhibitor (which may cause a chronic cough) alone may not experience incontinence; however, if the same patient is prescribed *both* of these medications, the combination may "tip the scales" and produce stress incontinence. This synergistic effect tends to hold true for any combination of potentially adverse substances, such as an evening cocktail and a nighttime dose of imipramine.

Psychological Factors. Behavioral factors can be among the most difficult to assess for their effect on continence. Psychological causes of incontinence have not been well studied for any age group,[1] and depression resulting from major surgery or the diagnosis of a serious illness can have a major influence on behavior, as can sleep deprivation during prolonged hospitalization. This depression may alter the patient's level of interest in self-care and in maintenance of continence. However, the patient dealing with depression may also be taking medications with potentially adverse effects on continence or may be dealing with reduced mobility or other medical problems affecting continence; thus, it is frequently hard to accurately measure the influence of psychological factors as a single entity. Depression is a major psychological disease that can tip the delicate balance of continence and can also negatively affect the management of UI,[26] and an association between depression and loss of bladder control has been reported by Steer and Lee.[27] Often health care providers and the patient's family fail to recognize depression, especially among the elderly; thus, it is imperative to screen actively for depression and to treat those who are depressed. For example, an elderly woman who lives alone and has a poor social support system may be at higher risk for depression and UI. Fortunately, pharmacologic treatment of depression has been found to be effective in the elderly population, with relapse rates of less than 80% for 6 to 18 months following treatment.[8]

Excess Urine Production. Conditions associated with production of large volumes of urine may produce transient incontinence if the patient is not able to reach the bathroom quickly enough to prevent leakage. The most common of these polyuria-producing conditions are as follows:

- uncontrolled diabetes mellitus with associated hyperglycemia and glycosuria, resulting in osmotic diuresis and rapid detrusor distension
- diabetes insipidus, which occurs as a result of dysfunction involving the posterior pituitary or hypothalamus and results in inability to concentrate urine (because of inadequate production of antidiuretic hormone)
- drug toxicity, such as lithium intoxication

- nephrogenic disorders resulting in excess urine production
- excessive water or fluid intake (a common finding in women following weight-reduction diets)
- diuretic therapy

In addition, congestive heart failure may produce nocturia, because the fluid built up in the lower extremities (especially the feet and ankles) is reabsorbed into the circulatory system when the patient is in the supine position and is then filtered and excreted by the kidneys once the patient assumes a recumbent position for sleep. In managing patients with excess urine production, the emphasis is on control or correction of the underlying disorder; this corrects the polyuria that is causing the incontinence. For the patient receiving diuretic therapy, simple modifications in the dosing schedule or provision of toileting aids such as bedside commodes may eliminate the problem with urinary leakage. Avoidance of excess fluid intake (more than 30 mL/kg weight) may be all that is needed for individuals who are consuming large amounts of fluid, and limiting fluid intake after the evening meal may help to reduce episodes of nocturia. Interestingly, a complex but common cause of nocturia is related to obstructive sleep apnea. In this condition, the diaphragm contracts against a closed upper airway, which increases intrathoracic pressures. This pressure produces a right atrial stretch and thereby stimulates the release of atrial natriuretic peptide (ANP), which causes vasodilation and sodium and water excretion (natriuresis). ANP also inhibits vasopressin (antidiuretic hormone) and the renin-angiotensin-aldosterone complex, which further contributes to increased urine production and possibly urinary leakage.[28]

Restricted Mobility. Many patients experience transient incontinence or temporary worsening of urinary leakage as a result of mobility restrictions or loss of manual dexterity, which compromises their ability to respond promptly to the urge to void. Altered mobility is a common causative or contributing factor to incontinence among individuals who are hospitalized for acute illness, injury, or major surgery, and for older individuals in long-term care facilities; mobility issues may also contribute to urinary leakage among community-dwelling elders.

Conditions that typically produce urgency but not incontinence, such as bladder infections, may produce incontinence in the patient who is unable to get to the toilet quickly or is unable to remove outer and inner garments in a timely manner. Simple interventions may facilitate continence in mobility-impaired individuals, such as bedside commodes or urinals, toileting schedules, and clothing that is easy to remove. Interventions to reduce functional incontinence are discussed further in Chapter 6.

Stool Impaction and Constipation. Bowel dysfunction is a common contributing factor to bladder dysfunction and UI, and fecal impaction is implicated as a causative factor for UI in up to 10% of elderly patients seen in acute-care settings or referred to incontinence clinics.[29] The hard mass of stool exerts pressure through the soft tissue of the perineum, which creates an outflow obstruction at the bladder neck[30]; this obstruction of flow may contribute to retention and overflow incontinence. A large fecal bolus in the rectum may also cause increased bladder contractility and "urge" pattern incontinence.

In reviewing the history of a patient with UI, it is common to find an association between the onset of problems with constipation and the onset or worsening of urinary leakage. Factors that commonly contribute to constipation include inadequate fluid intake and a large number of prescribed daily medications. The problem of inadequate fluid intake is further compounded by the tendency of many individuals with UI to restrict their fluid intake in an effort to prevent or reduce the leakage; this may cause worsening of the constipation in addition to increased bladder irritability and urinary leakage.

In addition to encouraging fluid intake (as discussed previously), the clinician needs to help the patient establish a daily regimen that promotes regular bowel elimination. Key components include adequate fiber intake and prompt response to the urge to defecate.[31] A recipe commonly used by continence nurses to provide fiber is a mixture of unprocessed bran or crushed bran flakes, prune juice, and applesauce, with the daily dose titrated to produce soft, formed stool. Gradual institution of fiber in the diet is mandatory to enhance compliance; otherwise, individuals may experience excessive gas and bloating, which typically result in discontinuation of the fiber regimen. Increasing fiber intake may take some creativity on the part of the patient and continence nurse. The goal is to establish an individualized plan that either provides sufficient fiber while addressing food/fluid preferences or provides fiber supplements in a form acceptable to the patient. Today, there are a wide variety of supplements in multiple forms, which tremendously facilitates the establishment of a "patient-friendly" fiber regimen. For most patients, laxatives other than bulking agents should be avoided. However, the use of bran mixtures or bulking agents alone may be inadequate to maintain regular bowel elimination in patients who have used laxatives or enemas regularly for many years; these patients may require the additional use of stool softeners, osmotic laxatives, stimulants such as Senokot, or enemas, although at a significantly reduced frequency. Bowel management is discussed in greater detail in Chapters 14 and 15.

Some patients with complaints of urinary leakage may find their urinary problems completely or significantly relieved simply by restoration of normal bowel function.

Factors Within the Urinary Tract

Pathologic conditions within the urinary tract itself may also cause acute incontinence; age-related changes in the urinary tract may predispose the elderly person to incontinence, and urinary tract infections (UTIs) and urogenital atrophy are additional factors that commonly cause or contribute to UI, especially in the elderly. Other "urinary tract" causes of acute UI include bladder outlet obstruction, conditions altering the position or innervation of the bladder and sphincter, and inflammatory conditions resulting in reduced compliance of the bladder wall.

Age-Related Changes in the Urinary Tract.
As noted earlier in this chapter, elderly persons are particularly prone to transient incontinence; this correlation is partially explained by the changes that normally occur within the urinary tract as a result of aging. The typical and "expected" changes include a reduced ability to delay urination, an increased frequency of involuntary detrusor contractions, decreased strength of detrusor contractions,

increased volume of postvoid residual urine, and an increase in the volume of urine produced at night.[32] There are also gender-related changes that affect continence in the elderly. In men, prostatic enlargement may produce progressive obstruction to urinary elimination, which is typically evidenced by a gradual worsening of symptoms such as frequency, urgency, and feelings of incomplete emptying; a few men with significant prostatic hypertrophy report no symptoms until they present clinically in acute urinary retention with overflow incontinence. In women, urogenital atrophy may cause urinary frequency, urgency, and dysuria, and it may also contribute to significant sphincter impairment; these women may have urge pattern incontinence, stress pattern incontinence, or mixed stress-urge incontinence.

Resnick and Yalla described several changes in bladder function affecting the elderly.[1] Detrusor overactivity is the most common and occurs in both men and women; this condition is characterized by increased spontaneous or involuntary contractions of the detrusor muscle. When detrusor overactivity occurs secondary to a neurologic disease or disorder, it is sometimes called "detrusor hyperreflexia"; common neurologic causes of detrusor overactivity in the elderly are cervical disk disease or spondylosis, Parkinson's disease, and stroke. When there is no neurologic cause for the detrusor overactivity, the condition is usually referred to as "detrusor instability" or "bladder overactivity"; the involuntary contractions produced by detrusor overactivity are frequently weak, and the patient may or may not be able to inhibit them. The patient with detrusor instability (overactive bladder) typically retains the ability to contract the detrusor voluntarily to urinate. A common form of bladder overactivity among the elderly population is the condition known as DHIC. In this condition, the detrusor muscle contracts spontaneously (involuntarily), but the contraction is too weak to effectively empty the bladder. The symptoms are similar to those produced by many dysfunctional conditions of the lower urinary tract; the patient perceives the involuntary contractions as the urge to void and complains of urgency and urge incontinence. In some patients, the involuntary contractions are triggered by increased abdominal pressure or even by changes in position; in these patients, the pattern of leakage may mimic stress incontinence. The clinician must be alert to the potential for DHIC among the elderly, because symptoms of urgency and urge incontinence are commonly treated with anticholinergic medications, and these medications can induce urinary retention in the patient with DHIC.[1]

In considering age-related factors that may contribute to transient or acute-onset UI, it is important to remember that in many situations there is not one single causative factor for the incontinence; rather, multiple contributing factors jointly produce the leakage. A thorough assessment of all possible reversible factors is therefore essential to the effective resolution of acute incontinence. It is very common to find multiple "reversible" causes in the elderly population; the initial treatment focus is then on correction of as many of these factors as possible. Correction of all reversible factors may totally eliminate the incontinence; failing resolution of the problem, most patients report tremendous improvement in the frequency and severity of leakage. At that point, a repeat evaluation can be done to determine the underlying pattern of incontinence and to intervene appropriately.

Urinary Tract Infection. UTI is a common and reversible cause of incontinence, and all patients reporting sudden onset or worsening of urinary leakage should undergo screening urinalysis (and urine culture when indicated). In older patients, symptomatic bladder infections may cause acute incontinence when the associated urgency and dysuria overcome the patient's ability to reach the toilet in time to prevent leakage.[20] Many older patients are found to have "asymptomatic urinary tract infection," that is, bacteriuria in the absence of reported dysuria. The continence nurse should remember that urinary leakage may be indicative of UTI in these patients even if no dysuria is reported, and treatment is usually indicated to rule out infection as a cause of the leakage. In some cases, treatment of the UTI with an appropriate antibiotic effectively resolves the incontinence.

A less common cause of UTI that should be considered in selected cases is candiduria, or fungal infection of the bladder. Candidal UTIs can cause a variety of symptoms, some of which are similar to bacterial bladder infections. The combination of recent hospitalization with indwelling catheterization and systemic antibiotic therapy represents a "high-risk" situation for fungal infections. Other risk factors include diabetes mellitus and steroid therapy.[33] In women, concurrent presentation of vulvovaginitis and signs and symptoms of a bladder infection should increase the clinician's index of suspicion that the infection may be fungal rather than bacterial. The diagnosis of candiduria is confirmed when a sterile urine specimen is obtained and is submitted for fungal culture. Oral therapy with fluconazole or ketoconazole will resolve most candidal UTIs; however, the patient must be monitored for response to therapy, and coexisting vulvovaginal infections may require topical treatment for symptomatic relief.

Atrophic Urethritis or Vaginitis. A common contributing factor to UI in the postmenopausal woman is atrophy of the urogenital tissues caused by the loss of estrogen. The urethra, trigone of the bladder, and vagina are rich in estrogen receptors, and these receptors are also found in the pelvic ligaments.[34] The development of urogenital atrophy affecting the lower urinary tract is described by some experts as an "intermediate" consequence of menopause, meaning that it occurs months to years after menopause.[32] Within the urinary tract, this atrophy results in thinning of the urethral epithelium, sclerosis of the periurethral tissues, and persistent or recurrent subjective complaints of urinary frequency, urgency, and dysuria. The vaginal pH increases, which increases the risk for recurrent vaginal infections; UTIs are more prevalent as well.[35,36]

Continence is often affected by urogenital atrophy. The thinning of the urethral epithelium results in a loss of urethral mucosal coaptation; this may cause reduced urethral resistance and urinary leakage when the bladder contains urine and the patient is upright and active. The risk for leakage is particularly significant when the individual suffers from weak pelvic floor and sphincter muscles in addition to the loss of mucosal coaptation. Estrogen deficiency may also increase bladder irritability and sensory urgency, and it may adversely affect the woman's ability to inhibit bladder contractions until she has reached the toilet; this may result in "urge" pattern incontinence. Thus, urogenital atrophy may play a contributing role in either stress incontinence or urge incontinence in the postmenopausal woman; however, urogenital atrophy develops slowly and does not, in and of itself, cause acute-onset UI.

It has been postulated that estrogen therapy may be useful in the prevention and management of incontinence in postmenopausal women. Treatment of atrophic vaginitis and urethritis has recently received increased attention because of the Women's Health Initiative study,[37] in which combination oral hormone therapy (HT) with conjugated equine estrogen and synthetic progestin (medroxyprogesterone acetate, or Prempro) was found to slightly increase the risk of heart disease, stroke, and blood clots.[37,38] The results of this study produced somewhat of a "hormone scare," and many women discontinued their HT as a result.[37] Likewise, the Heart and Estrogen/Progestin Replacement Study (HERS), a 4-year randomized, double-blinded, placebo-controlled trial, evaluated the effect of daily oral HT (Prempro) in subjects more than 80 years of age with a positive history of coronary artery disease and an intact uterus.[39] This study also addressed the ability of HT to reduce the severity of UI in subjects who reported UI at least weekly. Interestingly, in this study, oral combination HT *increased* the risk of urge and stress incontinence significantly in comparison with the placebo group.[39] It is not understood why treatment with oral combination HT seems to have a negative effect on continence because estrogen has been shown to improve the health of urogenital tissue.[40,41] It is possible that the progestin component or the specific type of estrogen used in the treatment regimen may cause this effect. In the light of these studies, oral combination HT is not recommended for the prevention or treatment of UI in older menopausal women.[39,42] Unfortunately, there have not been any randomized controlled trials to determine whether unopposed estrogen or vaginal estrogen may be of benefit in the prevention or treatment of UI. However, another type of medication *has* shown some initial promise for stress UI. Selective estrogen receptor modulators (SERMs) may have a protective effect on the pelvic floor as evidenced by data from three randomized controlled trials, which showed that raloxifene (a selective estrogen receptor modulator) significantly reduced the need for pelvic floor repair.[39] At this time, most clinical experts believe that application of local (topical) estrogen to atrophic urogenital tissues may help reduce vaginal dryness, improve vascularity, reverse atrophic changes, and reduce urge symptoms; topical agents are thought to carry minimal risk for adverse effects because systemic absorption is minimal as compared with oral HT.[40-44]

Bladder Outlet Obstruction. The most common cause of bladder outlet obstruction in men is benign prostatic hyperplasia (BPH). BPH begins to develop after 40 years of age and can result in significant obstructive symptoms even for men in their fifties. Less common causes of bladder outlet obstruction in men include prostate cancer, urethral strictures, and bladder neck contractures after prostatic surgery. Bladder outlet obstruction in women is usually caused by one of two conditions: (1) a surgical procedure that specifically compresses or tightens the bladder neck and urethra, such as an antiincontinence procedure, or (2) certain types of pelvic organ prolapse that alter the position of the bladder outlet.

Bladder outlet obstruction may produce two types of voiding symptoms: obstructive and irritative. Obstructive symptoms result from the mechanical obstruction of the urethra and include reduced force of the urinary stream, intermittent or interrupted urinary flow patterns, hesitancy, postvoid dribbling, and feelings of incomplete bladder emptying. The development of irritative symptoms is related to the changes that occur within the bladder as a result of prolonged obstruction. If the obstruction persists over time, the detrusor muscle gradually hypertrophies in response to the increased contractile force required to propel urine past the obstructed urethra.[45] Eventually, the hypertrophied detrusor muscle decompensates, resulting in involuntary bladder contractions (detrusor instability); bladder outlet obstruction secondary to BPH is believed to be the most common obstructive cause of detrusor instability.[46] When the hypertrophied detrusor becomes unstable (overactive), the patient may develop irritative symptoms such as frequency, urgency, and nocturia.[47]

This review of the normal progression of urethral obstructive disease helps to explain the various patterns of UI associated with BPH. A common presenting pattern in these patients is that of overflow incontinence, which usually follows an episode of acute urinary retention; however, the patient may also experience an "urge" pattern incontinence caused by detrusor instability or leakage caused by postvoid dribbling. It is significant that involuntary detrusor contractions in the patient with obstructive prostatic disease produce urinary leakage only if the contractions are strong enough to overcome the outlet obstruction; thus, some patients experience urgency and frequency but no leakage.

Management of the patient with UI secondary to BPH is not always a simple matter of removing excess prostatic tissue surgically; acute UI is a potential postoperative development for these patients. This can be explained by the fact that the bladder continues to function as it did before surgery, at least for a period of time; once the urethral obstruction is eliminated, continued detrusor instability results in urge pattern incontinence. This same sequence of events may occur in the patient with prostatic cancer producing bladder outlet obstruction; the bladder undergoes the same functional changes as have already been described in the discussion on BPH, and removal of the obstructing tissue then frequently results in transient acute incontinence.

Two other potential causes of bladder outlet obstruction in men deserve mention. Both are related to the growth of scar tissue within the urethra. Urethral strictures can result from transurethral surgery, long-term use of an indwelling catheter, traumatic urethral injuries, and some sexually transmitted diseases. Scar tissue can also develop at the bladder neck after radical prostatectomy for prostate cancer, a condition known as bladder neck contracture.[45] Progressive scarring at the bladder neck or within the urethra produces a steadily worsening outlet obstruction that may eventually result in urinary retention and in the development of a hypertrophic and overactive detrusor muscle.

When surgery is required to excise the scar tissue and relieve the obstruction, the patient may experience some degree of postoperative UI.

The effects of prolonged bladder outlet obstruction have been studied primarily in men; however, women can also develop urethral obstruction with similar sequelae. Urethral strictures are uncommon in women but can occur after childbirth, pelvic trauma, or vaginal surgery. Women undergoing surgery for the correction of stress incontinence may also develop urethral obstruction; one type of repair associated with occasional development of urethral obstruction is the pubovaginal sling, a procedure in which a strip of muscle or fascia is used to provide urethral compression and support. (Newer techniques utilize biocompatible materials for creation of the urethral sling.) If the sling creates excessive urethral compression, obstruction can occur, producing signs and symptoms of incomplete bladder emptying and obstructed voiding.

Another cause of bladder outlet obstruction following antiincontinence procedures is inappropriate placement or excessive tension on periurethral sutures.[48] Over time, the obstructed bladder decompensates in the same manner as has been previously described, resulting in detrusor overactivity, irritative voiding symptoms, and possibly urge incontinence. Women may also experience bladder outlet obstruction as a result of pelvic organ prolapse. Uterine prolapse can be quite obstructive to the bladder and urethra because a significant uterine descensus displaces the bladder and urethra anteriorly. Difficult urination is a symptom reported by many women who have both uterine prolapse and cystocele; it can also occur in women who have prolapse of either the bladder or the uterus. The position of the prolapsing organ in a prolapse extending past the introitus easily explains the bladder outlet obstruction; however, lesser-grade prolapses may also produce noticeable difficulty with voiding. For example, women with a cystocele extending to the introitus, either at rest or with straining, may report the need to "double void"; patients state that the urge to urinate returns when they stand after voiding. Usually, these women find that they can sit back down and again void; this need to double void presents the potential for incontinence if the individual is rushed and does not take time to void the second time. Patients with significant voiding dysfunction caused by pelvic organ prolapse may benefit from manual reduction of the prolapse and/or use of a correctly fitted pessary. (A pessary is a silcone device that is placed within the vaginal vault to correct pelvic prolapse and treat stress UI.) Many women can safely and effectively manage the pessary independently; alternatively, the pessary may be removed, cleaned, and replaced at regular intervals by a qualified clinician such as a continence nurse. Patients with pessaries should be monitored for complications such as vaginal erosion, infection, or poor fit and suboptimal outcomes. Some studies suggest that continued use of a pessary may reduce the severity of the prolapse over time, and pessaries can be used safely for long-term prolapse management.[49,50] Surgical correction of the prolapse is, of course, the definitive treatment for patients who are surgical candidates; however, recurrence is not uncommon.[51]

Conditions Altering the Position or Innervation of the Bladder and Sphincter. Voiding dysfunction and UI are potential complications after some surgical procedures involving the pelvic organs (the colon, rectum, prostate, or female reproductive organs). Actually, incontinence is not uncommon after gynecologic procedures such as radical hysterectomy, benign hysterectomy, antiincontinence procedures, and procedures to correct pelvic organ prolapse.[52] The effect of these procedures on continence may be explained partly by alterations in the position of the bladder but primarily by some degree of disruption in the nerve supply to the bladder or urethral sphincter (or both). For example, the voiding dysfunction that is sometimes seen after abdominoperineal resection for colorectal cancer is a result of damage to the nerve pathways that control bladder function.

The innervation of the urinary bladder and pelvic organs is complex and is described in detail in Chapter 2. A brief review is provided here to clarify the mechanisms by which pelvic surgery can produce bladder denervation and voiding dysfunction. Aronson and Sant described the nerve pathways succinctly: "The parasympathetic pelvic nerves arise from sacral segments S2-S4 and join branches

of the hypogastric nerve (sympathetic innervation) in the presacral area to form the inferior hypogastric plexus (mixture of sympathetic and parasympathetic fibers). This plexus is then oriented parasagittally on either side of the rectum, uterine cervix, vaginal fornix, and posterior aspect of the bladder, and extends into the base of the broad ligament of the uterus."[52] Any injury to the inferior hypogastric plexus (by surgery, tumor infiltration, infection, or inflammation) may produce varying degrees of denervation and voiding dysfunction.[53]

Voiding dysfunction secondary to nerve damage during pelvic surgery can result in several clinical "patterns," depending on the specific pathways damaged. Zimmern divided the clinical presentations into early, late, or delayed changes.[54] Early changes become evident within 1 week to 6 months postoperatively and are characterized either by urinary retention and overflow incontinence (when the nerve damage affects the parasympathetics supplying the bladder), or by stress incontinence (when the nerve damage affects the sympathetics supplying the bladder neck and urethra).

Late changes are manifest within 6 to 12 months postoperatively and are characterized either by urinary retention and overflow incontinence or by detrusor overactivity and urge incontinence. UI that occurs within the "late" period may be caused by disease recurrence, such as recurrence of malignancy, or by factors unrelated to the surgery. However, "late" changes are not usually caused by the surgical procedure itself.

One challenge in clinical practice is the development of acute incontinence in the patient who has undergone hysterectomy for benign disease or a procedure designed to correct stress incontinence. There is a growing body of evidence that hysterectomy is a risk factor for UI; recent studies have shown a twofold increase in risk for developing UI[55,56] and a 2.5-fold increase in risk for "bothersome urge" symptoms among women who have had a hysterectomy.[57] Although abdominal and vaginal approaches to these procedures specifically avoid the pelvic plexus, there is still the potential for denervation of the pelvic floor musculature, and this nerve damage may contribute to the development of acute incontinence following these procedures.[58]

Fortunately, these patients usually experience steady improvement as the nerve pathways repair themselves; however, behavioral management techniques and absorbent products may be required on a short-term basis.

Another challenge in clinical practice is management of the transient urinary retention that occurs in up to 41% of patients after bladder neck suspension procedures; these patients must either be taught intermittent catheterization or managed on a temporary basis with an indwelling urethral or suprapubic catheter. Fortunately, the problem usually resolves spontaneously as the nerve pathways recover normal function; approximately 95% of patients regain normal ability to void and to empty the bladder.[59] A more frustrating problem among patients undergoing antiincontinence procedures is the persistence of incontinence postoperatively.[52] For example, patients who have mixed stress and urge incontinence frequently report persistence of urge pattern incontinence following surgery, and a few patients with demonstrated genuine stress incontinence develop detrusor instability following surgery; these patients then require interventions to correct or manage the urge incontinence associated with detrusor instability.[60] (Strategies for management of urge incontinence are outlined in Chapter 5.) However, the most common reason for persistent incontinence following surgery is the failure to diagnose the type of incontinence accurately *before* surgery. Bladder neck suspension procedures do not correct or compensate for intrinsic sphincter deficiency, and procedures designed to correct stress incontinence will not eliminate detrusor overactivity. It is therefore essential to obtain a complete workup, including urodynamic studies, before planning any surgical intervention. Continence nurses have an opportunity to be patient advocates by presenting information to patients that is clear and accurate when surgical intervention is sought. Discussion of the absolute need for urodynamics to clearly define the etiology of the UI before surgical treatment may help to prevent inappropriate surgery and unrealistic expectations.

Another procedure associated with a high incidence of postoperative incontinence is radical prostatectomy,[61,62] which is caused by damage to the sphincters themselves or to the nerve pathways innervating the sphincters; postprostatectomy incontinence is one of the few types of acute incontinence for which there is a clear cause. Most patients and their families are poorly prepared for postoperative UI, partly because of limited preoperative discussion of postoperative complications, and partly because they are overwhelmed with the diagnosis of cancer and decisions regarding treatment options.[63] Most patients will regain bladder control; however, it may take several months to a year to acquire total continence.[64] Some of these patients respond well to pelvic muscle rehabilitation programs and to the beneficial influence of time on regeneration of damaged nerve fibers, whereas others require long-term use of absorptive or containment products or surgical intervention. The continence nurse has an opportunity to reduce anxiety dramatically and to improve the patient's quality of life by providing appropriate education and behavioral intervention both preoperatively and postoperatively.[62] Management of postprostatectomy incontinence is discussed further in Chapter 9.

Conditions Resulting in Reduced Compliance of the Bladder Wall. As explained in the discussion of normal bladder function in Chapter 2, intravesical pressure normally remains low through most of the "filling" phase of bladder function; it begins to rise as the bladder approaches capacity. This normal compliance, or "stretch," of the bladder wall prevents an early rise in bladder pressure with filling, and this "low pressure filling" is an important aspect in the preservation of renal function; it permits free flow of urine through the low-pressure ureteral system and into the bladder. Loss of normal bladder compliance places the individual at risk for upper tract damage. In addition, the elevated intravesical pressures in response to bladder filling produce voiding symptoms such as frequency, urgency, and urge incontinence.

Loss of compliance can be defined as loss of the bladder's normal ability to stretch with increasing volumes of urine and is evidenced urodynamically as a steady rise in intravesical pressure during bladder filling. Noncompliance may be caused by a structural alteration in the muscular or connective tissue elements of the bladder wall or by a functional change, such as an alteration in smooth muscle tone resulting from a neurologic lesion or process.[58,65] These changes in the bladder wall worsen over time, until the patient develops a "sudden" onset of UI. In most cases, it is clear that the acute onset of UI is actually caused by a worsening of preexisting alterations within the bladder wall, which results in a worsening of preexisting voiding symptoms.

The most common causes of noncompliance are inflammatory processes or fibrotic changes within the bladder wall; specific conditions include chemical cystitis, pelvic radiation therapy, and interstitial cystitis. Chemical cystitis may result from chemotherapeutic agents that are administered either intravenously or directly into the bladder (intravesically). Radiation damage to the bladder wall can occur after external or interstitial therapy for gynecologic, urologic, or colorectal malignancies. Interstitial cystitis is a poorly understood chronic inflammatory condition of the bladder that commonly produces loss of compliance.

The symptoms most commonly experienced by patients with reduced compliance of the bladder wall are excessive frequency, severe urgency (with or without urge UI), pain or burning on urination, and nocturia. These symptoms mimic those of UTI, but usually no bacterial infection is found; urinalysis and urine culture are typically negative. Urodynamic testing reveals a steady rise in intravesical pressure until leakage of urine occurs or the patient insists on voiding to relieve the pain; this picture is in sharp contrast to the sudden involuntary increase in intravesical pressure seen in patients with detrusor overactivity (detrusor instability). Urologic testing clearly demonstrates the diminished compliance; however, bladder distension can cause pain and bleeding in these patients. Therefore, this testing should be performed using anesthesia for patients whose symptoms include pain.

Management of the patient with altered bladder compliance is difficult. The initial goal is to correct the underlying condition causing reduced compliance. For example, patients with interstitial cystitis may benefit from a variety of therapies: bladder distension under anesthesia; intravesical instillation of agents such as dimethyl sulfoxide, heparin, lidocaine, bicarbonate, or hydrocortisone; oral medications such as sodium pentosan polysulfate (Elmiron), amitriptyline, and hydroxyzine; and dietary and fluid modifications, such as elimination of spicy foods and alcohol. These interventions provide variable levels of improvement in symptoms.[66]

Although the irritative symptoms associated with reduced bladder compliance are extremely distressing to the patient and may profoundly and adversely affect his or her quality of life, the most serious *organic* sequela of noncompliance is the potential for upper urinary tract dysfunction. The high pressures within the bladder eventually result in hydronephrosis and damage to the ureterovesical junction, which permits reflux; the final outcome is frequently renal insufficiency. Therefore, early intervention is indicated for any patient with evidence of reduced compliance; if the underlying condition cannot be corrected, the patient may require some form of urinary diversion to protect the upper tracts.

ASSESSMENT OF THE PATIENT WITH ACUTE-ONSET INCONTINENCE
Patient History

Assessment of the individual with new-onset or sudden worsening of incontinence begins with a careful history, during which the interviewer screens for recent changes or events that may be causing or contributing to the incontinence. It is helpful to remember the most common transient factors, as outlined in the mnemonic DIAPPERS, when the interview is being conducted. If the patient is unable to provide the history, the information should be obtained from a spouse or caregiver; if the patient is hospitalized, it may be helpful to review the chart and to discuss the patient's history and incontinence with the medical and nursing staffs. The history should include a thorough review of the patient's genitourinary, gastrointestinal, gynecologic, and past medical and surgical history as well as a complete review of all medications. A focused physical exam should then be performed, which should include a basic functional, abdominal, neurologic, gynecologic, and anorectal assessment.

It is beneficial to obtain a 3-day voiding diary to acquire precise data with regard to voiding habits, amounts of intake and output, types of fluids, and events associated with leakage. The continence nurse will find the "simple" voiding diary to be an invaluable tool in evaluating for common reversible factors; in addition, the diary provides "eye-opening" data for the patient on life style and toileting habits that may need to be altered. It is imperative to have the patient quantify the UI by recording frequency and volume of leakage and the type and quantity of absorptive products used to manage the leakage. The patient or caregiver should also be asked to record whether the pads are damp or saturated when changed and to note any activities that trigger the UI, such as coughing, laughing, or sneezing, or hurrying to the toilet because of an urgent need to void.

As has been discussed, recent changes in the patient's overall health status, medications, mental status, bowel function, or even daily routine may contribute to transient incontinence. Some recent events are obvious, such as urologic or gynecologic surgery or a neurologic injury or event; even a "mild" stroke or a slight worsening of Parkinson's disease may result in new-onset incontinence. For the hospitalized patient, the illness or injury that precipitated hospitalization may have altered the patient's normal function in a manner that compromises his or her continence status. For example, UI after orthopedic surgery may be related to restrictions in mobility. Similarly, patients who require short-term use of indwelling catheters after abdominal or thoracic surgery may develop bladder spasms or bacteriuria that triggers UI when the catheter is removed. Constipation and fecal impaction are common complications of many surgical procedures and are also common side effects of many commonly prescribed medications; therefore, the interviewer should always inquire about the patient's present and "usual" bowel function. The interviewer should also be alert to any evidence of compromised mental acuity. In elderly patients, a simple test of mental status or short-term memory may help to identify subtle degrees of confusion or delirium. The combination of altered mental status and age-related changes in the

urinary tract may be sufficient to trigger new onset of incontinence that will resolve if the changes in mental status can be reversed.

The interviewer should carefully explore recent changes in life style or medical treatment that may have precipitated the incontinence. If the changes are subtle and are not obviously related to urinary tract function, the patient or family may not identify them as potential causes of the incontinence. For example, changes in medications, the addition of new medications, or changes in the timing or dosage are common contributing factors to incontinence but are not typically recognized as part of the etiologic picture. In gathering data regarding medications, the interviewer should ask about over-the-counter medications and vitamin or nutritional supplements because many patients do not routinely include these when asked to list the medications they take. Dietary and fluid intake habits may also be contributory and should be addressed during the interview (or through a bladder diary that can quantify the problem and response to therapy with greater impartiality). The following examples illustrate the potential effect of medications, nutritional supplements, and fluids on continence:

- A 66-year-old woman begins an herbal diet plan for weight loss that requires high-volume fluid intake; shortly thereafter, she begins to experience frequency, nocturia, and episodes of urge incontinence.
- A 54-year-old woman begins taking high-dose calcium supplements and then begins to experience urgency, urge incontinence, and constipation.
- A 35-year old woman who drinks large volumes of soda is started on a diuretic for elevated blood pressure and is now experiencing increased urgency, frequency, and new onset of UI.
- A 75-year-old man begins using an over-the-counter nasal spray for seasonal allergies and suddenly finds himself unable to void in the middle of the night, although urine is dripping continually from his penis.

The patients in these examples may not recognize the negative effect of their "nonprescription" health care routines on their urinary tract and continence status.

Physical Examination

A focused physical examination is the next step in assessment of the individual with acute-onset UI. Abdominal inspection and palpation may reveal bladder distension, suprapubic tenderness, retained stool, or pelvic masses.[67] Rectal examination should be performed to determine anal sphincter tone, the presence or absence of the bulbocavernosus reflex and anal wink, the size and consistency of the prostate gland in men, and the presence or absence of fecal impaction. In women, at least a limited pelvic examination is indicated to assess pelvic muscle function and to identify any evidence of urogenital atrophy, pelvic floor prolapse, or urethral hypermobility (evidenced by leakage of urine in response to provocative maneuvers such as forceful cough). If there is vaginal discharge, the patient should be further examined for evidence of vaginitis or vulvitis. All patients should be assessed for any evidence of skin irritation or candidal rash, which must be addressed in the treatment plan.

Determination of postvoid residual volume should be included in the initial assessment of any patient with evidence of incomplete emptying and any patient "at risk" for retention, such as the man with BPH or the woman with a cystocele. Postvoid residual testing can be accomplished by ultrasonography (bladder scan) if this equipment is available and catheterization is not otherwise indicated. Although elevated postvoid residual does not typically cause incontinence, it is often a contributing factor; incomplete bladder emptying can exacerbate preexisting stress or urge incontinence, leading to increased frequency or volume of urinary leakage, and urinary retention may precipitate overflow incontinence.

Urinalysis. The initial evaluation of a patient with new-onset incontinence must include at least a urinalysis to rule out infection as a causative or contributing factor and to screen for hematuria, glucosuria, and proteinuria. This specimen can usually be obtained by the clean-catch midstream technique; however, catheterization should be considered when contamination of the clean-catch specimen is suspected (or confirmed by a previous urine culture) or when the presence of skin irritation or vaginal discharge is suggestive of fungal or bacterial infection. Urine culture and sensitivity testing need to be performed if the urinalysis indicates possible infection. See Chapter 12, Table 12-8.

TREATMENT OF THE PATIENT WITH ACUTE-ONSET INCONTINENCE

The initial goals in management of any patient with incontinence are identification and correction of reversible factors; specific interventions depend on the specific etiologic factors as discussed earlier in this chapter. A considerable amount of time may be needed to educate the patient regarding factors contributing to the problem and developing creative and flexible solutions that are acceptable to the patient. For example, the patient must understand how his or her six cups of coffee contribute to their bladder symptoms and must be assisted in developing a plan for gradually reducing caffeine intake. When all reversible factors have been corrected, the patient is reassessed; the pattern and cause of any residual incontinence can then be identified, and appropriate intervention based on the specific type and cause of the incontinence (that is, stress, urge, reflex, functional, overflow) can be initiated.

SUMMARY

Acute-onset incontinence and transient incontinence are not synonymous terms; acute-onset incontinence refers to sudden onset or worsening of urinary leakage, and it may be transient or persistent. Transient incontinence by definition is caused by reversible factors and resolves either spontaneously or with appropriate attention to the causative factors. Acute *or* transient incontinence can be caused by factors within the urinary tract or by factors outside the urinary tract. Factors outside the urinary tract commonly contribute to loss of continence in the elderly and include alterations in the cognitive and physical functions needed to maintain continence. Factors within the urinary tract are more commonly involved in acute-onset incontinence in younger individuals and postoperative patients.

Assessment of any individual with incontinence must include screening for reversible factors via a thorough history, focused physical examination, review of prescription and over the counter medications, and selected laboratory tests. Any reversible factors must then be addressed; correction of reversible factors actually eliminates the incontinence in many individuals and provides substantial improvement for many others. The individual whose incontinence persists following correction of reversible factors should be reassessed to identify the etiologic factors for the persistent incontinence; once reversible factors have been eliminated and the type of residual incontinence has been identified, an appropriately targeted treatment plan can be initiated to restore or maximize continence. Patient education is a key element of effective care for any individual with incontinence, and it is a primary intervention for the continence nurse.

SELF-ASSESSMENT EXERCISE

1. Differentiate between acute and transient incontinence in terms of onset, reversibility, and implications for management.

2. Explain why the assessment of a patient with chronic UI must include screening for reversible (transient) factors.

3. Identify the eight reversible factors reflected by the mnemonic DIAPPERS and explain the mechanism by which each contributes to incontinence.

4. Explain why a reversible factor (such as UTI) is more likely to cause incontinence in an older person than in a younger person.

5. Rate each of the following statements as true or false and explain your answers:

   _ Alpha-adrenergic agonists increase the risk for stress incontinence.

   _ ACE inhibitors may worsen stress incontinence because of the dry cough that is a common side effect.

   _ Calcium-channel blockers rarely affect bladder function or continence.

   _ Urinary retention is a potential side effect of medications with anticholinergic properties or components.

   _ When you are assessing the patient with acute-onset UI, urinalysis and culture should be done only if the patient has signs and symptoms of a UTI.

6. Explain the following statement: "The patient with BPH commonly has an 'overflow' pattern of incontinence; however, the patient may also have 'urge' pattern incontinence or urgency and frequency but no leakage."

7. Explain why the patient who undergoes TURP (transurethral resection of the prostate) for BPH may develop acute UI in the postoperative period.

8. Describe the mechanisms by which pelvic, colorectal, and gynecologic surgery may affect continence.

9. Explain why the patient with reduced bladder compliance is at risk for renal insufficiency.

10. Discuss briefly the guidelines for assessment and management of a patient with acute UI.

REFERENCES

1. Resnick NM, Yalla SV: Geriatric incontinence and voiding dysfunction. In Walsh PC, Retik AB, Vaughan ED, Wein AJ, editors: *Campbell's urology,* ed 7, Philadelphia, 1998, WB Saunders.
2. Kinchen K, Burgio K, Diokno A, et al: Factors associated with women's decisions to seek treatment for urinary incontinence, *J Womens Health* 12(7):687-698, 2003.
3. Diokno AC: Stress urinary incontinence: expanding the treatment options. Symposium held in Chicago, April 25, 2003; www.medscape.com/viewprogram/2484.
4. Serel S: The wet patient: understanding patients with overactive bladder and incontinence, *Curr Med Res Opin* 20(6):791-801, 2004; www.medscape.com/ viewarticle/ 481666.
5. Stewart WF, Van Rooyen JB, Cundiff GW, et al: Prevalence and burden of overactive bladder in the United States, *World J Urol* 20:327-336, 2003.
6. Fiers S, Thayer D: Management of intractable incontinence. In Doughty DB, editor: *Urinary and fecal incontinence: nursing management,* ed 2, St. Louis, 2000, Mosby.
7. Hunter K, Moore K: Diabetes-associated bladder dysfunction in the older adult, *Geriatr Nurs* 24(3): 138-147, 2003.
8. Kurlowicz L: Delirium and depression. In Cotter V, Stumpf N, editors: *Advanced practice nursing with older adults: clinical guidelines,* New York, 2002, McGraw-Hill.
9. Thom DH, Haan MN, van Den Eeden SK: Medically recognized urinary incontinence and risks of hospitalization, nursing home admission and mortality, *Age Ageing* 26:367, 1997.
10. Fantl JA, Newman DK, Colling J, et al: *Urinary incontinence in adults: acute and chronic management.* Clinical practice guideline no. 2, 1996 update, Rockville, Md, 1996, US Department of Health and Human Services,

Public health Service, Agency for Health Care Policy and Research, AHCPR Publication No. 96-0682.

11. Miller M: Nocturnal polyuria in older people, *J Am Geriatric Soc* 48:1321-1329, 2000.

12. Tan TL: Urinary incontinence in older persons: a simple approach to a complex problem, *Ann Acad Med Singapore* 32(6):731-739, 2003.

13. Hogan D: Revisiting the O complex: urinary incontinence, delirium and polypharmacy in elderly patients, *Can Med Assoc J* 157(8):1071-1077, 1997.

14. Lisi D: Definition of drug-induced cognitive impairment in the elderly, *Medscape Pharmacother* 2(1):2000; www.medscape.com/viewarticle/408593.

15. Flaherty JH: Commonly prescribed and over-the counter medications: causes of confusion, *Clin Geriatr Med* 14:101-127, 1998.

16. Dallosso HM, McGrother CW, Matthew RJ, et al: The association of diet and other lifestyle factors with overactive bladder and stress incontinence: a longitudinal study in women, *BJU Int* 92(1):69, 2002.

17. Newman DK: Urinary incontinence and overactive bladder: a focus on behavioral interventions, *Top Adv Pract Nurs eJ* 2001; www.medscape.com/viewarticle/408405.

18. Thorp JM Jr, Norton PA, Wall LL, et al: Urinary incontinence in pregnancy and the puerperium: a prospective study, *Am J Obstet Gynecol* 181:266-273, 1999.

19. Arya LA, Myers DL, Jacjson ND: Dietary caffeine intake and the risk for detrusor instability: a case-control study, *Obstet Gynecol* 96(1):85-89, 2000.

20. Resnick NM: Geriatric incontinence, *Urol Clin North Am* 23:55-74, 1996.

21. Bump R, McClish D: Cigarette smoking and pure genuine stress incontinence of urine: a comparison of risk factors and determinants between smokers and nonsmokers, *Am J Obstet Gynecol* 170:579-582, 1994.

22. Fleshner N, Garland J, Moadel A, et al: Smoking after bladder cancer: never too late to quit, *Cancer* 86(11): 2337-2345, 1999.

23. Donna M: Definition of drug-induced cognitive impairment in the elderly, *Medscape Pharmacother* 2(1):2000; www.medscape.com/viewarticle/408593

24. Staskin DR, Sand PK: Structural and functional differences in anticholinergics. Presented in: Quaternary and tertiary amines: is there a difference in drug options for the treatment of OAB? The SUNA Annual Symposium on Disorders of the Bladder, Bowel and Pelvic Floor, Chicago, March 2004.

25. Wein AJ, Barrett DM: *Voiding function and dysfunction: a logical and practical approach,* St. Louis, 1988, Mosby.

26. Koenig H, Blazer D: Depression, anxiety, and other mood disorders. In Cassel C, Leipzig R, Cohen H, et al, editors: *Geriatric medicine: an evidence-based approach,* ed 4, New York, 2003, Springer-Verlag.

27. Steers W, Lee K: Depression and incontinence, *World J Urol* 19:351-357, 2001.

28. Umlauf MG, Chasens ER: Sleep disordered breathing and nocturnal polyuria: nocturia and enuresis, *Sleep Med Rev* 7(5):403-411, 2003.

29. Resnick NM: Voiding dysfunction in the elderly: In Yalla SV, McGuire EJ, Elbadawi A, Blaivas JG, editors: *Neurourology and urodynamics: principles and practice,* New York, 1988, Macmillan.

30. Wells TJ: Nursing management. In O'Donnell PD, editor: *Urinary incontinence,* St. Louis, 1977, Mosby.

31. Newman DK: *The urinary incontinence sourcebook,* Los Angeles, 1997, Lowell House.

32. Belchetz PE: Hormonal treatment of postmenopausal women, *N Engl J Med* 330:1062-1071, 1994.

33. Wise GJ: Fungal infections of the urinary tract. In Walsh PC, Retik AB, Vaughan ED, Wein AJ, editors: *Campbell's urology,* ed 7, Philadelphia, 1998, WB Saunders.

34. Griebling TL, Nygaard IE: The role of estrogen replacement therapy in the management of urinary incontinence and urinary tract infection in postmenopausal women, *Endocrinol Metab Clin North Am* 26:347-360, 1997.

35. Josif CS, Bekassy Z: Prevalence of genitourinary symptoms in the late menopause, *Acta Obstet Gynecol Scand* 63:257-260, 1984.

36. Smith KPB: Estrogens and the urogenital tract: studies on steroid hormonal receptors and a clinical study on a new estradiol releasing vaginal ring, *Acta Obstet Gynecol Scand Suppl* 72:1-26, 1993.

37. Writing Group for the Women's Health Initiative Investigators: Risks and benefits of estrogen plus progestin in postmenopausal women: principal results from the Women's Health Initiative randomized controlled trial, *JAMA* 288:321-333, 2002.

38. Goldman JA: The women's health initiative 2004: review and critique, *Medscape Gen Med* 6(3): 2004; www.medscape.com/viewarticle/483902.

39. Willhite L, O'Connell MB: Urogenital atrophy: prevention and treatment, *Medscape Pharmacother* 21(4): 464-480, 2001; www.medscape.com/viewarticle/409697.

40. Hendrix S, McNeeley G: Urinary incontinence and menopause: update on evidence-based treatment, *Clin Update* Oct 28, 2002; www.medscape.com/viewprogram/2052.

41. Robinson D, Cardozo L: The role of estrogens in female lower urinary tract dysfunction, *Urology* 62(suppl 4A), 45-51, 2003.

42. Grady D, Brown JS, Vittinghof E, et al: Postmenopausal hormones and incontinence, *Obstet Gynecol* 185; 116-120, 2001.

43. Messenger-Rapport BJ, Thacker H: Prevention for the older woman: a practical guide to hormone replacement therapy and urogynecologic health, *Geriatrics* 56:32-34, 37-38, 40-42, 2001.

44. Hunskaar S, Arnold EP, Burgio K, et al: Epidemiology and natural history of urinary incontinence, *Int Urogynecol J Pelvic Floor Dysfunct* 11:301-319, 2000.

45. Carney S, Karlowicz KA, Meredith C, et al: Urinary tract obstructions. In Karlowicz KA, editor: *Urologic nursing: principles and practice,* Philadelphia, 1995, WB Saunders.

46. Jackson S, Abrams P: Etiology of urinary incontinence. In O'Donnell PD, editor: *Urinary incontinence,* St. Louis, 1997, Mosby.

47. Einhorn C: Diagnosing and treating benign prostatic hyperplasia, *Innovations Urol Nurs* 5:53-69, 1995.
48. Trockman BA, Leach GE: Complications of incontinence surgery. In O'Donnell PD, editor: *Urinary incontinence,* St. Louis, 1997, Mosby.
49. Handa V, Jones M: Do pessaries prevent the progression of pelvic organ prolapse? *Int Urogynecol J Pelvic Floor Dysfunct* 13(6):349-351;discussion 352, 2002.
50. Wu V, Farrell SA, Baskett TF, Flowerdew G: A simplified protocol for pessary management, *Obstet Gynecol* 90(6):990-994, 1997.
51. Cespedes R: Pelvic prolapse: diagnosing and treating uterine and vaginal vault prolapse, *Medscape Gen Med* 1(3):1999; www.medscape.com/viewarticle/408889.
52. Aronson MP, Sant GR: Urinary incontinence after pelvic surgery. In O'Donnell PD, editor: *Urinary incontinence,* St. Louis, 1997, Mosby.
53. Mundy AR: An anatomical explanation for bladder dysfunction following rectal and uterine surgery, *Br J Urol* 129:84-87, 1982.
54. Zimmern PE: Bladder dysfunction after radiation and radical pelvic surgery. In Raz S, editor: *Female urology,* ed 2, Philadelphia, 1996, WB Saunders.
55. Brown J, Sawaya G, Thom D, Grady D: Hysterectomy and urinary incontinence: a systematic review, Lancet 356:535-539, 2000.
56. Moallie PA, Jones I, Meyer LA, Zyczynski HM: Risk factors associated with pelvic floor disorders in women undergoing surgical repair, *Obstet Gynecol* 101:869-874, 2003.
57. Van der Vaart CH, Van der Bom JG, de Leeuw JR, et al: The contribution of hysterectomy to the occurrence of urge and stress urinary incontinence symptoms, *Br J Obstet Gynaecol* 109:149-154, 2002.
58. Smith ARB, Hosker GL, Warrel D: The role of partial denervation of the pelvic floor and the etiology of genitourinary prolapse and stress incontinence of urine: a neuro-physiologic study, *Br J Obstet Gynaecol* 96:24, 2989.
59. Raz S, Stothers L, Chopra A: Vaginal reconstructive surgery for incontinence and prolapse. In Walsh PC, Retik AB, Vaughan ED, Wein AJ, editors: *Campbell's urology,* ed 7, Philadelphia, 1998, WB Saunders.
60. Cardozo LD, Stanton SL, Williams JE: Detrusor instability following surgery for genuine stress incontinence, *Br J Urol* 51:204, 9279.
61. Herr HW: Quality of life in prostrate cancer patients, *Cancer J Clin* 47:202-217, 1997.
62. McGlynn B, Al-Saffar N, Begg H, et al: Management of urinary incontinence following radical prostatectomy, *Urol Nurs* 24(6):475-482, 2004.
63. Butler L, Downe-Wamboldt B, Marsh S, et al: Quality of life post-radical prostatectomy: a male perspective, *Urol Nurs* 21(4):283-288, 2001.
64. Moore KN, Dorey GF: Conservative treatment of urinary incontinence in men: a review of the literature, *Physiotherapy* 85(2):77-87, 1999.
65. Breslin DS, Staskin DR: Bladder noncompliance. In O'Donnell PD, editor: *Urinary incontinence,* St. Louis, 1997, Mosby.
66. Batra A: Interstitial cystitis update, *Infect Urol* 12(6): 155-158, 1999; www.medscape.com/viewarticle/417017.
67. Gallo ML, Fallon PJ, Staskin DR: Urinary incontinence: steps to evaluation, diagnosis, and treatment, *Nurse Pract* 22:21-44, 1997.

Pathology and Management of Stress Incontinence

DOROTHY B. DOUGHTY & PATRICIA A. BURNS

OBJECTIVES

1. Explain why stress incontinence is more common among women.
2. Describe the effects of each of the following on continence in women: loss of anatomic support; intrinsic sphincter weakness.
3. Explain the hammock theory of stress incontinence.
4. Outline critical parameters to be included in the assessment of an individual with suspected stress incontinence.
5. Describe the role of each of the following in the management of a patient with stress incontinence: alpha-adrenergic agonists, tricyclic antidepressants, estrogen, selective serotonin-norepinephrine reuptake inhibitors.
6. Identify indications for each of the following: retropubic colposuspension; tension-free midurethral slings; compressive suburethral sling; urethral bulking procedure.
7. Outline guidelines for instructing patients in pelvic muscle exercise programs.
8. Explain how biofeedback or vaginal weights can be used to facilitate pelvic muscle reeducation.
9. Explain the mechanism of action and indications or contraindications for electrical stimulation of the pelvic floor muscles.
10. Describe indications and guidelines for use of urethral inserts and pessaries.

Urinary incontinence is a very common health care problem, especially among women, and studies indicate that *stress urinary incontinence* is the most common type.[1,2] It is very difficult to accurately determine prevalence because most women do not report the condition, either because of embarrassment or the belief that nothing can be done; despite underreporting, stress incontinence is known to affect millions of women in the United States and to exact a significant toll in terms of cost of care and impact on lifestyle, sexual activity, and self-esteem.[1-3] Severe stress incontinence and mixed stress-urge incontinence have also been linked to increased incidence of panic disorder and depression.[4] Fortunately, stress incontinence is almost always correctable, through conservative behavioral therapy, pharmacotherapy, surgery, or combination therapy.

Stress incontinence is defined as urinary leakage that occurs during activities that cause increased intraabdominal pressure, such as coughing, sneezing, laughing, and exercising. The underlying problem is *inadequate urethral resistance;* when pressures rise in the abdomen, urine is forced past the urethral sphincter mechanism. It is important to understand that pure stress incontinence (genuine stress incontinence) occurs when the *bladder is relaxed.* The leakage is caused by sphincter dysfunction; the sphincter is unable to maintain a watertight seal when abdominal pressures are elevated.[1,2] This is in contrast to urge incontinence, which is caused by bladder dysfunction (inappropriate bladder contractions). Some women report a "combination pattern" of leakage; that is, they leak urine during activities that cause increased abdominal pressure but also experience leakage associated with urgency and the inability to delay voiding long enough to reach the toilet. This pattern of leakage is known as *mixed stress-urge incontinence.*

Although stress incontinence occurs primarily in middle-aged and elderly women, this type of incontinence can also occur in men following prostatectomy; postprostatectomy incontinence is addressed in Chapter 9. In addition, stress incontinence is fairly common among young women during pregnancy and the postpartum period, in young female athletes participating in "impact" sports such as gymnastics, and in female soldiers participating in rigorous exercise.[2,5]

RISK FACTORS

The etiology of stress incontinence is complex, and there is lack of consensus regarding the specific causes. However, most researchers and clinicians agree that vaginal delivery is the most significant risk factor, due to the potential for damage to the pelvic floor nerves, muscles, and ligaments. Large infants (larger than 4 kg), a prolonged second stage of labor (longer than 30 minutes), and forceps delivery seem to increase the risk for damage to the pelvic floor structures, as do multiple vaginal deliveries.[2,6,7] Nonobstetric risk factors include the following:

- Hysterectomy, probably because of partial denervation of the urethral sphincter mechanism; studies indicate that the impact is greater in radical hysterectomy and correlates at least in part to the length of vagina resected, but there is evidence of increased risk even among women undergoing simple hysterectomy.[2,8]
- Chronic straining at stool (as a result of stretch damage to the pudendal nerve, which innervates the striated muscles of the urethral sphincter and pelvic floor).[9]
- Menopause, because of loss of estrogen and a resultant loss of urethral coaptation.[6]
- Obesity, as a result of increased abdominal pressure and possibly compromised muscle function.[10,11]
- Pelvic organ prolapse (or previous repair of pelvic organ prolapse); pelvic organ prolapse significantly alters the anatomic and functional relationships of the bladder, sphincter, and pelvic floor, and surgical repair may cause denervation injury.[2,12] However, prolapse may also *mask* stress incontinence by causing outlet obstruction; this is particularly true of prolapse extending to the introitus or beyond.[2,12]
- Age, probably because of age-related deterioration in striated muscle contractility in addition to the negative effects of estrogen deficiency.[2,3]

- Collagen deficiencies in the periurethral and paravaginal tissues, resulting in reduced tensile strength of the pelvic floor structures and compromised support for the bladder, urethra, and vagina. Some studies suggest increased incidence of stress incontinence among women with benign joint hypermobility syndrome and increased incidence of collagen deficiency among women with stress incontinence.[9,12]

Other conditions associated with stress incontinence include smoking, pulmonary conditions that cause chronic cough, and neurologic processes that adversely affect innervation of the pelvic floor and urethral sphincter (such as myelodysplasia or spinal cord injury).[13] Race is also a significant risk factor; according to some studies, prevalence of stress incontinence is much lower among African-American women as compared with Asian, white, and Hispanic women (with Hispanic women having the highest prevalence).[14]

PATHOLOGY OF STRESS INCONTINENCE

Fluids such as urine move from areas of greater pressure to areas of lesser pressure; thus, urinary leakage occurs whenever pressures within the urethra fall below the pressures within the bladder. A normal bladder has the capacity to "stretch and store" moderate to large amounts of urine with minimal increases in pressure; this explains why stress incontinence does not usually occur "at rest" (because even a weak sphincter can usually maintain pressures that are higher than the minimal pressures exerted by the gradually distending bladder). When abdominal pressures rise as a result of coughing, sneezing, or lifting, these pressures are transmitted to the bladder, and the bladder and urethra are pushed down toward the pelvic floor. It is during these activities that a weakened sphincter mechanism "fails" and leakage occurs.

Continence during periods of increased abdominal pressure depends on a urethral sphincter mechanism that can "rise to the occasion" by generating urethral resistance that exceeds the elevated bladder pressures. Normally, the downward movement of the bladder and urethra is "countered" by contraction of the pelvic floor muscles; the "opposing lift" provided by pelvic muscle contraction serves to compress the urethra against the anterior vaginal wall, which significantly increases urethral resistance. Continence is further supported by contraction of the voluntary urethral sphincter muscles and by the normal softness and coaptation of the urethral walls.

The critical elements for "continence under stress" seem to be as follows: (1) sufficient anatomic support for the bladder neck, urethra, and anterior vaginal wall; and (2) normal innervation and function of the urethral and pelvic floor musculature. Normal urethral softness and coaptation comprise a third element contributing to urethral closure and urethral resistance.[2,3,15]

Role of Anatomic Support

Normal function of the urethral sphincter mechanism and prevention of urinary leakage depend in part on sufficient anatomic support for the bladder neck, urethra, and anterior vaginal wall. This is provided by the fascia, ligaments, and muscles of the pelvic floor. The fascia and ligaments secure and support the bladder, urethra, and vagina in their normal anatomic positions by attaching them to the symphysis pubis and the pelvic sidewalls. The pelvic floor muscles protect the pelvic ligaments against excessive stretch by supporting the weight of the pelvic organs; this support is particularly critical during periods of increased abdominal pressure and downward pressure on the pelvic organs and their supports. Key structures are illustrated in Fig. 2-6 and include the following:[3,15-17]

- The pubourethral ligament attaches the anterior urethra to the symphysis pubis (anterior support); this "anchors" the midportion of the urethra to a bony structure, which provides an important point of stability during periods of increased abdominal pressure.
- The urethropelvic ligaments anchor the urethra to the arcus tendineus fascia pelvis bilaterally (lateral support).
- The vesicopelvic (pubocervical) fascia attach the bladder, bladder neck, and vagina to the pelvic sidewalls (posterior support).
- The levator ani muscle complex forms the urogenital diaphragm and supports the pelvic organs in position. The two key components of

the levator complex are the pubovisceral and pubococcygeus muscles, which comprise a U-shaped band of muscles that pass around the anorectal junction posteriorly and attach to the symphysis pubis anteriorly (See Color Plate 1), and the ileococcygeus, which attaches to the arcus tendineus fascia pelvis on each side and provides primary support for the pelvic organs.

Loss of anatomic support is a major risk factor for stress incontinence, although the specific mechanism by which this occurs is controversial. In the past, it was believed that optimal sphincter function depended on maintenance of the bladder neck and proximal urethra in an intraabdominal position even when abdominal and bladder pressures were elevated. This intraabdominal position was thought to ensure a balanced transmission of abdominal pressures (that is, to the bladder *and* to the urethra) and also to ensure optimal function of the urethral and periurethral musculature (that is, optimal transmission of contractile pressures to the urethral lumen, with a resultant increase in urethral resistance). Loss of normal anatomic support as a result of tears, denervation, or laxity of the support structures (pelvic floor relaxation) is known to permit *urethral hypermobility*, that is, downward and outward displacement and rotation of the urethra and bladder neck during activities that increase intraabdominal pressure (Fig. 4-1). This downward displacement of the proximal urethra has been thought to cause stress incontinence. However, current studies suggest that many continent women demonstrate some degree of urethral hypermobility during stress maneuvers, and many antiincontinence procedures effectively correct stress incontinence without eliminating urethral hypermobility.[16,18] This has led to a reevaluation of the role of anatomic support in maintenance of continence and to development of the "hammock theory" by DeLancey. According to this theory, continence can be maintained even with downward movement of the urethra so long as the levator ani muscles provide sufficient counter pressure to compress the urethra against the fascia and the anterior vaginal wall; this theory emphasizes the importance of normal levator ani function (to provide counterpressure and to stabilize the pubocervical fascia)

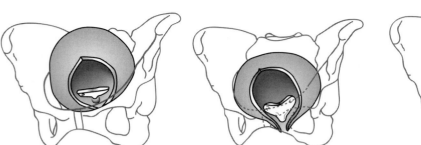
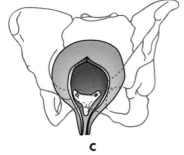

Fig. 4-1 Urethral hypermobility secondary to pelvic floor relaxation. **A,** At rest, bladder and bladder neck are situated above the superior margin of the symphysis pubis. **B** and **C,** with increased abdominal pressure, the bladder and urethra rotate and descend and the bladder neck opens to permit leakage.

as well as intact anatomic supports, specifically the pubourethral ligament.[3,15]

Current evidence (and the success of new "tension-free" sling procedures) suggests that the midurethra is particularly critical to continence during periods of increased abdominal pressure; fixation of the midurethra acts to "kink and compress" the proximal urethra against the vaginal wall. Data indicate that damage to the pubourethral ligament is associated with stress incontinence, because the midurethra moves out of position, and the platform for compression of the proximal urethra is lost. Loss of anatomic support for the anterior vaginal wall can also cause stress incontinence. This is because the anterior urethral wall is attached to the symphysis pubis at midpoint, but the posterior urethral wall is continuous with the anterior vaginal wall; therefore, displacement of the anterior vaginal wall causes the posterior urethral wall to "pull away from" the anterior urethral wall, with resultant loss of urethral coaptation and leakage.[15,16]

Role of Urethral Sphincter Function

The second major factor contributing to urethral resistance consists of the integrity, innervation, and contractility of the urethral sphincter and pelvic floor muscles. The urethral sphincter musculature is comprised of both smooth and striated muscle fibers within the urethral wall; the muscular sleeve

of the urethra contains both an inner layer of smooth muscle and an outer layer of striated muscle. The two contractile components of the urethral spincter mechanism are: (1) the smooth muscle component, which is under alpha-adrenergic control and is thought to maintain closure of the proximal urethra during bladder filling, and (2) the striated sphincter, which contributes to resting tone via reflex mechanisms and also provides for a rapid increase in urethral resistance via voluntary contraction; this is critical to maintenance of continence during periods of increased abdominal pressure.[1,15,19]

The role of the smooth muscle layer is somewhat controversial; some authors contend that the oblique orientation of the smooth muscle fibers at the bladder neck serves to constrict the bladder neck during filling and to open the bladder neck during voiding, whereas others point out that there is no "collar" of smooth muscle in women (as there is in men) and suggest that the smooth muscle fibers are more important to funneling of the bladder neck during voiding than to active support of continence.[15] The smooth muscle component of the urethral sphincter mechanism is innervated by sympathetic nerve fibers that originate in the lumbar region of the spinal cord; sympathetic stimulation of alpha-adrenergic receptors in the smooth muscle stimulates muscle contraction and is controlled by reflex arcs that are activated by bladder distension. The primary neuro-transmitters for smooth muscle innervation are serotonin and norepinephrine.

The striated sphincter includes several distinct muscles: the rhabdosphincter, which encompasses the urethra circumferentially and is most prominent at the midurethra, and a pair of muscular slings that provide support for the middle and distal urethra, that is, the compressor urethrae and the urethrovaginal sphincter (see Fig. 2-3). The rhabdosphincter is an intrinsic urethral muscle that "thins" posteriorly (in the area between the urethra and vagina); it is composed primarily of slow-twitch fibers, which provide sustained tonic support for the urethral lumen. The compressor urethrae and the urethrovaginal sphincter are periurethral muscle slings composed of fast-twitch fibers; contraction of these muscles provides for a rapid and marked increase in urethral resistance during periods of increased abdominal pressure.[15,19]

The striated muscle component of the urethral sphincter mechanism is unique in that it provides both resting tone, mediated by somatic reflex pathways, and voluntary contraction, mediated by the pudendal nerve. As the bladder fills, the increasing distension activates afferent pathways that, in turn, cause increased production of serotonin and norepinephrine by motor neurons; the end result is increasing sphincter tone in response to increasing bladder distension, a phenomenon known as the "guarding reflex."[1,19] Voluntary contraction of the sphincter mechanism is mediated via the pudendal nerve; normally, contraction of the sphincter provides a rapid marked increase in urethral resistance.

Intrinsic sphincter failure, or loss of contractility, may be caused by loss of innervation or by trauma to the muscles. For example, autonomic neuropathy can cause loss of innervation to the smooth muscle in the proximal portion of the urethra, and spinal cord lesions commonly cause denervation of the striated sphincter and the pelvic floor. Trauma can cause denervation injury or direct damage to the muscle itself; the most common source of injury is surgical trauma or trauma induced by long-term use of indwelling catheters. The result of such muscle damage or denervation is the development of a rigid, noncontractile urethra that is essentially "open" from the bladder to the meatus. This condition is sometimes referred to as a "drain pipe" or "lead pipe" urethra.[15,20]

Normal Urethral Softness and Coaptation

The female urethra is a 3- to 5-cm conduit composed of three layers: an inner mucosal layer, a midlayer composed of spongy vascular tissue, and an outer muscular sleeve containing both smooth and striated muscle layers. The inner layer is composed of squamous cell epithelium and contains numerous mucus-secreting glands; the mucus produced by these glands increases surface tension and helps provide a watertight seal within the urethra. The vascular midlayer contains abundant venous sinuses and arteriovenous connections; this vascular complex contributes its own compressive force and also serves as a conduit for transmission of intraabdominal pressure to the urethra. The submucosal vascular complex is thought to be responsible for as much as 30% of total urethral resistance. This is particularly significant in light of the finding that the urethral mucosa and vascular complex are highly influenced by estrogen and are known to atrophy significantly in the postmenopausal period.[12,15]

TYPES OF STRESS INCONTINENCE

In the past, stress incontinence was classified as being caused by *either* loss of anatomic support (that is,urethral hypermobility) *or* significant weakness of the urethral sphincter musculature (that is, intrinsic sphincter deficiency [ISD]). Stress incontinence associated with urethral hypermobility was termed "genuine stress urinary incontinence" and was sometimes classified as Type I and Type II. Patients were considered to have Type I stress incontinence if they lost the "posterior urethrovesical angle" during stress maneuvers but maintained the anterior support. Patients who lost both the posterior urethrovesical angle and the anterior support were considered to have Type II stress incontinence. Stress incontinence caused by weakness of the urethral sphincter musculature was known as ISD; in women, this was also sometimes called "Type III" incontinence to distinguish it from Type I and Type II incontinence, which were considered to be caused purely by urethral hypermobility.

Current evidence suggests that many patients present with some combination of the two primary mechanisms, that is, some loss of anatomic support coupled with some degree of muscle weakness; therefore, current thinking emphasizes a more integrated theory of stress incontinence as opposed to "either/or" thinking and management. In evaluating and treating any individual patient, the focus should always be on accurate identification and correction of the various factors contributing to *her* stress incontinence.[15]

CLINICAL PRESENTATION

The classic presentation of stress incontinence is leakage associated with increased abdominal pressure; leakage does not occur at rest and is not associated with any sense of urgency to void.[2] The severity of the incontinence varies, depending on the underlying etiologic factors. Women with mild stress incontinence typically report low-volume leakage associated with marked increases in abdominal pressure; common triggering activities include running, jumping, coughing, laughing, sneezing, golfing, and lifting. However, patients with very weak sphincter muscles may report significant leakage even with mild increases in abdominal pressure, such as rising from a sitting position (especially if this maneuver requires significant effort). (See Appendix B.)

As explained earlier, many women experience both stress incontinence and urge incontinence; these patients present with a combination of leakage with activity and leakage associated with urinary urgency.

EVALUATION

Assessment of the incontinent individual is covered in depth in Chapter 12. This section briefly addresses the parameters critical to the assessment of a woman with known or suspected stress incontinence. For these women, the goals of assessment include determination of the type(s) and severity of incontinence, identification of causative and contributing factors, and identification of associated and complicating conditions. Specifically, the workup must include assessment of the factors essential to "continence under stress": status of the urethral and vaginal tissues; innervation and contractile strength of the sphincter and pelvic floor muscles; and degree of anatomic support for the bladder, urethra, and vagina.[3]

History

The clinical evaluation of the client with stress incontinence begins with a complete history. This should include a symptom questionnaire that identifies the precipitating events for urinary leakage; that is, activities associated with incontinence. Typically, the patient with stress incontinence reports leakage during activities such as walking, coughing, and lifting, but denies leakage during sleep and quiet sitting. The positive predictive value of the "symptom" of stress incontinence (that is, leakage associated with activity and not accompanied by urgency) ranges from 0.56 to 0.79 in published studies comparing diagnoses based on patient reports with those based on urodynamic investigation; thus, the patient's report of activity-induced incontinence is of great significance.[21-23] The patient should also be questioned about factors associated with the onset of her incontinence, the frequency of her incontinent episodes, the volume of urine lost, and the impact on her quality of life. The patient should be specifically questioned regarding any impact on sexual relationships, because some women with stress incontinence report leakage during intercourse and significant interference with sexual activity.[2] The systems review should include specific questions regarding known risk factors for stress incontinence, that is, number of vaginal deliveries with particular focus on any difficult deliveries, menopausal status, urologic procedures (that is, "bladder tack" or other antiincontinence procedure), gynecologic procedures such as hysterectomy, history of chronic constipation, and smoking. In reviewing the patient's medication profile, the clinician should be alert to agents that may cause a chronic cough (such as angiotensin-converting enzyme inhibitors) and agents that may reduce sphincter tone (such as alpha adrenergic antagonists). The patient should be asked about previous treatments for incontinence (and response); if the patient is using pads, briefs, or protective devices, the type and volume should be determined and quantified.

The history should also contain questions to elicit any signs or symptoms of lower urinary tract dysfunction, such as hesitancy, poor or interrupted stream, straining, hematuria, nocturia, dysuria, or suprapubic or perineal pain. Any patient with signs or symptoms of lower urinary tract disease requires prompt referral for diagnosis and management.

Physical Examination

A careful physical examination helps to determine the cause and severity of the incontinence and must include a pelvic, rectal, and focused neurologic assessment. Ideally, the examination is conducted when the patient has a relatively full bladder; this allows the clinician to attempt to reproduce the incontinence by having the patient cough or perform other maneuvers that increase abdominal pressure. A *vaginal* or *pelvic examination* is then performed to assess the status of the vaginal mucosa, the innervation and contractility of the pelvic floor muscles, the degree of anatomic support (or evidence of diminished support), and evidence of pelvic organ prolapse. The perineal skin should also be assessed for any lesions, rashes, or evidence of skin breakdown. A *rectal examination* is performed to evaluate anorectal sensation and anal sphincter tone and to rule out any fecal impaction or perirectal mass. (In male patients, the rectal examination also includes palpation of the prostate gland to determine size and consistency.) A focused *neurologic examination* is performed to determine the client's overall cognitive status and the functional status of the sacral nerves innervating the bladder, urethra, and pelvic floor.

Cough Test. The cough test is an attempt to reproduce the patient's incontinence; the patient is placed in lithotomy position with a relatively full bladder and is instructed to cough vigorously while the examiner observes for loss of urine from the urethra.[24] If no urine loss is observed with the patient in the supine position, the test can be repeated in the upright position (typically following the pelvic examination). Loss of urine in small spurts occurring simultaneously with each cough supports a tentative diagnosis of stress incontinence. Many clinicians record the volume of urine lost with provocation, which helps to determine the severity of the incontinence. *Delayed* loss of urine, especially large-volume urine loss or complete emptying of the bladder, is suggestive of overactive bladder and urge incontinence. (In this case, the cough triggers an unstable bladder contraction, which is the causative factor for the incontinence.)

Inspection of Vaginal Mucosa and Urethral Position. The vaginal mucosa should be inspected for color, hydration, and the presence of rugae. The normal vagina is deep pink to red, moist, and rugated; a pale, thin, dry, and shiny mucosa or the loss of rugation indicate atrophic vaginitis secondary to low estrogen levels. A prominent cherry-red urethral meatus (urethral caruncle) is another indicator of estrogen deficiency. When the vaginal and urethral tissues are atrophic, topical estrogen therapy should be considered as a component of the overall treatment program (unless there are significant contraindications or the client is opposed to estrogen therapy).

When inspecting the perineum and pelvic tissues, the examiner should note the position of the urethra. A well-supported urethra should be midline; urethral deviation to the right or left of midline suggests loss of fascial supports on the contralateral side. (For example, deviation to the right suggests loss of fascial support on the left.)

Evaluation of Pelvic Muscle Strength. Evaluation of pelvic muscle control and vaginal wall support is a critical component of assessment for the individual with stress urinary incontinence. Pelvic muscle evaluation is typically conducted with the patient in both lithotomy and upright positions. While the patient is in lithotomy position, the examiner inserts one or two fingers into the vagina and places the other hand on the patient's abdomen; the patient is asked to contract her pelvic muscles (as if trying not to pass gas), and the examiner "grades" the contraction on a four-point scale based on strength, duration, and displacement[25] (Table 4-1). The examiner can also palpate the muscles at 5 o'clock and 7 o'clock by placing one finger in the vagina and the thumb on the perineum and asking the patient to tighten and lift. The standing component of the exam is conducted by having the patient place her right foot on a small stool or the footstep of the examining table while the examiner inserts

TABLE 4-1   Pelvic Muscle Strength Rating Scale

	1	2	3	4
Pressure	None	Slight pressure, not perceived around circumference of finger	Moderate pressure, perceived around circumference of finger	Strong pressure, perceived circumferentially
Duration	None	<1 second	1-3 seconds	>3 seconds
Displacement of finger	None	Slight incline, base of fingers slightly elevated	Greater incline, entire finger elevated	Fingers move up and inside, toward posterior vault

Adapted from Sampselle CM, Brink CA, Wells TJ: *Nurs Res* 38:135, 1989.

one or two fingers into the vagina; the patient is then asked to contract her vaginal muscles around the examiner's finger or fingers. (This component of the exam is typically conducted following the speculum exam and the rectal exam.)

Innervation of the urethral sphincter and pelvic floor muscles can be assumed to be intact when the patient is able to contract the muscles voluntarily on demand. If the patient is *unable* to contract the muscles on demand effectively, the clinician should verify intact nerve pathways by tapping or squeezing the clitoris and observing for contraction of the anal sphincter. (This response is known as a positive bulbocavernosus reflex and indicates intact nerve pathways between the sacral cord and the striated muscles of the pelvic floor.[24])

When conducting the vaginal examination, the clinician should also palpate the anterior vaginal wall and urethra; tenderness or discharge in response to palpation is suggestive of a urethral diverticulum, carcinoma, or inflammatory condition. Any patient with tenderness or discharge should be referred for further evaluation.

Assessment of Anatomic Support. The female patient with stress incontinence should also be examined for evidence of cystocele, rectocele, or pelvic organ prolapse. Ideally, this is accomplished by means of a speculum examination, which is within the scope of practice for nurse practitioners and other advanced practice nurses. The assessment of anatomic support for the pelvic organs is facilitated by the use of a Sims vaginal speculum; alternatively, the nurse may use the posterior blade

TABLE 4-2   Commonly Used Grading System for Cystoceles

GRADE	DESCRIPTION
I	Minimal bladder descensus
II	Bladder descensus to vaginal introitus with straining
III	Bladder descensus to vaginal introitus at rest
IV	Bladder prolapse through the labia at rest or with straining, or both

of an ordinary Graves speculum. To assess for a cystocele or urethrocele, the examiner retracts the posterior vaginal wall and inspects the anterior vaginal wall while the patient "bears down" to increase intraabdominal pressure. (A commonly used grading system for cystoceles is presented in Table 4-2.) To assess for a rectocele, the examiner retracts the anterior vaginal wall and inspects the posterior vaginal wall for bulging (in response to the "bearing-down" maneuver). The clinician should also be alert to urine loss occurring in response to the Valsalva maneuver; this is another positive indicator for stress incontinence.[24]

The primary continence care nurse who is not equipped or skilled in the speculum examination should perform a screening assessment for significant pelvic organ prolapse by having the patient stand and strain ("bear down") while the nurse observes for visible prolapse (that is, prolapse that extends past the introitus); patients with visible prolapse or other evidence of diminished anatomic support (such as urethral deviation) generally require referral for further evaluation and possible surgical intervention.

Q-Tip Test. The Q-Tip test is used by some practitioners to demonstrate urethral hypermobility objectively. To conduct the test, the clinician inserts a sterile, lubricated Q-Tip into the urethra to the level of the bladder neck (approximately 1 to 2 cm) and asks the patient to strain or perform a Valsalva maneuver. The examiner observes for upward movement of the Q-Tip, which indicates a downward movement of the bladder neck; upward movement of greater than 30 degrees is considered by many to be a "hypermobile urethra." This test is easily performed; however, the results are affected by patient effort, and the interpretation of upward movement is subjective and imprecise.[24] In addition, the importance of urethral hypermobility as an etiologic factor for stress incontinence is unclear, as discussed earlier. Therefore, this test is not routinely performed or recommended.

Marshall-Bonney Test. The Marshall-Bonney test is used by some clinicians to determine whether the patient's stress incontinence is caused by loss of anatomic support (urethral hypermobility) as opposed to intrinsic sphincter weakness. The test involves temporary elevation of the urethra and bladder neck into an anatomically correct position while the patient performs provocative maneuvers such as coughing. To elevate the bladder neck, the examiner places two fingers (or a rubber-shod clamp) on either side of the urethra, which pushes the bladder neck back into position; the patient is then asked to cough, and the examiner observes for any leakage. If no leakage is observed, the test is said to be positive, that is, indicative of urethral hypermobility as the cause of the incontinence. A positive test indicates that surgical repositioning of the bladder neck may be an appropriate treatment for the patient's stress incontinence.

Most clinicians believe that this test has limited value and that any patient considering surgical intervention should be evaluated by urodynamic studies. These clinicians point out that the maneuvers used to accomplish elevation of the bladder neck

may also produce mechanical compression of the urethra; this compression would tend to compensate for intrinsic urethral weakness and could produce a "false-positive" indication of urethral hypermobility as the sole cause of the incontinence.

Neurologic Examination. The neurologic examination for an incontinent patient should be focused on cognitive status and on the function of the nerve pathways innervating the bladder, urethra, and pelvic floor. The tool most commonly used to evaluate cognitive status is the Folstein Mini-Mental State Examination; this is a validated screen for cognitive decline. Scores between 23 and 30 indicate that the patient has the cognitive ability to participate in behavioral treatment.[26]

Tests to evaluate the nerve pathways innervating the bladder, urethra, and pelvic floor include the bulbocavernosus reflex and the anal wink; these tests should be carried out when there is any evidence that the patient's incontinence may be caused partly by sphincter denervation. The bulbocavernosus reflex test is described in the section on pelvic examination. The *anal wink test* is commonly used to evaluate the function of the sacral nerve roots (that is, the nerves exiting the spinal cord at S2 to S4); these nerve pathways innervate the external anal sphincter and the periurethral striated sphincter. The test is conducted by lightly stroking the mucocutaneous junction of the circumanal skin; an intact anal reflex is indicative of intact nerve pathways and is evidenced by visible contraction of the external anal sphincter (that is, the "anal wink"). Absence of the anal wink is suggestive of sacral disease and sphincter denervation in younger patients; in the elderly patient, the anal wink may be absent even without neurologic disease. The absence of both the anal wink and the bulbocavernosus reflex strongly suggests neurologic lesions causing sphincter denervation. Patients with known or suspected neurologic lesions should be referred to a neurologist for a complete workup.

Voiding Diary (Bladder Record). All patients should be asked to complete a bladder record (Fig. 4-2).[24,27] The bladder record should capture the following information: time (and, if possible, volume) of normal voids, time and approximate amount of urinary leakage, type of activity associated

VOIDING DIARY (BLADDER RECORD)

NAME: _____

DATE: _____

INSTRUCTIONS: Place a check in the appropriate column next to the time you urinated in the toilet or when an incontinence episode occurred. Note the reason for the incontinence and describe your liquid intake (for example, coffee, water) and estimate the amount (for example, one cup).

Time interval	Urinated in toilet	Had a small incontinence episode	Had a large incontinence episode	Reason for incontinence episode	Type/amount of liquid intake
6-8 AM					
8-10 AM					
10-noon					
Noon-2 PM					
2-4 PM					
4-6 PM					
6-8 PM					
8-10 PM					
10-midnight					
Overnight					

No. of pads used today: _____   No. of episodes: _____

Comments: _____

_____

_____

Fig. 4-2 Sample bladder record. (From *AHCPR Guidelines:* Managing acute and chronic urinary incontinence, Rockville, Md., 1996, US Dept. of Health and Human Services, Public Health Service, Agency for Health Care Policy and Research.)

with urine loss, type and number of pads or protective devices used in a 24-hour period, and type and volume of fluid intake. The data obtained from a bladder record are extremely beneficial to the clinician in determining the pattern and severity of the incontinence; even a "short-term" diary (that is, 1-to 3-day recording) can provide the needed information if the data are recorded accurately.[24,28,29]

Pad-Weight Tests. Pad-weight testing is a valuable tool in the evaluation of stress incontinence because it objectively quantifies the volume of urinary leakage. There are numerous approaches to pad-weight tests, ranging from a 15- to 20-minute "office" test to a 12- to 24-hour "home" test.[24] In a *12-hour pad-weight test,* preweighed perineal pads are placed in separate plastic bags with labels designating 2-hour intervals; the client wears each of the preweighed pads for the specified 2 hours and then reseals each pad in its plastic bag, recording all activities that occurred during the 2 hours the pad was worn. The *24-hour pad-weight test* is a variation on this approach; the patient is instructed to wear pads for 24 hours and to change them as needed based on wetness. (When the pad is changed, the used pad is replaced in its plastic bag and sealed.) The patient is instructed to maintain a voiding diary at the same time, with notations regarding activities and leakage. The pads are returned to the office (along with the voiding diary) and are weighed to determine the total volume of leakage during the test period.[24] The *1-hour "office" pad-weight test* provides quantification of urine loss during a specific set of incontinence-provoking maneuvers. The client is fitted with a perineal pad and an additional abdominal type of pad sufficient to contain large volumes of urine. Each of these pads is preweighed before use. The patient carries out all the incontinence-provoking maneuvers, and the pads are then reweighed on a calibrated scale. See Table 4-3 for a 1-hour pad-weight test protocol. In interpreting the results, an increase in pad weight of more than 1 g is considered indicative of urine loss; this is based on the finding that imprecision in weighing can account for a 1 g (more or less) deviation.

TABLE 4-3   Protocol for 1-Hour Pad-Weight Test

TIME (min)	PROCEDURE
0	Apply a preweighed pad
15	Drink 500 mL, sitting
30	Walk; walk up stairs
45-60	Alternate between sitting and standing (×10)
	Execute powerful coughs (×10)
	Jog in place for 1 minute
	Pick an object up off the floor (× 5)
	Wash hands for 1 minute
60	Remove pad; weigh it; calculate urine loss
	Void; determine voided volume

The interpretation of results should also take into consideration other potential sources of error, such as excessive perspiration, vaginal discharge, and measurement errors. (Evaporation has not been shown to be a significant factor in pad-weight test outcomes.) To minimize the potential for inaccurate results, pad-weight testing should not be performed immediately before or after the patient's menstrual period.

Additional Tests of Urologic Function. The assessment of the incontinent patient should routinely include studies to rule out conditions requiring treatment, that is, infection, retention, and malignancy. In addition, selected patients may require more complex studies to identify or clarify the cause of the urinary leakage.

Measurement of Postvoid Residual Volume. The assessment of postvoid residual urine volume (PVR) may be accomplished either by catheterization or by a bladder scan obtained with a portable ultrasound device.[30] A "normal" PVR is usually defined as 50 mL or less; however, PVRs in the range of 50 to 100 mL do not generally cause concern. The usual threshold for concern is a repeated PVR measurement of 100 to 200 mL or greater. An elevated PVR is indicative of voiding dysfunction, that is, the inability to empty the bladder effectively; this pattern is most commonly seen in patients with urethral obstruction or a neuropathic disorder affecting the bladder (such as the patient with a combination of stress incontinence and reflex incontinence caused by a spinal cord injury).

Urinalysis. An examination of the urine is an important aspect of any evaluation for urinary incontinence.[24] A clean-catch specimen is obtained after stringent cleansing to minimize contamination; careful technique is particularly important for female patients. The urine is initially examined by dipstick to test for glucose, ketones, blood, bilirubin, nitrites, protein, pH, and specific gravity. The dipstick evaluation may be followed by microscopic examination, which will reveal the presence of bacteria and white blood cells in concentrations of at least one or more white blood cells per high-power field. The dipstick urinalysis is used to screen for evidence of bacteriuria, renal calculi, diabetes, and renal disease; these conditions may all coexist with and contribute to urinary incontinence, and all require referral for further treatment.

Simple Cystometrogram. A cystometrogram (CMG) is a procedure in which sterile fluid is introduced into the bladder through a catheter to evaluate bladder capacity and the bladder's response to filling and to provocative maneuvers; it can help to differentiate between urge and stress incontinence when the clinical picture is unclear. Although a CMG is typically performed as an element of complex urodynamic testing, a simple CMG can be performed without electronic recording equipment. The patient is instructed to void, and a small catheter (12 to 16 Fr) is then inserted into the bladder; a 50-mL syringe is attached to the catheter, and the bladder is filled with sterile water or saline solution. The patient is instructed to report all sensations of bladder filling and the desire to void, and the clinician notes the volume at which these sensations are reported. The patient with overactive bladder typically reports a sense of fullness at low volumes and may experience unstable bladder contractions and urge incontinence in response to bladder filling. (Unstable bladder contractions and urge incontinence are manifest by a sudden rise in the level of fluid within the syringe accompanied by urinary leakage and patient reports of urgency).[24] If bladder filling is accomplished without leakage, the catheter is withdrawn and the patient is instructed to cough forcefully or to perform other provocative maneuvers. Leakage occurring immediately following provocative maneuvers is typically indicative of stress incontinence; delayed leakage is usually an indicator for urge incontinence.[31]

The test may be performed with the patient in the supine or standing positions; if the test is performed initially in the supine position and no leakage is elicited during filling or provocative maneuvers, the patient is asked to stand and repeat the provocative maneuvers with a full bladder (the filling catheter is removed before these maneuvers).

Multichannel Cystometrogram. Patients who are referred to a urologist for further workup to clarify or identify the cause of their incontinence typically undergo a CMG and possibly videourodynamics; these studies are extremely helpful in differentiating between stress and urge incontinence and may also help to differentiate between stress incontinence caused primarily by loss of anatomic support (that is, urethral hypermobility) and stress incontinence caused primarily by sphincter incompetence (intrinsic urethral weakness). A CMG measures changes in bladder pressure in response to bladder filling; data obtained include sensory status (volume at first sensation and at sensation of fullness), bladder capacity, intravesical pressures at baseline and in response to filling, and presence or absence of involuntary detrusor contractions. Involuntary detrusor contractions are evidenced by a sudden rise in intravesical pressure during bladder filling; involuntary contractions associated with urinary leakage are indicative of overactive bladder and urge incontinence.[32] Involuntary contractions may occur in response to provocative maneuvers such as cough or the Valsalva maneuver; in this case, the rise in abdominal pressure associated with the provocative maneuver triggers an involuntary bladder contraction and leakage that mimics stress incontinence. However, the CMG recording will clearly show that the leakage was caused by a bladder contraction as opposed to urethral relaxation in the absence of a detrusor contraction. Patients with mixed stress-urge incontinence typically exhibit evidence of both bladder overactivity and sphincter dysfunction; that is, leakage that *is* associated with unstable bladder contractions (urge incontinence) and leakage in response to provocative maneuvers that *is not* associated with unstable bladder contractions (stress incontinence). Videourodynamic studies combine fluoroscopic imaging with pressure/flow studies during bladder emptying; the combined study allows the clinician to correlate urinary leakage with visualized abnormalities such as urethral hypermobility, pelvic organ prolapse, or an open bladder neck (sphincter incompetence). Thus, videourodynamics are considered by some to be the "gold standard" for diagnosis of stress incontinence.[13,24]

To differentiate between stress incontinence caused simply by loss of anatomic support and stress incontinence caused by intrinsic urethral weakness (sphincter incompetence), it is necessary to measure the contractile force exerted by the sphincter muscles; that is, urethral resistance. The two tests commonly used to measure urethral resistance are the urethral pressure profile, which measures pressures exerted along the urethra either at rest or during provocative maneuvers, and the abdominal leak point pressure, which provides an indirect measure of urethral resistance during periods of increased abdominal pressure. Indicators of an incompetent sphincter include low resting pressures and low leak point pressures.

Urethral Pressure Profile Measurements. Urethral pressure studies may be conducted with the patient in the supine, sitting, or standing position, and under varying conditions of sphincter contraction: at rest, during voluntary contraction, during strain, and during voiding. However, urethral pressure profile measurements are generally obtained with the patient at rest, by pulling a pressure-sensitive catheter through the urethra at a fixed rate while simultaneously monitoring intravesical pressure. Data provided by these studies include maximum urethral pressure, maximum urethral closure pressure (the difference between urethral pressure and bladder pressure), functional urethral length, and pressure transmission ratios. At this time, there are no clearly defined "normal" values; maximum closure pressures lower than 20 cm H_2O are generally considered indicative of intrinsic urethral weakness, pressures between 20 and 30 cm H_2O are considered indeterminate (a "gray zone), and pressures greater than 30 cm H_2O are thought to "rule out" sphincter incompetence as the primary cause of the stress incontinence." The lack of consensus regarding "normal" values and the variability in pressures produced by different types of catheters significantly limit the value of this test.[18,24,33,34]

Abdominal Leak Point Pressure. Abdominal leak point pressure represents the amount of abdominal pressure required to force urine through the urethra; that is, to overcome urethral resistance. The test is conducted by having the patient perform a Valsalva maneuver with steadily increasing force; abdominal pressures are monitored via pressure-sensitive catheters placed in the vagina or rectum, and urinary leakage is determined via uroflow. The "abdominal leak point pressure" is the level of abdominal pressure at which urinary leakage occurs. In general, abdominal leak point pressures of less

than 60 cm H_2O are considered indicative of ISD, and pressures between 60 and 90 cm H_2O are considered the "gray zone." Medicare guidelines require a leak point pressure of less than 100 cm H_2O for a diagnosis of sphincter incompetence (intrinsic urethral weakness) and coverage for urethral bulking procedures.[13,35] The lack of clear consensus regarding normal and abnormal values underscores the importance of careful clinical correlation and the need for more research. Despite these limitations, the leak point pressure is currently considered more valid than the urethral pressure profile in diagnosing the specific etiologic factors for stress incontinence.[13]

Ultrasound. Transrectal, transvaginal, and transperineal ultrasound imaging can be used to assess a number of factors associated with stress incontinence: urethral mobility, pelvic organ prolapse, urethral vascularity, and pelvic muscle contraction. Ultrasound is rapidly becoming recognized as a valuable component of the continence workup and an alternative to radiologic imaging.[13,36,37]

MANAGEMENT OF STRESS INCONTINENCE

The patient with stress incontinence may be managed with monotherapy or with combination therapy; the management plan developed for any individual patient must be based upon the underlying cause of the incontinence as well as the patient's goals and preferences and other factors that could influence treatment outcomes. Treatment for all patients should be based on unbiased treatment protocols.

All treatment options for stress incontinence are designed to increase urethral resistance, by restoring anatomic support for the bladder neck and urethra, improving pelvic muscle contractility and/or endurance, and/or enhancing urethral tissue softness. Specific options include pelvic muscle reeducation (Kegel's exercises) with or without biofeedback, vaginal cone therapy, electrical stimulation, extracorporeal magnetic innervation therapy, pharmacologic therapy, surgical intervention, and the use of occlusive and absorptive devices. In general, the less expensive and less invasive treatments should be the first line of therapy; that is, pelvic muscle exercises would usually be a more appropriate "first intervention" than surgery. However, this is true only if weakness of the pelvic floor muscles is a significant contributing factor to this patient's incontinence and only if the pelvic muscles are sufficiently innervated and the patient is sufficiently motivated to make this a valid treatment approach. Patient preference, the severity of the incontinence, and comorbidities such as pelvic organ prolapse may alter the picture so surgical intervention is selected as initial therapy.

In addition to measures designed specifically to increase urethral resistance, individuals with stress incontinence may benefit from strategies that reduce intravesical pressures, such as routine voiding and fluid management. Although many of these measures offer variable degrees of improvement as opposed to a total "cure," they are all valid treatment options that can be used singly or in combination to manage a condition that is multifaceted and different for each patient. (See Appendix B.)

Behavioral Therapies

Behavioral therapy refers to any intervention in which the patient is taught to modify her or his usual behaviors to improve bladder control; this category includes dietary and fluid modifications, pelvic muscle exercises (with or without biofeedback or vaginal cone therapy), and instruction in strategies to increase urethral resistance during activities that increase abdominal pressure. Many clinicians also consider electrical stimulation to be behavioral therapy, because it is frequently used in combination with pelvic muscle exercise programs and can be used to help the patient identify the target muscle group; however, electrical stimulation can be used to strengthen the pelvic muscles without the patient's active involvement, and so some clinicians exclude it from the behavioral category.

Fluid Management and Scheduled Voiding. Stress incontinence occurs any time the pressure within the noncontracting bladder exceeds the pressures within the urethra. Although the primary triggers for leakage are activities that increase *abdominal* pressure, intravesical pressure is also affected by detrusor (filling) pressure; this means

that an overly full bladder also increases intravesical pressures and increases the risk for leakage during minor increases in abdominal pressure (such as bending or lifting). Thus, patients with stress incontinence frequently benefit from simple strategies to prevent excessive bladder distension: limited intake of diuretic fluids (such as caffeinated beverages), attention to patterns of fluid intake with the goal of spacing fluids fairly evenly throughout the day, and regularly scheduled voiding to prevent bladder distension.[38]

Pelvic Muscle Rehabilitation. Programs to strengthen the pelvic muscles are frequently considered to be the preferred "initial" approach to treatment of stress incontinence, and multiple studies have demonstrated subjective and objective improvement among women with stress incontinence who complete pelvic muscle exercise programs.[2,38,39] However, as Miller pointed out, "improvement" for many of these women means fewer incontinent episodes as opposed to elimination of incontinence; in addition, significant numbers of women fail to demonstrate *any* measurable improvement.[40] These data point to the importance of appropriately selecting those women most likely to benefit from pelvic muscle exercise programs.

Patient Selection Criteria. Until recently, many clinicians routinely prescribed pelvic muscle exercises as initial therapy for almost all patients with evidence of stress, urge, or mixed stress-urge incontinence. However, enhanced understanding of the etiologic factors for stress incontinence is changing this approach; we now realize that pelvic muscle exercise is *unlikely* to be of significant benefit for women whose incontinence is primarily the result of loss of anatomic support or whose incontinence is associated with significant pelvic organ prolapse. In addition, significant denervation or extreme muscle weakness may limit the therapeutic benefits derived from a pelvic muscle exercise program.[3,38,40] Thus, pelvic muscle rehabilitation programs should be prescribed only for women who are likely to benefit from them. Miller proposed the following specific criteria: evidence of intact anatomic support for bladder and urethra, absence of significant pelvic organ prolapse, and demonstrated ability to contract the pelvic floor muscles volitionally.

(Strategies for evaluating each of these criteria are outlined in Table 4-4.) In regard to the ability to contract the pelvic muscles "on command," some clinicians suggest that adequate baseline strength is a predictor of success in a pelvic muscle exercise program; however, other studies indicate that significant improvement can be obtained even when the pelvic muscles are very weak at baseline (so long as the patient retains the ability to contract the muscle voluntarily and is motivated to complete the training program).[40,41]

Principles of Exercise Physiology. Pelvic muscle exercises involve the repetitive contraction of the periurethral and pelvic floor striated muscles; if performed correctly and consistently over time, pelvic muscle exercises help to increase muscle bulk and muscle strength, which increase urethral resistance at rest and during contraction.[40,42-45] An effective exercise program must be individualized for the patient and must be based on an understanding of pelvic muscle physiology and strength training. Pelvic floor muscles are a blend of Type 1 (slow-twitch) and Type 2 (fast-twitch) fibers; the ratio is believed to be about 70% slow twitch and 30% fast twitch. Fast-twitch fibers provide the rapid strong contractions needed to increase urethral resistance significantly during sudden rises in abdominal pressure; however, fast-twitch fibers fatigue rapidly, and it is the slow-twitch fibers that provide sustained resistance (although at a lower level).[42-45] Normally, these two types of fibers work together to maintain urethral closure and prevent leakage. To increase the contractility and endurance of the pelvic floor muscles, they must be made to work beyond their usual limits but not past the point of fatigue.[43] Significant improvement usually requires 6 to 8 weeks of consistent exercise. Once the muscles are rehabilitated, the patient is typically instructed in a less demanding maintenance program for long-term support of continence.

Pelvic muscle exercises can be taught and performed with and without biofeedback; the obvious advantage of biofeedback is the visual or auditory feedback provided to the patient as she is

TABLE 4-4   Criteria For Effective Use of Pelvic Muscle Exercises[40]

CRITERION	ASSESSMENT STRATEGIES
Intact anatomic support	Midline position of urethra
	Intravaginal palpation of intact levator ani muscles (should be able to palpate muscle bilaterally as opposed to bony pelvic sidewalls)
Absence of significant pelvic organ prolapse	No prolapse or minimal prolapse during performance of Valsalva maneuver (any prolapse beyond hymenal ring is considered significant; levator ani contraction in these patients is likely to compress the posterior bladder wall as opposed to the urethra)
Sufficient innervation and muscle contractility	Ability to contract muscles voluntarily during digital examination
	Caudal movement of stick portion of obstetric/gynecologic cotton applicator (cotton tip positioned in upper vagina) when patient instructed to contract pelvic muscles
	Paper towel test: patient holds trifolded paper towel against perineum and coughs forcefully three times; then repeats test with new paper towel but contracts pelvic muscles during cough. (Positive test indicated by significant reduction in "wet area.")
	Perineal ultrasound demonstrating urethral hypermobility and ability of patient to momentarily stabilize urethra by contracting the pelvic floor muscles

contracting (or relaxing) her pelvic floor muscles. This is particularly advantageous with pelvic muscle exercises because these muscles are small and not easily identified. However, pelvic muscle exercises *can* be effectively taught without biofeedback; the challenge is to help the patient correctly identify the muscle to be contracted. Studies have shown that many women who believe that they are performing "Kegel's exercises" are in actuality contracting the gluteals, quadriceps, or abdominal muscles. Significant recruitment of the abdominal muscles can be particularly disadvantageous, because this increases intraabdominal pressure and the potential for leakage. When women are assisted to correctly identify and exercise the pelvic floor muscles, studies indicate a reduction in incontinent episodes ranging from 50% to more than 90%.[38]

Guidelines for Patient Instruction. There are at least two recognized approaches to helping the patient identify her (or his) periurethral muscles (other than the use of biofeedback equipment). The first is to perform a digital vaginal or anal exam while instructing the patient to lift and tighten the pelvic muscles ("as if trying not to pass gas or trying not to urinate"); the clinician may simultaneously monitor for abdominal muscle contraction by palpating the patient's abdomen with the other hand. The clinician then provides the patient with verbal feedback regarding her or his ability to contract the desired muscle groups, that is, effective (or at least identifiable) pelvic muscle contraction with minimal abdominal muscle contraction. The second approach is to instruct the patient to try to interrupt her or his urinary stream; the patient with weak periurethral and pelvic floor muscles will probably be unable to interrupt the urinary stream effectively, but this maneuver helps her or him to identify accurately the muscle group to be exercised.[45,46] (The patient should be cautioned *not* to attempt to interrupt the urinary stream routinely but to use the urinary stream interruption test as a periodic check for progress in pelvic muscle contractility.)

Once the patient is able to isolate the pelvic floor muscle group consistently, the clinician establishes an individualized exercise program based on the patient's initial strength and endurance.[44,45]

(For example, a patient with a contractility score of 2 and an endurance of less than 2 seconds could be started on a program of 10 contractions 3 times daily, with an endurance goal of 3 seconds.) As the patient's contractility and endurance progress, the number of repetitions and the endurance goal can be increased. Some data suggest that exercise protocols emphasizing endurance are as effective as those emphasizing contractile strength. For example, Johnson and colleagues conducted a study comparing the effects of submaximal force contractions to near maximal force contractions; for each group, the goal was continually adjusted based on the subject's current contractile strength. Interestingly, both groups demonstrated significant improvement, with no significant differences between the groups; outcome measures included pelvic muscle recruitment and endurance, and frequency and severity of leakage (per self-report and pad weight testing).[47]

Although the goals of a pelvic muscle exercise program are clear, the specifics (that is, the optimal number of repetitions per day and optimal exercise technique) have yet to be established.[38] Currently, most clinicians recommend a target range of 30 to 45 repetitions per day. One common approach is to divide the total number of daily repetitions into 3 exercise sessions; the patient performs one set of exercises in the reclining position, one set while sitting, and one set while standing. There is also variation in terms of specific exercise instructions; some clinicians use an exercise approach that combines strengthening for both Type 1 and Type 2 fibers, whereas others have the patient exercise the Type 1 and Type 2 fibers separately.[2,38,42,43] With the combined approach, the patient is instructed to perform a maximal contraction of the pelvic floor muscles and to hold the contraction for as long as possible (or for the prescribed "endurance" period); the muscle is then relaxed for at least 10 seconds.[45] The theory behind this approach is that the fast-twitch muscle fibers are exercised by the maximal-contraction component of the program, whereas the slow-twitch fibers are exercised by the endurance component of the exercise.[43] When the Type 1 and Type 2 fibers are exercised separately, the fast-twitch exercise is a "quick flick, maximal intensity" contraction, whereas the slow-twitch exercise is a slow (possibly submaximal) contraction that is held for the prescribed period of time. With this approach, the patient is assigned a certain number of "quick flick" and a certain number of "slowly contract and hold" exercises for each exercise period (such as 5 to 10 of each 2 to 3 times daily).[42] Studies have demonstrated both subjective and objective improvement in patients who correctly perform pelvic muscle exercises, regardless of specific technique; however, additional research is clearly needed to define the optimal approach. One approach to an individualized and physiologic pelvic muscle exercise program is outlined in Box 4-1.

Other Approaches to Strengthening the Pelvic Floor Muscles

One of the greatest obstacles to pelvic muscle reeducation is the difficulty encountered by many patients in correctly identifying and isolating the pelvic floor muscles. Biofeedback has demonstrated

---

BOX 4-1   Graduated Strength Training: A Pelvic Muscle Exercise Program

Level 1. Beginning Muscle Identification
Goal. Short, fast contractions (flicks). Use only the pelvic muscles. Avoid bearing down or straining. Avoid contracting abdominal, thigh, or buttock muscles.
Prescription. 10 short contractions per set; 5 sets per day. Allow 30 seconds rest between each set.
Minimum time. 5 minutes daily for 5 days per week.

Level 2. Advanced Muscle Identification
Goal. Identify higher muscle levels. Contraction, performed as three progressively higher shorter flicks. Count 1, 2, 3 as each level is quickly contracted.
Prescription. 10 graded contractions per set; 5 sets per day.
Allow 30 seconds rest between each set.
Minimum time. 5 minutes daily for 5 days per week.

Level 3. Beginning Strength Training
Goal. With each contraction, move smoothly through all levels of muscle. Direct the force inward and upward. Hold each contraction 3 seconds at the top (work up to holding for 6 seconds). While holding, contract the muscle as hard as you can.
Prescription. 10 contractions per set; 3 sets per day.
Allow 10 seconds rest between contractions; allow 30 seconds rest between sets.
Minimum time. 10 minutes daily per 5 days per week.

Level 4. Advanced Strength Training (Do not begin until you can solidly hold each level 3 contraction for 6 seconds.)
Goal. With each contraction hold at the top for 5 seconds, and then relax to midlevel and hold at midlevel for 5 seconds as well. Concentrate on high-intensity, powerful contractions.
Prescription. 5 contractions per set; 3 sets per day.
Allow 10 seconds rest between contractions; allow 30 seconds rest between sets.
Minimum time. 10 minutes daily for 5 days per week.

Level 5. Maintenance
Goal. Continue active pelvic muscle exercise in ongoing self-care. Concentrate on becoming aware of contracting the pelvic muscles preparatory to sneezing, coughing, lifting, etc. until this becomes second nature. Maintain optimum strength through practicing highly skilled, hard contractions.
Prescription. 5 contractions per set; 1 or 2 sets per week or more as able to fit into your routine.
Allow 10 seconds rest between contractions.
Minimum time. 5 to 10 minutes per week.

Modified from Miller J, Sampselle CM: *Urol Nurs* 14:95, 1994. Reprinted with permission of the publisher, Jannetti Publications. Inc., East Helly Avenue, Box 56, Pitman, NJ 08071-0056.

efficacy and is the "treatment of choice" in these situations; however, biofeedback is not available in all settings. Alternative approaches to strengthening the pelvic muscles include exercises to strengthen the thigh muscles that insert onto the pelvic floor, that is, abduction against resistance (using an exercise band), adduction against resistance (using an exercise ball held between the thighs), and standing plies (the ballet maneuver). Some physical therapists have reported success with the use of these maneuvers to improve pelvic muscle strength, and these reports are consistent with anecdotal reports by patients that their incontinence improved with use of the "Thighmaster" and similar exercise protocols. However, to date, these reports are anecdotal; no controlled trials are yet available to verify or dispute these reports.

Instruction in the "Knack." Patients should be taught to voluntarily contract the pelvic muscles immediately before activities that cause a significant increase in abdominal pressure, such as coughing, sneezing, or lifting; this mimics the reflex contraction of the pelvic floor muscles demonstrated in continent women in response to cough (and missing in women with stress incontinence.)[40] This purposeful contraction of the pelvic muscles to offset increased abdominal pressure has been termed the "knack" and has been shown to reduce the number of incontinent episodes significantly.[38] Instruction in appropriate use of the pelvic muscles to prevent incontinence involves several stages: the patient is first taught how to isolate and contract the muscles, is then instructed to practice sustained contraction during routine activities such as talking, turning, and bending, and is finally taught to incorporate the knack into activities of daily living.[40]

Pelvic Muscle Exercises with Biofeedback. Biofeedback is frequently used to assist patients in learning to isolate and contract the pelvic muscles; this technology provides the patient with visual or auditory feedback regarding contraction of the desired muscle groups. Arnold Kegel developed the first vaginal perineometer for biofeedback treatment of urinary incontinence in the late 1940s.[48] This early biofeedback device consisted of a vaginal chamber attached to a manometer that measured pelvic muscle contractions and provided visual feedback.

Kegel's initial study of the effectiveness of biofeedback for stress incontinence demonstrated a 90% reduction in symptoms of urine loss.[48] Despite these promising results, no further studies were conducted until the late 1970s. Shepherd treated 11 community-dwelling women with genuine stress incontinence (incontinence secondary to urethral hypermobility); the treatment group received visual biofeedback, and 91% were cured or improved, as compared with 55% cured or improved in the control group, who did not receive visual reinforcement.[49] Since that time, numerous studies have been conducted comparing the benefits of biofeedback-assisted pelvic muscle exercise programs with exercise alone, with conflicting results. Some studies show superior outcomes in the biofeedback-assisted group, whereas other studies demonstrate comparable outcomes between the two groups.[38,50-53] It seems reasonable that biofeedback would improve outcomes among women who have difficulty identifying and isolating the pelvic muscles, but would provide no additive benefit to exercise alone for women who are able to identify and isolate these muscles effectively at the beginning of treatment. Payne suggested use of pelvic muscle exercises alone for women who are motivated and able to contract the pelvic muscles but demonstrate poor strength and biofeedback-assisted exercises for patients who have very limited ability to isolate and contract the muscles at baseline or limited motivation to complete a self-directed exercise program.[38,54]

Biofeedback equipment. Biofeedback equipment is chosen by the clinician on the basis of cost, ease of use, and intended application (that is, home versus office use). It is critical to choose equipment that supports the patient in learning to contract the pelvic muscles while maintaining relaxation of the abdominal muscles. To provide the patient with feedback on both of these muscle groups (abdominal and pelvic), it is essential to obtain equipment that has at least two biofeedback channels. Another consideration is the method used to "measure" pelvic muscle contractions; some systems use pressure-sensitive probes (either vaginal or anal), whereas others use electrodes (usually skin electrodes) to pick up the electrical signals generated by muscle contraction. The decision regarding selection is governed by clinician and patient preference; for example, some patients are much more comfortable using skin electrodes than intravaginal or intraanal probes. When possible, a multichannel system should be obtained; these systems provide channels for pressure biofeedback *and* for electromyographic (EMG) biofeedback regarding pelvic muscle contraction, in addition to the channel for measurement of abdominal muscle contraction. Multichannel systems are somewhat more expensive, but they can be very helpful in effectively managing patients with stress incontinence because they provide feedback regarding both the pelvic floor and the abdominal muscles.

One of the many biofeedback units available is shown in Fig. 4-3. This particular system is equipped to provide pressure biofeedback or EMG biofeedback; muscle activity can be monitored with vaginal or anal probes or with surface electrodes, depending on the clinician's and patient's preference. The system is also equipped to provide electrical stimulation. This system is available in "home trainer" units as well as office-based units; these home units permit patients to continue their biofeedback or electrical stimulation therapy at home.

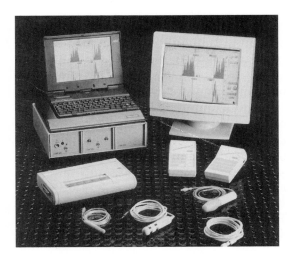

Fig. 4-3 Sample biofeedback equipment. (Courtesy of InCare Medical, Libertyville, Ill.)

Biofeedback procedure. Biofeedback therapy has no direct effect on pelvic muscle contractility or endurance; rather, it is a training technique that helps the patient learn to exercise the pelvic floor muscles effectively while relaxing the abdominal muscles. (The patient does the work!) It is therefore important to conduct biofeedback sessions in a quiet, comfortable environment that assists the patient to concentrate on the therapy.

As noted in the previous section, biofeedback should be conducted with a dual-channel or multichannel system that provides visual feedback regarding both abdominal muscle activity and pelvic muscle activity. Feedback regarding abdominal muscle contraction is provided by two active surface electrodes placed 1 inch apart just below the umbilicus; a ground electrode is placed on a convenient bony prominence.

As noted earlier, there are two approaches to providing feedback about pelvic muscle contraction: EMG feedback and pressure feedback. EMG biofeedback can be provided via sensor probes placed in the vagina or anorectum but is most commonly provided via active surface electrodes applied to the perianal skin at the 10 o'clock and 2 o'clock positions; the ground lead is then placed on a bony prominence (such as the iliac crest). Manometric (pressure) biofeedback is provided by pressure-sensitive probes placed in the patient's vagina or anorectum. The sensors (either EMG or pressure) are connected to transducers that produce a visual display of pelvic muscle activity on the computer monitor. The *advantage* to using pressure biofeedback is that the intravaginal or intraanal probe provides resistive pressure to pelvic muscle contraction; this provides sensory feedback to the patient regarding her (or his) success in contracting the pelvic muscles. The main *disadvantage* to pressure biofeedback is that the patient must purchase a personal vaginal or rectal probe, whereas the surface electrodes typically used for EMG biofeedback are disposable, convenient, and easily used in both office and home settings.

Before initiating biofeedback, the clinician should assess the patient's ability to identify, isolate, and contract the pelvic muscles; this is typically done during the pelvic or rectal examination, when the patient is instructed to contract the pelvic muscles around the examiner's fingers while relaxing the abdominal, thigh, and buttock muscles. These assessment data assist the clinician to individualize the biofeedback therapy appropriately, based on the patient's baseline performance. Typically, the first step in the biofeedback procedure is to have the patient relax her (or his) pelvic muscles while observing the visual "feedback" displayed on the computer screen. The patient is then instructed to contract the pelvic muscles (and to relax the abdominal muscles) while observing the visual display. The therapist coaches the patient in identifying the correct muscle group and in performing lifting and tightening contractions as opposed to pushing contractions. (For example, the therapist may remind the patient to "lift and tighten as if trying not to pass gas or trying to interrupt the urinary stream.")

Once the patient can correctly isolate and appropriately contract the pelvic muscles, the clinician programs the biofeedback equipment to provide an appropriate training session based on the patient's "baseline" function. Variables that the clinician can control include the height of the visual display (which may need to be augmented during the early stages of therapy, when the contractile force is minimal), the number of contractions to be performed during each session, and the length of the contracting (work) phase and of the relaxation (resting) phase. The goals are advanced as the patient gains control, strength, and endurance.

No absolute norms exist for biofeedback parameters; rather, the patient serves as her or his own control, and progress is measured against the patient's baseline values. There is also no agreement regarding the optimal number of training sessions; some clinicians advocate a limited number of office sessions (to assist the patient in learning to identify, isolate, and contract the appropriate muscles) followed by pelvic muscle exercises without biofeedback, whereas others recommend more extended training sessions and the use of home trainers to support compliance with therapy and to optimize each training session. More research is needed to resolve these issues; it is likely (and logical) that the optimal use of biofeedback will vary from patient to patient.

Pelvic Muscle Reeducation Using Vaginal Weight Cone Therapy. Vaginal weight cone therapy was introduced by Plevnik as a means of evaluating and strengthening the pelvic floor muscles.[55] Intravaginal weights are available in sets of five smooth cones that range in weight from 20 g (0.7 oz) to 70 g (2.5 oz). Each has a silicone removal cord. The patient is taught to insert one of the weights into the vagina and to attempt to retain the weight for approximately 15 minutes while ambulating normally. The weights function by providing sensory feedback; that is, the patient senses when the weight begins to slip out of the vagina and is thus reminded to contract the pelvic muscles. In addition, it is believed that the presence and weight of the cone may stimulate reflex contraction of the pelvic muscles.

The patient is instructed to begin with the lightest cone and to graduate to heavier and heavier cones until she finds a cone that is difficult to retain; the best starting cone is one that she can initially retain for only 1 minute. The patient is instructed to insert this cone twice daily for 15 minutes; as her muscles become stronger and she gains the ability to retain the cone, she should move on to a heavier weight. It should be emphasized that vaginal cones should not be inserted during menses, and the patient must have sufficient muscle strength to retain at least the lightest cone for brief periods of time for this therapy to be effective.

Studies on vaginal weight therapy have yielded variable data regarding cure and improvement rates. Peattie and colleagues found that 43% of the women studied demonstrated increased pelvic muscle strength and satisfaction with treatment.[56,57] Herbison and colleagues recently conducted a systematic review of controlled trials involving vaginal cones, some of which compared the effects of cone therapy with no treatment and some of which compared cone therapy with other treatment modalities. Their review included 15 studies and 1126 subjects, 466 of whom received cone therapy. The review was complicated by small studies, high dropout rates, and variable outcomes measures. The reviewers concluded that data currently available support cone therapy as superior to no treatment for women with stress incontinence; the data available are inconclusive in terms of differences in outcomes for women treated with cone therapy and those treated with pelvic floor muscle exercises or electrical stimulation. These findings support the need for further research; until additional data are obtained, cone therapy should be presented to women as one possible treatment option.[58]

Electrical Stimulation. Huffman and colleagues introduced electrical stimulation for the treatment of urinary incontinence,[59] and it has now been used for the treatment of multiple lower urinary tract disorders, including stress urinary incontinence, urge incontinence, mixed stress-urge incontinence, urgency and frequency, and painful bladder syndrome. Its use is based on the following effects of stimulation with nonimplanted electrodes: the electrical impulses activate afferent pudendal nerve fibers; this causes reflex activation of sympathetic and pudendal efferent fibers; the end results are contraction of the smooth and striated muscles in the urethral and pelvic floor and reflex inhibition of the detrusor muscle. Because electrical stimulation "works" by activating sacral autonomic and somatic nerve pathways, therapeutic response depends on intact nerve pathways between the sacral cord and the pelvic floor.[60]

The most common form of electrical stimulation for stress incontinence involves delivery of a high-intensity stimulus (the maximum stimulus tolerated without pain) over short periods of time, typically 15- to 30-minute sessions one to three times per week. Electrical stimulation therapy employs a short burst of stimulation alternated with rest; the ratio of stimulation time to rest time is called the "duty cycle" and is typically in the range of 1:2. The stimulus can be delivered via vaginal or anal probes or via surface electrodes.

The goal of electrical stimulation therapy for the patient with stress incontinence is to improve the function of the pelvic floor and sphincter muscles, including both smooth and striated muscle fibers and both fast-twitch and slow-twitch fibers. Most nerve fibers supplying the urethral musculature operate at a relatively high frequency of 50 to 100 Hz; therefore, high frequencies (such as 50 Hz) are typically used for treatment of stress incontinence.[61] (Low frequencies, that is, approximately 10 to 20 Hz,

are typically used for treatment of detrusor instability and urge incontinence; patients with mixed stress-urge incontinence may benefit from stimulation in the range of 20 to 50 Hz.)

Studies comparing pelvic floor electrical stimulation (PFES) with sham PFES for the treatment of stress incontinence have demonstrated better outcomes with PFES. However, studies comparing PFES with pelvic muscle exercise training have suggested either comparable results or superior outcomes with pelvic muscle exercises.[46] In a recent randomized controlled study, Goode and colleagues compared the results of an 8-week protocol involving behavioral therapy plus electrical stimulation with behavioral therapy alone; the behavioral therapy program included biofeedback-assisted pelvic muscle exercises, home exercises, instruction in bladder control strategies, and self-monitoring via bladder diaries. In addition, women in the electrical stimulation group were provided with a home PFES unit and instructed to use the unit for 15 minutes every other day. (On alternate days, patients were instructed to perform three sessions of pelvic muscle exercises.) The PFES units were programmed to provide biphasic pulses at a frequency of 20 Hz; intensity was adjusted by the patient to a maximum of 100 mA. The control group in this study received a self-help booklet that contained guidelines for a "do-it-yourself" behavioral treatment program. Interestingly, all three groups demonstrated a marked reduction in incontinent episodes, but behavioral therapy and behavioral therapy plus PFES were significantly more effective than the self-help booklet (71.9% reduction for behavioral therapy plus PFES, 68.6% reduction for behavioral therapy alone, and 52.5% reduction with the self-help booklet). Although no significant difference was reported between the two treatment groups in the primary outcome measure (reduction in incontinent episodes), women who received PFES in addition to behavioral therapy reported significantly greater *perceived progress* and satisfaction with care.[46] Thus, this study suggests that there is no objective difference in outcomes but there *is* a subjective difference when PFES is added to behavioral therapy programs. Jeyaseelan and Oldham suggested that the disappointing results provided by PFES in terms of objective outcomes may relate to the type of electrical frequency used; they contended that the uniform frequencies typically used in human studies have been shown to be ineffective in animal studies, and they suggested that different patterns of stimulation may be more effective in building strength and endurance without causing fatigue.[62] It is clear that more research is needed to clarify the role of PFES in the treatment of stress incontinence.

Extracorporeal Magnetic Innervation Therapy. The newest tool for pelvic muscle strengthening is extracorporeal electromagnetic therapy. The US Food and Drug Administration (FDA) has recently approved the NeoControl chair (Neotonus, Marietta, Ga.), which incorporates a powerful electromagnet into the seat; the magnet is controlled by an external power source. When the magnet is activated, it induces electrical depolarization of the nerves and muscles within the magnetic field (the pelvic floor), thus producing a strong contraction of the pelvic muscles.[63] One advantage of this therapy is its noninvasive nature; the patient simply sits, fully clothed, in the chair. Preliminary studies, based on a 6-week course of treatment with two treatments per week, demonstrated a significant reduction in the number of incontinent episodes, pad use, and volume of urine lost (as measured by pad-weight testing) but no significant change in urodynamic parameters.[63,64]

Pharmacologic Therapy

Pharmacologic agents for stress incontinence are most commonly used as adjuncts to behavioral therapy; the types of medications most often prescribed are alpha-adrenergic agonists, tricyclic antidepressants, and estrogens. Currently, a new drug is being evaluated for management of stress incontinence, a combined serotonin-norepinephrine reuptake inhibitor.

Alpha–Adrenergic Agonists. Smooth muscle tone within the proximal portion of the urethra and the bladder neck is maintained primarily by sympathetic stimulation via the alpha-adrenergic receptors; stimulation of these receptors increases smooth muscle tone, which increases urethral resistance (as measured by maximum urethral pressure and

urethral closure pressure).[17] This effect may be enhanced by concurrent use of topical estrogen.[4] The most commonly used alpha-adrenergic agonist is pseudoephedrine, which stimulates the alpha-adrenergic receptors within the proximal portion of the urethra and the bladder neck; the results are increased urethral tone and reduced risk for stress incontinence.

Alpha-adrenergic agonists are associated with numerous side effects, such as weakness, insomnia, drowsiness, anxiety, and elevated blood pressure. The clinician should be alert to the fact that women with stress incontinence are at greatest risk for leakage during episodes of strenuous activity, such as aerobic exercise; thus, any pharmacologic agent designed to reduce episodes of stress incontinence is most likely to be taken just before planned "high risk" activities. Because exercise is associated with elevated heart rate and blood pressure, and given that alpha-adrenergic agonists also cause these effects, the combined effects of the activity and the medication could be clinically significant. Therefore, these agents should be used with extreme caution, especially in elderly patients and those with hypertension, cardiovascular disease, or hyperthyroidism.[2,4]

Tricyclic Antidepressants. Tricyclic antidepressants have both anticholinergic and alpha-adrenergic agonist activity; they increase smooth muscle tone within the bladder neck and proximal portion of the urethra, thereby increasing urethral resistance. Imipramine (Tofranil) is a commonly used drug that has both alpha-adrenergic stimulating and anticholinergic effects; it therefore increases tone within the urethra and bladder neck while simultaneously reducing detrusor contractility. This dual effect makes imipramine particularly useful in the treatment of patients with mixed stress-urge incontinence.[4]

Tricyclic antidepressants cause numerous adverse effects: nausea, insomnia, weakness, hypotension and fatigue, dry mouth, ataxia, hallucinations, and tachycardia. The dose of the drug should therefore be titrated based on patient response and the occurrence of side effects; elderly patients should be monitored especially carefully for changes in mental function or other adverse effects.[4]

Estrogen. The female urethra and trigone of the bladder are richly supplied with estrogen receptors, and estrogenic influences on the urethral mucosa and the submucosal vasculature contribute significantly to mucosal thickness and coaptation and to engorgement of the underlying blood vessels.[2,65,66] In addition to these primary effects on the urogenital tissues, estrogen increases the sensitivity of the proximal portion of the urethra and bladder neck to alpha-adrenergic stimulation, which further increases urethral resistance.[65,66] In the premenopausal woman, estrogenic effects account for 30% of urethral resistance.[65] The decline in circulating estrogens after menopause produces urogenital atrophy, which may produce irritative symptoms such as dysuria, urgency, frequency, and nocturnal incontinence (urge incontinence) as well as reduced urethral resistance and stress incontinence.[4,65,66] Randomized trials involving *systemic* hormone replacement have demonstrated no benefit in the treatment of stress incontinence[4,67]; however, topical estrogen therapy may be of benefit (in combination with behavioral therapy) for postmenopausal women with stress, urge, or mixed incontinence who have atrophic changes on pelvic examination and no contraindications to estrogen.[2] *Contraindications* include undiagnosed vaginal bleeding, breast cancer or other estrogen-dependent malignancy, thromboembolic disease, and acute liver disease.[66]

Topical application of estrogen is the route of choice for treatment of urogenital atrophy; topical agents provide greater local absorption but significantly less systemic absorption.[65] Most clinicians recommend an initial course of intravaginal cream 2 to 4 g administered nightly for 1 to 2 weeks, or 1 g every other night for 1 month followed by a maintenance regimen of 0.5 to 1 g 2 or 3 times a week. For women with atrophic urethritis but no symptomatic vaginitis, a pea-sized amount of estrogen cream can be applied directly to the periurethral tissues (as opposed to an applicator of cream delivered intravaginally); this approach reverses atrophic urethritis while minimizing absorption and significantly reducing the cost of therapy. Another option, which is particularly beneficial in the long-term care setting, is the ESTring (Pharmacia Upjohn); this is a silicone intravaginal ring that delivers a daily dose of 8.0 mcg of 17 beta-estradiol for 90 days.[2,61,65]

Duloxetine. Duloxetine is a new drug under investigation by the FDA for the treatment of stress incontinence; it acts as a balanced norepinephrine and serotononin reuptake inhibitor.[1] As noted earlier in this chapter, these neurotransmitters are important mediators for the smooth and striated muscles within the urethra; thus, duloxetine promotes enhanced tone and contractility of the sphincter and increases urethral closure pressure.[1,4,68,69] In double-blind, randomized, placebo-controlled trials, duloxetine demonstrated a dose-dependent reduction in frequency of incontinent episodes among women aged 18 to 65 years who had stress incontinence; reduction in incontinent episodes was 41% for placebo, 54% for duloxetine 20 mg/day, 59% for duloxetine 40 mg/day, and 64% for duloxetine 80 mg/day. (Results were even more impressive among a subset of women with more severe stress incontinence; the duloxetine-treated group had a 49% to 64% reduction in incontinent episodes as opposed to a 30% reduction in the placebo group.) Nausea was the most common reason for discontinuation of the drug; in Phase III trials, nausea occurred in 62% of the subjects but was usually mild and transient. There were no clinically severe adverse effects.[1,4]

Surgical Management

Surgical intervention is frequently recommended as initial therapy for patients with coexisting pelvic organ prolapse, patients with loss of anatomic support and significant leakage, or patients with severe sphincter weakness resulting from muscle damage or denervation. In contrast, patients with urethral hypermobility uncomplicated by prolapse and patients with pelvic muscle weakness resulting in mild to moderate leakage *may* elect surgery as initial intervention or may begin with behavioral therapy and resort to surgery only if conservative measures prove ineffective. The type of procedure selected is determined by the specific etiologic factors, that is, pelvic muscle weakness and urethral hypermobility versus sphincter incompetence caused by muscle damage or denervation versus pelvic organ prolapse and loss of anatomic support. All procedures for stress incontinence are designed to increase urethral resistance, but the specific procedures have different mechanisms of action and different effects on bladder and sphincter function; for example, procedures designed to stabilize a hypermobile urethra may actually cause worsening of incontinence in the patient with coexisting sphincteric incompetence. It is therefore critical for any patient contemplating surgical intervention to have a complete workup, including physical examination, CMG with urethral pressure profile (to determine the contractility and stability of the bladder and the adequacy of intrinsic urethral resistance), and ultrasonography or cystoscopy. These data facilitate selection of the most appropriate surgical procedure.

Procedures to Correct Urethral Hypermobility. The objective of surgical intervention for the patient whose stress incontinence is primarily the result of urethral hypermobility is to improve anatomic support for the sphincter unit without creating obstruction. The two procedures most commonly used for these patients are retropubic colposuspension procedures and midurethral sling procedures. In the past, needle suspensions and anterior vaginal repairs were also used; however, these procedures are no longer recommended because of very poor long-term outcomes and, in the case of needle suspensions, higher complication rates.[70,71] Anterior vaginal repair *is*, of course, indicated for the patient with an anterior vaginal defect and cystocele, but it is not recommended for management of stress incontinence caused by urethral hypermobility.

Retropubic suspension. The goal of retropubic colposuspension procedures is to elevate and stabilize the tissues surrounding the bladder neck and proximal urethra in a retropubic and intraabdominal position; stabilization prevents urethral descent and promotes compression of the urethra against the underlying (suburethral) tissues. This type of procedure is *not* recommended for patients with sphincter damage or denervation because it provides no urethral compression and no baseline increase in urethral resistance.

The two most commonly known of these procedures are the Burch and the Marshall-Marchetti-Krantz; the Burch procedure is the "most studied" and most commonly performed

retropubic suspension.[70,72-75] In 33 trials involving 2403 women, reported cure rates for retropubic suspension procedures ranged from 69% to 88%; these results are durable, as evidenced by a 5-year cure rate of approximately 70%.[72] Currently, retropubic colposuspensions are considered *the most effective* procedure for stress incontinence resulting from urethral hypermobility; although initial cure rates for the newer midurethral sling procedures are comparable, the long-term results are not yet known. One major advance in the area of retropubic colposuspensions is the development of a laporoscopic approach. Following a systematic review of studies comparing the laparoscopic with the open approach, Moehrer and colleagues reported that the laparoscopic approach was associated with a lower complication rate, and there was no statistically significant difference in outcomes (although the evidence did *suggest* better outcomes with the open approach); these investigators concluded that more data are needed before any recommendations can be made.[74] The most common complication of retropubic suspensions is transient urinary retention, which typically resolves within about 7 days.[72,75]

Midurethral sling procedures. Midurethral slings are the newest approach to surgical correction of stress incontinence; they have rapidly gained popularity, as evidenced by the fact that this technique is now the most common surgical approach to management of stress incontinence *worldwide*. This category includes a number of minimally invasive procedures designed to stabilize and support the urethra via placement of a tension-free sling at the midurethra; the best known of these procedures are the tension-free vaginal tape and the transobturator tape procedures. These procedures "work" by recreating the effects of the pubourethral ligament; a strip of polypropylene mesh tape is placed at the level of the midurethra via a transvaginal or similar approach. The tissue reaction to the tape strip stimulates collagen production along the tape, and this newly synthesized collagen acts to "secure and fix" the midurethra to the pubic bone. This does not stabilize the proximal urethra and does not "correct" urethral hypermobility in the classic sense; rather, it is theorized that midurethral stabilization may limit downward descent of the urethra and may cause "kinking" of the urethra at the point of stabilization.[16,70,75-77] This procedure is currently used and recommended for women with urethral hypermobility and normal pelvic muscle/sphincter contractility and also for women with a combination of urethral hypermobility and some degree of sphincteric incompetence. Most clinicians and investigators recommend a compressive sling for patients with significant urethral incompetence (suburethral sling as described below).[18]

Early results of these procedures are very impressive; a systematic review comparing the tension-free vaginal tape procedure to laporoscopic and open retropubic suspensions, traditional suburethral slings, and urethral bulking agents found that the tension-free tape procedure produced cure rates of 83-87%, which are comparable to those provided by retropubic colposuspension and traditional slings and superior to those reported for bulking agents.[70] These results have led some investigators to consider that these procedures may become the new "gold standard" for management of urethral hypermobility with or without some degree of sphincteric incompetence.[18] However, it must be noted that we lack randomized control trials on long-term results. Some early studies on patients 5 years following tension-free vaginal tape report "success" rates of 85% with an additional 10% of patients reporting improvement, but these are not randomized controlled trials.[75] Thus, definitive recommendations regarding the role of these procedures must await further studies.[16]

The most common reported complication for tension-free midurethral slings is transient retention. There are also reports of serious complications, the most common of which is bladder perforation[16,78]; some authors suggest that the incidence of bladder perforation will probably diminish as surgeons gain experience with the surgical technique. Modifications in approach, such as the transobturator approach, may also reduce the incidence of bladder injury.[76]

Procedures to Correct Sphincteric Incompetence (Intrinsic Sphincter Deficiency). Surgical options for the management of ISD include periurethral bulking injections, suburethral sling procedures, and artificial urinary sphincter implantation. Periurethral bulking injections are

sometimes recommended as first-line treatment for women with ISD who have no coexisting hypermobility; however, the ideal bulking agent has not yet been developed, and these procedures do not typically provide long-term benefit. Sling procedures may also be used as first-line therapy for ISD and are appropriate for women who have ISD with coexisting hypermobility. Artificial urinary sphincters are recommended only for patients with severe ISD that is unresponsive to other surgical interventions.

Periurethral bulking injections. Periurethral bulking procedures are one option for women with a noncontractile sphincter muscle and minimal urethral resistance resulting from sphincter damage or denervation; some clinicians also recommend these procedures for management of incontinence caused by urethral hypermobility.[79] These procedures are designed to improve urethral resistance by creating urethral "cushions" that reduce the size of the urethral lumen. Several different agents have been used for periurethral bulking; glutaraldehyde cross-linked collagen (Contigen) and pyrolytic carbon-coated zirconium oxide beads (Durasphere) are the agents most commonly used in the United States. Unfortunately, none of the currently available agents meet the criteria for an ideal agent: nonimmunogenic, hypoallergenic, biocompatible, and durable. Contigen is degraded within 2 years following injection, and there are limited long-term data regarding Durasphere. In general, 50% to 70% of patients treated with bulking agents report "significant improvement," but only 30% to 50% are dry. In addition, success rates drop to 26% to 65% 2 years following treatment.[20,79] Positive aspects of this treatment are that it can usually be done as an outpatient procedure and there are usually no serious complications. Based on a systematic review of the currently available research, Pickard and colleagues stated that current evidence is insufficient to recommend injection therapy as an alternative to an open surgical procedure unless the patient is not a surgical candidate.[80]

Sling procedures. Sling procedures are so named because they involve the placement of strips of autologous fascia, allografts, xenografts, or synthetic material underneath the urethra; the strips are then anchored to retropubic or abdominal structures to elevate the urethra (the sling effect). The goal is to restore sufficient urethral resistance to prevent leakage without creating obstruction; slings "work" partly by restoring the normal anatomic position of the proximal urethra and partly by compressing the urethra sufficiently to provide resistance "at rest."[18,20] Outcomes data support slings as being both effective and durable; the overall reported "success" rates for these procedures range from 85% to 97%, and continence rates at 10 years after sling procedures are comparable to continence rates at 1 year after these procedures. Although "success" is defined differently by different investigators, the mean continence rate for the suburethral sling is generally considered to be about 94%.[18,20,75] The most common adverse effect of the sling procedure is acute transient retention; de novo urgency and persistent retention do occur but are uncommon.

Artificial urinary sphincter. The first artificial urinary sphincter was introduced in 1947[81]; the device currently in use is the American Medical Systems (AMS) 800 artificial sphincter by American Medical Systems. This device is constructed of a wear-resistant, biocompatible, silicone elastomer and consists of three components connected by special kink-resistant color-coded silicone tubing: a soft, pliable, dip-coated silicone cuff placed around the urethra or bladder neck, a pressure-regulating balloon (reservoir) placed into the abdominal cavity, and a pump placed into the scrotum or labia. When the cuff is inflated, it mechanically compresses the urethra to prevent leakage; the patient uses the pump to deflate the cuff for voiding or catheterization. (The fluid is displaced into the pressure-regulating balloon.) The fluid then slowly flows back into the cuff; a flow resistor within the pump acts to slow cuff-refill time sufficiently to permit adequate time for voiding or catheterization. A deactivation button can be engaged to prevent cuff refill, that is, to maintain cuff deflation. Fig. 4-4 illustrates the AMS 800 prosthesis with the artificial sphincter, pump, and deactivation button.

Postoperative complications include infection, erosion, and mechanical malfunction. Early complications are usually caused by urethral or bladder injury during implantation of the device, whereas

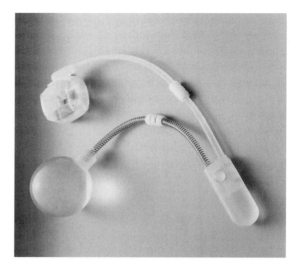

Fig. 4-4 Artificial urinary sphincter. (Courtesy of American Medical Systems, Inc, Minnetonka, Minn.)

delayed complications relate to device malfunction, cuff-induced atrophy, incomplete urethral compression, or urethral erosion.[82] Improvements in the device have resulted in a significant reduction in mechanical failures and improved long-term outcomes.[83] Artificial sphincters are most commonly used for patients with ISD after prostatectomy.[83]

Devices Used in the Management of Stress Incontinence

Patients with stress incontinence may benefit from the use of devices to reduce or prevent urinary leakage; typically devices are used as an alternative to absorptive products and in conjunction with therapies designed to correct the underlying problem. Currently available devices for women include a urethral insert and a wide variety of pessaries.

Urethral Occlusion Insert. The first urethral occlusion insert was approved by the FDA in July 1996 (Reliance, UroMed, Inc., Needham, Mass.). This device was a 14-French soft balloon-tipped catheter that was inserted into the urethra; after insertion, the balloon was inflated to maintain device position. The Reliance insert prevented leakage by passively occluding the bladder neck and urethra. Although the device was found to be effective, there was a high discontinuation rate related to insertion and handling difficulties, discomfort (foreign body sensation) when the device was in place, and recurrent urinary tract infection.[61]

The Femsoft urethral plug (Rochester Medical, Rochester, Minn.) is a urethral insert that works on the same principles as the Reliance device; the insert prevents leakage by passively occluding the urethra and bladder neck (Fig. 4-5). However, the Femsoft device is constructed of silicone and is extremely soft, which is thought to be the basis for improved patient tolerance. A recent multicenter study evaluated the long-term results for the Femsoft device; outcome measures included pad weight tests, voiding diaries, quality of life measures, and satisfaction questionnaires. Results showed both device efficacy and patient satisfaction; there were significant reductions in incontinence episodes and volume of urine loss per pad weight testing, and 93% of the subjects were "dry" at 12 months (by pad weight testing). In addition, study participants reported that the device was easy to use and comfortable; there were significant improvements in quality of life scores. Only minor adverse effects were reported, and these required minimal or no treatment. The investigators concluded that the device should be considered a valid option for the treatment of stress incontinence in women.[84]

Vaginal Pessaries. Pessaries are intravaginal devices commonly used for the nonsurgical management of pelvic organ prolapse. Pessaries can also be used to support the urethrovesical junction in a more anatomic position, thereby reducing stress incontinence.[85,86] Pessaries are available in a variety of forms and sizes; the most commonly used pessaries are the ring and the donut, but there are many other varieties (Fig. 4-6). Pessaries must be selected and sized for the individual patient based on the patient's particular problem, such as presence or absence of cystocele or rectocele and presence and severity of prolapse. Pessary fitting involves "trial and error"; the clinician estimates width and length of the vaginal vault via digital exam, inserts a trial pessary of the estimated size, evaluates fit (by having the patient bear down and ambulate and then checking for dislodgement, and by questioning the patient regarding discomfort), and then makes adjustments as necessary. An appropriately fitted pessary should not cause any discomfort, should not interfere with urination or defecation, should not damage the vaginal walls, and should reduce the symptoms for which it was placed.[85,86] Most clinicians have patients return within 48 hours following pessary fitting for repeat evaluation; this precaution permits early detection of any problems such as damage to the vaginal mucosa. It is essential to assess for atrophic vaginitis before pessary placement and to delay pessary placement until the tissues are well estrogenized; estrogen improves the integrity of the vaginal wall and reduces the potential for irritation, ulceration, or infection.[85]

Patients who are capable of self-care are instructed in routine removal, cleansing, and replacement of the pessary; patients who are unable to do this themselves are scheduled for routine follow-up in the office or home on a monthly basis.[85,86]

SUMMARY

Stress urinary incontinence is extremely common among women and may also occur in men after prostatectomy. The leakage associated with stress incontinence occurs during activities that cause increased abdominal pressure and is the result of compromised sphincter function; the most common etiologic factors are pelvic muscle weakness/loss of support for the proximal urethra (urethral hypermobility) and damage or denervation affecting the

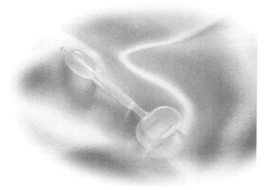

Fig. 4-5 FemSoft Urethral Insert. (Courtesy of Rochester Medical, Rochester, Minn.)

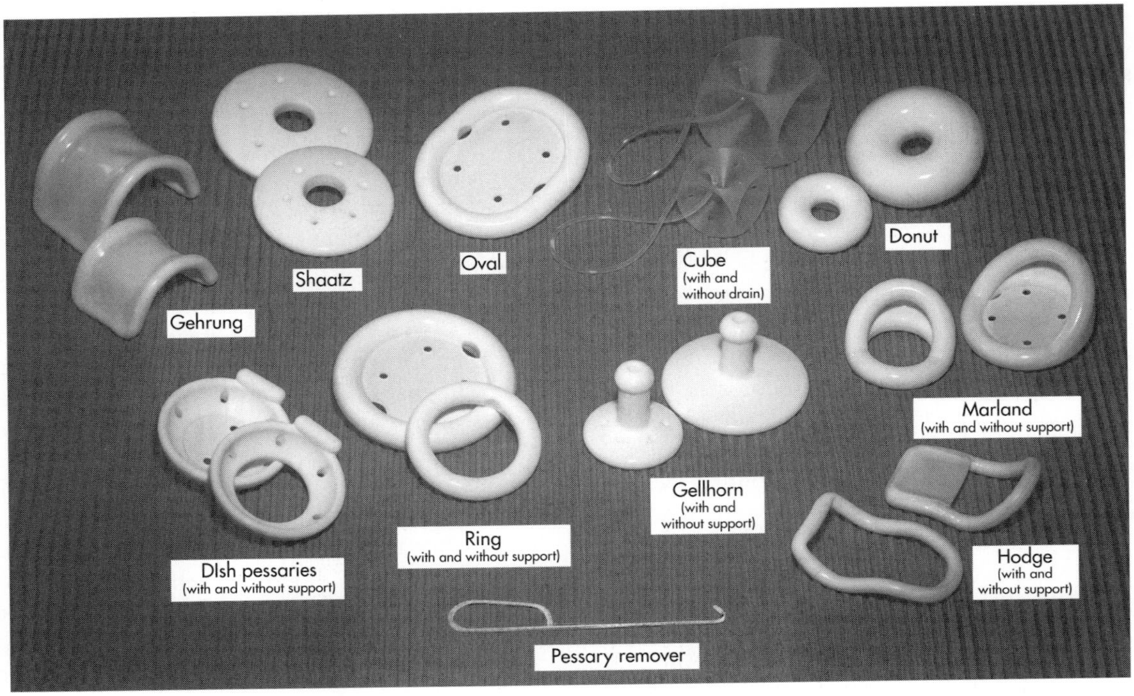

Fig. 4-6 Various types of vaginal pessaries. (Courtesy of Mentor, Santa Barbara, Calif.)

sphincter muscles. Effective management depends on the specific etiologic factors, the severity of the leakage, and patient preference. In most situations, the leakage is mild to moderate, and behavioral therapies are typically considered first-line interventions for these patients. Behavioral therapies are designed to reduce bladder pressures and to increase urethral resistance via strategies such as fluid management, timed voiding, pelvic muscle exercises, and volitional contraction of the pelvic floor muscles during activities that cause a sudden increase in abdominal pressure. Pharmacologic agents may also be of benefit; topical estrogen can be used to correct atrophic urethritis, and a serotonin-norepinephrine reuptake inhibitor (duloxetine) may soon be prescribed for treatment of stress incontinence. In addition, several surgical options exist; surgery is particularly appropriate for the patient with coexisting pelvic organ prolapse or total loss of sphincter function resulting from denervation, and new minimally invasive procedures (such as the

tension free midurethral sling) provide excellent results for the patient with leakage caused by urethral hypermobility. Finally, patients may benefit from the adjunctive use of devices to reduce or eliminate urinary leakage.

SELF-ASSESSMENT EXERCISE

1. Explain the following statement: "Incontinence caused by urethral hypermobility occurs only in women, but incontinence caused by intrinsic sphincter weakness may occur in either women or men."

2. Identify the relevance of each of the following in the assessment of a woman with stress incontinence:
   a. Bladder chart
   b. Pad-weight testing
   c. Pelvic exam in women
   d. Anal wink and bulbocavernosus reflex

e. Cystometrogram/videourodynamics

f. Urethral pressure profile

g. Leak point pressure

h. Ultrasound

3. Outline guidelines for a pelvic muscle exercise program *without* biofeedback, to include criteria for patient selection.

4. Explain how biofeedback can facilitate pelvic muscle reeducation.

5. Explain the role of electrical stimulation and magnetic therapy in the treatment of stress incontinence.

6. Identify indications and options for surgical intervention in the management of stress incontinence.

7. Explain why most clinicians consider urodynamic studies to be a critical component of the workup for a patient considering surgical intervention.

8. Explain the rationale for use of the following pharmacologic agents in the treatment of stress incontinence: topical estrogen; duloxetine.

9. List devices that may be recommended to women as adjunctive therapy to reduce or eliminate urinary leakage.

REFERENCES

1. Fraser MO, Chancellor MB: Neural control of the urethra and development of pharmacotherapy for stress urinary incontinence, *BJU Int* 91(8):743-748, 2003.
2. Newman D: Stress urinary incontinence in women: involuntary urine leakage during physical exertion affects countless women, *Am J Nurs* 103(8):46-55, 2003.
3. Ashton-Miller J, Howard D, DeLancey J: The functional anatomy of the female pelvic floor and stress continence control system, *Scand J Urol Nephrol Suppl* 207:1-7, 2001.
4. Huggins M, Bhatia N, Ostergard D: Urinary incontinence: newer pharmacotherapeutic trends, *Curr Opin Obstet Gynecol* 15(5):419-427, 2003.
5. Greydanus D, Patel D: The female athlete before and beyond puberty, *Pediatr Clin North Am* 49:553-580, 2002.
6. Cannon T, Damaser M: Pathophysiology of the lower urinary tract: continence and incontinence, *Clin Obstet Gynecol* 47(1):28-35, 2004.
7. Peeker I, Peeker R: Early diagnosis and treatment of genuine stress urinary incontinence in women after pregnancy: midwives as detectives, *J Midwifery Womens Health* 48(1):60-66, 2003.
8. Zullo MA, Manci N, Angoli R, et al: Vesical dysfunctions after radical hysterectomy for cervical cancer: a critical review, *Crit Rev Oncol Hematol* 48(3):287-293, 2003.
9. Manning J, Korda A, Benness C, Solomon M: The association of obstructive defecation, lower urinary tract dysfunction, and the benign joint hypermobility syndrome: a case-control study, *Int Urogynecol J* 14(2): 128-132, 2003.
10. Cummings JM, Rodning LB: Urinary stress incontinence among obese women: review of pathophysiology and therapy, *Int Urogynecol J* 11(1):41-44, 2000.
11. Dallosso H, McGrother C, Matthews R, et al: The association of diet and other lifestyle factors with overactive bladder and stress incontinence: a longitudinal study in women, *BJU Int* 92(1):69-77, 2003.
12. Romanzi L: Management of the urethral outlet in patients with severe prolapse, *Curr Opin Urol* 12(4):339-344, 2002.
13. Betson LH, Siddiqui G, Bhatia N. Intrinsic urethral sphincter deficiency: critical analysis of various diagnostic modalities. Current opinion in *Obstetrics and Gynecolgy* 15(5):411-417, 2003.
14. Duong TH, Korn AP: A comparison of urinary incontinence among African-American, Asian, Hispanic, and white women, *Am J Obstet Gynecol* 184(6):1083-1086, 2001.
15. Plzak L, Staskin D: Genuine stress incontinence: theories of etiology and surgical correction, *Urol Clin North Am* 29:527-535, 2002.
16. Boustead GB: The tension-free vaginal tape for treating female stress urinary incontinence, *BJU Int* 89(7): 687-693, 2002.
17. Sampselle C, DeLancey J: Anatomy of female continence, *J Wound Ostomy Continence Nurs* 25:63-74, 1998.
18. Bemelmans B, Chapple C: Are slings now the gold standard treatment for the management of female urinary stress incontinence and if so which technique? *Curr Opin Urol* 13(4):301-307, 2003.
19. Sullivan M, Yalla S: Physiology of female micturition, *Urol Clin North Am* 29:499-514, 2002.
20. Wilson T, Lemack G, Zimmern P: Management of intrinsic sphincteric deficiency in women, *J Urol* 169(5): 1662-1669, 2003.
21. Diokno AC, Wells TJ, Brink CA: Urinary incontinence in elderly women: urodynamic evaluation, *J Am Geriatr Soc* 35: 940-946, 1987.
22. Jensen JK, Nielsen R, Ostergard D: The role of the patient history in the diagnosis of urinary incontinence, *Obstet Gynecol* 85(5): 904-909, 1994.
23. Harvey M, Versi E: Predictive value of clinical evaluation of stress urinary incontinence: a summary of the published literature, *Int Urogynecol J* 12(1):31-37, 2001.
24. Flisser A, Blaivas J: Evaluating incontinence in women, *Urol Clin North Am* 29:515-526, 2002.
25. Sampselle C, Brink C, Wells T: Digital measurement of pelvic muscle strength in childbearing women, *Nurs Res* 38:134-138, 1989.
26. Folstein M, Folstein S, McHugh P: Mini-mental state: a practical method for grading the cognitive state of

patients for the clinician, *J Psychiatr Res* 12:189-198, 1975.

27. Fantl J, Newman D, Colling J, et al: *Urinary incontinence in adults: acute and chronic management.* Clinical practice guidelines no. 2, Rockville, Md, 1996 update, US Department of Health and Human Services, Public Health Service, Agency for Health Care Policy and Research.

28. Wyman J, Choi S, Harkins S, et al: The urinary diary in evaluation of urinary incontinent women: a test-retest analysis, *Obstet Gynecol* 71(6):812-817, 1988.

29. Nygaard I, Holcomb R: Reproducibility of the seven-day voiding diary in women with stress urinary incontinence, *Int Urogynecol J* 11:15-17, 2000.

30. Ouslander J, Simmons S, Tuico E, et al: Use of a portable ultrasound device to measure postvoid residual volume among incontinent nursing home residents, *J Am Geriatr Soc* 42(11):1189-1192, 1994.

31. Ouslander J, Leach G, Staskin D: Simplified tests of lower urinary tract function in evaluation of geriatric urinary incontinence, *J Am Geriatr Soc* 37(8):706-714, 1989.

32. Kolton D: *The fundamentals of female urodynamic study interpretation.* MedAmicus, 1997, Minneapolis, Minn.

33. Miller J, Kasper C, Sampselle C: Review of muscle physiology with application to pelvic muscle exercise, *Urol Nurs* 14(3):92-97, 1994.

34. Weber A: Is urethral pressure profilometry a useful diagnostic test for stress urinary incontinence? *Obstet Gynecol Surv* 56(11):720-735, 2001.

35. Weber A: Leak point pressure measurements and stress urinary incontinence, *Curr Womens Health Rep* 1(1):45-52, 2001.

36. Dietz HP: Ultrasound imaging of the pelvic floor: Part II: Three-dimensional or volume imaging, *Ultrasound in Obstetrics and Gynecolgy* 23(6):616-625, 2004.

37. Tunn R, Petri E: Introital and transvaginal ultrasound as the main tool in assessment of urogenital and pelvic floor dysfunction; and imaging panel and practical approach. *Ultrasound in Obstetrics and Gynecology*, 22(2):205-213, 2003.

38. Gormley EA: Biofeedback and behavioral therapy for the management of female urinary incontinence, *Urol Clin North Am* 29:551-557, 2002.

39. Siu LS, Chang AM, Yip SK: Compliance with a pelvic muscle exercise program as a causal predictor of urinary stress incontinence amongst Chinese women, *Neurourol Urodyn* 22(7):659-663, 2003.

40. Miller J: Criteria for therapeutic use of pelvic floor muscle training in women, *J Wound Ostomy Continence Nurs* 29(6):301-311, 2002.

41. Swart AM, Hegerty J, Corstiaans A, Rane A: Management of the very weak pelvic floor: is there a point? *Int Urogynecol J* 13(6):346-348, 2002.

42. Dougherty M: Current status of research on pelvic muscle strengthening exercises, *J Wound Ostomy Continence Nurs* 25(2):75-83, 1998.

43. Johnson V: How the principles of exercise physiology influence pelvic floor muscle training, *J Wound Ostomy Continence Nurs* 28(3):150-155, 2001.

44. Laycock J: Pelvic muscle exercises: physiotherapy for the pelvic floor, *Urol Nurs* 14(3):136-140, 1994.

45. Kegel AH: Progressive resistance exercise in the functional restoration of the perineal muscles, *Am J Obstet Gynecol* 56:238, 1948.

46. Goode P, Burgio K, Locher J, et al: Effect of behavioral training with or without pelvic floor electrical stimulation on stress incontinence in women: a randomized controlled trial, *JAMA* 290(3):345-352, 2003.

47. Johnson V: Effects of a submaximal exercise protocol to recondition the pelvic floor musculature, *Nurs Res* 50(1):33-41, 2001.

48. Kegel AH: Stress incontinence of women: physiologic treatment, *J Int Coll Surg* 25:484, 1956.

49. Shepherd AM: Treatment of genuine stress incontinence with a new perineometer, *Physiotherapy* 69(4):113, 1983.

50. Berghmans LC, Hendricks HJ, Bo K, et al: Conservative treatment of stress urinary incontinence in women: a systematic review of randomized clinical trials, *Br J Urol* 82:181-191, 1998.

51. Weatherall M: Biofeedback in pelvic floor muscle exercises for female genuine stress incontinence: a meta-analysis of trials identified in systematic review, *BJU Int* 83:1015-1016, 1999.

52. Aukee P, Immonen P, Penttinen J, et al: Increase in pelvic floor muscle activity after 12 weeks' training: a randomized prospective pilot study, *Urology* 60(6):1020-1023, 2002.

53. Aksac B, Aki S, Karam A, et al: Biofeedback and pelvic floor exercises for the rehabilitation of urinary stress incontinence, *Gynecol Obstet Invest* 56(1):23-27, 2003.

54. Payne CK: Biofeedback for community dwelling individuals with urinary incontinence, *Urology* 51(suppl 2A):35-39, 1998.

55. Plevnik S: New methods for testing and strengthening of pelvic floor muscles. In *Proceedings of the 15th Annual General Meeting of International Continence Society* 27:268, 1985.

56. Peattie AB, Plevnik S: Cones versus physiotherapy as conservative management of genuine stress incontinence, *Neurourol Urodyn* 7(3):72-73, 1998.

57. Peattie AB, Plevnik S, Stanton SL: Vaginal cones: a conservative method of treating genuine stress incontinence, *Br J Obstet Gynecol* 95:1049-1053, 1988.

58. Herbison P, Plevnik S, Mantle J: Weighted vaginal cones for urinary incontinence, *Cochrane Database Syst Rev* 1:CD002114, 2002.

59. Huffman JW, Osborne SL, Sokol JK: Electrical stimulation in treatment of intractable stress incontinence, *Arch Phys Med* 33:674, 1952.

60. Vodusek DB, Plevnik S, Vrtacnik P, Janez J: Detrusor inhibition on selective pudendal nerve stimulation in the perineum, *Neurourol Urodyn* 6:389-393, 1988.

61. Junemann K: The management of female urinary stress incontinence II: the use of devices, *BJU Int* 87(5):449-455, 2001.

62. Jeyaseelan S, Oldham J: Electrical stimulation as a treatment for stress incontinence, *Br J Nurs* 9(15):1001-1007, 2000.

63. Galloway N, El-Galley R, Appell R, et al: Multicenter trial: extracorporeal magnetic innervation (ExMI) for the treatment of stress urinary incontinence. Abstract presented at International Continence Society Meeting, Monaco, June 1998.
64. Rovner ES: Treatment of urinary incontinence, *Curr Urol Rep* 1(3):235-244, 2000.
65. Bernier F, Jenkins P: The role of vaginal estrogen in the treatment of urogenital dysfunction in post-menopausal women, *Urol Nurs* 17(3):92-95, 1997.
66. Maloney C: Estrogen in urinary incontinence treatment: an anatomic and physiologic approach, *Urol Nurs* 17(3): 88-91, 1997.
67. Al-Badr R, Ross S, Soroka D, Drutz H: What is the available evidence for hormone replacement therapy in women stress urinary incontinence? *J Obstet Gynecol Can* 25(7):565-574, 2003.
68. Viktrup L, Bump R: Pharmacological agents used for the treatment of stress urinary incontinence in women, *Curr Med Res Opin* 19(6):485-490, 2003.
69. Zinner N: Duloxetine: a serotonin-noradrenaline reuptake inhibitor for the treatment of stress urinary incontinence, *Expert Opin Invest Drugs* 12(9):1559-1566, 2003.
70. Agarwala N, Liu C: Minimally invasive management of urinary incontinence, *Curr Opin Obstet Gynecol* 14(4): 429-433, 2002.
71. Glazener C, Cooper K: Bladder neck needle suspension for urinary incontinence in women, *Cochrane Database Syst Rev* 2:CD003636, 2002.
72. Lapitan M, Cody D, Grant A: Open retropubic colposuspension for urinary incontinence in women, *Cochrane Database Syst Rev* 1:CDOO2912, 2003.
73. Nguyen J: Diagnosis and treatment of voiding dysfunction caused by urethral obstruction after anti-incontinence surgery, *Obstet Gynecol Surv* 57(7): 468-475, 2002.
74. Moehrer B, Carey M, Wilson D: Laparoscopic colposuspension: a systematic review. *Br J Obstet Gynecol* 110(3):230-235, 2003.
75. Walters M, Daneshgari F: Surgical management of stress urinary incontinence, *Clin Obstet Gynecol* 47(1):93-103, 2004.
76. Cody J, Wyness L, Wallace S, et al: Systematic review of the clinical effectiveness and cost-effectiveness of tension-free vaginal tape for treatment of stress urinary incontinence, *Health Technol Assess* 7(21):iii, 1-189, 2003.
77. Merlin T, Arnold E, Petros P, et al: A systematic review of tension-free urethropexy for stress urinary incontinence: intravaginal slingplasty and the tension-free vaginal tape procedures, *BJU Int* 88(9):871-880, 2001.
78. Boublil V, Ciofu C, Traxer O, et al: Complications of urethral sling procedures, *Curr Opin Obstet Gynecol* 14(5):515-520, 2002.
79. Lightner D: Review of the available urethral bulking agents, *Curr Opin Urol* 12(4):333-338, 2002.
80. Pickard R, Reaper J, Wyness L, et al: Periurethral injection therapy for urinary incontinence in women, *Cochrane Database Syst Rev* 2:2004.
81. Foley FB: An artificial urinary sphincter, *J Urol* 50:250, 1947.
82. Wang Y, Hadley HR: Management of persistent or recurrent urinary incontinence, *J Urol* 146:1005-1006, 1991.
83. Haab F, Trockman BA, Zimmern PE, Leach GE: Quality of life and continence assessment of the artificial urinary sphincter in men with minimum 3.5 years of followup, *J Urol* 158:435-439, 1997.
84. Sirls LT, Foote JE, Kaufman JM, et al: Long-term results of the FemSoft urethral insert for the management of female stress urinary incontinence, *Int Urogynecol J* 13(2):88-95, 2002.
85. Bash K: Review of vaginal pessaries, *Obstet Gynecol Surv* 55(7):455-460, 2000.
86. Palumbo MV: Pessary placement and management, *Ostomy Wound Manage* 46(12):40-45, 2000.

Pathology and Management of the Overactive Bladder

MARTA KRISSOVICH

OBJECTIVES

1. Define the following terms: urge urinary incontinence (UUI), overactive bladder (OAB), and detrusor hyperactivity with impaired contractility (DHIC).
2. List five factors outside the lower urinary tract associated with OAB symptoms.
3. List four classic symptoms of overactive bladder.
4. Describe three factors that must be investigated during the history of individuals presenting with OAB symptoms.
5. Explain two major goals of the evaluation of OAB.
6. List potential findings from the OAB evaluation that warrant further investigation.
7. List at least three types of behavioral therapy for OAB not including bladder training and urge suppression.
8. Define bladder training and outline its key components.
9. Define urge suppression and outline its key components.
10. Explain the proposed mechanism of action of anticholinergic medications for OAB.
11. List two surgical procedures that may be used for overactive bladder.
12. Explain the evidence base for a combined approach to treatment of OAB and urge incontinence.
13. Given an actual or hypothetical patient with urge incontinence, develop an appropriate treatment program.

For many years, overactive bladder (OAB) and urge urinary incontinence (UUI) were very poorly understood, and management was largely empiric. Fortunately, a recent plethora of studies significantly increased our understanding of this condition and provided the basis for a much more evidence-based approach to management of these patients. We now have new information on the epidemiology and etiology of OAB and new insights into its impact on quality of life. This enhanced understanding has provided the basis for development of an internationally accepted definition of OAB and for guidelines for diagnosis of OAB and urge UI. Concurrently, the scientific base for behavioral, pharmaceutical, and surgical treatments has greatly expanded. Instead of telling patients "there are a few things we can try," we can now offer a variety of management strategies that are scientifically based (see Appendix B). Although numerous questions remain, a new era has dawned for patients and clinicians dealing with OAB. These advances are especially important to nurses involved in continence care because nurses are ideally suited to administer and/or monitor most of the first-line therapies recommended for OAB.

This chapter provides a review of OAB and urge UI, in terms of epidemiology, impact, pathophysiology, diagnosis, and management. Throughout the chapter, the importance of nursing intervention is emphasized.

DEFINITIONS

As described in Chapter 1, the International Continence Society (ICS) has updated its report on standardization of terminology for the lower urinary tract (LUT).[1] The definitions included in this terminology report have gained wide acceptance among clinicians, including the Second International Consultation on Urinary Incontinence (ICI2).[2] Definitions pertinent to this chapter are outlined in Table 5-1; points of particular importance include the following:[1]

- "Overactive bladder syndrome" is the term used to describe urinary urgency, *with or without urge UI,* and typically combined with urinary frequency and nocturia; the term "overactive bladder" is synonymous with the terms "urge syndrome" and "urgency-frequency syndrome."
- Urgency is defined as "a sudden compelling desire to pass urine which is difficult to defer."

Text continued on p. 115

TABLE 5-1   **International Continence Society (ICS) Definitions Pertinent to the Syndrome of Overactive Bladder**

STORAGE SYMPTOMS	
These symptoms experienced during the storage phase of the bladder, including daytime frequency and nocturia (NEW)	
Increased daytime frequency	The complaint by the patient who considers that he or she voids too often by day. (NEW) This term is equivalent to pollakiuria used in many countries.
Nocturia	The complaint of waking at night one or more times to void (NEW)
Nighttime frequency	The total number of voids during the night, while awake or asleep. (The term nighttime frequency differs from that for nocturia, because it includes voids that occur after the individual has gone to bed, but before he or she has gone to sleep, and the voids that occur in the early morning and prevent the individual from getting back to sleep as he or she wishes. These voids before and after sleep may need to be considered in research studies, for example, in nocturnal polyuria. If this definition were used, then an adapted definition of daytime frequency would need to be used with it.)
Urgency	The complaint of a sudden compelling desire to pass urine that is difficult to defer (CHANGED)
Urinary incontinence	The complaint of any involuntary leakage of urine (NEW) (In each specific circumstance, urinary incontinence should be further described by specifying relevant factors such as type, frequency, severity, precipitating factors, social impact, effect on hygiene and quality of life, the measures used to contain the leakage, and whether or not the individual seeks or desires help because of urinary incontinence. Urinary leakage may need to be distinguished from sweating or vaginal discharge.)
Urge urinary incontinence	The complaint of involuntary leakage accompanied by or immediately preceded by urgency. (CHANGED) Urge incontinence can present in different symptomatic forms, for example, as frequent small losses between micturitions or as a catastrophic leak with complete bladder emptying.
Mixed urinary incontinence	The complaint of involuntary leakage associated with urgency and also with exertion, effort, sneezing, or coughing (NEW)
Enuresis	Any involuntary loss of urine. If it is used to denote incontinence during sleep, it should always be qualified with the adjective "nocturnal." (ORIGINAL)

TABLE 5-1 **International Continence Society (ICS) Definitions Pertinent to the Syndrome of Overactive Bladder—cont'd**

STORAGE SYMPTOMS—cont'd	
Continuous urinary incontinence	The complaint of continuous leakage (NEW)
Polyuria	A 24-hour urine volume of more than 40 mL/kg body weight. Polyuria can be caused by diabetes mellitus and diabetes insipidus, and such possibilities should be excluded using the appropriate specialized tests.
Nocturnal enuresis	The complaint of loss of urine occurring during sleep (NEW)
Nocturnal polyuria	Production of excessive volumes of urine during sleep. Nocturia will result if nocturnal urine volume exceeds the functional bladder capacity. In patients with normal 24-hour urine output, the ICS committee recommends expressing the nocturnal urine output as a percentage of the total 24-hour volume. This percentage will be lower in the young (less than 20%) than in the elderly (more than 33%), and interindividual variation is also to be expected.
BLADDER SENSATION REPORTS ACQUIRED DURING HISTORY ACQUISITION	
Normal	The individual is aware of bladder filling and increasing sensation up to a strong desire to void. (NEW)
Increased	The individual feels an early and persistent desire to void. (NEW)
Reduced	The individual is aware of bladder filling but does not feel a definite desire to void. (NEW)
Absent	The individual reports no sensation of bladder filling or desire to void.(NEW)
Nonspecific	The individual reports no specific bladder sensation but may perceive bladder filling as abdominal fullness, vegetative symptoms, or spasticity. (NEW) These nonspecific symptoms are most frequently seen in neurologic patients, particularly those with spinal cord trauma and in children and adults with malformations of the spinal cord.)
SYMPTOM SYNDROMES SUGGESTIVE OF LOWER URINARY TRACT DYSFUNCTION	
Overactive bladder syndrome Urge syndrome Urgency-frequency syndrome	Interchangeable terms for syndromes that describe urgency, with or without urge incontinence, usually with frequency and nocturia (NEW) (These symptom combinations are suggestive of urodynamically demonstrable detrusor overactivity but can be caused by other forms of urethrovesical dysfunction. These terms can be used if there is no proven infection or other obvious pathologic features.)
TYPES OF VOIDING DIARIES (BLADDER CHARTS)	
Micturition time chart	Records only the times of micturitions, day and night, for at least 24 hours(NEW)
Frequency volume chart (FVC)	Records the volumes voided as well as the time of each micturition, day and night, for at least 24 hours
Bladder diary	Records the times of micturitions and voided volumes, incontinence episodes, pad usage, and other information such as fluid intake, the degree of urgency, and the degree of incontinence. (NEW) (It is useful to ask the individual to make an estimate of liquid intake. This may be done precisely by measuring the volume of each drink or crudely by asking

Continued

TABLE 5-1 **International Continence Society (ICS) Definitions Pertinent to the Syndrome of Overactive Bladder—cont'd**

TYPES OF VOIDING DIARIES (BLADDER CHARTS)—cont'd	
	how many drinks are taken in a 24-hour period. If the individual eats significant quantities of water-containing foods [vegetables, fruit, salads], then an appreciable effect on urine production will result. The time that diuretic therapy is taken should be marked on a chart or diary.)
ITEMS THAT CAN BE ABSTRACTED FROM FREQUENCY VOLUME CHARTS AND BLADDER DIARIES	
Daytime frequency	Number of voids recorded during waking hours; includes the last void before sleep and the first void after waking and rising in the morning (NEW)
24-hour frequency	Total number of daytime voids and episodes of nocturia during a specified 24-hour period (NEW)
24-hour production	Measured by collecting all urine for 24 hours. (NEW) This is usually commenced *after* the first void produced after rising in the morning and is completed by including the first void on rising the following morning.
Polyuria	Measured production of urine of more than 40 mL / kg body weight in 24 hours in adults (2.8 liters for a 70-kg person). (NEW). It may be useful to look at output over shorter time frames (van Kerrebroeck et al., 2002). (The causes of polyuria are various and reviewed elsewhere but include habitual excess fluid intake.)
Maximum voided volume	The largest volume of urine voided during a single micturition, determined either from the frequency volume chart or bladder diary. (NEW) The maximum, mean, and minimum voided volumes over the period of recording may be stated. (Functional bladder capacity is a confusing term and is no longer recommended.)
Night	The period of time between going to bed with the intention of sleep and waking with the intention of arising.
Nocturia	The complaint that the individual has to wake at night one or more times to void. The number of voids recorded during a night's sleep: each void is preceded and followed by sleep
Nocturnal enuresis	The complaint of loss of urine occurring during sleep (NEW)
Night-time voiding	All micturitions during the night whether the person is awake or asleep
Nocturnal urine volume	The total volume of urine passed between the time the individual goes to bed with the intention of sleeping and the time of waking with the intention of arising. (NEW) Therefore, it excludes the last void before going to bed but includes the first void after arising in the morning.
Nocturnal polyuria	Present when an increased proportion of the 24-hour output occurs at night (normally during the 8 hours while the patient is in bed). (NEW) The nighttime urine output excludes the last void before sleep but includes the first void of the morning and should be expressed as a percentage of the total 24-hour urine volume. (The precise definition is dependent on age. Nocturnal polyuria is present when more than 20% [young adults] to more than 33% [over 65 years] of the 24-hour urine volume is produced at night.)

TABLE 5-1   **International Continence Society (ICS) Definitions Pertinent to the Syndrome of Overactive Bladder—cont'd**

ITEMS THAT CAN BE ABSTRACTED FROM FREQUENCY VOLUME CHARTS AND BLADDER DIARIES—cont'd	
Functional bladder capacity	This term is no longer recommended, because "voided volume" is a clearer and less confusing term, particularly if qualified, such as maximum voided volume. (If the term "bladder capacity" is used, it implies that this has been measured in some way, if only by abdominal ultrasound. In adults, voided volumes vary considerably. In children, the "expected volume" may be calculated from the formula (30+ [age in years $\times$ 30] in ml). Assuming no residual urine, this will be equal to the "expected bladder capacity.")

DATA OBTAINED DURING URODYNAMIC STUDIES

Urodynamic observations are observations made during urodynamic studies. (NEW) For example, an involuntary detrusor contraction (detrusor overactivity) is a urodynamic observation. In general, a urodynamic observation does not represent a definitive diagnosis of a disease or condition and may occur with a variety of symptoms and signs, or in the absence of any symptoms or signs.

BLADDER SENSATIONS THAT MAY BE REPORTED DURING FILLING CYSTOMETRY	
Normal bladder sensation	Can be judged by three defined points noted during filling cystometry (first sensation, normal desire, strong desire) and evaluated in relation to the bladder volume at that moment and in relation to the patient's symptomatic complaints
First sensation of bladder filling	The feeling the patient has when he or she first becomes aware of the bladder filling (NEW)
First desire to void	The feeling that would lead the patient to pass urine at the next convenient moment, but voiding can be delayed if necessary (CHANGED)
Strong desire to void	The persistent desire to void without the fear of leakage (ORIGINAL)
Bladder pain	A self-explanatory term and an abnormal finding (NEW)
Urgency	A sudden compelling desire to void. (NEW) (The ICS no longer recommends the terms "motor urgency" and "sensory urgency." These terms are often misused and have little intuitive meaning. Furthermore, it may be simplistic to relate urgency just to the presence or absence of detrusor overactivity when there is usually a concomitant fall in urethral pressure.)
The vesical/urethral sensory threshold	The least (lowest) current that consistently produces a sensation perceived by the subject during stimulation at the site under investigation (ORIGINAL)

DETRUSOR FUNCTION DURING FILLING CYSTOMETRY	
Normal detrusor function	A bladder that allows filling with little or no change in pressure. No involuntary phasic contractions occur despite provocation. (ORIGINAL)
Detrusor overactivity	A urodynamic observation characterized by involuntary detrusor contractions during the filling phase which may be spontaneous or provoked. (CHANGED)*
Involuntary detrusor activity	Any detrusor activity before permission to void is given (In everyday life, the individual attempts to inhibit detrusor activity until he or she is in a position to void. Therefore, when the aims of the filling study have been achieved, and when the patient has a desire to void, "permission to void" is normally given. That moment is indicated on the urodynamic tracing.)

*The phrase "which the patient cannot completely suppress" has been deleted from the old definition. There is no lower limit for the amplitude of an involuntary detrusor contraction, and confident interpretation of low pressure waves (amplitude less than 5 cm of H_2O) depends on "high quality" urodynamic technique.

Continued

TABLE 5-1   **International Continence Society (ICS) Definitions Pertinent to the Syndrome of Overactive Bladder—cont'd**

DETRUSOR FUNCTION DURING FILLING CYSTOMETRY—cont'd	
Phasic detrusor overactivity	A characteristic wave form that may or may not lead to urinary incontinence. This activity is not always accompanied by sensation or may be interpreted as a first sensation of bladder filling or as a normal desire to void by the patient.
PATTERNS OF DETRUSOR OVERACTIVITY	
Terminal detrusor overactivity	A single, involuntary detrusor contraction, occurring at cystometric capacity, which cannot be suppressed and which results in incontinence (usually complete bladder emptying, that is, voiding). (NEW) (Overactivity may be associated with reduced or absent bladder sensation; for example, in the elderly stroke patient, urgency may be felt as the voiding contraction occurs, and the patient with complete spinal cord injury may have no sensation whatsoever.)
Detrusor overactivity incontinence	Incontinence resulting from an involuntary detrusor contraction. (NEW) In a patient with normal sensation, urgency is likely to be experienced just before the leakage episode.
Motor urge incontinence, reflex incontinence	The ICS recommends that these terms should no longer be used because they have no intuitive meaning and are often misused.
ADDITIONAL TERMS FOR QUALIFYING DETRUSOR OVERACTIVITY ACCORDING TO CAUSE	
Neurogenic detrusor overactivity	Detrusor overactivity when there is a relevant neurologic condition. This term replaces the term "detrusor hyperreflexia." (NEW) (It is likely that the proportion of neurogenic to idiopathic detrusor overactivity will increase if a more complete neurologic assessment is carried out.)
Idiopathic detrusor overactivity	Detrusor overactivity with no defined cause. (NEW) This term replaces "detrusor instability."
Other patterns of detrusor overactivity	Example: The combination of phasic and terminal detrusor overactivity, and the sustained high-pressure detrusor contractions seen in patients with spinal cord injury when attempted voiding occurs against a dyssynergic sphincter
TERMS RELATED TO URODYNAMIC TECHNIQUE	
Provocative maneuvers	Techniques used during urodynamics in an effort to provoke detrusor overactivity, for example, rapid filling, use of cooled or acid medium, postural changes, and hand washing (NEW)
TERMS RELATED TO TREATMENT	
The following definitions were published in the seventh ICS report on lower urinary tract rehabilitation techniques[188] and republished unchanged in the 2002 report:	
Lower urinary tract rehabilitation	Nonsurgical, nonpharmacologic treatment for lower urinary tract function
Pelvic floor training	Repetitive selective voluntary contraction and relaxation of specific pelvic floor muscles
Biofeedback	Technique by which information about a normally unconscious physiologic process is presented to the patient and/or the therapist as a visual, auditory, or tactile signal

TABLE 5-1 **International Continence Society (ICS) Definitions Pertinent to the Syndrome of Overactive Bladder—cont'd**

TERMS RELATED TO TREATMENT—cont'd	
Behavioral modification	Analysis and alteration of the relationship between the patient's symptoms and his or her environment for the treatment of maladaptive voiding patterns. This may be achieved by modification of the behavior and/or environment of the patient.
Electrical stimulation	Application of electrical current to stimulate the pelvic viscera or their nerve supply. The aim of electrical stimulation may be to induce a therapeutic response directly or to modulate lower urinary tract, bowel, or sexual dysfunction.

Data from references 24, 85, 188, and 189.

- Urge urinary incontinence is defined as "the complaint of involuntary leakage accompanied by or immediately preceded by urgency." (Urge UI may present clinically either as frequent episodes of low-volume leakage between voluntary voids or as major high-volume leakage associated with complete bladder emptying.)
- Nocturia. In 2002, the ICS defined nocturia as "the number of times a person wakes to void," whereas the current definition of nocturia is "the *complaint* of waking at night one or more times to void." Although these definitions are essentially the same, the first is simply a numeric measure, whereas the current definition interjects the concept of "bother." Either way, it is important to qualify the word nocturia with a number, such as "nocturia × 3," and it is also important to assess the degree to which the patient is bothered by the need to void during the night.

EPIDEMIOLOGY

The National Overactive Bladder Evaluation (NOBLE) program explored the prevalence and impact of OAB using a telephone survey of 5204 persons who were representative of the US adult population in terms of gender, age, and geographic region.[3] The survey found the overall prevalence of OAB to be similar between men (16%) and women (16.9%) across all age groups; however, women were more likely than men to experience urge UI. In fact, 55% of women with OAB reported at least three episodes of urinary leakage in the previous

month that did not appear to be related to stress UI. Age seemed to be another important risk factor for urge UI; as participants aged, the prevalence of urge UI increased from 2% to 19%, with a marked increase after 44 years of age. (For men, the marked increase in prevalence did not occur until age 64.)

Prevalence in Europe appears to be similar to that in the United States. Milsom and colleagues collected data using a telephone survey of a representative sample of 16,773 men and women in six European countries.[4] In this study, 1963 people (16.6%) with symptoms of OAB were identified and further interviewed. Rates of OAB were 12% in France and Italy, 19% in the United Kingdom, and 22% in Spain; overall prevalence increased from 6% in the 40 to 44-year olds to 35% in those 75 years of age or older. Not surprisingly, urinary frequency was the most commonly reported symptom, occurring in 85% of the OAB population; urgency was reported by 54% of the participants and urge UI by 36%. As has often been found in the United States, 60% of symptomatic respondents had consulted a physician, but only 27% were currently receiving treatment.

Although these were both very large, well-designed studies, the numbers could have been higher still if subjects had been interviewed in person,[5] a finding that points out the need for more studies related to prevalence of OAB and urge UI. In addition, studies are needed in the areas of *incidence* (newly developing cases over an established period of time) and *remission* (cure of the condition). We do have limited data regarding remission rates.

For example, Nygaard and Lemke followed 2025 elderly female residents in rural Iowa over 6 years (a longitudinal cohort study). At baseline, the prevalence was 36.3% for urge UI and 40.3% for stress UI. The 3-year incidence and remission rates for urge UI (measured during the third and sixth years) were 28.5% and 22.1%, respectively. For stress UI, the incidence and remission rates for the same periods were 28.6% and 25.1%, respectively. Not surprisingly, as the subjects' ages advanced, so did the incidence of urge UI; however, improvements in functional status were associated with reductions in urge UI.[6]

Impact of Overactive Bladder and Urge UI on Quality of Life

OAB, both with and without urge UI, has repeatedly been found to be associated with emotional distress, reduced social and recreational activity, and sexual dysfunction.[7] In addition, the NOBLE program found that individuals with OAB reported a significantly negative impact on general health-related quality of life, emotional stability, and sleep (as compared with controls).

Several investigators have found that OAB, with or without urge UI, imposes a greater burden on health-related quality of life than stress UI. Hunskaar and Vinsnes utilized the Sickness Impact Profile to investigate the impact of types of leakage and duration of symptoms on quality of life. Subjects were randomly selected from an incontinence clinic and were stratified by age group and symptoms. These investigators found that elders seemed to tolerate stress UI symptoms better than younger cohorts. More importantly, patients complaining of urge symptoms were more severely impaired than those with stress UI in all age groups; the areas of greatest impact were sleep and rest, emotional stability, mobility, social interaction, and participation in recreational activities.[8]

Coyne and colleagues conducted a nested, case-controlled study of NOBLE participants utilizing the Overactive Bladder Health Related Quality of Life questionnaire (OAB-q), the Medical Outcomes Study Short Form-36, the Medical Outcomes Study Sleep Scale, and the Center for Epidemiological Studies Depression scale.[9,10] Of the 919 participants (82.5% female, mean age 55.9), 171 reported incontinence; 69 reported urge UI, 62 reported stress UI, and 40 reported mixed UI. These investigators found little difference in health-related quality of life scores between the groups with mixed UI and urge UI, but both groups reported significantly higher levels of bother from symptoms and lower satisfaction with sleep ($p = .001$) than counterparts suffering from stress UI alone. In another study, these investigators found that nocturia was common, increased with age, affected men and women equally, and had a direct effect on health-related quality of life; as the number of bladder-related sleep interruptions increased, the health-related quality of life decreased.[11]

Relationship of Overactive Bladder and Urge UI to Comorbidities

OAB symptoms are commonly associated with urinary tract and genital skin infections, falls and fractures, and depression and sleep disturbances (as outlined earlier).[12] The risk for falls and resulting hip fracture is particularly increased among individuals experiencing both urinary frequency and urge UI, because this combination causes the person to rush to the bathroom frequently in attempts to avoid leakage.[13] Brown and Vittinghoff followed 6049 community-dwelling women for falls and fractures; these investigators sent postcards every 3 months with a query regarding any falls or fractures, and all fractures were confirmed radiologically. Utilizing logistic and proportional hazard models, the risk of a fall or fracture was independently associated with urge UI occurring at least weekly.[13]

In 2002, Wagner and Hu and their colleagues published information gathered from the NOBLE study on the medical consequences of OAB.[14] They found that persons with OAB reported more frequent urinary tract infections (UTIs), injurious falls, and physician visits than age- and gender-matched controls, at an annual cost of $1.8 billion (2000 dollars).

Economic Burden of Overactive Bladder and Urge UI

Hu and Wagner have followed the costs of urinary incontinence in elders living in the United States and have classified these costs into direct and indirect categories. They have recently expanded the study population to all adults living in the United States and have included OAB in their analysis. These investigators describe the direct costs of OAB as those associated with treatment, diagnosis, routine care, and medical consequences and indirect costs as lost wages and productivity, pain and suffering, and impaired quality of life.[15] Utilizing these definitions and data gleaned from the NOBLE program, Hu and Wagner have estimated the total direct cost of OAB to be $12.02 billion; 76% of these costs are community based, and 23% reflect institutional costs.[16] In 2004, the same team utilized a complex economic framework to estimate that the total cost of OAB (treatment, diagnosis, routine care, and medical consequences) in the United States was $12.6 billion in the year 2000.[17]

NORMAL BLADDER FUNCTION

Because bladder function is often manipulated via conservative therapies, the continence care clinician must have a solid understanding of normal bladder function and the changes associated with OAB. Normal bladder function is described in detail in Chapter 2. In summary, the bladder stores urine via elastic and neuromuscular properties in the detrusor muscle that allow filling at low pressures; storage is further supported by the fact that the "normal" bladder stays relaxed and does not initiate significant contractile activity until voiding is voluntarily initiated.[18] (This characteristic of normal bladder function is known as "stability.") As described by de Groat in 1997, urine storage requires a relaxed detrusor, which is mediated by stimulation of the sympathetic and somatic pathways, coupled with suppression of the parasympathetic pathways.[19] (Sympathetic stimulation causes bladder relaxation and increased sphincter tone, whereas parasympathetic stimulation causes bladder contraction.) Conversely, effective voiding is dependent on bladder contraction and urethral relaxation, which is mediated by stimulation of the parasympathetic pathways and inhibition (suppression) of the sympathetic and somatic pathways. This activity at the level of the bladder and sphincter is controlled by the cerebral cortex, coordinated by the pons, and communicated via the spinal cord and its multiple pathways (sympathetic, parasympathetic, and somatic). Disorders of any of these structures may contribute to the symptoms of OAB.[19]

Bladder Capacity and Sensory Awareness of Bladder Filling

Interestingly, there has been no consensus on how much the "normal" bladder holds and how often "normal" people urinate, especially during waking hours. Current evidence is insufficient to accurately define "normal" bladder capacity; however, the combined results from the artificial setting of urodynamic testing and the surveys of "asymptomatic" individuals provide ranges that will assist the continence care clinician when assessing and managing patients. In a survey of 300 racially diverse, asymptomatic women, Fitzgerald and colleagues found that subjects voided a mean of eight times/ 24 hours.[20] The median number of voids per liter of *intake* was four (one void for each 250 mL of intake), and the median number of voids per liter of *output* was five (for an average voided volume of 200 mL). Linear regression analysis showed that both diurnal and nocturnal urinary frequency increased with age and fluid intake; of note, average voided volumes tended to be lower for black women. Fitzgerald also reported on findings from a retrospective chart review of 200 women who had submitted frequency volume charts and Urological Distress Inventories.[21] Although the degree of distress was correlated with daytime and nighttime voiding frequency and with average voided volume, 90% of the participants reported at least minor bother related to their urinary frequency (including 76% of the 34 women who reported voiding fewer than eight times in 24 hours). Average voided volumes may be somewhat higher for men; Mueller and colleagues surveyed asymptomatic men in regard to their voiding habits and found a mean volume per void of 300 mL ($p = .04$).[22]

Until clear definitions of "normal" capacity and voiding frequency are established, the parameters described by Jackson and Abrams may prove useful for patient counseling.[23] The "first sensation" (awareness) of bladder filling is usually felt at approximately half of capacity (150 to 200 mlL). About 1 to 2 hours later, depending on activity and fluid intake, the "normal desire" to void is reported;

this typically occurs at 75% of capacity (250 to 450 mL). If voiding is inconvenient, that desire should fade from consciousness, returning at ever-increasing intervals and becoming very strong and fairly persistent as the bladder nears capacity (300 to 600 mL). Sensory awareness of bladder filling that occurs earlier than the parameters described earlier is described as "increased sensory awareness;" sensory awareness that occurs later than these parameters is described as "reduced sensation," and the total absence of sensation related to bladder filling is referred to as "absent sensation" (according to ICS terminology).[24] The differences between "increased sensory awareness" and "urgency" are discussed further under bladder diary interpretation.

Micturition Reflex

Urinary storage and bladder emptying are mediated primarily by the autonomic nervous system but are subject to voluntary control via the cerebral cortex and somatic nerve pathways. As explained in Chapter 2, micturition can be divided into two major phases: bladder filling/storage, and voiding/emptying:[25,26]

- The bladder-filling phase is a mostly passive event characterized by slow filling from the kidneys via the ureters with little resistance or change in bladder wall pressure. The urethra is closed, and the pelvic floor provides passive support. Cerebral inhibition of bladder contractility is mostly automatic, and the individual feels only a vague awareness of filling.
- The urge to void occurs when the detrusor muscle fibers stretch (distend) sufficiently to activate sensory afferent pathways; this stimulates the cerebral cortex and leads to a conscious decision regarding voiding. If the decision is made to delay voiding, the cerebral cortex inhibits the automatic voiding centers, and the sympathetic nervous system is activated; alpha-adrenergic stimulation augments urethral resistance, and beta-adrenergic stimulation suppresses bladder contractility. In addition, the pudendal (somatic) nerve pathways mediate increased tone within the voluntary sphincter and pelvic floor muscles (PFMs).

- Voiding (emptying) is a mostly active event where increased sensory (afferent) stimulation of the cerebral cortex leads to a decision to void and movement to an acceptable location. Once there, cerebral inhibition of the bladder ceases, and the outlet is opened via pelvic floor and urethral relaxation. As sympathetic stimulation to the bladder ceases, parasympathetic (cholinergic) activity increases, and bladder contraction is initiated.

Behavioral therapy for OAB capitalizes on both the cerebral and the pudendal/pelvic floor components of the micturition reflex. Pharmaceutical therapy primarily affects bladder and sphincter function via modulation of autonomic nervous system neurotransmitters.[27]

PATHOLOGY OF OVERACTIVE BLADDER AND URGE UI

The OAB typically contracts inappropriately, sometimes with little provocation and often when only partially full; these inappropriate contractions occur during the storage phase of micturition when the bladder is normally relaxed and quiet.[28] Individuals with OAB typically experience a strong sensation of urgency, which may be followed by leakage (urge UI); they usually report frequency and nocturia as well.

Although more research into the pathology of OAB is clearly needed,[29] our current understanding suggests that the primary causes of bladder overactivity can be classified as idiopathic, neurogenic, myogenic, or a combination of neurogenic and myogenic. Idiopathic OAB is the term that is used when the specific cause is unknown; it is likely that idiopathic OAB is caused by a variety of conditions that have a final common pathway.[30]

Because the voluntary control of micturition depends on the neural connections between the cerebral cortex and the brainstem, disruption of these pathways (brain tumor, stroke, head trauma, Parkinson's disease, etc.) impairs the ability to suppress and control bladder contractions. As indicated in Table 5-1, the ICS describes OAB associated with a known and relevant neurologic disease as "neurogenic detrusor overactivity." The neurogenic classification of OAB is based on the recognition that both known neurologic conditions and subtle central neurologic injuries may reduce cerebral inhibition of the bladder and may adversely affect sensory awareness of bladder filling. Specific etiologic factors include alterations in neurotransmitter levels, changes in nerve growth factors, or the emergence of primitive reflex C-afferent pathways; all of these conditions could serve to increase detrusor contractility.[31] The emergence of primitive reflex pathways appears especially promising as one of the mechanisms contributing to detrusor overactivity following spinal cord disruption.

The myogenic classification of OAB is based on actual changes in the detrusor smooth muscle cells as a common final pathway resulting in OAB.[32] These changes include partial denervation, cellular hypoxia, and ultrastructural changes that cause increased cellular excitability and enhanced propagation of activity among cells; these changes in the smooth muscle can result in involuntary detrusor contractions.

A weak pelvic floor also seems to be an etiologic factor for OAB. Although the exact mechanisms are poorly understood, the pelvic floor normally serves to facilitate storage and prevent leakage, and contraction of the PFMs causes reflex inhibition of bladder contractility. Ouslander and many others have suggested that sphincter and pelvic floor weakness may permit urine to leak into the proximal urethra, thus precipitating urgency, and the weakened PFMs and sphincter muscles are unable to contract effectively enough to inhibit bladder contractions when this occurs.[33]

The relationship between bladder overactivity and bladder outlet obstruction also deserves special mention. Although the relationship may not be direct, is likely multifactorial, and requires more study, bladder outlet obstruction may be a causative factor for OAB.[34] One proposed mechanism is ultrastructural changes in the smooth muscle cells of the detrusor.[35] The theory is that detrusor cell hypertrophy (in response to outlet obstruction) may reduce elasticity and increase excitability, thus leading to reduced capacity and overactivity.[18] If the condition progresses, bladder wall compliance and contraction velocity may also be reduced, resulting in an OAB that does not empty well.[36] Neil Resnick assigned the term "detrusor hyperactivity with impaired contractility" (DHIC) to overactive but poorly contractile bladders; this term is appropriately used to refer to any condition in which there is a combination of overactivity and reduced contractility, and bladder outlet obstruction is not a necessary part of the definition. In actuality, DHIC is seen more commonly in elders who have no evidence of outlet obstruction.[37]

RISK FACTORS FOR OAB
Extraurinary Tract Factors

In 1989, Neil Resnick popularized the theory that urinary incontinence could be caused by factors other than detrusor or urethral dysfunction and suggested that these be addressed before or coincident with treatment for LUT dysfunction.[38] Research indicates that this is also true for symptoms of OAB. Table 5-2 summarizes the genitourinary, neurologic, systemic, functional, and psychologic factors associated with OAB symptoms, along with their mechanism or effect and implications for management. Table 5-3 lists pharmaceutical factors associated with OAB symptoms. Some of the extraurinary tract risk factors deserve special mention, as follows.

Life-Style Factors. Several life-style factors, including obesity, smoking, diet, and fluid intake have been identified as being factors relevant to the development or exacerbation of OAB symptoms; some factors increase the risk for OAB symptoms, whereas others seem to reduce the risk.

Dietary Intake. Dallosso and associates reported on the impact of dietary intake and the onset of OAB symptoms by using logistic regression analysis of postal survey responses. These investigators mailed questionnaires regarding urinary symptoms, diet, and lifestyle to a random sample of community-dwelling individuals 40 years of age or older, at baseline and again 1 year later. The first survey set was returned by 6424 women; results indicated that obesity, smoking, and carbonated drinks were associated with a significant *increase* in risk for OAB symptoms, whereas a higher consumption of vegetables, bread, and chicken were associated with *reduced* risk.[39] The second set of surveys focused on nutrients rather than food groups and was returned by 5816 women. These results indicated that higher

TABLE 5-2   **Conditions Associated with Symptoms of Overactive Bladder**

CONDITIONS	MECHANISMS OR EFFECT	IMPLICATIONS FOR MANAGEMENT
Genitourinary Conditions		
Both sexes		
Urinary tract infection	Inflammation occurs, with activation of sensory afferent pathways and increased urgency and frequency.	Treat infection before other interventions are considered.
Obstruction: iatrogenic, bladder neck dysfunction, sphincter dyssynergia, benign prostatic hypertrophy, or pelvic organ prolapse	Obstruction can alter smooth muscle sensitivity and can contribute to both detrusor overactivity and urinary retention.	Address etiologic factors for obstruction.
Impaired bladder contractility	Impaired bladder emptying and increased postvoid residual urine contribute to increased urinary frequency and can challenge an irritable bladder	Avoid drugs that decrease bladder contractility. Teach patients techniques to enhance voiding and reduce retention (such as scheduled voiding and double voiding). Consider intermittent catheterization if the above methods are ineffective.
Bladder abnormalities or inflammation (such as tumors, calculi, interstitial cystitis)	Intravesical abnormalities can precipitate detrusor overactivity.	Sterile hematuria and risk factors for bladder cancer should prompt further evaluation; persistent severe urgency and pain require referral for further evaluation.
Pelvic floor dysfunction	Loss of reflexive bladder control occurs; that is, loss of ability to use pelvic floor muscle contraction to inhibit detrusor activity.	Pelvic muscle reeducation is indicated.
Painful bladder syndrome or interstitial cystitis	Increased voiding is used to manage pain.	Treat medically and behaviorally.
Women		
Estrogen deficiency	Inflammation from atrophic vaginitis or urethritis can contribute to symptoms.	Topical estrogen may ameliorate symptoms.
Sphincter weakness/ stress incontinence	Leakage of urine into the proximal urethra may precipitate urgency or increase chance of leakage with uninhibited contractions.	Topical estrogen and pelvic muscle exercises may help strengthen the sphincter.
Pelvic floor weakness/overactive bladder	The ability to inhibit detrusor by pelvic muscle contractions may be diminished.	Periurethral injections or surgical procedures may be helpful in selected patients.

TABLE 5-2   **Conditions Associated with Symptoms of Overactive Bladder—cont'd**

CONDITIONS	MECHANISMS OR EFFECT	IMPLICATIONS FOR MANAGEMENT
Men		
Prostate enlargement	Benign or malignant prostate enlargement can cause obstructed voiding and detrusor overactivity.	Evaluation and treatment for prostate cancer should be considered. Alpha-adrenergic blockers may improve symptoms. 5-Alpha-reductase inhibitors may reduce prostate size. Surgical removal of obstructing prostate may be indicated.
Neurologic Conditions		
Brain		
Stroke, Alzheimer's disease, multiinfarct dementia, other dementias, Parkinson's disease, multiple sclerosis	Cortical inhibition of the bladder is impaired, causing neurogenic detrusor overactivity.	Management must include strategies to compensate for impaired cognition, impaired mobility, or both.
Spinal cord		
Multiple sclerosis, cervical or lumbar stenosis or disk herniation, spinal cord injury, myelodysplasia	It results in loss of voluntary control of voiding; it typically causes neurogenic detrusor overactivity; it may cause sphincter dyssynergia and/or urinary retention.	Urodynamic testing is essential for definitive determination of bladder and sphincter response to bladder filling and for establishment of an appropriate management plan.
Peripheral innervation		
Diabetic neuropathy, nerve injury	It may cause loss of bladder contractility and urinary retention.	Management is based on clinical presentation; it may require intermittent catheterization.
Systemic Conditions		
Congestive heart failure, venous insufficiency	Volume overload can contribute to urinary frequency and nocturia when supine.	Proper timing of diuretics may ameliorate symptoms. Elevation, support hose, and salt restriction may help.
Diabetes mellitus	Poor blood glucose control can contribute to osmotic diuresis and polyuria.	Improved blood glucose control may ameliorate symptoms.
Sleep disorders (sleep apnea, periodic leg movements)	Sleep disorders may contribute to nocturia or nocturnal polyuria.	Sleep disruption or heavy snoring may require further evaluation.
Abnormalities of vasopressin	Impaired secretion or action of vasopressin may cause polyuria and nocturia.	Carefully selected patients may benefit from desmopressin therapy.

Continued

TABLE 5-2   Conditions Associated with Symptoms of Overactive Bladder—cont'd

CONDITIONS	MECHANISMS OR EFFECT	IMPLICATIONS FOR MANAGEMENT
Functional and Behavioral Conditions		
Excess intake of caffeine, alcohol, and other fluids, especially over short periods	Caffeine directly stimulates the bladder. Alcohol may reduce awareness of filling and acts as diuretic. All three may increase urine production.	Educate the patient regarding the impact of excess fluid intake and the potential effects of caffeine and alcohol on bladder function.
Poor bowel habits and constipation	Fecal impaction can contribute to symptoms by causing partial outlet obstruction and by compressing the bladder and thus reducing bladder capacity.	An appropriate bowel regimen will reduce the incidence of fecal impaction and constipation.
Impaired mobility	Impaired mobility can interfere with toileting ability and can contribute to urge incontinence.	Measures to improve mobility are recommended, including the use of assistive devices and physical therapy evaluation, as well as the use of bedside commodes and urinals if indicated.
Psychologic Conditions		
Chronic anxiety learned Voiding dysfunction	These conditions can cause symptoms of overactive bladder.	Voiding dysfunction may cause anxiety or vice versa. Rule out other disorders before assigning a psychogenic cause.

Data from references 33, 99, 116, and 190.

TABLE 5-3   Medications that May Contribute to Overactive Bladder Symptoms

DRUG CLASS	EFFECTS	RECOMMENDATIONS
Diuretics, especially rapid-acting agents	Some diuretics rapidly increase bladder volume, which may precipitate urgency and detrusor overactivity by activating stretch receptors.	Changing to a longer-acting diuretic, altering the timing of the dose, or discontinuing the drug, if appropriate, may ameliorate symptoms.
Anticholinergics, antiparkinsonians, antihistamines, antipsychotics, tricyclic antidepressants, calcium-channel blockers and beta blockers, narcotics, sedative hypnotics	These drugs may decrease bladder contractility and impair emptying.	If the postvoid residual (PVR) is increased, such drugs should be reduced or discontinued if feasible. A mildly elevated PVR may challenge, but not limit, treatment outcomes.
Acetylcholinesterase inhibitors	These drugs may cause polyuria or contribute to urgency and frequency by increasing acetylcholine levels.	This is only theoretic, but consider it in patients whose symptoms develop after the initiation of one of these agents.

Data from references 33 and 175.

intake of vitamin D, protein, and potassium were associated with a significant *reduction* in risk for OAB symptoms ($p = .008, .03$, and $.05$ respectively). The investigators acknowledged the need for confirmation of these results as well as research into the methods by which these substances may affect the risk for OAB.[40]

The third set of dual surveys, returned by 4887 men, failed to demonstrate any clear association between various foods and OAB symptoms; the possible exception was a very high intake of potatoes, which was correlated with increased risk for OAB ($p = .05$). Interestingly, men who seldom or never drank beer had a significantly greater risk of developing OAB symptoms over the year studied. In this study, physical activity, smoking, and obesity were *not* significantly associated with OAB symptom onset. The researchers concluded that some component of beer may have a protective role in terms of OAB onset, and further study is needed before any conclusions or recommendations can be made.[41]

Obesity. The relationship between obesity in women and all types of incontinence including urge UI has been demonstrated in several studies.[42-44] The NOBLE survey indicated that the prevalence of OAB among women whose body mass index (BMI) exceeded 30 was more than double the prevalence among women of ideal weight. (BMI of 30 or higher was the indicator for obesity).[45]

Smoking. Nicotine has been shown to increase intravesical pressure in anesthetized cats[46] and to produce a phasic contraction in anesthetized guinea pigs.[47] Nuotio and associates also found that smoking was associated with OAB symptoms in elderly persons. These findings were based on population-based interviews of 1059 community-dwelling elderly individuals (60 to 89 years old). Using age-adjusted, logistic regression models, these investigators found that current smokers had a greater risk of urgency (odds ratio [OR], 2.76) than never-smokers and former smokers (OR, 1.63).[48] Two studies demonstrated an association between smoking and increased prevalence of urinary symptoms, including urge UI, among men.[49,50] Although a causal relationship cannot be inferred by any of the studies, these findings are consistent with those of other studies in regard to the relationship among smoking, OAB, and urge UI in adults, both male and female. In summary, the relationship between smoking and all types of incontinence, including urge UI and OAB, is consistent across the life span and for both men and women; current data suggest that current smokers are at greatest risk. These risks continue long after smoking has stopped but do lessen somewhat over time.[42,51-54]

Alcohol. Continence care clinicians have typically counseled patients with OAB symptoms, especially elderly patients, to avoid alcohol. These instructions were based on concerns that alcohol could delay or blunt sensory awareness of bladder filling (because of sedation), could reduce mobility and thus lengthen the time required to reach the bathroom and disrobe for voiding, could cause polyuria from diuresis, and could cause increased urinary frequency and urgency (as a result of polyuria and bladder distension).[55] Recently, Ouslander and Dutcher reviewed oral substances that could potentially affect bladder control;[56] in their report, substances associated with OAB symptoms included diuretics, alcohol, caffeine, and even skeletal muscle relaxants (via urethral sphincter relaxation). Conversely, in three European population-based, postal surveys of 3143 men, 1059 elders, and 27,939 women, no relationship between alcohol and symptoms of OAB was found.[42,50,57] This finding is supported by the study performed by Dallosso and colleagues, in which beer appeared to be protective against OAB for men living in the United Kingdom.[41]

Reduced Reserves Related to Aging. Although normal aging does not cause urinary dysfunction, it does deplete reserves, and this leaves frail elders even more vulnerable to the genitourinary effects of certain medications, altered cognition, and impaired mobility. Infection, atrophic vaginitis, pharmaceuticals, psychologic issues, excessive urine production, reduced mobility, and stool impaction have all been shown to be reversible etiologic factors for OAB in women,[58] and they probably have a negative impact on LUT function in men as well. Any of these factors can exacerbate symptoms and further challenge continence in an individual who already has some degree of bladder overactivity;

however, infection, urogenital atrophy, selected pharmaceuticals, excessive urine production, stool impaction, and functional impairments are especially pertinent to OAB. Guidelines for assessment and correction of reversible and functional factors contributing to incontinence are addressed in greater detail in Chapters 3 and 6.

The estrogen question. The urethra, trigone of the bladder, and vagina are all embryonically related and all include receptors for estrogen, and numerous positive physiologic effects have been ascribed to estrogen and demonstrated in both animal and tissue models.[59] In clinical trials, however, the relative benefits of estrogen have been more difficult to determine. The conflict appears to be at least partly related to the type of incontinence and the route of estrogen administration. In a review article published in 1990, Cardozo questioned the role of estrogen replacement for stress UI but found support for its role in management of the constellation of symptoms that accompanies OAB. Since then, a significant body of evidence has accumulated that suggests that oral estrogen provides no benefit in the treatment of stress UI and may even increase the risk for development of the condition.[60-63] Ouslander and associates found no effect on the severity of incontinence in elderly women with stress and/or urge UI who were treated with oral estrogen combined with progesterone,[63] and Klingele and colleagues found no urodynamic difference in women with stress and urge UI when they were treated with estrogen.[64] In contrast, Fitzgerald and colleagues reported that postmenopausal women receiving hormone replacement therapy (HRT) recorded fewer nighttime voids in their bladder diaries than subjects who were not receiving HRT.[21] Further research is clearly needed to identify the role of HRT in treatment of OAB, stress UI, and mixed stress-urge UI and to clearly differentiate the benefits and adverse effects of oral versus topical therapy.

In a 2003 Cochrane review, Moehrer, Hextall, and Jackson found evidence that HRT (varying combinations of estrogen, dose, treatment duration, and follow-up times) was more useful for urge UI than for stress UI.[65] The effect was not a panacea, however; the overall difference in improvement was only 25% for HRT treatment groups over placebo, and a small difference in the number of voids per 24 hours. There was no statistically significant difference in frequency, nocturia, or urgency among subjects receiving HRT and those who did not. Cardozo and Robinson conducted a literature review in 2003 and found stronger support for the use of estrogen replacement for irritative voiding symptoms (urgency, frequency, and urge UI); however, these investigators suggested that the effect may be related more closely to the reversal of urogenital atrophy than to any direct effect on the LUT. This review found clear support for low-dose, vaginally administered estrogens in the treatment of urogenital atrophy and suggested that such therapy may be efficacious for recurrent UTIs as well.[58] At this point, Ouslander and Greendale suggest that future studies of estrogen for urinary incontinence in frail nursing home residents utilize a topical instead of an oral preparation and include UTI as an outcome measure.[63] This author would extend that recommendation to studies on younger women.

Excess Urine Output. As noted earlier, detrusor distension and the resulting activation of stretch receptors in the muscle fibers serve to initiate the micturition cycle. In an OAB that contracts without the owner's permission and with little notice, excess urine output may be especially troublesome. As explained in Chapter 3, numerous substances and conditions can dramatically increase urine output; these include diuretics, excess fluid intake, and metabolic abnormalities (such as hyperglycemia, hypercalcemia, or diabetes insipidus). Consumption of large amounts of fluids that act as bladder irritants is particularly likely to exacerbate the symptoms of OAB because of the dual effects of excess urine production (which causes detrusor distension) and irritant substances (which cause exaggerated sensory awareness). Nocturnal UI may result from mobilization of fluid that has been sequestered in the lower extremities as a result of venous insufficiency or congestive heart failure;[66] nocturnal UI may also be caused by increased urine production related to hormonal and renal responses to sleep apnea.[67] Many individuals consume their largest quantity of fluid in the morning and may take their diuretic in the morning as well; in these individuals, a diuretic administered with or just before breakfast can be a double insult to a bladder that is already prone to inappropriate contractions.[56]

Relationship to Functional Impairments. As described in Chapter 6, urinary continence requires adequate mobility, mentation, motivation, and manual dexterity in addition to integrated control of the LUT. Again, these issues are especially important for the patient who experiences severe urgency and has limited time to reach the toilet before leakage occurs. Leakage related to altered mobility is one type of functional UI. In a population-based, cross-sectional cohort study of women 20 to 45 years old, van der Vaart and colleagues found a positive relationship between OAB and limited mobility, but no association between limited mobility and stress UI.[68]

Alternative Causes for Specific Symptoms. When an individual presents with symptoms commonly produced by OAB, it is easy to assume that the symptoms are caused by a bladder that is contracting inappropriately, that is, without its owner's permission. Although this is often the case, the clinician must always be alert to evidence of other pathologic conditions that can produce specific LUT symptoms. For example, the patient with urinary retention may present with frequency, urgency, and urge UI and may or may not be aware of incomplete emptying. Another common condition

consists of urgency and frequency caused by excessive fluid intake; this may result from a medical condition or may be a self-induced weight loss strategy. Table 5-4 highlights factors other than OAB that may cause the specific symptoms of frequency, urgency, nocturia, and urge UI.

EVALUATION OF THE PATIENT WITH SUSPECTED OAB

The evaluation of incontinence is discussed in detail in Chapter 12; therefore, this section is limited to aspects that are especially pertinent to OAB and urge UI. As explained in Chapter 12, assessment of any patient with urinary tract dysfunction or UI includes a history, physical examination, and additional tests as indicated; this is true for the patient with OAB as well. Because OAB is essentially a diagnosis of exclusion,[69] the evaluation is designed to identify contributing factors and to assess for conditions other than OAB that could produce the reported symptoms. Box 5-1 summarizes goals for assessment of the patient with suspected OAB.

In July 2001, the ICI2 met in Paris. This international group of experts was organized by the ICS and the International Consultation on Urological Diseases (ICUD) in collaboration with the World Health Organization. One of the results of this important collaboration was evidence-based recommendations for the diagnostic evaluation and

---

TABLE 5-4   Potential Alternative Causes of Specific Overactive Bladder Symptoms

Increased urinary frequency	Behavioral, psychological, environmental issues causing excess fluid intake
	Diurnal or 24-hour polyuria; polyuria/polydipsia syndromes (such as diabetes mellitus, primary polydipsia, diabetes insipidus, hypercalcemia); diuretics
Urgency	Cystitis, estrogen deficiency (atrophic vaginitis/urethritis), decreased bladder capacity, reduced bladder compliance, benign prostatic hypertrophy, bladder cancer, fecal impaction
Nocturia	Sleep-related issues (such as sleep disturbance, sleep apnea, hypnotics or sedatives) Nocturnal polyuria related to daytime fluid retention, venous insufficiency, hypoalbuminemia, diuretic therapy, congestive heart failure, renal disease, neurologic dysfunction, sleep apnea
Urge UI	Detrusor overactivity in the presence of a weak or underactive pelvic floor/urethral sphincter mechanism

Data from references 191 to 193.

BOX 5-1 Goals for Evaluation of Patients with Overactive Bladder Complaints

• •

- Identification and characterization of symptoms
- Identification of transient or reversible factors contributing to bladder Inflammation or impaired emptying (urinary tract infection, atrophic vaginitis/urethritis, fecal impaction)
- Identification of any medical conditions contributing to overactive bladder symptoms that require additional evaluation and management (such as multiple sclerosis, diabetes, Parkinson's disease, cognitive decline, past cerebrovascular accident)
- Screening for other conditions resulting in overactive bladder symptoms (see Tables 5-2 and 5-3)

From Payne CK: Epidemiology, pathophysiology, and evaluation of urinary incontinence and overactive bladder, *Urology* 51(2A suppl):3-10, 1998.

BOX 5-2 Components of the History for Patients with Overactive Bladder Symptoms

• •

Nature and **duration** of genitourinary and lower alimentary tract symptoms

Previous surgical procedures, especially those affecting the genitourinary tract

Environmental issues, including the social and cultural environment

Patient mobility and self-care ability, which may affect management

Mental status, including ability to understand proposed management and participate in treatment plan decisions; formal testing essential when cognitive function in doubt

Disease status: coexisting diseases possibly having profound impact on lower urinary tract function

Medications, including review of every medication and analysis of potential impact on lower urinary tract function

Lower genitourinary symptoms, including those of pelvic organ prolapse

Sexual function: although scientific correlates lacking, sexual function and satisfaction to be assessed when appropriate (depending on age)

Bowel function, which often has considerable influence; fecal incontinence or bowel dysfunction possible in conjunction with LUT dysfunction

Patient's goals or expectations of treatment

Patient's fitness for possible surgical procedures

From Abrams P, Andersson KE, Artibani W, et al. Second International Consultation on Incontinence recommendations of the International Scientific Committee: evaluation and treatment of urinary incontinence, pelvic organ prolapse and faecal incontinence: *http://www.congress-urology.org/image/content.in.pdf,* 2002.

treatment of urinary incontinence.[2] The ICI2 recommendations are divided into highly recommended, recommended, optional, and not recommended. The group highly recommends that all patients who complain of urinary incontinence should receive the following:

- An initial evaluation including a general history
- A symptom review including a simple frequency volume chart
- An assessment of both impact on quality of life and desire for treatment
- A physical examination
- A urinalysis

These recommendations are consistent with those of the ICS. In fact, one of the reasons the ICS accepted the term "overactive bladder" was recognition that empiric diagnoses are often used as the basis for initial management.[24]

History

By definition, the diagnosis of OAB is empiric and is based on a thorough investigation of the patient's presenting symptoms. The four cardinal symptoms of OAB are the following:

- Frequency
- Nocturia
- Urgency
- Leakage after the sensation of urgency[70]

Although a diagnosis cannot be made by history alone, a good history is essential to a comprehensive assessment and should serve to focus the physical examination and to guide selection of additional tests.

The ICI2 stressed the importance of a holistic approach to patient assessment and patient management; this is reflected in their recommendations regarding elements to be included in the history.[2] These elements are listed in Box 5-2.

Symptom Survey and Quality of Life Questionnaires. Several tools have been developed that facilitate the assessment of LUT symptoms and the impact of these symptoms on patients' quality of life (QoL). These tools are helpful in documenting both baseline status and response to treatment, which permits clinicians to monitor efficacy of therapy and helps patients to appreciate how far they have come in terms of improvement. Naughton and colleagues analyzed a number of validated questionnaires currently in use for the evaluation of OAB and urinary incontinence,[71] and they recommended three types of questionnaires for use in clinical practice and research: (1) questionnaires to assess symptoms, (2) generic health-related quality of life tools, and (3) condition-specific measures to assess impact on quality of life. Numerous tools have been developed in each of these categories for the condition of urinary incontinence, and some have been validated specifically for OAB.

Symptom Questionnaires. A thorough and accurate description of symptoms is critical to baseline assessment; these data facilitate diagnosis, help to ensure that treatment goals are consistent with patient goals, and provide the baseline data that permit assessment of treatment response. The Urge-Urinary Distress Inventory measures symptoms and distress specific to OAB and urge UI in women.[72,73] This tool was developed by modifying the well-validated Urological Distress Inventory to focus only on items associated with urge UI and OAB. A four-point scale is used to quantify the degree of "bother" (distress) produced by symptoms such as urinary frequency, urgency, difficulty postponing urination, various types of leakage, nocturia, and nocturnal enuresis. The scores provided by this tool help to differentiate patients with OAB from those with "mixed" symptoms resulting from mixed urinary incontinence.

The King's Health Questionnaire (KHQ), developed in Britain, includes questions about 10 different domains related to health-related quality of life and urinary symptoms. These domains include the following: impact on role, physical, and social performance; personal relationships; emotions; sleep and energy; symptom severity and coping measures; and general health perceptions. Thus, the KHQ serves both to measure symptoms and to provide condition-specific data regarding impact on quality of life.[74] The KHQ has demonstrated good reliability and validity for incontinence-related symptoms and impact on quality of life; it continues to undergo cultural adaptations and international language translations.[71] Recently, the KHQ has also been shown to be a reliable and valid tool for measuring the impact of OAB on health-related quality of life.[75,76] Although "urgency" is the cornerstone symptom of OAB, the term is troublesome for two reasons: (1) some patients use "urgency" or "urge" to describe "normal desire," and (2) the sensation labeled "urgency" may vary among patients.[77] One option is to attempt to differentiate between "urgency" and "desire" (and to agree to avoid the word "urge" early in the evaluation phase). Another option is to use a validated tool that characterizes levels of urgency to facilitate communication about this important symptom. One such tool uses a three-level scale:

- Level 1: "I am usually not able to hold urine."
- Level 2: "I am usually able to hold urine until I reach the toilet if I go immediately."
- Level 3: I am usually able to finish what I am doing before going to the toilet."[78]

  Another tool uses a four-point scale:
- 0: No urgency
- 1: Awareness of urgency but easily tolerated
- 2: Enough urgency/discomfort that it interferes with usual tasks
- 3: Extreme urgency/discomfort that abruptly stops all activity/tasks[79]

Generic Quality of Life Questionnaires. Health-related quality of life tools measure general physical, social, and psychological well-being. Rather than symptoms, they investigate dimensions such as personal productivity, pain, sleep, overall life satisfaction, spirituality, and neuropsychological, cognitive, or sexual function. They can be used to compare the impact of disparate conditions but tend to be relatively insensitive to changes in a specific condition.[71] The Medical Outcomes Study Short – Form-36 is the most commonly used general quality of life tool,[80] and it has been used several times in clinical trials related to OAB.[9,10,45,81,82]

Disease/Condition-Specific Questionnaires. Condition-specific measures can be used not only to measure the burden imposed by a particular condition,[71] but also to predict readiness for treatment and to measure the effect of that treatment.[71,83] Validated quality of life questionnaires specific to OAB and urge UI include the Urge-Urinary Distress Inventory and the KHQ (as described previously), and the OAB-q. The OAB-q is a 33-item, self-administered tool that includes measures of symptom distress (bother) and a health-related quality of life scale; this tool has been shown to discriminate reliably and validly between normal controls and persons with OAB and urge UI.[9]

Bladder Diary: Considerations in Analysis

As discussed in Chapter 12, the bladder diary is an important tool in the evaluation of voiding dysfunction because it reflects the severity of the problem and provides hints regarding patient motivation. The bladder diary is particularly important to the diagnosis of OAB, because this is a symptom-based diagnosis; the bladder diary provides critical data regarding symptom type and symptom severity. Bladder diaries are highly recommended by the ICI2 for determination of urinary frequency, voided volumes, leakage (including antecedent or coincident events, quantity, and frequency), and pad usage. Studies have demonstrated the validity of results obtained by bladder diary when the patient is also provided with written instructions. It is frequently beneficial to send the diary before the first visit; this serves both to reduce the treatment impact of the first encounter and to help focus that first visit.[84] Fig. 5-1 illustrates a bladder diary and instructions designed for this purpose.

In selecting a bladder diary for the patient with OAB, the clinician must consider the various types of diaries/charts available and the data provided by each, the optimal duration of the record, and clear definitions of the terms "urge" and "urgency." (As seen in Table 5-1, urgency is defined as "a sudden compelling desire to pass urine which is difficult to defer," in contrast to normal desire, which is defined as awareness of bladder filling and desire to urinate that *can* be deferred.) Classic "bladder diary" findings for the patient with OAB include voiding more than eight times/24 hours, two or more episodes of nocturia, and episodes of urgency that may or may not lead to leakage.

The ICS has identified three tools for quantifying (LUT) symptoms that are especially useful for documenting baseline status for patients with OAB and also for monitoring response to OAB therapy. As noted earlier, the bladder diary provides a record of voluntary voids, incontinent episodes, and pad usage; many diaries also include information such as types and volumes of fluid intake, the degree of urgency, and events/conditions associated with leakage. It is the gold standard for documenting OAB symptoms at baseline, partly because it allows correlation between type and volume of fluid intake and symptoms; however, it is generally considered too burdensome for ongoing monitoring of symptoms during treatment. Frequency volume charts are a less burdensome approach to monitoring symptoms and response to therapy; data to be recorded are limited to time and volume of voids throughout the 24-hour period (day and night). A 24- to 72-hour frequency volume chart is also recommended for differentiating between nocturnal polyuria and other causes of increased nighttime voiding frequency.[85] To identify nocturnal polyuria, data regarding time and volume of voids must be recorded for a full 24-hour period, and daytime volumes must be differentiated from nighttime volumes;[86] either a bladder diary or a frequency volume chart could be used for this purpose. The simplest type of tool is a micturition time chart; recorded data are limited to the time of micturition throughout a 24-hour period (both day and night). This type of chart may be used to monitor response to treatment if increased urinary frequency is the symptom of major interest, and it offers an alternative for patients who find the frequency volume chart too burdensome.

Electronic Diaries. Quinn, Goka, and colleagues utilized a randomized, crossover design to compare the efficacy of portable electronic diaries to 7-day paper diaries in 35 patients with OAB. These investigators found that the two methods provided similar results, with two exceptions: daily micturitions (7.3 electronic versus 8.5 paper diary) and urgency (5.8 electronic versus 4.7 paper). According to the authors, subjects reported acceptable ease of use for the electronic diaries, and the electronic approach provided the following specific advantages: rapid clinician interpretation, easier comparison of data points (which enhanced assessment of treatment response), and easier communication of data during clinical trials.[87]

Increased Daytime Frequency. Although "normal" voiding frequency has not yet been clearly established, most clinical investigators use the criterion of more than eight voids/24 hours as indicative of increased daytime frequency.[26] In contrast, the ICS uses a patient-based, qualitative definition for increased daytime frequency, that is, "the complaint by the patient who considers that he/she voids too often by day" (see Table 5-1). Although qualitative definitions can be problematic for clinicians and researchers when monitoring outcomes, some researchers consider the standard quantitative definition (more than eight voids in 24 hours) to be too restrictive.[21] The continence clinician is therefore advised not only to consider voiding frequency and the patient's opinion about his or her voiding frequency, but also to consider usual voided volumes; if they are consistently less than expected (less than 250 to 300 mL in adults), intervention is probably indicated.

Although urgency is a key "subjective" indicator of OAB, urinary frequency is an important *objective* indicator. When considering the four cardinal symptoms of OAB, van Brummen and colleagues found that urinary frequency was the symptom most highly correlated with objective parameters from the bladder diary and filling cystometry. These researchers utilized a retrospective review of charts from women with OAB to explore the association between the four cardinal symptoms of OAB and more objective parameters,[88] including bladder diaries, standardized QoL questionnaires, and filling cystometry. Using univariate and multivariate (ANOVA) analysis, the investigators found that the reported *symptom* of urinary frequency was positively correlated with increased 24-hour frequency and lower maximum and mean voided volumes on bladder diaries, and with increased sensory awareness of bladder filling (at lower volumes) and greater propensity to unstable bladder contractions on filling cystometry. Thus, frequency was positively associated with multiple indicators of OAB syndrome.

As noted earlier, bladder diaries are a critical tool in the diagnosis of OAB; therefore, it is essential to assess their validity and reliability.

Brown, McNaughton, and colleagues examined the test-retest reliability and validity of 3- and 7-day bladder diaries in 21 men and 133 women with OAB.[89] These investigators found that a diary exhibited good to excellent reliability and validity for documenting both baseline and posttreatment status in terms of strong urge, diurnal and nocturnal micturitions, total incontinence, and urge UI episodes (for both men and women). They suggested using 3- or 4-day diaries because the data indicated only slight reduction in reliability (as compared with the 7-day diary), which was offset by the reduction in burden for the patients. These investigators also strongly emphasized the importance of providing detailed instruction on diary use. These findings agree with those of Ku and colleagues.[90]

Physical Examination and Basic Testing

The physical exam of the patient with OAB is essentially the same as the examination for any patient with voiding dysfunction and is described in Chapter 12. No physical findings are specific to OAB. Rather, the physical examination is focused on identification of any indicators of medical conditions that could cause or contribute to OAB symptoms (Tables 5-2 and 5-3). Indicators of bladder inflammation, impaired bladder emptying, or neurologic dysfunction are particularly important; therefore, the neurologic, pelvic, and rectal examinations are of special significance in the evaluation of a patient with OAB.

In conducting the neurologic exam, the clinician should pay special attention to any signs of peripheral neuropathy and to mental status. Treatment of OAB frequently involves behavioral therapies; therefore, assessment of cognitive function is an essential element of the initial evaluation. For most patients, the history and bladder diary process provide adequate indicators of cognitive function, but the clinician should not hesitate to include mental status testing if there is any concern regarding cognitive impairment. (Patients are quite accepting of cognitive testing as a component of initial "standard" evaluation, but they may become upset if this testing is done "after the fact," that is, after treatment has been initiated.) In addition to the correlates mentioned under pathophysiology, impaired orientation to time has special relevance, especially when

BLADDER DIARY (Nights and columns 1 and 4 are optional)

Mark here each time you change a pad _____

INSTRUCTIONS: It is very helpful if we know something about your fluid intake, your toileting habits, and if you have it, leakage. Please complete *at least 2 days* worth of this diary; 3 would be better.

Any more than 3 days is not necessary but is quite helpful. If you do only 3 days, be sure to record every urination or wetting carefully.

The columns are as follows:

FLUIDS—Each time you drink something, write down what it was & *about* how much in ounces. If it takes you more than 1 hour to finish, write the amout when started & draw an arrow down to when finished.

URINE—Each time you urinate in the toilet, commode, or urinal: Please mark it in the column marked "Urinated" next to the appropriate hour. Please write the amount either in ounces (preferred) or by estimating and writing "Sm." if it's less than 1/2 a cup, "Med" if it's 1/2 to 1 cup, or "Lg" if it's more than a cup.

BOWEL MOVEMENTS—Please write down each time you have a bowel movement.

LEAKAGE & leakage amount—Each time urine or stool accidentally leaked out, soiled or wet on your underwear, a pad, or on your bed, clothes, furniture, or floor, please estimate the amount and mark it next to the time it happened, under "Leakage" (first column). If you aren't sure when you leaked, please guess the time and place the mark there. For the amount, please jot down whether drops, a squirt, or a gush came out or was it enough to wet or soil your underwear, your clothing, the furniture, or the floor. (D = drops; S = squirt; G = gush; W = wet)

DAY # 1 DATE ------ TIMES →	1. FLUIDS type & amount (in ounces if possible)	2. URINE Amount in oz (Sm, Med, Lg. & / or BM)	3. LEAKAGE Estimated amount (Sm., Med., Lg., or D, S, G, W)	4. ACTIVITY during leakage (lift, stand, cough, sneeze, walk, after urgency, etc.
6 A.M. – 7 A.M.				
7 A.M. – 8 A.M.				
8 A.M. – 9 A.M.				
9 A.M. – 10 A.M.				
10 A.M. – 11 A.M.				
11 A.M. – Noon				
Noon – 1 P.M.				
1 P.M. – 2 P.M.				
2 P.M. – 3 P.M.				
3 P.M. – 4 P.M.				
4 P.M. – 5 P.M.				
5 P.M. – 6 P.M.				

6 P.M. – 7 P.M.						
7 P.M. – 8 P.M.						
8 P.M. – 9 P.M.						
9 P.M. – 10 P.M.						
10 P.M. – 11 P.M.						
11 P.M. – 12 Mid						
12 Mid – 1 A.M.						
1 A.M. – 2 A.M.						
2 A.M. – 3 A.M.						
3 A.M. – 4 A.M.						
4 A.M. – 5 A.M.						
5 A.M. – 6 A.M.						

ACTIVITY—With leakage of urine or stool, jot down what you were doing as you leaked (standing, coughing, sneezing, lifting, walking, on the way to the bathroom, doing nothing at all, etc).

Be sure to note whether your bladder gave you a warning before the urine leaked out (even if only a few seconds before) and if so, was it a normal "DESIRE" or "URGENT"?

With BMs or leakage of stool, note if hard, firm, soft, not formed, etc.

SUGGESTIONS:

1. Keep the diary and a pen very handy. It's tough to remember things like toileting/urinating, so mark your record right away.

2. If marking in this record is difficult, *mark only columns 3 & 4.*

3. If marking in this record will disturb your sleep, don't mark it during bedtime hours, but try to remember what happened the next morning.

4. If still a problem, make up your own diary and don't use this one.

Fig. 5-1 This sample bladder diary illustrates one day's bladder activity. A 3-day diary should be given to the patient because 3 days of data are needed for evaluation.

bladder overactivity is combined with blunted sensation of bladder filling.[91]

In addition to factors discussed in Chapter 12, the pelvic and rectal examinations for the patient with OAB include several aspects of special interest: vaginal vault support and tissue integrity, evidence of fecal impaction, and PFM function. Special attention is paid to assessment of vaginal vault support and rectal fullness because moderate to severe pelvic organ prolapse and fecal impaction can both result in partial bladder outlet obstruction. The clinician must also assess the female patient with OAB for evidence of atrophic vaginitis or urethritis, because atrophic urethritis may contribute to irritative voiding symptoms (urgency and increased detrusor irritability). PFM tone and function may be etiologic factors for the development of OAB and are important in therapy; thus, it is important to evaluate the patient's ability to isolate the PFMs and to assess both contractile strength and endurance. Although pelvic floor weakness and poor endurance have long been considered risk factors for urinary incontinence and OAB,[92] recent data suggest that *high* PFM tone may be related to OAB.[93] Careful palpation of the vaginal and perineal tissues and the anal sphincter may reveal areas of spasticity or tenderness, which are indicators of high PFM tone.

Advanced Testing: Urodynamics. Urodynamic testing provides dynamic assessment of the mechanical and physiologic activity of the bladder and its outlet. Its aim is to "reproduce symptoms whilst making precise measurements in order to identify the underlying causes for the symptoms, and to quantify the related pathophysiological processes. By doing so, it should be possible to establish objectively the presence of a dysfunction and understand its clinical implications."[94] According to the ICI2, key objectives of the routine urodynamic evaluation are as follows:

- Detecting detrusor overactivity
- Assessing urethral competence during filling
- Determining detrusor function during voiding
- Measuring residual urine

As described in Chapter 12, urodynamic studies usually include filling cystometry (with provocation, and tailored to the individual patient's requirements) and voiding cystometry.[2] Urodynamic testing is *not* routinely indicated for the patient with OAB; ICI2 indications for urodynamic testing in these patients are limited to the following: patients in whom primary treatment has failed, patients in whom invasive therapies are being considered, and patients with neurogenic LUT dysfunction and complicated UI (as part of a long-term surveillance program). See the discussion on situations warranting referral or specialized testing (Box 5-3).

Filling cystometry can be accomplished via simple (also called "bedside" or "eyeball") or complex multichannel techniques. Simple cystometry may be single channel utilizing a urethral catheter connected to an open syringe or a manometer,[95,96] or it may be dual channel, in which a rectal balloon catheter is placed to provide monitoring of abdominal pressure.[97] (see Chapter 12). Multichannel cystometry allows simultaneous monitoring of detrusor pressures, rectal pressures, sphincter electromyography (EMG), and possibly urethral pressures during the filling phase; these data provide thorough insight into outlet function during bladder filling. (Technical aspects of complex urodynamics are thoroughly described by the ICS in the article entitled "Good Urodynamic Practice."[94]) Irrespective of the method used, detrusor function is monitored in terms of capacity, compliance, and stability, and the patient is queried as to sensory awareness. Bladder stability is a particularly important element of assessment for the patient with OAB; therefore, provocative measures are typically included in the filling study for these patients. (Provocative measures include rapid filling, exposing the patient to the sound of running water, and placing the patient's hands in warm water; in the patient with OAB, these maneuvers typically prompt severe urgency and frequently cause urinary leakage.)

The pressure flow study (voiding cystometry) provides thorough assessment of the emptying phase via multichannel cystometry; data gathered include detrusor pressure, abdominal pressure, and sphincter activity as well as urinary flow rate and voided volume. For the patient with impaired bladder emptying, simultaneous monitoring of urinary flow rate, detrusor pressure, and striated sphincter function (via EMG) during voiding allows the clinician to determine whether the problem results from an underactive detrusor (impaired contractility) or an overactive outlet (bladder outlet obstruction).

Typical urodynamic findings for the patient with OAB include hypersensitivity to bladder filling (sensory awareness of bladder filling at low bladder volumes) and involuntary detrusor contractions during filling that either lead to leakage or are spontaneously suppressed via PFM activity (as shown on the EMG). Because mixed (stress and urge) urinary symptoms are so common, urethral sphincter integrity is typically also determined via the leak point pressure. If the patient leaks with cough or Valsalva maneuver during the leak point pressure study, it is important to analyze the coincident detrusor pressure because the leakage may actually have been caused by an involuntary detrusor contraction rather than a weak urethral sphincter mechanism. In addition, because impaired or prolonged emptying may accompany OAB symptoms, the voiding cystometrogram should be assessed for evidence of impaired emptying. Low flow rates despite high detrusor pressures are indicative of bladder outlet obstruction, whereas low flow rates accompanied by low detrusor pressures suggest impaired detrusor contractility. As noted earlier, bladder overactivity may coexist with impaired contractility, especially in older adults; this condition is known as DHIC.[37] Table 5-5 lists common and potential findings from the evaluation of patients with OAB.

TABLE 5-5   **Common or Potential Findings in the Evaluation of Patients with Symptoms of Overactive Bladder**

PORTION OF EVALUATION	COMMON OR POTENTIAL FINDING	CONSIDERATIONS
Patterns	Insidious onset	Difficult to pinpoint, often "years ago"
	Gradual progression	Possible periods of partial remission
	Response to past treatments (medical and self-care) often less than satisfactory	Past history of several different treatments possible
Symptoms	Urinary frequency	Usually more than eight voids/ 24 hours
	Urinary urgency	A strong and sudden desire to void
	Urinary urge incontinence: leakage shortly after, or in concert with, the sensation of urgency	If the urgency cannot be suppressed or "can't reach toilet in time"
	Amount of urine lost possibly large	Bladder may empty completely
	Nocturia: complaints of voiding during the night	0 to 1 times/night is normal
	Nocturnal enuresis (bedwetting)	Difficult to tolerate
	May have "unconscious incontinence;" (leakage related to bladder overactivity in absence of urgency or even an awareness of the leakage)	May herald neurologic disease
	Leakage with activity: may indicate an involuntary bladder contraction that was stimulated by movement or stress urinary incontinence related to a weak urethral sphincter	Mixed incontinence refers to stress and urge together

Continued

TABLE 5-5 **Common or Potential Findings in the Evaluation of Patients with Symptoms of Overactive Bladder—cont'd**

PORTION OF EVALUATION	COMMON OR POTENTIAL FINDING	CONSIDERATIONS
Review of symptoms: focus on consequences of OAB symptoms and factors potentially related to etiology	Voiding symptoms: urinary hesitancy, weak or intermittent stream, sensation of incomplete emptying	Bladder outlet obstruction or weak detrusor
	Fatigue/low energy/daytime sleepiness	Nocturia or nocturnal enuresis
	Blurred vision, double vision; excess fluid intake, polyuria, increased appetite	Glaucoma, multiple sclerosis, diabetes, behavioral
	Dry eyes or dry mouth	May limit use of anticholinergics
	Voice or breath changes when supine, sleep apneic episodes, sleep disturbance	
	Pedal edema, nocturnal cough, or paroxysmal nocturnal dyspnea	Consider congestive heart failure
	Sexual concerns	Orgasm may stimulate bladder contraction
	Perineal redness, odor, rash or itching	Diaper dermatitis or candidiasis; assess containment products and skin care
	Low back pain, general muscle weakness, paresthesias, transient paralysis, radicular pain, tremors, or altered perineal sensation	Consider neurologic disorder
	Mood lability, anxiety, poor concentration	Consider impaired quality of life, depression, or cognitive decline
Medications and substances	Diuretics, alcohol	Sudden diuresis, activates stretch fibers and may cause involuntary bladder contraction
	Tricyclic antidepressants, alpha agonists, beta antagonists, narcotic analgesics, sedatives, anticholinergics	Enhanced urethral tone or reduced bladder activity may impair emptying
Medical history	Cerebrovascular accident, spinal cord injury, multiple sclerosis, dementia	Consider neurologic cause for OAB
	Prior pelvic or abdominal surgery	Assess for weak pelvic floor or subtle BOO
	Benign and malignant diseases of the prostate	BOO
Physical exam:		
Digital rectal exam and the appropriate utilization of prostate-specific antigen testing	Enlarged prostate; fecal impaction	BOO
Abdominal exam	Full bladder and colonic distension	Assess for retention/BOO
Neurologic assessment (perineum and lower extremities)	Normally intact	If abnormal, consider neurologic etiology OAB
Vaginal exam in women	Evidence of prolapse or hormonal deficiency	Contributing factors to OAB
Anterior vaginal wall prolapse during Valsalva's maneuver in women	Check for cystocele and urethral hypermobility	Contributing factors to OAB

TABLE 5-5   **Common or Potential Findings in the Evaluation of Patients with Symptoms of Overactive Bladder—cont'd**

PORTION OF EVALUATION	COMMON OR POTENTIAL FINDING	CONSIDERATIONS
Pelvic floor muscle function: isolation, strength, endurance, tenderness, spasticity	Check visually and during vaginal and/or rectal exam	May be normal, weak, or spastic; weak or spastic PFMs may contribute to OAB
BASIC TESTING RECOMMENDED BEFORE INITIAL TREATMENT		
Urinalysis, urine microscopy and culture, diagnostic gold standard.	Pyuria and/or bacteriuria: possible UTI, do culture and sensitivity if symptomatic	UTI may cause OAB-type symptoms via increased bladder sensitivity
Reagent strip testing for screening (sensitive and less expensive)	If microscopic hematuria:- cytology for lower urinary tract cancer (may cause urgency, frequency, and BOO)	Avoid OAB treatment until hematuria is worked up
	Glucosuria	Consider diabetes
	Proteinuria	Consider renal pathology
Postvoid residual measurement by ultrasound or catheter	Should be done for pt with voiding symptoms (see review of symptoms), recurrent or persistent UTIs, complicated neurologic disease, or suspicion of distended bladder on physical examination	More than 100 mL is positive but clinical impact of 100 to 200 mL unclear. Check medication side effects
ADVANCED TESTING RESERVED FOR SPECIFIC INDICATIONS		
Urodynamic studies (see below)	Demonstrates bladder versus outlet causes of leakage and poor emptying. Indicated for complicated urinary incontinence, uncertain diagnosis resulting from mixed symptoms, or failed initial treatment	With OAB, detrusor overactivity (involuntary contractions) often seen during filling cystometry
Endoscopic evaluation of the lower urinary tract	Cystourethroscopy	Evaluate possible neoplasms, inflammation, or anatomic obstruction
Serum lab tests	Creatinine	Check renal function
	Prostate-specific antigen	Check for prostatic cancer
	Urine cytology if hematuria, new-onset urgency, or pain	To identify or rule out urinary tract neoplasm
Radiographic imaging.	Voiding cystourethrogram, magnetic resonance imaging, intravenous pyelography, renal ultrasound, spine imaging, computed tomography, myelography done only when indicated and only if results may alter treatment plan	Suspected pelvic, lower urinary tract, or neurogenic cause of OAB (such as significant postvoiding residual, flank pain, severe untreated pelvic organ prolapse (POP)

BOO, bladder outlet obstruction; OAB, overactive bladder; UTI, urinary tract infection.
Data from references 2, 33, and 194.

Situations Warranting Referral or Specialized Testing. In most patients with symptoms of OAB, a presumptive diagnosis can be made following a careful history, physical, and bladder diary assessment. If the initial assessment reveals evidence of serious medical disorders or complicated UI, further testing and referrals are indicated. The ICI2 recommends further testing (which may include urodynamics) or specialty referral in the situations noted in Box 5-3.[2]

Putting the Evaluation in Perspective

In selected situations, primary assessment findings reveal evidence of a significant problem that mandates further testing and evaluation; however, in the majority of cases, the primary assessment serves to support the clinical diagnosis of OAB. In these situations, it is safe to begin conservative therapy following the basic evaluation. Most clinicians and researchers (including the ICS) recognize that it is safe to initiate empiric therapy once a basic assessment has been completed, especially since we now have numerous therapies available that are fairly low risk.[24,98]

BOX 5-3 **International Consultation on Urinary Incontinence Recommendations for Further Testing**

Either sex
  Recurrent incontinence
  Incontinence associated with:
    Pain
    Hematuria
    Recurrent infection
    Voiding symptoms
    Radical pelvic surgery
Male patients
  Prostate irradiation
Female patients
  Incontinence associated with:
    Pelvic irradiation
    Suspected fistula
    Other abnormality
    Significant postvoid residual
    Significant pelvic organ prolapse
    Pelvic mass

Mostwin emphasized this by pointing out that, with the exception of the serious medical disorders listed in Box 5-3, first-line therapeutic choices may not require diagnostic precision.[99] The critical priorities are to complete a basic evaluation, start conservative therapy, closely monitor patient response, and then adjust, adjust, adjust as needed or refer as indicated. There are now many scientifically based options available for the treatment of OAB. What is important is to get the patient started.

NURSING'S ROLE IN MANAGEMENT OF PATIENTS WITH OAB

Nurses integrate a substantial amount of scientific knowledge and technical skill into their efforts to help people cope with difficulties in daily living associated with health problems. Continence nurses utilize a holistic approach,[100] which fully recognizes the psychoneurologic aspects of OAB pathophysiology and is based on using behavioral interventions to meet the patient's goals.[101] Although nurses are adept at helping patients *manage* many alterations in health status, OAB is one area in which *cure* may be realized by approaches fully in the realm of nursing. Continence nurses are able to evaluate individuals with incontinence and to assist patients in effecting their own cure via behavioral interventions. Continence nurses also help patients to manage OAB symptoms with products and devices, and they may provide counseling regarding pharmaceutical therapies. (Advanced practice nurses may also prescribe medications when indicated.) The foundation of present-day continence care includes a strong focus on multidisciplinary collaboration,[102] and the complexity of OAB certainly demands a multidisciplinary approach.

Orem's Self-Care Theory of Nursing and OAB

Nursing theory provides a context and justification for professional nursing and guides not only practice but knowledge acquisition and research.[103] One such theory, the Self-Care Deficit Theory of Nursing developed by Dorothea Orem, Ph.D., is especially useful as a guide to nurses who manage patients with OAB and urge UI.[104] According to Orem, self-care is an intentional act, usually self-directed, that maintains life and supports healthful functioning. Because OAB involves neurourology that can sometimes be controlled by patients,[105] and because behavioral strategies are often suggested as first-line therapy,[2] nurses are uniquely prepared to manage patients with OAB, and Orem's Self-Care Theory provides the context and guidance for that care. Bernier provides insight into the relevance of Orem's Self-Care Theory to continence care; she describes the demands placed on the patient by bladder dysfunction and addresses nursing's ability to reduce the demand by bolstering the patient's ability to take control (self-care agency).[103] Because behavioral therapies are critical to successful treatment, Orem's theory is especially pertinent for nurses working with patients affected by OAB. Bernier suggested that Orem's Self-Care Deficit Theory of Nursing serves as a practical guide that encourages strong patient responsibility.[106]

Health behavior change theory may also be applicable to continence care; specific theories included in this category include Social Cognitive Theory, Health Belief Model, and the Transtheoretical and Stages of Change Model.[107] One area of commonality among these theories is the concept of self-efficacy or confidence in one's ability, similar to the "self-care agency" concept described earlier. Bernier reminds us that patient motivation is critical to the success of behavioral therapy, and that the continence nurse acts as facilitator, educator, resource person, and cheerleader and bolsters motivation by enhancing both patient confidence and ability. Palmer makes an eloquent argument that integration of health behavior change theories into continence research should ultimately reduce the incidence and prevalence of incontinence.

TREATMENT OF OAB AND URGE UI

The ICI2 recommends noninvasive therapies (behavioral and pharmaceutical therapies) as first-line treatment for patients with urge UI and OAB; they recommend that surgery be considered only if these treatments fail. (See Appendix B.)

Specific therapies recommended for men with OAB include the following:
- Pelvic floor exercises
- Bladder training
- Antimuscarinic drugs if detrusor overactivity is suspected
- Alpha-adrenergic antagonists (alpha blockers) if bladder outlet obstruction is suspected

Specialty referral is highly recommended for men who fail to demonstrate significant improvement after 8 to 12 weeks.

Specific therapies recommended by this group of international experts for women include the following:
- Life-style interventions
- PFM training (PFMT)
- Bladder training with or without antimuscarinic therapy

Life-style interventions include weight reduction, smoking cessation, dietary modifications, fluid management, and, when indicated, treatment for estrogen deficiency and UTI. When symptoms of both stress UI and OAB/urge UI are present, the group recommends that initial treatment be directed to the predominant symptom. If response is inadequate after 8 to 12 weeks, the ICI2 recommends reassessment and consideration of specialty referral.[2]

Before beginning any treatment specific to OAB symptoms, it is important to evaluate for and address as many of the factors listed in Tables 5-2 and 5-3 as possible.

Behavioral Therapies: Overview

Behavioral therapies include life-style interventions, bladder training (including urge suppression strategies), and PFMT. These therapies are designed to prevent or reduce the occurrence of OAB symptoms and to provide the patient with tools to suppress urgency when it does occur. Dr. Kathryn Burgio describes behavioral treatment as a group of therapies that involve learning new skills or strategies and changing one's behaviors or environment to improve bladder control. For urge UI, the goal is "improving the patient's ability to inhibit detrusor contractions using pelvic muscle training, urge suppression strategies, or timed voiding schedules such as bladder training."[105] For OAB, PFMT, urge inhibition techniques, and bladder training are related strategies that can be viewed as a continuum of care and that can be used in a stair-step approach.

With the exception of dietary modifications, there is significant overlap in the behavioral therapies recommended for patients with stress UI and urge UI, a fact that is convenient considering the prevalence of mixed symptoms. There are some differences, however, in the underlying mechanisms, goals, techniques, and efficacy of these therapies when used for OAB as opposed to stress UI. Some overlap also exists between strategies used for management of OAB and those used for patients with functional UI. Behavioral therapies for stress UI and functional UI are addressed in Chapters 4 and 6, respectively. This section explores the use of behavioral therapies for OAB and urge UI.

Life-Style Interventions

Dietary modifications. Dietary modifications for patients with OAB involve modifying the intake of food and fluids that may affect the irritability, sensitivity, or motor activity of the bladder. Based on anecdotal evidence, many authors suggest the following as being potentially problematic for the patient with OAB: caffeine; coffee and tea (even if decaffeinated, for some patients); alcohol; chocolate; carbonation; citrus juices and fresh citrus fruits; fresh or cooked tomatoes; cola drinks; and other substances such as honey, sugar and artificial sweeteners.[108] Unfortunately, only a few of these have been investigated scientifically.[109] As explained in the section on "risk factors", life-style factors that have been investigated include carbonation, caffeine, vegetables, bread, chicken, alcohol, fluid intake, obesity, and smoking. As noted in Table 5-2, constipation is an important life-style factor. A high intake of vegetables, bread, and chicken *may* delay the onset of OAB in women, and a low intake of beer may hasten its onset for men, but the impact of these agents may not pertain to persons who already have OAB symptoms. In addition, there are conflicting data about the impact of alcohol consumption on OAB symptoms. For now, the best evidence we have is regarding the relationship of OAB symptoms and caffeine, constipation, fluid intake, obesity, and smoking.

For the other potential irritants, such as alcohol, chocolate, carbonation, citrus in juice or fresh fruit, cold (fresh) or cooked tomatoes, and other substances such as honey, sugar, and artificial sweeteners, it seems reasonable to notify patients with OAB that these substances may increase symptoms, so personal experimentation is an option. Fig. 5-2 is a patient education sheet that lists the many ways in which caffeine can slip into the diet and suggests personal monitoring for the effects of other possible irritants.

Caffeine intake management. Caffeine is associated with symptoms of OAB;[52] fortunately for patients, it appears to be a dose-related response. Arya and colleagues found that women with high levels of caffeine intake (484 ± 123 mg/day) demonstrated more detrusor instability on cystometry than women with lower levels of caffeine intake (194 ± 84 mg/day).[110] (A 5-ounce cup of brewed coffee has 100 to 164 mg of caffeine.) Creighton and Stanton found that the administration of 200 mg of caffeine citrate before cystometry significantly increased the incidence of uninhibited contractions in 20 women known to have detrusor instability (OAB); interestingly, administration of caffeine to asymptomatic women produced no such change in detrusor activity.[111] Bryant and colleagues assessed the impact of caffeine reduction in a prospective, randomized trial involving 95 adults; both groups received bladder training, and the experimental group also reduced caffeine intake to less than 100 mg/day. The group who also reduced caffeine intake had no greater reduction in episodes of leakage but did report a significant decline in urgency and frequency as compared with the control group.[112]

The pharmacology and effects of caffeine and its role in urinary incontinence were addressed in an Evidence-Based Report Card (EBRC) published in the *Journal of Wound, Ostomy and Continence Nursing* in 2001.[113] Findings were as follows:
- Caffeine affects smooth muscle contractility in the human detrusor by mobilizing intracellular stores of calcium ions.
- This effect is altered by neurotransmitters affecting the LUT and by the extracellular pH (concentration of hydrogen ions).

DIETARY CHANGES AND BLADDER IRRITANTS

Some foods have a tendency to make bladders overactive. If your bladder is irritable, consider reducing or at least experimenting with some of the items below. If the reduction helps, continue for a while, then add items back SLOWLY, carefully & in moderation.

Dietary changes may help improve bladder control. Reducing alcohol, sugar substitutes, and *caffeine may be* very helpful.

With the exception of caffeine, response to these items is *very* individual, so experiment: stop the items for 3–5 days then try a little, then try more, when keeping a diary of frequency, urgency, & leakage.

Limit the items that increase urinary frequency or urgency and enjoy the others.

Keep urine dilute—most need ½ oz fluid for every 1 lb. of body weight/day but most come from food.

Shoot for 48 – 64 oz/day = 6 – 8, 8 oz cups

1/2 should be clear liquids you can see.

Citrus juice (fruit is OK)—Bladder irritant for some.

Limit alcohol—May increase night bladder problems

Colas & soda pop—Carbonation alone irritates some bladders. Dark colas usually the worst.

Artificial sweeteners—Aspartame and possibly saccharine, *may* irritate some bladders.

Tomatoes & spicy foods—more often a problem if not a regular part of diet.

Space fluids evenly throughout the day.
If you urinate too often during the night, try *filling* your tanks early in the day (before 6 pm). Then limit evening & night time fluids.

Keep stool regular & soft but formed
Constipation from low fluid & *fiber* leads to:
• enlarged bowel & sometimes difficult urination
• bladder instability (overactivity)

Limit caffeine, the most universal blader stimulant
Substitutes for caffeinated tea & coffee
• Decaf coffee or tea; some decaf processes add irritating chemicals. If decaf is too stimulating for you, try European Water Process decaf.
• Pero coffee substitute (health food stores)
• Sun-brew tea to decrease acidity
• Experiment with herbal teas. (There are 100s). Some are very robust and satisfying such as: Good Earth Herbal Sweet & Spicy Blend or Republic of Tea - Cardamon Cinnamon

More than 200 mg/day (or in a short interval) of caffeine irritates many a bladder. Although often not on labels, caffeine is often found in many processed foods and over-the-counter medications.

Caffeine can be found in surprising places.

Source (milligram)	Serving	Caffeine (mg)
Coffee: Brewed	5 oz	100-164
Instant	5 oz	50-75
Decaffeinated	5 oz	2-4
Tea: 1-Minute brew	5 oz	20-34
3-Minute brew	5 oz	35-46
5-Minute brew	5 oz	39-50
Iced Tea	12 oz	67-76
Chocolate Milk	5 oz	2-15
Hot Chocolate	5 oz	2-15
Soft Drinks:		
Coca-Cola	12 oz	46
Diet Coke	12 oz	46
Tab	12 oz	46
Pepsi-Cola	12 oz	38
Diet Pepsi	12 oz	36
Jolt Cola	12 oz	71
Dr Pepper	12 oz	40
Mountain Dew	12 oz	54
Chocolate Desserts:		
Brownie (w/nut)	1.25 oz	8
Cake	1/16 of 9"	14
Ice Cream	cup	5
Pudding	cup	6
Chocolate Candy:		
Milk Chocolate	1 oz	1-15
Dark Chocolate	1 oz	20
Baking Chocolate	1 oz	25-35
Pain killers:		
Anacin	2 tablets	64
Excedrin	2 tablets	130
Vanquish	2 tablets	66
Midol	2 tablets	64
Aspirin (plain)	2 tablets	0
Cold/Allergy:		
Coryban-D	1 tablet	30
Dristan	2 tablets	32
Sinarest	1 tablet	30
Stimulants:		
No-Doz	2 tablets	200
Vivarin	1 tablet	200

Fig. 5-2 Evaluating bladder irritants. A patient education tool. (Courtesy Marta Krissovich.)

- In the clinical setting, the net effect of caffeine administration appears to be an increase in detrusor muscle tone.
- Little evidence exists to substantiate claims that caffeine acts as a diuretic.

Based on the foregoing, it is reasonable to suggest that patients with OAB limit their total caffeine intake to 200 mg/day or less. Patients who report nocturia should, of course, eliminate caffeine later in the day.

Bowel management. The relationship between bladder function and bowel function is irrefutable. Fecal and urinary incontinence often occur together, especially in the older adult,[114] and OAB and constipation are associated with the same risk factors[115] and comorbidities,[58] at least in women. In addition, detrusor overactivity and functional bowel disorders may share the same pathophysiology in terms of afferent mechanisms.[116] Furthermore, constipation may cause or contribute to bladder overactivity via outlet obstruction,[117] and OAB may contribute to constipation because a common coping mechanism among patients with OAB is fluid restriction.[118] There are also similarities in the personal and physiologic impact of bowel and bladder dysfunction, and the side effects of antimuscarinic medications can affect both the bowel and the bladder.[119,120] Finally, bowel and bladder dysfunction sometimes respond comparably to similar therapies.[121]

The treatment of constipation is described in detail in Chapters 14 and 15. In summary, the age-old "prescription" of fluid, fiber, and activity remains appropriate as initial management. The continence clinician should assess all patients with bladder dysfunction for evidence of constipation and should assist patients to find acceptable ways to increase their fiber, fluid, and activity to the recommended levels. Patients who fail to respond to these strategies require further evaluation and more aggressive management, as discussed in Chapter 14.

Fluid management. Continence clinicians have long suggested fluid management as an important strategy for enhancing bladder control, and they carefully monitor intake via bladder diaries or fluid volume charts. The theory is that both inadequate and excess levels of fluid intake can be problematic. Fluid reduction has been described as a common coping technique that is often deemed useful by patients with OAB;[122-124] however, inadequate intake may result in concentrated urine, which is thought to act as a bladder irritant and to produce increased urgency and frequency. Inadequate intake may also cause constipation, which can partially block the bladder outlet and thus contribute to the symptoms of OAB (via increased activity of the local afferent pathways). Excessive intake can also be problematic, in that excess intake causes increased urine production, which contributes to urinary frequency; in addition, if the bladder fills rapidly because of fluid boluses, the sudden bladder distension can trigger detrusor overactivity. Excessive intake is becoming more common because of the increased emphasis on water intake ("the more water the better"); this is reflected by the fact that water bottles have become ubiquitous. Intake is sometimes increased in an attempt to elevate the urinary pH; this maneuver is based on the incorrect belief that acidic urine increases urinary urgency and frequency and that increased fluid intake will alkalinize the urine.[118] In reality, increased fluid intake typically *lowers* the urinary pH, thus resulting in *more* acidic urine; this is beneficial in that acidic urine causes less odor, is less damaging to the perineal skin, reduces the risk of UTI, and is more physiologic than alkaline urine. However, *excess* amounts of fluid intake can cause urgency, frequency, and leakage, as described earlier. A strong link has been demonstrated between volume of fluid intake and both nocturnal urine production in men[125] and nocturnal urinary leakage in impaired elders with urge UI and detrusor instability (documented by cystometry);[126] however, the impact of increased fluid intake on diurnal voiding patterns is less clear.

Fluid intake does, of course, correlate to urine production and therefore to urinary frequency;[127,128] however, research has yet to show a direct correlation between fluid intake (either increased or decreased) and either urinary urgency or diurnal urge UI.

This subject was explored in an EBRC in the *Journal of Wound, Ostomy and Continence Nursing.*[129] Current evidence supports the following as optimal daily fluid intake, whether or not the individual is incontinent: 30 mL/kg of body weight/day, or

1500 to 2500 mL/day.[130,131] The EBRC also suggested that increased fluid intake could reduce the occurrence of UTI and bladder cancer, two causes of urgency and frequency. This recommendation is particularly relevant for elders, because they are at increased risk for dehydration and constipation, and their sense of thirst as a warning sign of dehydration is less reliable.[132] Because sudden bladder distension can cause or contribute to uninhibited detrusor contractions, it seems reasonable to counsel patients to spread their intake more evenly throughout the day. In addition, the literature does support counseling those who suffer from nocturia to reduce fluids 2 hours before bed. Patients with nocturia who complain of excess evening thirst can be counseled to "fill their tanks" earlier in the day. If the complaint is one of continual thirst, the clinician should rule out diabetes mellitus and should review their medications for anticholinergic side effects and their total fluid intake for adequacy.

Weight management. BMI is measured as weight in kilograms/height in meters;[133,134] the range for ideal/normal is 18.5 to 24.9, the range for overweight is 25.0 to 29.9, and the range for obese is 30.0 and greater.[135] BMI ranges are based on the effect of body weight on disease and death. As BMI increases, especially to 30 or higher, the risk for premature death, cardiovascular disease, high blood pressure, osteoarthritis, some cancers, and diabetes all increase as well.[136] We now have some evidence that the risk for incontinence also increases. In a small study of morbidly obese women, bariatric surgery significantly reduced both urge UI and stress UI.[137] Using both subjective and objective measures (including cystometry), there was a significant reduction in incontinence among these patients; only 25% of the 12 patients who complained of urinary leakage before surgery reported leakage after surgery, and only one of those believed that her urinary incontinence required treatment. The improved control persisted at 1-year follow-up. Although this finding was expected for stress UI because of the mechanical impact of obesity on the LUT, the mechanism for the improvement in urge UI is more elusive. In another small study ($n = 10$) of significantly overweight women (mean BMI, 38.3 ± 10.1), even a 5% weight loss resulted in 51%

reduction in leakage episodes.[138] The picture is less clear, however, regarding the impact of weight loss in men and in overweight, as opposed to obese, women.[139] Although "ideal" body weight is a laudable goal, patients who are able to reduce their BMI to less than 30, or perhaps by just 5%, can significantly reduce their risk of OAB symptoms (as well as their risk for cardiovascular disease and premature death).

Smoking cessation. The impact of smoking cessation on OAB has not been directly studied, but the data suggest a benefit. Nicotine is thought to be stimulating to bladder smooth muscle, and former smokers have a lower risk for urgency than current smokers. This finding supports the assumption that smoking likely enhances bladder overactivity in men and women. Although the effect of smoking cessation may not be felt as quickly or dramatically as weight loss, patients should be counseled that OAB is one more reason to reduce or eliminate tobacco use.

Bladder Training. The term "bladder training," also known as bladder drill, bladder reeducation, or bladder retraining, was first introduced as "bladder discipline" by Jeffcoate and Francis in the 1960s.[140] Some use the term "bladder training" as an umbrella term for all scheduled voiding regimens including timed voiding, prompted voiding, habit training, and patterned urge response toileting; however, each of these is a separate entity. All five of these programs fit better under the umbrella classification of "scheduled voiding regimens."[141] Bladder training is a specific program designed to increase bladder capacity and reduce urinary frequency; it is indicated for motivated and cognitively intact individuals with OAB symptoms and is discussed in this chapter. The other types of scheduled voiding regimens are indicated primarily for individuals with functional incontinence and are therefore discussed in Chapter 6.

Bladder training is recommended for the initial management of OAB and urge, stress, and mixed urinary incontinence in both men and women.[2] It is most often utilized for management of OAB symptoms and urge UI, especially when the patient also experiences frequency. The determination of abnormal frequency must be based on usual voided volumes. For example, patients often say, "Yes, I urinate often but that's because I drink so much." The accuracy of this statement must be determined by analysis of the bladder diary. If voided volumes are significantly greater than "average" (more than 500 to 600 mL), and the patient is complaining of LUT symptoms such as urgency, the patient may benefit either from a timed voiding program in which he or she voids by the clock (if she or he is voiding infrequently) or from a reduction in fluid intake (if she or he is voiding large volumes on a frequent basis). In contrast, the patient with urinary frequency whose voided volumes are much less than average (less than 250 to 300 mL) is likely to benefit from bladder training, assuming that she or he is motivated and cognitively intact.

The specific mechanisms by which bladder training "works" is unknown but may include improved cortical control over LUT function.[142] Potential goals for bladder training include extended voiding intervals, increased functional bladder capacity, improved bladder control, and resumption of normal activities. Bladder training serves to guide patients in reestablishing bladder control via the following interventions: comprehensive patient education with a focus on strategies for controlling urgency and delaying voiding, scheduled voiding programs with progressive extension of the voiding interval, and positive reinforcement.[143,144] The comprehensive education includes items such as basic genitourinary anatomy, the phases of micturition (in lay terms), an explanation of the patient's specific bladder control disorder(s), and the principles underlying the bladder training program.

A patient instruction sheet for bladder training is shown in Fig. 5-3. A fluid volume chart that may be used during bladder training is shown in Fig. 5-4. If this proves too burdensome for the patient, the clinician may elect to omit the least important portions; for example, the record of fluid intake may be omitted if fluid intake is not an issue for that particular patient.

There are several key steps the clinician must follow to initiate a bladder training program.[145] First, the clinician must analyze a bladder diary that has been completed by the patient; ideally this is a 3-day bladder recording though a 1-day recording

can be used if that is the only data available. The clinician uses the bladder diary data to determine the patient's shortest comfortable voiding interval and uses this as the initial voiding interval for the bladder training program. The clinician must then instruct the patient in the bladder training program, emphasizing the following points:

1. Void soon after rising in the morning and then begin voiding at the established interval (based on your shortest comfortable voiding interval) for 1 to 2 weeks. (Urinate by the clock, not by the urge.)
2. Urinate just before bed and urinate based on need, not the voiding schedule, during the night.
3. Increase the voiding interval by 15 to 20 minutes each time the previous voiding interval is "successfully" achieved. ("Successfully achieved" can be interpreted as either your comfort and readiness to move on, when fewer than 25% of your scheduled voiding intervals are interrupted by urgency, when the number of leakage episodes are reduced by at least 10% as compared with the previous week, or some combination of these.)
4. If you feel a strong urge to void before the scheduled time, use relaxation/deep breathing and distraction techniques to help delay voiding.
5. Continue with this process until you are satisfied with your voiding interval and level of bladder control; normally your goal should be a 3- to 4-hour voiding interval.
6. If you are struggling to achieve a certain voiding interval, you may need to return to a shorter voiding interval for a week or two, or you may need to stay at the "difficult" level for a longer period of time; you should not try to advance to a longer interval until you feel comfortable with your control at the current interval.

Obviously, a bladder diary is a critical aspect to both the patient's learning and the clinician's analysis. The clinician should explain to the patient that nighttime voiding intervals tend to increase as diurnal intervals increase. If this does not occur, the nocturia should be evaluated separately.[146,147]

Positive reinforcement is critical to success. This is a tedious process that may take several months. It is important to work with the patient to make steps achievable and realistic. Patients often forget how severe their symptoms were as they progress with

BLADDER TRAINING (AKA Bladder Retraining or Bladder Drill)

Bladders learn good behavior when young but can forget over time, especially when overactive. Bladder training helps re-teach those good habits, such as urinating no more often than necessary. It involves working with a healthcare professional to learn how to resist or inhibit an early desire to go or to postpone voiding by urinating according to a timetable (rather than to early bladder messages). Your current pattern, lifestyle, and preferences will help us work with you to determine a program.

Normal bladder messages

During normal bladder filling the bladder sends several signals to the brain.
The first is simply an awareness of early filling—the bladder says "Hi, I'm here, just checking in."
We'll call that the **First Awareness of Bladder Filling.**
Later, the bladder sends another message—"Hello again, just want to let you know that I could empty now, if you have the time. Otherwise, don't worry about it; I can wait."
Let's call this the **First Desire to Void/Urinate.**
Later still, the bladder sends another message saying—"It's getting pretty full in here, I'd really like to go soon. If it is not possible, however, I can wait a bit longer." This is called a **Strong Desire to Void.**
Finally, the bladder calls back and says—"Sorry, I've been patient but I am completely full now; please find a place to go as soon as possible." Walking to the bathroom might be uncomfortable, as if the bladder might burst so it makes you want to walk slowly to avoid increasing the discomfort. We can call this **Capacity or Full.**

Notice how the bladder has been patient and courteous during these normal sensations.
Some people have an abnormal sensation, called **Urinary Urgency.** In this case the bladder says, "Whatever you are doing, drop it and go to the bathroom NOW or I'll make you pay; even make you leak." Urgency makes people want to rush/run to the bathroom, but that usually only makes matters worse. Urgency is NOT courteous. It is pushy, insistent, and usually means the bladder is contracting/squeezing inappropriately. Urgency is NOT normal, even if voiding has been delayed.

Bladder retraining teaches normal voiding patterns and how to stretch the times between urinations/voiding and, maybe, increase bladder capacity (the amount it will hold).

Goal: Void no more often than every 3 to 4 hrs or no more than every 2½ to 3 hrs if greater than 65 to 70 yrs old.

What we need to do first:
1. A bladder diary so we can determine both your starting (baseline) intervals and your ultimate goal.
2. Bladder training is easier for those who exercise their Kegel muscles regularly.
3. If you get urgency, learn to suppress it before beginning bladder training.

EARLY or SIMPLIFIED BLADDER TRAINING
To get a head start, try these simple techniques:
1. When you get an early desire to urinate, wait an extra 1, then 5, then 10, then 15, and finally 20 minutes from the time you'd first like to go until the time you actually go to the bathroom.
2. Once you get to 10 to 20 minutes, you may forget you even needed to go.

FORMAL BLADDER TRAINING (refers to daytime only; void as needed during the night, at first)
1. Urinate at your shortest comfort level for at least one week.
2. If able to keep to schedule fairly well and leakage isn't too bad, increase interval by 15 minutes.
3. Each time you get comfortable at one interval, increase the time by another 15 minutes, but don't increase intervals more often than every 5 to 7 days.
4. Your goal is to urinate no more often than every 3 to 4 hours and to urinate at least 1 to 2 cups at most voids.
   Be patient. An entire bladder training program usually takes at least 6 to 12 weeks to produce results. If it is too tough, add Kegel exercises and/or bladder relaxing medications. If you get urgency, be sure to learn and use the **Urgency Suppression** technique. This combination of all techniques is often VERY helpful.

DOES IT WORK?
Yes, research has shown that 75% of women with stress and urge incontinence who followed a bladder retraining program significantly reduced both trips to the bathroom and urinary leakage (incontinence).

Fig. 5-3 Bladder training patient education tool. (Courtesy Marta Krissovich.)

PATIENT'S NAME_____   DATE STARTED_____

INSTRUCTIONS: Please complete for one perfect day (measuring ALL intake & output) or three good days (measuring some).

INTAKE (time & amounts of fluids you drink)			OUTPUT (time & amounts of urinations or accidents)		
Date	Time	Amount & type of fluid	Time of void	Amount voided (oz)	Accidents (ACTIVITY: [cough, sneeze, etc.] or urgency

Fig. 5-4 Fluid-in and volume-out charting provides helpful information for bladder training.

the training, and a review of past bladder diaries or a quantitative analysis of symptoms can be exceptionally motivating.

Bladder training has been systematically evaluated, and a Cochrane review of its efficacy was recently updated.[148] Of 36 potentially relevant trials, only 10 were randomized or quasirandomized and therefore eligible for inclusion. The included trials provided data for 1366, predominantly female, subjects. The studies addressed the efficacy of bladder training in the management of urinary incontinence; although patients with OAB were included in these trials, the studies did not focus on OAB exclusively, and the data on OAB patients were not separately reported. The questions addressed by the Cochrane review are as follows:

1. Is bladder training better than no bladder training for the management of urinary incontinence?

2. Is bladder training better than other treatments such as medications, other behavioral/physical psychological treatments, surgical management, medical devices or other interventions?

In addition, this Cochrane review explored whether bladder training in combination with another treatment (such as conservative or pharmacologic) is better than the other treatment alone. A large body of evidence has amassed over the years showing consistently positive results for bladder training, but the quality of studies has been variable, the sample sizes small, and the confidence intervals wide. Therefore, the reviewers were limited to the following tentative conclusion: "bladder training may be helpful for the treatment of urinary incontinence."

Urgency Suppression Training. Urgency, the cornerstone symptom of OAB,[77] is defined as "the complaint of a sudden compelling desire to pass urine which is difficult to defer"[24] and is typically associated with a sudden increase in detrusor pressure (overactivity). Strategies for directly suppressing or inhibiting the sensation of urgency and, presumably, the uninhibited bladder contraction causing that sensation, have been described numerous times in the clinical literature, but the technique is usually considered under the category of bladder training.[118,148] In 1985, Burgio and colleagues described this volitional use of the PFMs for urgency suppression as a separate entity; they used instrumentation to teach patients this strategy, and their technique is described later in this chapter.[149] Although some clinicians automatically include urgency suppression as part of bladder training programs, it is not technically a component and is often not included in clinical trials involving bladder training.[148] Urgency suppression is considered separately here because of both its potential clinical efficacy and the utility of introducing it separately in a clinical setting.

Urgency suppression involves contraction of the PFMs in an attempt to reduce the sensation of urgency and to inhibit the bladder overactivity that caused it.[105] Several authors have suggested a mechanism of action for this bladder inhibition. For example, Petros and Ulmsten suggested that the loss of bladder neck support caused by pelvic muscle laxity and weakness could cause stimulation of the stretch receptors at the bladder base, which could inappropriately activate the micturition reflex.[150]

In 2003, Shafik and Shafik studied the role of PFM contractions in the inhibition of involuntary bladder contractions (overactivity) in a group of 28 men and women with OAB (mean age 44.8 years), and 17 asymptomatic volunteer controls (mean age 42.6 years).[151] The investigators filled the subjects' bladders twice during cystometry. The initial filling was used to establish a baseline point associated with involuntary voiding (urge incontinence) in patients with OAB and the desire to void in asymptomatic controls. The bladders were then refilled to that point and subjects were asked to contract the pelvic floor for 10 seconds. The investigators reported a significant increase in urethral pressure with contraction and, concomitantly, a significant decline in detrusor pressure for both patients with

OAB and controls ($p = .01$); subjects with OAB were able to suppress leakage, and asymptomatic controls were able to suppress the desire to void. These investigators referred to this response as the "voluntary urinary inhibition reflex." Interestingly, the increase in urethral pressure with PFM contraction was far greater for controls (122.1 ± 17.4 cm H_2O) than for patients (69.3 ± 7.9 cm H_2O).

In 2004, Ouslander suggested that leakage of urine into the proximal urethra resulting from urethral *sphincter weakness* could both precipitate urgency and diminish the ability to inhibit bladder contractions once the urgency is felt.[33] Also in 2004, Clare Fowler, a neurologist with a long-standing interest in neurourology, questioned why the universal and daily activity of suppressing inconvenient desires to urinate and defecate had not been labeled and studied more diligently. She proposed the umbrella term "procontinence reaction" for the sometimes-subconscious act of contracting the urethral or anal sphincter to postpone elimination. Experimental evidence points to an inhibitory effect on the detrusor and presumably the lower rectum resulting from pelvic floor and anal or urethral sphincter contraction. Fowler concurred with others that sphincter contraction serves both to increase outlet resistance and to reduce pressure within the associated viscus (bladder and/or rectum); the reduced pressure within the involved organ results in reduced sensation of urgency. Fowler further suggested that this inhibition may well be the result of a segmental reflex that can be voluntarily initiated, and that this voluntary initiation of reflex activity is the basis for urgency suppression/inhibition strategies taught for control of both urinary and defecatory urgency.[116]

Various techniques for urgency suppression have been described by different authors, but all involve volitional contraction of the PFMs.[33,105,145,152,153] In summary, cognitively intact patients are taught to respond to the sensation of urgency by discontinuing all movement (whether sitting or standing) and repeatedly contracting their PFMs. Some techniques also integrate intermittent deep breathing with a very slow, prolonged exhalation in an attempt to further focus the mind and relax the body. Once the urge subsides, patients are instructed either to walk slowly to the bathroom and void or to use distraction strategies to delay voiding until the predetermined time (if they are participating in a bladder training program). One approach that blends urgency suppression training and bladder training is to gradually increase the time from suppression of urgency to volitional voiding from 1 to 10 or 20 minutes. Obviously, the ability to contract the pelvic floor without increasing intraabdominal pressure is an important prerequisite for effective use of this urgency suppression technique. Burgio and Goode suggest that patients learn to identify the pelvic floor and practice pelvic muscle isolation for at least a week before beginning urgency suppression training.[105] See Fig. 5-5 for a sample Urgency Suppression Patient Education Sheet.

Urgency suppression has been recently and appropriately classified as a "cognitive behavioral" technique.[148] Because it is only natural to head toward the bathroom when the desire to void is strong, this technique is counterintuitive and requires a significant amount of support and encouragement. A few supportive explanations may be helpful for patients, such as the following:

- The natural response to urgency, that is, rushing to the bathroom, may actually stimulate additional bladder activity both by movement (increased abdominal pressure) and by thoughts of urinating. In addition, movement may reduce concentration and impair the ability to contract the pelvic floor, both of which are needed for inhibition of bladder contractions.[105]
- The bladder is only a muscle and can contract only so long before it fatigues. (You can illustrate this concept by demonstrating voluntary contraction and involuntary relaxation of the deltoid; although this comparison is not physiologically perfect, because of differences between the smooth muscle of the detrusor and the striated muscle of the deltoid, it is easy to demonstrate and understandable to patients).
- Urgency may return as the person approaches the bathroom because the toilet is a powerful bladder trigger. In this case, the patient should be instructed to repeat the strategies for urgency suppression. (Caution is advised if emptying is impaired.)

- Urgency is not considered normal and should be suppressed any time it is felt; this includes urgency that is felt when it is time to urinate based on a bladder training schedule. Once the urgency is controlled/eliminated, the patient should be instructed to void on schedule.

In talking with patients regarding urgency suppression, terminology is important. Good terms to use are "desire to void" or "normal desire to void," "strong desire to void," and "urgency," because these terms help to differentiate normal sensations (desire to void) from abnormal sensations (urgency).

Pelvic Floor Muscle Training. According to the ICI, PFMT is appropriate for several types of voiding dysfunction in men and women.[2] For men, PFMT is indicated for the initial management of postmicturition dribble, OAB and urge UI, and postprostatectomy stress and mixed UI. For women, PFMT is indicated for the initial management of OAB and urge UI, stress UI, and mixed UI. PFMT can be facilitated by verbal instruction (although verbal instruction alone is often considered inadequate), digital palpation, biofeedback, vaginal cones/weights, electrical stimulation, or a combination of these. The use of PFMT for stress urinary incontinence is described in Chapter 4. This section reviews PFMT for OAB symptoms, including urge UI.

PFM function plays an important role in detrusor control.[105] The goals of PFMT for the patient with OAB are the prevention and suppression of urinary urgency until appropriate toileting is possible.[154] The theoretic basis for use of PFMT in the management of OAB is based on normal function during the storage/filling phase of the micturition cycle. During storage, bladder contractility is normally suppressed both by cerebral inhibition and by enhanced reflex tone in the PFMs. Very little has been written on how approaches to PFMT differ for stress UI versus OAB/urge UI. Johnson suggests that PFMT be directed toward the clinical disorder; for patients with OAB, she recommends a focus on strengthening of the fast-twitch fibers, which provide a strong, quick contraction in response to urgency.[154] (This strong contraction causes reflexive relaxation of the detrusor muscle.)

SUPPRESSING URGENCY

WHAT IS URGENCY?

A sudden, strong urge to urinate (void) is called urgency.

    It means your bladder is contracting (squeezing). When your bladder squeezes, it sends a message to your urethra (tube you urinate through) to relax (open). Therefore, when you feel urgency, your bladder is trying to push the urine out, and meanwhile your urethra is opening to help it come out.

If you move, the urine will just fall out.

SO WHEN YOU FEEL URGENCY:

1. **STOP** and sit or stand very still. Don't move. You need to stay very still to keep control over your bladder.

2. **SQUEEZE!** If you have been taught to do pelvic muscle exercises, do 3 to 4 squeezes. Hold each one for a count of 3 to 4; then relax for a count of 1 before squeezing again.

3. **BREATHE:**
TAKE A DEEP BREATH (inhale thru your nose, hold 1 second) Then **EXHALE VERY SLOWLY** through pursed lips.

4. **RELAX!** Think of anything other than your bladder AND think tough.

If the urge doesn't go away, **REPEAT** the steps above until it does.

FINALLY: When the urge goes away completely, wait at least 30 seconds (slowly building up to 5 minutes) then walk slowly to the bathroom. **If the urge returns on the way or while removing your clothes, REPEAT** steps 1 through 3.

Once you get the hang of it, it's OK to mix and match steps 2 and 3.

It is difficult to learn these techniques. It takes time, practice, and a positive attitude. Try not to get discouraged even if you leak a bit at first

***How we store urine* 1.** The bladder sends a gentle message to the brain that it is starting to fill with urine. **2.** The brain decides if it is an OK time to urinate. If it is not time, the brain sends a message to your bladder to wait, relax, and allow more filling and to the muscles around the urethra to tighten up (squeeze) to close the door tighter. **3.** When the muscles around the urethra tighten, another message is sent to the bladder to relax and wait.

Normally, these are both done without your thinking much about it. Your bladder starts squeezing (contracting) anytime it even has a little urine in it (you feel this as urgency) and your brain allows your bladder to squeeze too soon, even when it's not an appropriate time.

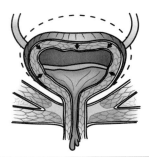 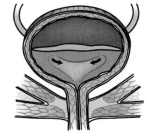

When you feel urgency, it doesn't mean your bladder suddenly got REALLY full. Instead, it means your bladder is suddenly and inappropriately contracting (squeezing). When the bladder is contracting and the urethra is open, the risk of leakage is high. Movement (walking) will only make it worse.	With Urgency Suppression techniques your bladder relaxes, making the sensation of urgency go away. Once the bladder relaxes, the urethra closes. Once urgency subsides/goes away, it is safe to walk to the bathroom.

REMEMBER: WHEN URGENCY STRIKES

FREEZE   SQUEEZE   BREATHE

Fig. 5-5 Guidelines for suppressing urgency. A patient education tool. (**Courtesy:** Marta Krissovich.)

In contrast, Madersbacher suggests that the "physiological organization of Onuf's nuclei and of the levator ani motor neurons as well as the reflex control of a tonic activity, essential for the generation of maintained force in slow twitch muscle fibers, is an important part of the normal function of the system."[155] The result of maintained slow-twitch muscle fiber force, which could be subconscious, is an inhibition of bladder contractility and prevention of overactivity. This activity is sometimes seen as a very slow increase in the EMG activity during filling cystometry (the guarding reflex). The importance of PFM function is supported by one study in which patients with the most severe urgency were found to have the weakest PFMs (according to periurethral measurements).[156] Burgio and Goode recommend no difference in PFMT for stress UI versus urge UI but do suggest a difference in utilization of the strengthened muscles; specifically, they suggest that individuals with stress UI utilize volitional muscle contraction to counteract the impact of increased intraabdominal pressure on the urethra, whereas individuals with OAB utilize the same contraction to inhibit detrusor contractions and calm the bladder.[105]

A recent systematic Cochrane review of PFMT in women confirms a wide variability in approaches to PFMT for stress UI.[157] Most trials utilized prescriptions focusing both on short ("quick flick") contractions for strength and "held"/sustained contractions of up to 30 to 40 seconds for endurance. Although most included a daily home exercise program, there was little consistency in terms of approach, that is, variables such as contraction and relaxation times, exercise positions, and duration of treatment. Some exercise prescriptions were based on time, such as 5 minutes twice daily. Others prescribed a specific number of repetitions (contraction/relaxation cycles) per day, which ranged from 36 to 200, with 50 being the most common number of recommended repetitions. The length of training varied from 1 week to 9 months, with 12 weeks being the most common. Only a third of the trials reported confirmation of proper PFM contraction and relaxation techniques before training began.

The ICI2 suggests that, irrespective of type of incontinence, PFMT should be continued for 8 to 12 weeks before any advanced management/treatment is considered.[2] In a recent review, Sampselle recommended the following protocol, with a target goal of 24 to 45 repetitions per day:[158]

- Find the pelvic muscles by tightening as if holding urine or flatus back or the action that would grasp a penis during coitus while keeping surrounding muscle groups (abdomen, buttocks, and thighs) quiet. An upward and inward movement should be felt at the pelvic floor, not a bearing-down or pushing.
- Attempt to maintain contractions at moderate to near-maximum intensity, because these provide the greatest benefit.
- Completely relax the pelvic muscles after each contraction for a period of time at least equivalent to the "contraction" time.
- Build over time to 10-second contractions with a minimum of 10-second rest periods.

A patient education sheet to facilitate PFMT is found in Fig. 5-6, pp. 150–151.

The question of efficacy of PFMT for OAB (including urge UI and detrusor instability) was addressed by the Cochrane review mentioned earlier.[157] The authors stated they were not able to make a determination regarding efficacy of PFMT for OAB because most trials focused on stress and/or mixed UI; when patients with OAB were included, their results were not reported separately but were typically mixed into the results of women with stress or mixed UI. These investigators suggested that the current best evidence for PFMT in women with OAB are the studies reported by Nygaard and colleagues in 1996, Wyman and associates in 1998, and Burgio and associates in 1998.[97,153,159] Nygaard and colleagues conducted a prospective randomized trial of PFMT in 71 women with stress, urge, or mixed UI.[159] Patients' ability to contract the PFMs properly was confirmed by digital examination, and patients were instructed to perform the exercises with up to 8-second contractions (and 8 – 10 second periods of relaxation) for 5 minutes twice a day for 12 weeks. The individual assessing outcomes was blinded to group allocation. Subjects who completed the full 12-week course experienced a decline in episodes of urge UI from 2.8 to 0.5. Follow-up results were reported 6 months after treatment for all women with urge UI, regardless of whether or not they completed the full course of treatment. Seven of 17 women reported continued satisfaction with their results, but two had begun treatment with anticholinergic agents.[159] Burgio and colleagues compared efficacy of behavioral management (including PFMT) with pharmacologic management in a randomized placebo-controlled trial and found the outcomes of behavioral therapy to be superior to those produced by pharmacologic management.[97] This study is discussed further under the section on pharmaceutical therapies. The Wyman group investigated the efficacy of individual versus combined behavioral therapies; this study is discussed in the section on combination therapy.[153]

Biofeedback-assisted pelvic floor muscle training. PFMT can be difficult for patients because they cannot "visualize" pelvic muscle contractions; when the PFMs are weak, they may also be unable to "feel" the muscles. As a result, patients may struggle to identify (find) or isolate the correct set of muscles. In addition, it may be difficult for clinicians to quantify strength, endurance, fine motor control, quality of contraction release, and resting tone utilizing only digital vaginal or anal palpation. In the 1950s, Arnold Kegel, M.D. developed the perineometer to measure the intravaginal pressure generated by pelvic muscle contractions. Today, clinicians have a choice between monitoring the electrical activity of pelvic floor nerves and muscles via EMG and determining the pressure generated by actual muscle contraction via manometry. Biofeedback therapy may be delivered during clinic visits or via devices designed for home use. Irrespective of type, a two-channel device that allows concomitant monitoring of accessory muscle activity (typically abdominal muscles, thighs, or buttocks) is important for patients who struggle with identification or isolation of the PFMs. For patients with OAB, biofeedback can be used both to improve general pelvic muscle function (addressing either hypotonicity/weakness or, if present, hypertonicity) and to allow practice/modeling of urgency suppression strategies.

Trials demonstrating the efficacy of biofeedback in the treatment of OAB are limited, because most trials over the years have focused on either stress UI

or stress-predominant mixed UI.[157] One trial comparing the efficacy of PFMT with biofeedback versus PFMT without biofeedback did report separately on outcomes for patients with detrusor instability/OAB. In a study of 450 female soldiers, Sherman and colleagues conducted further evaluation on 46 of the 150 women who reported urinary leakage during exercise and field training activities. The mean age of the women was 39.9 years, with a standard deviation of 7.8 years. The subjects were stratified by type of incontinence (stress UI or mixed UI), with diagnosis based on symptoms and urodynamic testing; there was no stratification based on PFM function at baseline. Subjects were then randomized to either an 8-week intervention of pelvic muscle exercises alone or pelvic muscle exercises with urethral biofeedback. (Urethral biofeedback required instrumentation.) Both groups were instructed to practice exercises at home for 20 minutes twice daily with a goal of five sets of five 10-second contractions followed by 10 seconds of relaxation. In this study, all patients improved significantly, with very few desiring further treatment. The patients with detrusor instability (overactivity) at baseline were reported to have stable bladders on repeat cystometry at the study's end.[160]

In 2002 Burgio, Goode, and colleagues examined the impact of behavioral training with and without biofeedback in a prospective, randomized controlled trial with a volunteer sample of 222 community-dwelling women aged 55 to 92 years with urge or urge predominant mixed UI.[161] Patients were stratified by race, type of incontinence (urge versus urge predominant mixed UI), and frequency of incontinent episodes, but not by baseline PFM function. The two treatment groups received an 8-week trial of either biofeedback-assisted behavioral training ($n = 73$) or behavioral training alone (including instruction on pelvic muscle exercises during vaginal palpation). The control group received a self-help booklet on behavioral therapies. At the end of treatment, results indicated significant improvement for all three groups (biofeedback, verbal feedback, and self-help) in terms of quality of life, and the difference in mean reduction of leakage episodes (based on bladder diaries) did not reach significance ($p = 23$). There was, however,

Pelvic Muscle/Kegel Exercises for Pelvic Floor Training

What are pelvic muscle exercises? Exercises designed to make the important pelvic muscles perform more effectively. Pelvic muscles often get weak. Since most people don't know they have them, most don't exercise them. They also can get damaged during things such as childbirth and straining with BMs.

Why should I do pelvic muscle exercises? Healthy pelvic muscles help to:
- reduce and help to control the sensation of urinary and rectal urgency.
- reduce the desire to go to the bathroom too frequently.
- control urinary and rectal/fecal leakage/incontinence.
- control pelvic pain and improve one's ability to empty completely during bowel movements.
- enhance the sexual experience for men and women and their partners.

Finding the right muscle? See the pictures.
- The muscle is deep inside and not part of or even near the abdomen, buttocks, thighs, or chest.
- Think of the sensation of contracting the muscles during the physical examination or the computerized muscle evaluation when you were in our office. Try to recreate this.
- Imagine you are in an elevator and trying not to pass gas/wind and squeeze that muscle.
- Women can slip a finger inside the vagina and tighten around it.
  Men will see the penis rise just slightly during a correct pelvic muscle contraction.

We *don't* recommend using the muscle to slow the urinary stream because this may confuse the bladder.

Best positions (see Figure 5-6, B). At first when it is difficult to find the muscle, try:
- Half sitting up in bed or placing a pillow behind your neck or upper back with your knees bent.
- Getting down on all fours (hands & knees) with your abdomen hanging down loosely (see the pictures?)

Once the muscles are stronger, you can progress to doing pelvic exercises sitting up with your feet well supported. When the muscles are even stronger, do some exercises while standing—the position of most leaks.

Tips for success: Many have tried them but have been doing them incorrectly.
1. Squeeze your pelvic muscles as hard as you want, *as long as you are able to:*
   - Keep your abdomen, buttocks, and thighs quiet the whole time. Monitor these with your hand. If you feel them relax at the end of the contraction, they must have been tight. If the abdomen, buttocks, thighs or chest move with the pelvic muscles, don't squeeze so hard.
   - Breathe, at least shallowly, during the contractions.
   - Hold the contractions for the whole time that we suggest. If you don't feel the muscle relax at the end of a contraction, it means that it gave out before it should have.
2. Be sure to relax for the same length of time between contractions as you squeezed during the contraction, i.e., if you squeezed for a count of 4, try to relax for a count of 4
3. To help you remember, attach the exercises to something else you already do 3 to 4 times/day.
4. *Don't give up!* It takes a while to tighten and strengthen the muscle, but *virtually everyone* with weak pelvic muscles achieves great benefit rather quickly when they do them regularly.

Frequently Asked Questions:
1. *Do I have to do these exercises forever?* YES, but much less frequently than during training.
   Most who follow our plan achieve their goals within 3 months. Others will benefit more from continuing another 3 months. After that, exercising once a day or just 3 to 5 times/week will be enough to maintain your good progress. We will guide you on the decision when the time comes.
2. *The exercises are difficult to do. Are aides or assistive devices available?* YES. Biofeedback training, as in our office, is the "gold standard." Other aides, such as vaginal weights, home biofeedback, and even electrical stimulation, help specific patients but typically aren't covered by insurance companies. It is important to remember that research shows that Kegel exercises often do not work unless done under the guidance of a specially trained healthcare professional. If they aren't working, don't stop. Get help.

Fig. 5-6 A, Guidelines for pelvic muscle exercise.

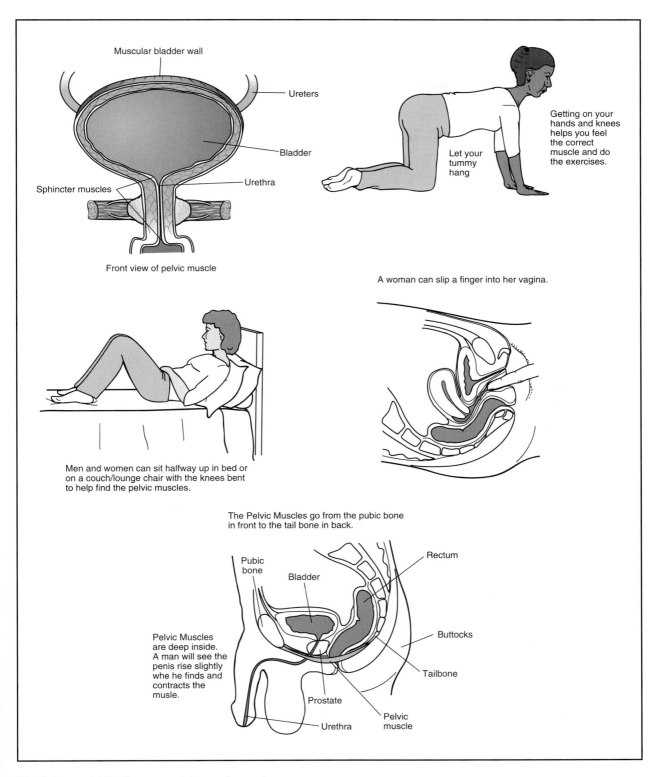

Muscular bladder wall

Ureters

Bladder

Urethra

Sphincter muscles

Front view of pelvic muscle

Getting on your hands and knees helps you feel the correct muscle and do the exercises.

Let your tummy hang

A woman can slip a finger into her vagina.

Men and women can sit halfway up in bed or on a couch/lounge chair with the knees bent to help find the pelvic muscles.

The Pelvic Muscles go from the pubic bone in front to the tail bone in back.

Pubic bone

Bladder

Rectum

Buttocks

Tailbone

Pelvic Muscles are deep inside. A man will see the penis rise slightly whe he finds and contracts the musle.

Prostate

Urethra

Pelvic muscle

Fig. 5-6, cont'd. B, Illustrates pelvic muscle exercise.

a significant difference among the groups in terms of patient reports of "complete" satisfaction with the therapies: biofeedback, 75%; verbal feedback, 85.5%; and self-help, 55.7%. The investigators concluded that behavioral therapy with either computer-assisted *or* verbal feedback is effective, and, in this study, these approaches generated greater patient satisfaction over a self-help program for the treatment of urge UI in community-dwelling older women.

Vaginal cones. Vaginal cones or weights are available over the counter and are sometimes recommended to women as an adjunct for PFMT; this approach is based on the theory that the cones may improve PFM identification via enhanced proprioception[118] and may contribute to the development of enhanced PFM strength. The cones are commonly plastic and tampon shaped, but they may be stainless steel and either hourglass shaped or spheric; they typically range in weight from 10 to 70 g. Women are instructed to wear the heaviest cone that they are able to retain for 15 to 20 minutes twice daily, while walking about. These devices have the advantage of simplicity and economy and are well tolerated, with the exception of women with significant obesity or vaginal atrophy, prolapse, or stenosis. Although the evidence included in a recent systematic Cochrane review supported their use in women with mild to moderate stress UI,[162] no randomized controlled trials could be located studying their use specifically for patients with OAB symptoms. However, any strategy that improves a woman's PFM strength has the potential to improve her ability to inhibit detrusor overactivity via voluntary PFM contraction (see Chapter 4).

Electrical stimulation. Pelvic floor electrical stimulation (PFES)has been utilized for treatment of urinary incontinence since 1963, via a number of approaches: vaginal or anal probes, surface "patch" electrodes, "electric" vaginal pessaries, implanted radiofrequency-controlled pelvic floor electrodes, and indirect sacral stimulation.[163] Although electrical stimulation is a passive therapy and therefore not technically a "behavioral" therapy, PFES is typically discussed under behavioral therapy because, for most patients, the ultimate goal is independent PFM exercises or PFMT.

A substantial body of evidence has been collected since the 1960s that supports the role of electrical stimulation in treatment of urgency, frequency, painful bladder syndrome, urinary and fecal incontinence, and chronic constipation. Unfortunately, the exact role and benefit of electrical stimulation have yet to be fully defined because the studies conducted to date have utilized a number of different approaches, with significant variability in application of the various approaches. As a result, it is not possible at this point to consider the data in aggregate form and to conduct a meaningful metaanalysis.[163]

Payne described three ways in which PFES could contribute to improved bladder function and continence:

- Enhanced structural support for the urethra and bladder neck
- Improved resting and active closure of the proximal urethra
- Enhanced reflex inhibition of bladder contractions[163]

The first two mechanisms relate primarily to stress urinary incontinence and are discussed in Chapter 4. The third mechanism is germane to this discussion on OAB, in which the goal is reflex inhibition of bladder contractions via stimulation of afferent nerves to the pelvic organs.

In continence centers, three groups of patients with OAB are typically offered electrical stimulation therapy:

- Patients who are unable to identify the PFMs despite digital palpation and feedback from a trained provider and computerized biofeedback; electrical stimulation provides these patients with proprioceptive feedback that facilitates muscle identification.
- Patients in whom an adequate trial of PFMT has failed
- Patients with a chronic neurologic disorder that predicts long-term detrusor overactivity.

The first group of patients typically need only one or two clinic sessions to identify the PFMs. Patients in whom PFMT has failed frequently benefit from short-term treatment with a home unit in addition to clinic sessions; the electrical stimulation provides continued feedback regarding muscle identification and also contributes to strengthening of very weak muscles. Patients with chronic neuro-logic disorders usually require long-term therapy that is self-administered via home devices. In any of these scenarios, low frequencies of 10 to 20 Hz are most commonly delivered to pudendal nerve affer-ents (via vaginal or anal probes) in an alternating pattern of 5 to 10 seconds on/5 to 20 seconds off over a period of 15 to 30 minutes. A review of normal voiding physiology helps to explain why therapies such as electrical stimulation may work during the time they are being delivered; however, the longer-term "carryover" effect is more difficult to understand. The best explanation currently avail-able suggests that the long-term benefits may relate to "some type of reorganization of the micturition reflex that results in facilitation of existing bladder inhibition."[163]

As noted, it is difficult to compare studies on the efficacy of any type of electrical stimulation because of the marked variability in the approach to delivery of electrical stimulation. In addition, most studies have been small and not controlled, or they have focused on either the neuropathic OAB or on patients with stress or stress-predominant mixed UI. Three randomized studies published in English explored the effect of direct PFES on nonneuro-pathic OAB. In 1997, Brubaker and colleagues conducted a prospective, double-blind, randomized clinical trial of PFES with a sham-device control group; the subjects were 121 women with urody-namically proven detrusor instability (overactivity) and/or stress UI. Repeat urodynamics conducted at the end of the study demonstrated elimination of bladder overactivity for 49% of the women with bladder overactivity ($p = .0004$); there was no statistically significant difference on postinterven-tion urodynamics for the women with stress UI or women in the sham device groups.[164] Also in 1997, Siegel and colleagues compared daily versus alter-nate-day PFES in a group of 68 women with urge or mixed UI over 20 weeks.[165] Although these investi-gators found no statistically significant difference between the women receiving two 15-minute sessions of PFES daily and those receiving two 15-minute sessions of PFES every other day, they did find that both groups experienced a significant decrease in total leaks ($p = .001$), nocturnal

episodes ($p = .001$), pad count ($p = .002$), and total voids per 24 hours ($p = .003$). Subjects reported 93% compliance and 72% were satisfied with the therapy. In 2004, Wang and colleagues reported on a single-blind, randomized trial exploring the rela-tive efficacy of PFMT, biofeedback-assisted PFMT (BAPFMT), and PFES in 103 women with OAB.[166] In this study, a therapist who was blinded to progress and outcome administered either individ-ualized PFMT ($n = 34$), BAPFMT ($n = 34$), or PFES ($n = 35$) at 10 Hz, a 10/5-second duty cycle, and an intensity that achieved contraction without patient discomfort. All patients followed a home exercise program individualized to their pelvic floor function. At the study's end, differences were reported in three quality of life domains between BAPFMT and PFES but the difference in the total quality of life score for these two groups, as measured by the KHQ, was not significant ($p = .952$). However, there *was* a significant difference in quality of life between the BAPFMT and PFES groups as compared with the PFMT group ($p = .0004$ and .003, respectively). The difference in patient reports of cure/improve-ment of OAB symptoms was also insignificant for the BAPFMT and PFES groups (50.0% and 51.4%, respectively), but there *was* a significant difference in the cure/improvement rates for these two groups as compared with the group receiving PFMT alone (38.2%; $p = .567$). All of these studies support the efficacy of PFES in the treatment of OAB.

Passive Therapies to Improve Pelvic Floor Function and Lower Urinary Tract Symptoms

Therapies that are more passive than active cannot be considered "behavioral," but several of them merit discussion because of their potential impact on pelvic floor and bladder function. They include extracorporeal magnetic stimulation, percutaneous afferent neuromodulation of the tibial nerve, and acupuncture. Although anecdotal evidence is increas-ing regarding each of these therapies, we currently lack the randomized controlled investigations that provide objective data regarding efficacy. Each of these therapies can be evaluated in comparison with sham controls, so we hope that these trials will be forthcoming.

Extracorporeal Magnetic Innervation. Extracorporeal magnetic innervation is thought to "work" by inducing electrical currents in the pelvis that activate the nerve pathways controlling the bladder and pelvic floor. The magnetic stimulation of sacral nerve pathways is reported to suppress detrusor overactivity[167] and thus to reduce OAB symptoms. Extracorporeal magnetic innervation is typically delivered while patients sit, fully clothed, in a chair for 15 to 20 minutes two times a week over 8 to 20 weeks. One small randomized controlled trial of 37 women with OAB symptoms (including urge UI) demonstrated positive preliminary outcomes in the treatment group as compared with the placebo group.[168] The group receiving extracorporeal magnetic innervation reported increased mean voided volumes ($p = .04$), improved quality of life scores ($p = .01$), and reduced incontinence episodes ($p = .04$). The authors suggest that magnetic stimulation may be useful for treatment of urinary frequency and urge UI; however, these results need to be confirmed in a larger trial with greater numerical power.

Percutaneous Afferent Neuromodulation of the Tibial Nerve. Percutaneous afferent neuromodulation of the tibial nerve (PANTN) is performed by administering electrical current via a 34-gauge stainless steel needle (similar to those used in acupuncture) at a point 5 cm above the medial malleolus for approximately 30 minutes per week over 8 to 12 weeks;[169] the theorized benefits are based on the fact that the tibial nerve and the nerves controlling the bladder and pelvic floor all exit the spinal cord at the sacral level. Although this therapy is intriguing, randomized controlled trials of sufficient power have yet to provide guidance on its use. Only the abstract was available from one small study of women 45 to 63 years of age with OAB ($n = 28$).[170] According to the abstract, patients were randomized to receive PANTN, oral oxybutynin 5 mg three times daily, or no treatment. The authors reported significant improvements in symptom and quality of life scores for the two treatment groups (PANTN and oxybutynin) but not for the control group. Information about the durability of these effects was not available, and the small group size makes it difficult to draw conclusions, but these positive preliminary results encourage larger trials.

Acupuncture. Acupuncture without electrical current has also been reported to reduce OAB symptoms, but, again, trials have been small, and no randomized controlled trials were found that addressed the use of acupuncture in this group of patients. One approach to measuring the effects of therapy, which has been utilized with extracorporeal magnetic innervation and PANTN, is to assess bladder function via urodynamic studies before and immediately following treatment.[171] However, in the absence of a control group, it is difficult to judge whether the improvements in urodynamic results were the result of the treatment, increased patient comfort with the test, or some other testing-related factor (such as increased bladder accommodation to retrograde filling unrelated to the therapy).

Pharmaceutical Therapies

The primary pharmacologic options for management of OAB are anticholinergic agents; until recently, however, use of these drugs has been severely limited by problems with efficacy and with side effects (especially dry mouth and constipation) that have made therapeutic dosing difficult.[172] For many years, the mainstay of anticholinergic therapy was oxybutynin; other agents sometimes used included imipramine and hyoscyamine. The introduction of tolterodine in the late 1990s represented the first major advance in pharmaceutical therapy for OAB and urge urinary incontinence in more than a decade. Since the introduction of tolterodine, both oxybutynin and tolterodine have been made available in long-acting formulations, and oxybutynin is now also available in a transdermal patch. In addition, three other anticholinergic medications have recently come to market: trospium chloride, solifenacin, and darifenacin (Table 5-6). Each of these agents is designed to improve bladder stability and to reduce overactivity at least as well as generic oxybutynin while significantly reducing the adverse effects that compromise patient adherence.

During bladder storage, the bladder normally remains relaxed and noncontractile as a result of beta-adrenergic (sympathetic) stimulation at the level of the bladder, alpha-adrenergic (sympathetic)

TABLE 5-6   **Medications Used to treat Overactive Bladder and Urge Urinary Incontinence**

MEDICATION: GENERIC/TRADE	USUAL DOSAGE	COMMENTS
darifenacin/Enablex	7.5 to 15 mg once daily, orally	New to United States market; appears to be more selective for M3 receptors
hyoscyamine/Levsin	0.375 mg twice daily, orally	Consider sublingual, rapid-release form for intermittent (special event) use; otherwise, side effects limit use
oxybutynin, generic (immediate-release, oral)	2.5 to 5.0 mg two to three times daily, orally	Side effects may limit use or therapeutic titration
oxybutynin/ Ditropan XL	5 to 15 mg once daily, orally; 10 mg is most common	Long-acting formulation appears to have a better efficacy and tolerability profile over short-acting formulation
oxybutynin/Oxytrol	Transdermal formulation; 3.9-mg/day; patch changed every 3 to 4 days	Local skin irritation may limit use in some patients
propantheline/ Pro-Banthine	7.5 to 15 mg four times daily, orally	Use limited by anticholinergic side effects
solifenacin/Vesicare	5 to 10 mg once daily, orally	New to United States market; appears to be more selective for M3 receptors
tolterodine/Detrol	1 to 2 mg twice daily, orally	Short-acting "immediate-release" formulation
tolterodine/Detrol LA	4 mg once daily, orally	Long-acting formulation appears to have a better efficacy and tolerability profile over short-acting formulation
trospium chloride/ Sanctura	20 mg twice daily, orally	A quaternary amine; may not cross blood-brain barrier, possibly reducing cognitive side effects
imipramine, desipramine, and nortriptyline	10 to 25 mg three times daily but typically given at bedtime for nocturia	May be helpful for mixed urinary incontinence but limited evidence, and cognitive and cardiac side effects may limit use
desmopressin/DDAVP	20- to 40-mcg intranasal spray at bedtime; 0.1 to 0.4 mg orally 2 hours before bedtime	For nocturnal polyuria may cause hyponatremia in first 3 weeks; monitor serum sodium
Vaginal estrogens	Indicated for symptomatic vaginal atrophy including recurrent urinary tract infection	May reduce urgency and frequency; clinical trials needed
estradiol/Estring	2-mg intravaginal estradiol ring, changed every 90 days	Especially useful when regular vaginal applications are problematic; low systemic effects
estradiol or Premarin creams	0.5 - 2 g per vagina nightly for 10 to 14 days, then 2 to 3 times/week	Cream sometimes soothing to irritated vaginal tissues
estradiol/Vagifem	One tablet once daily per vagina for 10 to 14 days; then 2 times/week	Well accepted by women, especially if at risk of forgetting ring and considers the cream "messy"

Data from references 33, 174, 175, and 180.

stimulation of the bladder outlet, and parasympathetic (cholinergic) blockade. In theory, the currently available antimuscarinic (anticholinergic) medications decrease bladder contractility during storage by blocking the muscarinic (cholinergic) receptors in the detrusor muscle. Five types of muscarinic receptors have been identified (M1 to M5) throughout the body; both M2 and M3 receptors have been found on detrusor smooth muscle cells, but the M3 receptors are thought to be the ones primarily responsible for bladder contractility during voiding.[119,173] The goal in development of pharmacologic agents is to identify a medication that effectively blocks the M3 receptors responsible for bladder overactivity while minimizing any blockade of the receptors controlling normal salivation and colonic motility. (This concept is known as uroselectivity.) Although the concept is logical and clear, it has been difficult to find an agent that is truly uroselective; thus, all currently available medications are associated with some level of adverse effects, although the newer agents generally produce much less severe side effects than the original anticholinergic drugs.[174]

Of the more established antimuscarinic therapies, both oxybutynin and tolterodine have demonstrated efficacy in numerous trials, and, in their long-acting forms, both are better tolerated than the immediate release oral oxybutynin. Oxybutynin is now also available in a transdermal patch, which also demonstrates a better side effect profile than the immediate release oral form.[33] One concern with use of these medications is the potential for subtle impairments in cognitive function, which is of particular concern for patients in cognitively challenging careers (such as airline pilots) and cognitively vulnerable older adults. It has been suggested that tolterodine and trospium chloride may have less potential impact on cognitive function than immediate-release oxybutynin; however, this has not been adequately tested.[33] Darifenacin and solifenacin are now available for clinical use, and both reportedly have greater selectivity for M3 receptors; it is hoped that these agents will provide both improved efficacy and a better side effect profile.

A systematic Cochrane review of OAB medications with direct anticholinergic action was recently completed;[174] the review included randomized

controlled trials (published before January 2002) that permitted comparison among the following agents: emepronium bromide, emepronium carrageenate, darifenacin, dicyclomine chloride, oxybutynin chloride, propantheline bromide, propiverine, tolterodine, and trospium chloride. (Emepronium bromide, emepronium carrageenate, and propiverine are not currently available in the United States.) In all, 32 trials involving 6800 subjects (including at least 1529 men and 3938 women) were included in the review. Although not all information was reported in every trial, the reviewers concluded that anticholinergic therapy consistently provided small but significant improvements in urgency, frequency, bladder control, and, when tested, urodynamic measures as compared with placebo. Although dry mouth of variable severity was a consistent side effect, postvoid residual urine was not significantly elevated. As with other trials looking at OAB, both control and treatment subjects experienced a marked improvement in symptoms; this improvement accounts for the relatively small, although significant, treatment effect.

Topical Estrogen. Although the efficacy of oral estrogen therapy for urge urinary incontinence and OAB has been questioned, local vaginal therapy appears to significantly improve day and night time frequency, bladder control, volume at first sensation to void, and bladder capacity; topical estrogen therapy is therefore recommended for patients who present with signs of atrophic vaginitis in addition to OAB symptoms.[61]

Agents with Dual Effects. Tricyclic antidepressant agents, such as imipramine, nortriptyline, and desipramine, may be of benefit for patients with mixed stress and urge UI because these drugs exert dual effects on the LUT; they act both to reduce bladder contractility and to increase urethral resistance. However, there are limited data regarding efficacy, and some agents (such as imipramine) can cause cardiac side effects such as postural hypotension and conduction abnormalities; thus, their use should be restricted to patients in whom behavioral therapy has failed. Patients receiving these medications must be carefully monitored for any adverse effects.[175]

Combination Therapy: Alpha-Adrenergic Antagonists and Anticholinergics. As explained earlier in this chapter, even mild bladder outlet obstruction can result in bladder overactivity; this situation is often seen in men with benign prostatic hypertrophy. In the past, clinicians were hesitant to prescribe anticholinergic medications for these patients because of concerns regarding severe urinary retention. It now appears that these patients may benefit from a combination of alpha-adrenergic antagonists to reduce urethral resistance and anticholinergics to reduce bladder overactivity. Treatment algorithms have been suggested in which alpha-adrenergic blockade is established initially, followed by the addition of anticholinergic therapy.[176, 177, 178]

Vasopressin Analogs. When nocturia is related to an overproduction of urine that is limited to the nighttime hours, desmopressin (DDAVP) may be useful. DDAVP is an analog of vasopressin (antidiuretic hormone), which reduces urine production by promoting tubular reabsorption of sodium chloride and water.[179] Until recently, this medication was used only in children, primarily because of concerns related to side effects such as hyponatremia; however, a recent international consensus statement suggests that it is well tolerated in healthy adults, and, although the risk of hyponatremia is greater in persons more than 65 years of age, this effect usually occurs early in treatment.[180]

Pharmaceutical versus Behavioral Therapy

Burgio and colleagues conducted a placebo-controlled trial in which 197 women (age 55 to 92 years) with urge or urge-predominant mixed UI were randomized into three treatment groups: biofeedback-assisted behavioral treatment (four sessions over 8 weeks); oxybutynin chloride, 2.5 to 5 mg three times daily; and placebo.[97] For all three treatment groups, incontinence was most notably improved early in treatment, but improvement continued gradually thereafter. The biofeedback-assisted behavioral therapy group achieved the best results, with an 80.7% reduction in leakage as compared with 68.5% for the oxybutynin group ($p = .04$); both treatment groups achieved significantly greater improvement than the placebo group, which experienced a 39.4% reduction in leakage ($p = .001$ and .009, respectively). Patient perception

of improvement as "much improved" was 74.1%, 50.9%, and 26.9% for the biofeedback, oxybutynin, and placebo groups, respectively. Only 14.0% of patients in the behavioral group were interested in further treatment versus 75.5% of participants in the other two groups. The investigators suggested that behavioral treatment was safe and effective and should be considered as first-line treatment for urge and mixed incontinence.

Surgical Therapies

Behavioral therapies and pharmacologic therapy provide significant improvement for most patients with OAB, with or without urge UI; thus, these therapies are typically considered first-line and second-line interventions. When these therapies are ineffective in providing sufficient symptom control to permit patients to resume their usual activities, surgical procedures such as neuromodulation and augmentation cystoplasty may be indicated.

Implanted Neuromodulation. Although mechanisms of action have not been clearly described, it is likely that most of the behavioral therapies have a psychoneurologic component. Implanted neuromodulator technology capitalizes on much of the knowledge that has been gained in the field of neurourology regarding the role of the pelvic neuromuscular system in LUT dysfunction. The therapy involves surgical implantation of wires along the sacral nerve pathways; following implantation, the wires are attached to a stimulator. The initial indication for use of this device (the InterStim Device) was intractable urgency and frequency; the device is now being used for management of other LUT symptoms as well. One key advantage to the implanted sacral nerve stimulator is that patients can be evaluated for efficacy before undergoing the surgical implantation by having temporary wires inserted under local anesthesia; in addition, patients can control their own therapy and can determine continued need for therapy by turning the device on and off. In a recent review of randomized controlled trials that evaluated the effects of neuromodulation on urge UI, Abrams and Blaivas and their colleagues reported that sacral neuromodulation is effective, has good durability, and, considering that the therapy is indicated for refractory patients, demonstrates an acceptable benefit risk profile.[133]

Bladder Augmentation. Bladder augmentation (augmentation cystoplasty) is the last therapy to be presented in this chapter; this is appropriate because it is viewed as a last resort for patients with severe detrusor overactivity (typically resulting from a neurologic disorder) or markedly reduced bladder compliance.[181] This procedure involves incising the bladder wall and attaching a detubularized segment of ileum, colon, or ureter. In addition to enlarging the bladder and increasing bladder capacity, this procedure renders the bladder noncontractile by interrupting the muscle fibers of the detrusor and thus interfering with propagation of contractile messages between the muscle cells. Although this procedure does increase bladder capacity and eliminate bladder overactivity, it also places the patient at high risk for urinary retention and lifelong dependence on intermittent catheterization for bladder emptying.[182] In addition, especially when ileum is used, mucus production can be problematic.[183] Because so many other therapies now exist, this procedure is usually reserved for patients who have high-pressure low-capacity bladders resulting from neurologic disorders, and it is unlikely that the patient with nonneurogenic OAB would require this procedure.

The Case for a Stepped Approach and Combining Therapies

The preceding discussion on treatment of OAB demonstrates that many worthwhile therapies are available. Unfortunately, it also demonstrates that there are no "silver bullets" or panaceas; that is, no methods that provide easy and rapid cure, or even a dramatic reduction in symptoms, when used as solo therapy. However, there *is* evidence to support combination therapy based on the individual patient's need, lifestyle, and preferences. For example, Wyman and colleagues compared the efficacy of bladder training, biofeedback-assisted pelvic muscle exercise, and a combination of the two in a randomized controlled trial with 204 women, 59 of whom had been diagnosed with detrusor overactivity.[153] Each group received six office visits and six mail/telephone contacts over a 12-week period.

At the end of treatment, the combined behavioral therapy group had significantly better outcomes as compared with the other two groups in terms of bladder control, quality of life, and treatment satisfaction. At 3-month follow-up, however, there were no discernible differences in terms of those outcomes among the three groups. The researchers concluded that, although combination therapy enjoyed good early outcomes, education, counseling and frequent patient contact may be the critical variables. Several randomized controlled trials have demonstrated the benefit of combining behavioral and pharmaceutical therapies for OAB with or without urge UI. In a 1995 double-blind, dose-adjusted, crossover trial ($n = 63$), Ouslander and colleagues found that the addition of oxybutynin to prompted voiding provided a small but beneficial improvement for a group of nursing home residents.[184] In a 2000 modified crossover randomized controlled trial extension study ($n = 197$), Burgio and colleagues found that subjects treated with biofeedback-assisted behavioral therapy showed greater improvement than those treated with oxybutynin alone, but subjects who received both biofeedback-assisted behavioral therapy *and* oxybutynin had the best results.[185] Similarly, Mattiasson explored the impact of combining behavioral therapy with short-acting tolterodine (2 mg twice daily) and demonstrated improved outcomes with the addition of a simplified bladder training program to the drug therapy (multicenter, single-blind study; $n = 505$).[186] In contrast, Millard and colleagues found that the only benefit derived from the addition of simplified PFM exercises to a tolterodine treatment program was patient perception regarding improvement.[187]

Other trials have explored the impact of combining various pharmacologic agents for selected groups of patients. For example, recent studies have addressed the potential benefits of combined anticholinergic and alpha-adrenergic antagonist therapy for patients with a combination of OAB and bladder outlet obstruction. As noted earlier, bladder outlet obstruction is often associated with bladder overactivity; although alpha blockade is commonly prescribed for these patients, most clinicians have been hesitant to use anticholinergics to control OAB symptoms, because of concerns regarding urinary retention. Although caution is appropriate in this situation, it appears that the addition of anticholinergic therapy is safe once urethral resistance has been at least partially reduced by alpha-adrenergic antagonists.[107] Two recent review articles describe approaches to balancing these two types of medications in the patient with both OAB and bladder outlet obstruction.[176,178]

Although at present there are no "easy answers" to the management of OAB, current evidence suggests that the best approach for most patients is a combination of various behavioral therapies, and, when indicated, judicious use of medications (with careful monitoring and diligence in terms of drug and dosage adjustment). This approach is supported by most clinicians and expert review panels, including the ICI2.[2]

SUMMARY

In summary, this is a new era in the management of OAB. The epidemiology, etiology, and impact of OAB are much clearer, and there is now a good deal of diagnostic guidance, which enjoys broad international accord. In addition, clinicians now have a variety of treatment options from which to choose in managing any individual patient. However, no single treatment is a panacea. Rather, maximal benefit is derived from stepped approach to therapy and from combination therapy that balances safety with efficacy. Most importantly, clinicians no longer need to design treatment programs based on anecdotal evidence alone. Although many questions remain, a deep and growing body of knowledge allows an evidence-based approach to patient care. The complexity of the physiology of OAB and of its treatments, however, demands a multidisciplinary approach, and the continence care nurse is a critical part of that team.

SELF-ASSESSMENT EXERCISE

1. Define the following terms: urge urinary incontinence; overactive bladder; and detrusor hyperactivity with impaired contractility.
2. List five factors outside the lower urinary tract associated with OAB symptoms.
3. List the four classic symptoms of overactive bladder.
4. Describe three factors that must be investigated during the history of an individual complaining of OAB symptoms.
5. List two major goals for the evaluation of an individual with OAB.
6. List at least four potential findings from the OAB evaluation that warrant further investigation.
7. List at least three types of behavioral therapy for OAB not including bladder training and urgency suppression.
8. Define bladder training and outline its key components.
9. Define urge suppression and outline its key components.
10. Briefly explain the proposed mechanism of action of anticholinergic (specifically antimuscarinic) medications for OAB.
11. List two surgical therapies for overactive bladder.
12. Explain why the evidence base for treatment of OAB suggests that a combined approach should be the most effective.
13. Given an actual or hypothetical patient with urge incontinence, develop an appropriate treatment program.

REFERENCES

1. Abrams P, Cardozo L, Fall M, et al: The standardisation of terminology of lower urinary tract function: report from the standardisation sub-committee of the International Continence Society, *Neurourol Urodyn* 21(2):167-178, 2002.
2. Abrams P, Andersson KE, Artibani W, et al: Second International Consultation on Incontinence recommendations of the International Scientific Committee: evaluation and treatment of urinary incontinence, pelvic organ prolapse and faecal incontinence: *http://www.congress-urology.org/image/content.in.pdf,* 2002.
3. Stewart WF, Van Rooyen JB, Cundiff GW, et al: Prevalence and burden of overactive bladder in the United States, *World J Urol* 20(6):327-336, 2003.
4. Milsom I, Abrams P, Cardozo L, et al: How widespread are the symptoms of an overactive bladder and how are they managed? A population-based prevalence study, *BJU Int* 87(9):760-766, 2001.

5. Thom D: Variation in estimates of urinary incontinence prevalence in the community: effects of differences in definition, population characteristics, and study type, *J Am Geriatr Soc* 46(4):473-480, 1998.

6. Nygaard IE, Lemke JH: Urinary incontinence in rural older women: prevalence, incidence and remission, *J Am Geriatr Soc* 44(9):1049-1054, 1996.

7. Jackson S: The patient with an overactive bladder: symptoms and quality-of-life issues, *Urology* 50(6A suppl):18-22; discussion 23-24, 1997.

8. Hunskaar S and Vinsnes A. The quality of life in women with urinary incontinence as measured by the sickness impact profile. *J Am Geriar Soc* 39(4):378-382, 1991.

9. Coyne K, Revicki D, Hunt T, et al: Psychometric validation of an overactive bladder symptom and health-related quality of life questionnaire: the OAB-Q, *Qual Life Res* 11(6):563-574, 2002.

10. Coyne KS, Zhou Z, Thompson C, et al: The impact on health-related quality of life of stress, urge and mixed urinary incontinence, *BJU Int* 92(7):731-735, 2003.

11. Coyne KS, Zhou Z, Bhattacharyya SK, et al: The prevalence of nocturia and its effect on health-related quality of life and sleep in a community sample in the USA, *BJU Int* 92(9):948-954, 2003.

12. Brown JS, McGhan WF, Chokroverty S: Comorbidities associated with overactive bladder, *Am J Manag Care* 6(11 suppl):S574-S759, 2000.

13. Brown JS, Vittinghoff E, Wyman JF, et al: Urinary incontinence: does it increase risk for falls and fractures? Study of osteoporotic fractures research group, *J Am Geriatr Soc* 48(7):721-725, 2000.

14. Wagner TH, Hu TW, Bentkover J, et al: Health-related consequences of overactive bladder, *Am J Manag Care* 8(19 suppl):S598-S607, 2002.

15. Hu TW, Wagner TH: Economic considerations in overactive bladder, *Am J Manag Care* 6(11 suppl):S591-S598, 2000.

16. Hu TW, Wagner TH, Bentkover JD, et al: Estimated economic costs of overactive bladder in the United States, *Urology* 61(6):1123-1128, 2003.

17. Hu TW, Wagner TH, Bentkover JD, et al: Costs of urinary incontinence and overactive bladder in the United States: a comparative study, *Urology* 63(3):461-465, 2004.

18. Zimmern PE, McConnell JD: Voiding dysfunction, incontinence and bladder pain. In Braunwald E, Fauci AS, Kasper DL, et al, editors: *Harrison's principles of internal medicine*, vol 2, New York: McGraw-Hill Professional, 2001, sect 7.

19. de Groat WC: A neurologic basis for the overactive bladder, *Urology* 50(6A suppl):36-52; discussion 53-56, 1997.

20. Fitzgerald MP, Stablein U, Brubaker L: Urinary habits among asymptomatic women, *Am J Obstet Gynecol* 187(5):1384-1388, 2002.

21. FitzGerald MP, Butler N, Shott S, et al: Bother arising from urinary frequency in women, *Neurourol Urodyn* 21(1):36-40; discussion 41, 2002.

22. Mueller E, Latini J, Lux M, et al: Gender differences in 24-hour urinary diaries of asymptomatic North American adults, *J Urol* 173(2):490-492, 2005.

23. Simon J, Abrams P. The cystometrogram. In O'Donnell PD, editor: *Urinary incontinence*, St. Louis, 1997, Mosby-Year Book.

24. Abrams P, Cardozo L, Fall M, et al: The standardisation of terminology of lower urinary tract function: report from the standardisation sub-committee of the International Continence Society, *Neurourol Urodyn* 21(2):167-178, 2002.

25. de Groat WC. Central nervous system control of micturition. In O'Donnell PD, editor: *Urinary incontinence*, St. Louis, 1997, Mosby-Year Book.

26. Mattiasson A. Physiology of continence. In O'Donnell PD, editor: *Urinary incontinence*, St. Louis, 1997, Mosby-Year Book, pp 25-33.

27. Wein AJ, Barrett DM. Normal lower urinary tract filling/storing and emptying: simple overview, extrapolation, and application of the two days concept. In *Voiding function and dysfunction: a logical and practical approach*, Chicago, 1988, Year Book Medical Publishers, pp 114-136.

28. O'Donnell P: Volume-interval relationship of incontinence episodes in elderly inpatient men, *Urology* 41(4):334-337, 1993.

29. Garnett S, Abrams P: Clinical aspects of the overactive bladder and detrusor overactivity, *Scand J Urol Nephrol Suppl* 210:65-71, 2002.

30. Artibani W: Diagnosis and significance of idiopathic overactive bladder, *Urology* 50(6A suppl):25-32; discussion 33-35, 1997.

31. de Groat WC: A neurologic basis for the overactive bladder, *Urology* 50(6A suppl):36-52; discussion 53-56, 1997.

32. Brading AF: A myogenic basis for the overactive bladder, *Urology* 50(6A suppl):57-67; discussion 68-73, 1997.

33. Ouslander JG: Management of overactive bladder, *N Engl J Med* 350(8):786-799, 2004.

34. Thomas AW, Abrams P: Lower urinary tract symptoms, benign prostatic obstruction and the overactive bladder, *BJU Int* 85(suppl 3):57-68; discussion 70-71, 2000.

35. Elbadawi A, Yalla SV, Resnick NM: Structural basis of geriatric voiding dysfunction. IV: bladder outlet obstruction, *J Urol* 150(5):1681-1695, 1993.

36. Semins MJ, Chancellor MB: Diagnosis and management of patients with over-overactive bladder syndrome and abnormal detrusor activity, *Nat Clin Pract Urol* 1(2):2004.

37. Resnick NM, Yalla SV: Detrusor hyperactivity with impaired contractile function: an unrecognized but common cause of incontinence in elderly patients, *JAMA* 257(22):3076-3081, 1987.

38. Resnick NM: Diagnosis and treatment of incontinence in the institutionalized elderly, *Semin Urol* 7(2):117-123, 1989.

39. Dallosso HM, McGrother CW, Matthews RJ, et al: The association of diet and other lifestyle factors with overactive bladder and stress incontinence: a longitudinal study in women, *BJU Int* 92(1):69-77, 2003.

40. Dallosso HM, McGrother CW, Matthews RJ, et al: Nutrient composition of the diet and the development of overactive bladder: a longitudinal study in women, *Neurourol Urodyn* 23(3):204-210, 2004.

41. Dallosso HM, Matthews RJ, McGrother CW, et al: The association of diet and other lifestyle factors with the onset of overactive bladder: a longitudinal study in men, *Public Health Nutr* 7(7):885-891, 2004.

42. Hannestad YS, Rortveit G, Daltveit AK, et al: Are smoking and other lifestyle factors associated with female urinary incontinence? The Norwegian Epincont Study, *Bjog* 110(3):247-254, 2003.

43. Parazzini F, Chiaffarino F, Lavezzari M, et al: Risk factors for stress, urge or mixed urinary incontinence in Italy, *Bjog* 110(10):927-933, 2003.

44. Teleman PM, Lidfeldt J, Nerbrand C, et al: Overactive bladder: prevalence, risk factors and relation to stress incontinence in middle-aged women, *Bjog* 111(6): 600-604, 2004.

45. Stewart WF, Van Rooyen JB, Cundiff GW, et al: Prevalence and burden of overactive bladder in the United States, *World J Urol* 20(6):327-336, 2003.

46. Koley B, Koley J, Saha JK: The effects of nicotine on spontaneous contractions of cat urinary bladder in situ, *Br J Pharmacol* 83(2):347-355, 1984.

47. Hisayama T, Shinkai M, Takayanagi I, et al: Mechanism of action of nicotine in isolated urinary bladder of guinea-pig, *Br J Pharmacol* 95(2):465-472, 1988.

48. Nuotio M, Jylha M, Koivisto AM, et al: Association of smoking with urgency in older people, *Eur Urol* 40(2):206-212, 2001.

49. Haidinger G: Risk factors for lower urinary tract symptoms in elderly men: for the prostate study group of the Austrian Society of Urology, *Eur Urol* 37(4):413-420, 2000.

50. Koskimaki J, Hakama M, Huhtala H, et al: Association of dietary elements and lower urinary tract symptoms, *Scand J Urol Nephrol* 34(1):46-50, 2000.

51. Bump RC, McClish DK: Cigarette smoking and urinary incontinence in women, *Am J Obstet Gynecol* 167(5):1213-1218, 1992.

52. Holroyd-Leduc JM, Straus SE: Management of urinary incontinence in women: scientific review, *JAMA* 291(8):986-995, 2004.

53. Koskimaki J, Hakama M, Huhtala H, et al: Association of smoking with lower urinary tract symptoms, *J Urol* 159(5):1580-1582, 1998.

54. Tampakoudis P, Tantanassis T, Grimbizis G, et al: Cigarette smoking and urinary incontinence in women: a new calculative method of estimating the exposure to smoke, *Eur J Obstet Gynecol Reprod Biol* 63(1):27-30, 1995.

55. Resnick NM. Geriatric medicine. In Tierney LM, McPhee SJ, Schroeder SA, et al, editors: *Current medical diagnosis and treatment*, vol 32, Stamford, Conn., 1993, Appleton & Lange, pp 45-68.

56. Ouslander JG, Dutcher JA: Overactive bladder: assessment and nonpharmacologic interventions, *Consult Pharmacist* 18(suppl B):13-20, 2003.

57. Nuotio M, Tammela TL, Luukkaala T, et al: Urgency and urge incontinence in an older population: ten-year changes and their association with mortality, *Aging Clin Exp Res* 14(5):412-419, 2002.

58. Cardozo L, Robinson D: Special considerations in premenopausal and postmenopausal women with symptoms of overactive bladder, *Urology* 60(5 suppl 1): 64-71; discussion 71, 2002.

59. Nigro DA, Wein AJ. Pharmacologic therapy. In O'Donnell PD, editor: *Urinary incontinence*, St. Louis, 1997, Mosby-Year Book, pp 277-286.

60. Bjornsdottir LT, Geirsson RT, Jonsson PV: Urinary incontinence and urinary tract infections in octogenarian women, *Acta Obstet Gynecol Scand* 77(1):105-109, 1998.

61. Cardozo L, Lose G, McClish D, et al: A systematic review of the effects of estrogens for symptoms suggestive of overactive bladder, *Acta Obstet Gynecol Scand* 83(10):892-897, 2004.

62. Grady D, Brown JS, Vittinghoff E, et al: Postmenopausal hormones and incontinence: the heart and estrogen/progestin replacement study, *Obstet Gynecol* 97(1):116-120, 2001.

63. Ouslander JG, Greendale GA, Uman G, et al: Effects of oral estrogen and progestin on the lower urinary tract among female nursing home residents, *J Am Geriatr Soc* 49(6):803-807, 2001.

64. Klingele CJ, Carley ME, Hill RF: Patient characteristics that are associated with urodynamically diagnosed detrusor instability and genuine stress incontinence, *Am J Obstet Gynecol* 186(5):866-868, 2002.

65. Moehrer B, Hextall A, Jackson S: Oestrogens for urinary incontinence in women, *Cochrane Database Syst Rev* (2):CD001405, 2003.

66. Weiss BD: Diagnostic evaluation of urinary incontinence in geriatric patients, *Am Fam Physician* 57(11): 2675-2684, 2688-2690, 1998.

67. Umlauf M, Kurtzer E, Valappil T, et al: Sleep-disordered breathing as a mechanism for nocturia: preliminary findings, *Ostomy Wound Manage* 45(12):52-60, 1999.

68. van der Vaart CH, de Leeuw JR, Roovers JP, et al: The effect of urinary incontinence and overactive bladder symptoms on quality of life in young women, *BJU Int* 90(6):544-549, 2002.

69. Abrams P, Cardozo L, Fall M, et al: The standardisation of terminology in lower urinary tract function: report from the standardisation sub-committee of the International Continence Society, *Urology* 61(1):37-49, 2003.

70. Abrams P: Describing bladder storage function: overactive bladder syndrome and detrusor overactivity, *Urology* 62(5 suppl 2):28-37; discussion 40-42, 2003.

71. Naughton MJ, Donovan J, Badia X, et al: Symptom severity and QOL scales for urinary incontinence, *Gastroenterology* 126(1 suppl 1):S114-S123, 2004.

72. Brown JS, Posner SF, Stewart AL: Urge incontinence: new health-related quality of life measures, *J Am Geriatr Soc* 47(8):980-988, 1999.

73. Lubeck DP, Prebil LA, Peeples P, et al: A health related quality of life measure for use in patients with urge urinary incontinence: a validation study, *Qual Life Res* 8(4):337-344, 1999.

74. Kelleher CJ, Cardozo LD, Khullar V, et al: A new questionnaire to assess the quality of life of urinary incontinent women, *Br J Obstet Gynaecol* 104(12):1374-1379, 1997.

75. Homma Y, Uemura S: Use of the short form of King's Health Questionnaire to measure quality of life in patients with an overactive bladder, *BJU Int* 93(7):1009-1013, 2004.

76. Reese PR, Pleil AM, Okano GJ, et al: Multinational study of reliability and validity of the King's Health Questionnaire in patients with overactive bladder, *Qual Life Res* 12(4):427-442, 2003.

77. Brubaker L: Urgency: the cornerstone symptom of overactive bladder, *Urology* 64(6 suppl 1):12-6, 2004.

78. Freeman R, Hill S, Millard R, et al: Reduced perception of urgency in treatment of overactive bladder with extended-release tolterodine, *Obstet Gynecol* 102(3):605-611, 2003.

79. Dmochowski R, Heit M, Sand P. The effect of anticholinergic therapy on urgency severity in patients with overactive bladder: clinical assessment of a newly validated tool. In International Continence Society, October 5-9, 2003, Florence.

80. Brazier JE, Harper R, Jones NMB: Validating the SF-36 Health Survey Questionnaire: a new outcome measure for primary care, *BMJ* 305:160-164, 1992.

81. Kelleher CJ, Kreder KJ, Pleil AM, et al: Long-term health-related quality of life of patients receiving extended-release tolterodine for overactive bladder, *Am J Manag Care* 8(19 suppl):S616-S630, 2002.

82. Kelleher CJ, Reese PR, Pleil AM, et al: Health-related quality of life of patients receiving extended-release tolterodine for overactive bladder, *Am J Manag Care* 8(19 suppl):S608-S615, 2002.

83. Kelleher CJ, Pleil AM, Reese PR, et al: How much is enough and who says so? *Bjog* 111(6):605-612, 2004.

84. Robinson D, McClish DK, Wyman JF, et al: Comparison between urinary diaries completed with and without intensive patient instructions, *Neurourol Urodyn* 15(2):143-148, 1996.

85. Van Kerrebroeck P: Standardization of terminology in nocturia: commentary on the ICS report, *BJU Int* 90(suppl 3):16-17, 2002.

86. Weiss JP, Blaivas JG: Nocturnal polyuria versus overactive bladder in nocturia, *Urology* 60(5 suppl 1):28-32; discussion 32, 2002.

87. Quinn P, Goka J, and Richardson H. Assessment of an electronic daily diary in patients with overactive bladder. *BJU Int'l* 91(7):647-652, 2003.

88. van Brummen HJ, Heintz AP, van der Vaart CH: The association between overactive bladder symptoms and objective parameters from bladder diary and filling cystometry, *Neurourol Urodyn* 23(1):38-42, 2004.

89. Brown JS, McNaughton KS, Wyman JF, et al: Measurement characteristics of a voiding diary for use by men and women with overactive bladder, *Urology* 61(4):802-809, 2003.

90. Ku JH, Jeong IG, Lim DJ, et al: Voiding diary for the evaluation of urinary incontinence and lower urinary tract symptoms: prospective assessment of patient compliance and burden, *Neurourol Urodyn* 23(4):331-335, 2004.

91. Griffiths DJ, McCracken PN, Harrison GM, et al: Urinary incontinence in the elderly: the brain factor, *Scand J Urol Nephrol Suppl* 157:83-88, 1994.

92. Di Benedetto P: Female urinary incontinence rehabilitation, *Minerva Ginecol* 56(4):353-369, 2004.

93. Hunskaar S, Vinsnes A: The quality of life in women with urinary incontinence as measured by the sickness impact profile, *J Am Geriatr Soc* 39(4):378-382, 1991.

94. Schafer W, Abrams P, Liao L, et al: Good urodynamic practices: uroflowmetry, filling cystometry, and pressure-flow studies, *Neurourol Urodyn* 21(3):261-274, 2002.

95. Ouslander J, Leach G, Abelson S, et al: Simple versus multichannel cystometry in the evaluation of bladder function in an incontinent geriatric population, *J Urol* 140(6):1482-1486, 1988.

96. Rayome RG: Simple urodynamic techniques, *J Wound Ostomy Continence Nurs* 22(1):17-26, 1995.

97. Burgio KL, Locher JL, Goode PS, et al: Behavioral vs drug treatment for urge urinary incontinence in older women: a randomized controlled trial, *JAMA* 280(23):1995-2000, 1998.

98. Rovner ES, Wein AJ: Evaluation of lower urinary tract symptoms in females, *Curr Opin Urol* 13(4):273-278, 2003.

99. Mostwin JL: Pathophysiology: the varieties of bladder overactivity, *Urology* 60(5 suppl 1):22-26; discussion 27, 2002.

100. Gray M: Continence nursing at the dawn of the 21st century: a futurist perspective, *Urol Nurs* 22(4):233-236, 2002.

101. Thompson DL, Smith DA: Continence nursing: a whole person approach, *Holist Nurs Pract* 16(2):14-31, 2002.

102. Heywood J: Continence: the science, art, and charity of decency, *J Wound Ostomy Continence Nurs* 29(2):63-64, 2002.

103. Bernier F: Relationship of a pelvic floor rehabilitation program for urinary incontinence to Orem's self-care deficit theory of nursing: part 1, *Urol Nurs* 22(6):378-383, 390; quiz 391, 2002.

104. Orem DE: *Nursing: concepts of practice,* 4 ed, St. Louis, 1991, Mosby-Year Book.

105. Burgio KL, Goode PS. Behavior therapy. In O'Donnell PD, editor: *Urinary incontinence,* St. Louis, 1997, Mosby-Year Book.

106. Bernier F: Applying Orem's self-care deficit theory of nursing to continence care: part 2, *Urol Nurs* 22(6):384-390, 2002.

107. Palmer MH: Use of health behavior change theories to guide urinary incontinence research, *Nurs Res* 53(6 suppl):S49-S55, 2004.

108. Carcio H: Comprehensive continence care: the nurse practitioner's role, *Adv Nurse Pract* 11(10):26-35; quiz 35-36, 2003.

109. Wyman JF: Management of urinary incontinence in adult ambulatory care populations, *Annu Rev Nurs Res* 18(10):171-194, 2000.

110. Arya LA, Myers DL, Jackson ND: Dietary caffeine intake and the risk for detrusor instability: a case-control study, *Obstet Gynecol* 96(1):85-89, 2000.

111. Creighton SM, Stanton SL: Caffeine: does it affect your bladder? *Br J Urol* 66(6):613-614, 1990.

112. Bryant CM, Dowell CJ, Fairbrother G: Caffeine reduction education to improve urinary symptoms, *Br J Nurs* 11(8):560-565, 2002.

113. Gray M: Caffeine and urinary continence, *J Wound Ostomy Continence Nurs* 28(2):66-69, 2001.

114. Chiang L, Ouslander J, Schnelle J, et al: Dually incontinent nursing home residents: clinical characteristics and treatment differences, *J Am Geriatr Soc* 48(6):673-676, 2000.

115. Chen GD, Hu SW, Chen YC, et al: Prevalence and correlations of anal incontinence and constipation in Taiwanese women, *Neurourol Urodyn* 22(7):664-669, 2003.

116. Fowler CJ: The perspective of a neurologist on treatment-related research in fecal and urinary incontinence, *Gastroenterology* 126(1 suppl 1):S172-S174, 2004.

117. Schroder A, Uvelius B, Newgreen D, et al: Bladder overactivity in mice after 1 week of outlet obstruction: mainly afferent dysfunction? *J Urol* 170(3):1017-1021, 2003.

118. Newman DK. Urinary incontinence and overactive bladder: a focus on behavioral interventions. In © 2001 Medscape Portals I, editor: *Top Adv Pract Nurs eJ* 1, 2001.

119. Chapple CR, Yamanishi T, Chess-Williams R: Muscarinic receptor subtypes and management of the overactive bladder, *Urology* 60(5 suppl 1):82-88; discussion 88-89, 2002.

120. Miner PB, Jr.: Economic and personal impact of fecal and urinary incontinence, *Gastroenterology* 126(1 suppl 1):S8-S13, 2004.

121. Ganio E, Masin A, Ratto C, et al: Short-term sacral nerve stimulation for functional anorectal and urinary disturbances: results in 40 patients: evaluation of a new option for anorectal functional disorders, *Dis Colon Rectum* 44(9):1261-1267, 2001.

122. Diokno AC, Burgio K, Fultz NH, et al: Medical and self-care practices reported by women with urinary incontinence, *Am J Manag Care* 10(2):69-78, 2004.

123. Dowd TT, Campbell JM, Jones JA: Fluid intake and urinary incontinence in older community-dwelling women, *J Commun Health Nurs* 13(3):179-186, 1996.

124. Fitzgerald ST, Palmer MH, Berry SJ, et al: Urinary incontinence: impact on working women, *AAOHN J* 48(3):112-118, 2000.

125. Matthiesen TB, Rittig S, Mortensen JT, et al: Nocturia and polyuria in men referred with lower urinary tract symptoms, assessed using a 7-day frequency-volume chart, *BJU Int* 83(9):1017-1022, 1999.

126. Griffiths DJ, McCracken PN, Harrison GM, et al: Relationship of fluid intake to voluntary micturition and urinary incontinence in geriatric patients, *Neurourol Urodyn* 12(1):1-7, 1993.

127. Al-Mulhim AA, Al-Gazzar SA, Bahnassy AA: Conservative treatment of idiopathic detrusor instability in elderly women: physiotherapy, *Saudi Med J* 23(5):543-545, 2002.

128. Fitzgerald M, Stablein U, Brubaker L: Urinary habits among asymptomatic women, *Am J Obstet Gynecol* 187:1384-1388, 2002.

129. Gray M, Krissovich M: Does fluid intake influence the risk for urinary incontinence, urinary tract infection, and bladder cancer? *J Wound Ostomy Continence Nurs* 30(3):126-131, 2003.

130. Iqbal P, Castleden CM: Management of urinary incontinence in the elderly, *Gerontology* 43(3):151-157, 1997.

131. Wells TJ. Nursing management. In O'Donnell PD, editor: *Urinary incontinence,* St. Louis, 1997, Mosby-Year Book.

132. Pearson BD: Liquidate a myth: reducing liquid intake is not advisable for elderly with urine control problems, *Urol Nurs* 13(3):86-87, 1993.

133. Abrams P, Blaivas JG, Fowler CJ, et al: The role of neuromodulation in the management of urinary urge incontinence, *BJU Int* 91(4):355-359, 2003.

134. Flegal K, Carroll M, Kuczmarski R, et al: Overweight and obesity in the United States: prevalence and trends, 1960-1994, *Int J Obes Rel Metab Disord* 22:39-47, 1998.

135. World Health Organization (WHO). Physical status: the use and interpretation of anthropometry. In Organization WH, editor: WHO Technical Report Series. Geneva, 1995, World Health Organization.

136. Calle EE, Thun MJ, Petrelli JM, et al: Body-mass index and mortality in a prospective cohort of US adults, *N Engl J Med* 341(15):1097-1105, 1999.

137. Bump RC, Sugerman HJ, Fantl JA, et al: Obesity and lower urinary tract function in women: effect of surgically induced weight loss, *Am J Obstet Gynecol* 167(2):392-397; discussion 397-399, 1992.

138. Subak LL, Johnson C, Whitcomb E, et al: Does weight loss improve incontinence in moderately obese women? *Int Urogynecol J Pelvic Floor Dysfunct* 13(1):40-43, 2002.

139. Milne JL: Behavioral therapies at the primary care level: the current state of knowledge, *J Wound Ostomy Continence Nurs* 31(6):367-378, 2004.

140. Rigby D: The overactive bladder, *Nurs Stand* 17(39):45-52; quiz 54, 56, 2003.

141. Wyman JF: Treatment of urinary incontinence in men and older women: the evidence shows the efficacy of a variety of techniques, *Am J Nurs* 103 (suppl):26-35, 2003.

142. Elser DM, Wyman JF, McClish DK, et al: The effect of bladder training, pelvic floor muscle training, or combination training on urodynamic parameters in women with urinary incontinence: continence program for women research group, *Neurourol Urodyn* 18(5):427-446, 1999.

143. Quinn P, Goka J, Richardson H: Assessment of an electronic daily diary in patients with overactive bladder, *BJU Int* 91 (7):647-652, 2003.

144. Wyman JF: Managing urinary incontinence with bladder training: a case study, *J ET Nurs* 20(3):121-126, 1993.

145. Fantl JA, Wyman JF, McClish DK, et al: Efficacy of bladder training in older women with urinary incontinence, *JAMA* 265(5):609-613, 1991.

146. Weiss JP, Blaivas JG: Nocturnal polyuria versus overactive bladder in nocturia, *Urology* 60(5 suppl 1):28-32; discussion 32, 2002.

147. Weiss JP, Blaivas JG, Stember DS, et al: Nocturia in adults: etiology and classification, *Neurourol Urodyn* 17(5):467-472, 1998.

148. Wallace SA, Roe B, Williams K, et al: Bladder training for urinary incontinence in adults, *Cochrane Database Syst Rev* (1):CD001308, 2004.

149. Burgio KL, Whitehead WE, Engel BT: Urinary incontinence in the elderly: bladder-sphincter biofeedback and toileting skills training, *Ann Intern Med* 103(4):507-515, 1985.

150. Petros PE, Ulmsten UI: An integral theory of female urinary incontinence: experimental and clinical considerations, *Acta Obstet Gynecol Scand Suppl* 153: 7-31, 1990.

151. Shafik A, Shafik IA: Overactive bladder inhibition in response to pelvic floor muscle exercises, *World J Urol* 20(6):374-377, 2003.

152. Burgio KL: Current perspectives on management of urgency using bladder and behavioral training, *J Am Acad Nurse Pract* 16(10 suppl):4-7, 2004.

153. Wyman JF, Fantl JA, McClish DK, et al: Comparative efficacy of behavioral interventions in the management of female urinary incontinence: continence program for women research group, *Am J Obstet Gynecol* 179(4): 999-1007, 1998.

154. Sampselle C: Behavioral interventions in young and middle-aged women: simple interventions to combat a complex problem, *Am J Nurs* (suppl):9-19, 2003.

155. Madersbacher H: Neurourology and pelvic floor dysfunction, *Minerva Ginecol* 56(4):303-309, 2004.

156. Cucchi A, Siracusano S, Di Benedetto P, et al: Urgency of voiding and abdominal pressure transmission in women with mixed urinary incontinence, *Neurourol Urodyn* 23(1):43-47, 2004.

157. Hay-Smith EJ, Bo Berghmans LC, Hendriks HJ, et al: Pelvic floor muscle training for urinary incontinence in women, *Cochrane Database Syst Rev* (1):CD001407, 2001.

158. Sampselle C. Behavioral interventions in young and middle-aged women: Simple interventions to combat a complex problem. *Am J Nurs* (suppl):9-19, 2003.

159. Nygaard IE, Kreder KJ, Lepic MM, et al: Efficacy of pelvic floor muscle exercises in women with stress, urge, and mixed urinary incontinence, *Am J Obstet Gynecol* 174(1):120-125, 1996.

160. Sherman RA, Davis GD, Wong MF: Behavioral treatment of exercise-induced urinary incontinence among female soldiers, *Mil Med* 162(10):690-694, 1997.

161. Burgio KL, Goode PS, Locher JL, et al: Behavioral training with and without biofeedback in the treatment of urge incontinence in older women: a randomized controlled trial, *JAMA* 288(18):2293-2299, 2002.

162. Herbison P, Plevnik S, Mantle J: Weighted vaginal cones for urinary incontinence, *Cochrane Database Syst Rev* (1):CD002114, 2002.

163. Payne CK. Electrostimulation. In O'Donnell PD, editor: *Urinary incontinence,* St. Louis, 1997, Mosby-Year Book.

164. Brubaker L, Benson JT, Bent A, et al: Transvaginal electrical stimulation for female urinary incontinence, *Am J Obstet Gynecol* 177(3):536-540, 1997.

165. Siegel SW, Richardson DA, Miller KL, et al: Pelvic floor electrical stimulation for the treatment of urge and mixed urinary incontinence in women, *Urology* 50(6):934-940, 1997.

166. Wang AC, Wang YY, Chen MC: Single-blind, randomized trial of pelvic floor muscle training, biofeedback-assisted pelvic floor muscle training, and electrical stimulation in the management of overactive bladder, *Urology* 63(1):61-66, 2004.

167. Takahashi S, Kitamura T: Overactive bladder: Magnetic versus electrical stimulation, *Curr Opin Obstet Gynecol* 15(5):429-433, 2003.

168. Fujishiro T, Takahashi S, Enomoto H, et al: Magnetic stimulation of the sacral roots for the treatment of urinary frequency and urge incontinence: an investigational study and placebo controlled trial, *J Urol* 168(3):1036-1039, 2002.

169. Govier FE, Litwiller S, Nitti V, et al: Percutaneous afferent neuromodulation for the refractory overactive bladder: results of a multicenter study, *J Urol* 165(4):1193-1198, 2001.

170. Svihra J, Kurca E, Luptak J, et al: Neuromodulative treatment of overactive bladder—noninvasive tibial nerve stimulation, *Bratisl Lek Listy* 103(12):480-483, 2002.

171. Chang PL: Urodynamic studies in acupuncture for women with frequency, urgency and dysuria, *J Urol* 140(3):563-566, 1988.

172. Smith DA. Urge incontinence. In Doughty DB, editor: *Urinary and fecal incontinence: nursing management,* ed 2 ed, St. Louis, 2000, Mosby, pp 91-104.

173. Andersson KE: The overactive bladder: pharmacologic basis of drug treatment. *Urology* 50(6A suppl):74-84; discussion 85-89, 1997.

174. Herbison P, Hay-Smith J, Ellis G, et al: Effectiveness of anticholinergic drugs compared with placebo in the treatment of overactive bladder: systematic review, *BMJ* 326(7394):841-844, 2003.

175. Lackner TE: Innovations and strategies for achieving urinary continence in the elderly, *Clin Consult* 16(suppl 2):1-20, 2001.

176. Gonzalez RR, Te AE: Overactive bladder and men: indications for anticholinergics, *Curr Urol Rep* 4(6):429-435, 2003.

177. Lee JY, Kim HW, Lee SJ, et al: Comparison of doxazosin with or without tolterodine in men with symptomatic bladder outlet obstruction and an overactive bladder, *BJU Int* 94(6):817-820, 2004.

178. Reynard JM: Does anticholinergic medication have a role for men with lower urinary tract symptoms/benign prostatic hyperplasia either alone or in combination with other agents? *Curr Opin Urol* 14(1):13-16, 2004.

179. Hunsballe JM, Hansen TK, Rittig S, et al: The efficacy of DDAVP is related to the circadian rhythm of urine output in patients with persisting nocturnal enuresis, *Clin Endocrinol (Oxf)* 49(6):793-801, 1998.

180. Wein A, Abrams P: Statement from the first international consultation on nocturia: reaching for a consensus, *BJU Int* 90(suppl 3):37, 2002.

181. Sullivan J, Abrams P: Overactive detrusor, *Curr Opin Urol* 9(4):291-296, 1999.

182. Churchill BM, Aliabadi H, Landau EH, et al. Ureteral bladder augmentation, *J Urol* 150 (2):716-720, 1993.

183. Landau EH, Jayanthi VR, Khoury AE, et al: Bladder augmentation: ureterocystoplasty versus ileocystoplasty, *J Urol* 152(2):716-719, 1994.

184. Ouslander JG, Schnelle JF, Uman G, et al: Does oxybutynin add to the effectiveness of prompted voiding for urinary incontinence among nursing home residents? A placebo-controlled trial, *J Am Geriatr Soc* 43(6): 610-617, 1995

185. Burgio KL, Locher JL, Goode PS: Combined behavioral and drug therapy for urge incontinence in older women, *J Am Geriatr Soc* 48(4):370-374, 2000.

186. Mattiasson A, Blaakaer J, Hoye K, et al: Simplified bladder training augments the effectiveness of tolterodine in patients with an overactive bladder, *BJU Int* 91(1):54-60, 2003.

187. Millard RJ: Clinical efficacy of tolterodine with or without a simplified pelvic floor exercise regimen, *Neurourol Urodyn* 23(1):48-53, 2004.

188. Andersen JT, Blaivas JG, Cardozo L, et al: ICS 7th report on the standardisation of terminology of lower urinary tract function: lower urinary tract rehabilitation techniques, *Neurourol Urodyn* 11:593-603, 1992.

189. van Kerrebroeck P, Abrams P, Chaikin D, et al: The standardisation of terminology in nocturia: report from the standardisation sub-committee of the International Continence Society, *Neurourol Urodyn* 21(2):179-183, 2002.

190. Goldberg RP, Sand PK: Pathophysiology of the overactive bladder, *Clin Obstet Gynecol* 45(1):182-192, 2002.

191. Flisser AJ, Walmsley K, Blaivas JG: Urodynamic classification of patients with symptoms of overactive bladder, *J Urol* 169(2):529-533; discussion 533-534, 2003.

192. Payne CK: Epidemiology, pathophysiology, and evaluation of urinary incontinence and overactive bladder, *Urology* 51(2A suppl):3-10, 1998.

193. Wein A, Lose GR, Fonda D: Nocturia in men, women and the elderly: a practical approach, *BJU Int* 90(suppl 3):28-31, 2002.

194. Rovner ES, Wein AJ: The treatment of overactive bladder in the geriatric patient, *Clin Geriatr* 10(1): 20-35, 2002.

CHAPTER 6

Pathology and Management of Functional Factors Contributing to Incontinence

DONNA L. THOMPSON

OBJECTIVES

1. Define the term "functional incontinence."
2. Describe the relationship between changes associated with aging and risk for the development of functional incontinence.
3. Relate the four major barriers to continence to the development of functional incontinence.
4. Describe how the environment of care contributes to functional incontinence.
5. Discuss the importance of a cognitive assessment (including the specific mental impairments that occur with dementia) when planning interventions for functional incontinence.
6. Integrate elements of an assessment that focus on functional incontinence into the comprehensive continence evaluation.
7. Name six different interventions that can be made that will modify barriers to continence.
8. Compare and contrast the following toileting programs in terms of indications, guidelines for implementation, and limitations:
   a. Routine scheduled toileting
   b. Habit training
   c. Prompted voiding

Functional incontinence can be defined as loss of urine and/or stool caused by factors outside the urinary and/or gastrointestinal tract that interfere with the ability to respond in a socially appropriate way to the urge to void or defecate. The lower urinary tract and bowel produce normal sensations of urge, and the ability to inhibit urge is intact but other factors precipitate the loss of control. Functional incontinence is often associated with cognitive impairment and/or loss of the ability to perform behaviors needed for independent toileting. The end result is the inability to respond to bladder or bowel urge, which results in varying degrees of incontinence.

ETIOLOGY OF FUNCTIONAL INCONTINENCE

To maintain continence, there must be intact sensory and motor function of the urinary tract and bowel as well as the ability and desire to respond appropriately to urge. The central nervous system must process stimuli effectively so that the individual can recognize the sensation of urge, determine the appropriate response, and carry out the sequence of psychomotor activities necessary for controlled voiding or defecation. The individual must be motivated to maintain continence and must be able to use a toilet or a toilet alternative such as a urinal or bedpan. Mobility and coordination must be such that the sequence of gross and fine motor skills required for toileting can be executed. Finally, the environment must provide cues and toileting facilities that support continence. In summary, an individual is at risk for functional incontinence if he or she has cognitive impairment, diminished motivation, a loss of mobility and/or coordination, and/or environmental barriers to toileting. Box 6-1 lists patients at risk for functional incontinence.

Frail older adults, adults with multisystem and multidimensional impairments,[1] and adults who are developmentally disabled have a greater risk for the development of functional incontinence resulting from physical and/or cognitive impairments.[2] Some changes in bladder function associated with aging also contribute to increased risk in this population. These changes are highlighted in Table 6-1; those of greatest significance to the development of

167

BOX 6-1 Individuals at Risk for Developing Functional Incontinence

Cognitive Impairment
Dementias (Alzheimer's disease)
Delirium
Cerebrovascular accident or transient ischemic attacks
Huntington's disease

Motivational Issues
Depression
Bipolar disease
Schizophrenia
Psychosis

Compromised Mobility/Coordination/Manual Dexterity
Rheumatoid arthritis
Stroke
Parkinson's disease
Multiple sclerosis
Musculoskeletal trauma
Osteoarthritis
Acute and chronic pain syndromes
Weakness, deconditioning

Environmental Factors
Inaccessible toilet facilities
Toilet seats that are too low
Clothing that is difficult to remove
Limited privacy
Crowded toileting facilities
Use of incontinence containment products
Use of restraints
Caregiver issues and education

TABLE 6-1 Normal Changes That Occur in the Genitourinary System with Aging

Bladder capacity	Decreased
	Decreased ability to delay voiding
Residual urine	Increased
Bladder contractility	Increased involuntary detrusor contractions
	Increased risk for urge incontinence
Female urogenital tissues	Thinning of vascular cushion
	Reduced coaptation of urethal mucosa
	Reduced mucus production
	Increased risk for urinary tract infection
	Increased risk for stress and urge incontinence
Urine production	Increased urine production at night
Prostate	Enlarged
	Increased risk for urinary outlet obstruction

functional *urinary* incontinence (UI) include the following:

1. In the older adult, there is a decrease in bladder size and an increase in postvoid residual urine. These normal changes reduce functional bladder capacity and cause an increase in voiding frequency. In the presence of impaired mobility, increased voiding frequency can increase the risk of incontinence because the individual may not be able to reach the toilet in time.

2. Older adults can also experience increased urine production at night (that is, nocturnal polyuria);

this is usually a normal finding but can also be symptomatic of disease such as renal failure, hypercalcemia, or diabetes.[3,4] Frequent nighttime urination contributes to functional UI when an older adult has difficulty getting out of bed or takes excessive time to do so.

3. Older adults can also experience increased frequency of uninhibited bladder contractions, which produce urinary urgency and frequency.[5,6] When these "normal" changes are compounded by impaired cognition or reduced mobility, the end result is a complex UI that can be difficult to diagnose as well as treat.

Cognitive Impairment

Cognitive impairment is a common cause of functional incontinence and has been identified along with immobility as a critical contributing factor in the development of incontinence in nursing home residents.[2,7-9] Intact cognitive function is crucial to the effective execution of the series of behaviors required for maintenance of continence. The individual must be able to recognize the sensation of urge, determine the appropriate response, locate a bathroom or socially acceptable substitute, remove clothing, perform personal hygiene, and flush the toilet or empty the waste receptacle. Cognitive impairment can limit the individual's ability to activate this complex sequence of behaviors.

The origin of cognitive impairment ranges from the acute impairment caused by traumatic brain injury to the gradual steady decline in cognition that characterizes most dementias. Cognitive skills guide interaction with one's environment, and when compromised, the individual will experience some degree of loss in the ability to perform self-care and to cope with the environment in a socially acceptable manner. Alzheimer's disease is the most common form of dementia among people 65 years old and and older, with prevalence doubling every 5 years beyond the age of 65.[10] Dementia always causes loss of memory plus one or more additional mental impairments that include the following:

- Loss of use of words (aphasia)
- Loss of seeing things as they are (perceptual confusion)
- Loss of ability to recognize things (agnosia)
- Loss of movement coordination (apraxia)
- Loss of the ability to perform sequential tasks (executive dysfunction), as described earlier

These mental impairments or cognitive deficits are listed in Table 6-2, with examples of how

TABLE 6-2   Cognitive Deficits and Incontinence

COGNITIVE DEFICIT	EFFECT ON CONTINENCE
Learning and information retention deficit Memory loss	Difficulty learning how to remove and apply continence containment products Difficulty adjusting to a new environment and learning the location and use of the bathroom Poor attention and concentration No memory of culturally mandated guidelines for appropriate urination
Agnosia (unable to recognize or identify objects)	Inability to recognize a toilet or urinal (thus will not use it for voiding)
Apraxia (loss of movement or coordination of hands, arms, legs or mouth)	Inability to manage clothing during toileting Difficult gait and ambulation
Executive function deficit	Difficulty following multistep instructions Inability to sequence the steps required to use a toilet
Reasoning deficit	Inability to solve problems such as what to do with a wet containment product or how to flush a toilet Problems with responding appropriately to the urge to void (may void in a trashcan or corner instead of a toilet)
Perceptual confusion (spatial sense and orientation)	Inability to find the bathroom Inability to locate supplies needed for hygiene when in the bathroom
Aphasia (loss of words)	Inability to communicate the need to use a toilet Calling the bathroom by other names
Personality and mood changes	Apathy: loss of interest in being continent Aggressiveness with caregivers during toileting Anxiety that can be exacerbated when toileted

each deficit affects continence. It is important to understand that cognitive impairment is a complex problem that requires careful assessment to identify the area(s) and degree of impairment as well as the areas of residual ability that can be supported.

Motivation

Functional incontinence can be caused in total or in part by lack of motivation to maintain continence. As discussed earlier, continence requires a complex series of psychomotor skills that may demand an exceptional exertion of effort. A diagnosis of depression may result in impaired physical, mental, and social functioning, which can affect the desire and ability to be continent,[11] and studies have shown that incontinence has a negative impact on psychologic health.[12-14] Thus, a vicious cycle can be created, in which depression causes or contributes to incontinence, which then exacerbates the depression. Health care providers often underdiagnose and undertreat depression in older adults because the older adult does not manifest typical symptoms such as depressed mood; instead, depression in the elderly may be manifest by symptoms such as social withdrawal, isolation, and decline in activities of daily living, which can include toileting and self-care activities.[15,16] Fortunately, both incontinence and depression are usually treatable, and studies indicate that treatment of incontinence results in an improved sense of psychologic well-being.[12-14]

There are situations when incontinence may be a conscious choice because the physical effort required to use the toilet is valued as being too burdensome. Persons with acute or chronic pain, weakness and fatigue, or debilitating dyspnea may be incontinent until their pain and/or energy levels are manageable enough to permit toileting. Frail older adults may also forego continence because of the effort required to be continent. Some may fear toileting because of a recent fall or injury and out of this fear will refuse to use the toilet until they feel secure in their ability to transfer to the toilet safely. The clinician must intervene to modify factors that contribute to poor motivation (such as fear or fatigue) while respecting the autonomous wishes of the individual.

Compromised Mobility or Manual Dexterity

Functional incontinence can be caused by any factor that interferes with the ability to perform the sequence of fine and gross motor skills required for independent toileting. The culturally mandated response to a full bladder involves moving to an appropriate toileting facility and executing a number of fine motor skills such as clothing removal and personal hygiene. Any compromise in mobility or manual dexterity can result in the inability to respond to a full bladder or rectum "fast enough" to prevent incontinence. Musculoskeletal trauma, joint contractures, and deconditioning have the potential to cause incontinence because they affect the mobility and motor skills necessary for independent toileting. A common example of this type of functional incontinence occurs in the older adult following hip or shoulder fracture. Hip fracture interferes with independent ambulation to a toilet, and a fracture of the shoulder interferes with some of the motor skills needed for clothing management and personal hygiene. Individuals with preexisting "stress" UI, "urge" UI, or fecal urgency may experience a significant increase in their incontinence after musculoskeletal trauma because the ability to quickly reach the bathroom is compromised.

Any condition that interferes with manual dexterity can cause or contribute to functional incontinence. For example, the joint deformities and pain caused by arthritis can interfere with the ability to open bathroom doors, manage clothing, perform hygiene, or flush a toilet. Individuals with neuromuscular diseases or disorders such as multiple sclerosis, Parkinson's disease, spinal cord injury, or cerebrovascular accident are all high risk for incontinence, in part because of the neurologic impairment and in part because of motor skill disabilities that compromise their ability to use the toilet independently. Thus, these patients should be carefully assessed for functional as well as neurologic contributors to their incontinence.

Environmental Factors

Anything that creates a barrier to reaching a toilet or toilet substitute in a timely manner contributes to functional incontinence. This is especially true in patients with impaired cognition, mobility, or manual dexterity. Toileting barriers include elements in the physical environment that interfere with toileting and a care environment where continence is dependent on caregivers.

Continence depends on the ability to reach the appropriate place to void or defecate in a timely manner. Easily accessible toilets or toileting substitutes such as commodes or urinals are essential. Persons who use wheelchairs, crutches, or walkers may have increased difficulty with toilet access because not all bathrooms are "wheelchair or walker accessible." Poorly lit bathrooms and access hallways can act as a barrier for the person with decreased visual acuity. Bathrooms and access hallways may be unsafe because of uneven floors, throw rugs, and wet floors (caused by leaking plumbing or urine); all of these factors can impede independent toileting. Toilet seats that are too low, the absence of grab bars, or bathrooms that are too small to accommodate wheel chair transfers or walkers can create significant barriers for both independent and dependent toileting. Bathrooms that are located at a distance from living areas, bathrooms that require climbing or descending stairs, and bathrooms with pathways blocked by furniture, trash, or equipment all increase the time needed to reach the toilet and can all interfere with independent or assisted toileting. There may also be instances when bathroom accessibility is impeded by crowded conditions and too few toilets for the number of people. This is a well-founded fear of incontinent people when they travel, visit public places, or are in institutions. Individuals who are unable to reach or hold a urinal in a secure manner are also dealing with a barrier to continence. In all these instances, continence is possible if bathrooms and/or equipment are modified to accommodate needs.

An often-overlooked environmental barrier to continence is the inappropriate use of incontinence containment products. Containment products are an essential component of continence management but should not interfere with timely access to toileting. Products that are difficult to remove such as pads with buttons and belts, adult briefs, or external catheters create incontinent episodes because the product cannot be removed quickly enough to use

a toilet, bedpan, or urinal. Individuals with impaired manual dexterity are at higher risk to experience functional incontinence caused by an inability to manage an incontinence containment product independently.

Preventing falls in individuals with impaired mobility and coordination is an important aspect of providing care, and there is some evidence that urinary incontinence and urgency contribute to falls.[16,17] Unfortunately, some of the techniques and products used to prevent falls can contribute to functional incontinence. With good intentions, individuals identified at risk for falls are placed in chairs and beds that are purposely designed to prevent easy rising, such as recliners, chairs with wedges that make it difficult to rise from a sitting position, soft foam removable restraints, and removable tables. Side rails on beds are raised, and bed mattresses are placed on the floor. These measures may decrease falls, but they also impede continence.

Cognitively impaired persons encounter environmental barriers to continence that are linked to their inability to identify appropriate toileting facilities. Depending on the degree and type of impairment, some of these individuals could remain independently continent if bathrooms were clearly labeled and adequately illuminated. Unfortunately, in some situations, cognitively impaired persons have been told by caregivers to use the adult incontinence brief as a toilet, and thus the adult brief has become a psychological barrier to continence. In confused and agitated older adults, medications used to treat agitation become a pharmacologic barrier to continence by causing excessive lethargy and decreasing awareness of urge.

Certain barriers to continence are specific to the environment of care, such as an environment where continence is dependent on caregivers. Nursing staff members in long-term care facilities have been caring for incontinent persons under a burden of limited staffing resources for a long time.[18] Staff in long-term care facilities may be committed to addressing continence, but long-term effectiveness and sustainability are difficult. Specific problems include inadequate numbers of registered nurses skilled in completing the continence assessment and developing a treatment plan, heavy workloads, and an inconsistent assignment of caregiver staff. Thus, residents in long-term care facilities may experience functional incontinence purely because they cannot obtain toileting assistance in a timely manner.[19] In long-term care, programs that promote continence may not succeed because of heavy workloads, high absenteeism, and high staff turnover.[20]

Nursing assistants provide the majority of direct care to incontinent residents, and issues related to nursing assistants can be the greatest barriers to achieving or maintaining continence. Because of heavy workloads, nursing assistants may not be available to respond promptly to toileting requests or schedules. In addition, nursing assistants may be inadequately educated about the causes of incontinence and interventions to prevent incontinence. Lack of understanding about the components and goals of toileting programs may create significant barriers to continence, especially for residents who are cognitively impaired or who have reduced mobility. An effective continence program must therefore include education for the nursing assistants regarding caregiver behaviors that support continence and the importance of a patient-encouraging attitude. A resident may not request help from a nursing assistant who displays impatience or lack of respect during the toileting process.

Barriers to continence are also present in the acute care setting. Because of short staffing and a lack of understanding concerning the causes of incontinence, acute care staff frequently turn to indwelling urinary catheters[22] or containment devices rather than toileting programs, which are vital to the continence of individuals with mobility and/or cognitive impairments. In addition, use of indwelling urinary catheters increases the risk of urinary tract infection, which is a common cause of transient urinary incontinence in the elderly.[21,22] Delirium, an acute, reversible impairment of cognition, is another cause of transient urinary incontinence in older adults and is common in the acute care setting. Older adults admitted to an acute care facility may exhibit new-onset incontinence that is caused by their sudden alteration in mental status. Unfortunately, these individuals are then frequently "labeled" as incontinent. As a result, the staff may fail to provide toileting support even when the

delirium has been resolved; thus, the care environment actually contributes to persistent (chronic) incontinence.

When continence is dependent on a caregiver, the risks for developing functional incontinence increase. In the home, it may be difficult to contract with a caregiver for 24 hour a day care. Dependent individuals who are left home alone can remain continent only if they have the cognition, mobility, and dexterity to toilet independently. In addition, caregivers in the home who fail to understand the importance of timely toileting create a barrier to continence. Cognitively impaired individuals and their home-based caregivers may lack access to health care providers who understand and can facilitate the implementation of a toileting program. Even when such expertise is available, home caregivers may not be motivated or physically able to implement such a labor-intensive program as toileting.

In all settings, the clinician must consider the environment of the patient or resident and include the caregiver (family or nursing assistant) in the development of individual goals and modification of barriers.

ASSESSMENT

The assessment of functional incontinence should include an evaluation of all factors that could influence timely access to a toilet (or toilet substitute) and effective toileting. When the clinician suspects functional incontinence, either alone or in combination with other types of incontinence, the evaluation should include a careful assessment of cognition, other mental impairments, motivation, fear, mobility and coordination, manual dexterity, the living environment, clothing, use of containment products, devices or equipment that restrain independent movement, and the ability, motivation, and education of caregivers to promote and support continence. One of the greatest challenges in assessing functional incontinence is that there is no definitive set of diagnostic tests or presenting symptoms that clearly identifies the problem as "functional incontinence." The diagnosis of functional incontinence is most often presumptive; the individual has some functional impairment, and other causes of incontinence are excluded. The diagnosis can be further complicated when the incontinent individual presents with vague symptoms and a "mixed type" of incontinence is suspected. Initial management includes modifying identified barriers to continence and initiating a toileting program. If there is significant improvement of the incontinence with these modifications, functional incontinence can be presumed. If some improvement occurs but the incontinence continues, the patient should be further evaluated and treated for the coexisting form of incontinence. The assessment for functional factors contributing to incontinence should be an integral part of the assessment of any incontinent individual.

Cognitive Assessment

An evaluation of cognition and function is an essential component in the assessment and treatment of the incontinent person who is cognitively impaired. Numerous mental status exams are available that measure different aspects of cognition including alertness, attention, cooperation, orientation, memory, language, apraxia, logic, and mood. A frequently used test is the Folstein Mini-Mental Status Exam, which includes questions about the following: the year, season, day, and date; memory and math questions; and language questions that assess the ability to understand and follow spoken and written instructions.[23] If a standardized tool is not available, the clinician should be sure to evaluate orientation (person, place, time), memory (short-term and long-term), and the ability to read and follow simple directions. Mental status exams are not perfect measures of memory loss or mental decline. An individual's level of education, native language, hearing or vision problems, psychiatric problems (such as depression), and many other factors may influence the results of these tests.

High-functioning incontinent individuals may be candidates for higher-level interventions that require them to follow written instructions, practice pelvic floor exercises, and keep track of their progress. If an individual has poor short-term memory but can read and follow directions, techniques such as written signs and instructions may be of benefit. This illustrates one benefit of cognitive tests that isolate the specific problems; the results allow the clinician to build on the patient's residual abilities while compensating for those that are lost.

Cognitively impaired individuals may or may not be aware of their incontinence, depending on the level of impairment; in addition, many may deny or be unable to describe their problems in holding urine or stool. This makes it more difficult to accurately evaluate any coexisting forms of incontinence, such as stress UI or urge UI. The clinician must be alert to clues in patients' statements, such as "it always drips," or references to wetness and a need to "rush" to the bathroom. In addition, the clinician should search for clues that indicate the frequency and severity of the incontinence: wet, stained clothing; hidden clothing that is urine or stool stained; stains or wetness on chairs or bed pads; drips or puddles in the bathroom or on the floor leading to the bathroom; urine odor; and the use of paper towels, tissues, and/or more traditional products to contain incontinence. Because it is not unusual for the cognitively impaired individual to deny a problem with continence, an interview with the caregiver is essential to gather appropriate information. The clinician obtaining the health history should ask the caregiver to describe incontinent episodes as completely as possible, including behaviors and events before and after the occurrence of incontinence. A complete description helps to shed light on the origin of the incontinence and is the first step in planning appropriate interventions. Caregivers should be asked about habits or behaviors associated with toileting or incontinence such as restlessness, increased confusion, or aimless wandering. These behaviors could mean that the cognitively impaired individual senses a full bladder or an urge to defecate but has difficulty remembering the appropriate response or the location of the toileting facilities.

Motivation Assessment

When addressing issues of motivation, it is important to identify factors that could interfere with the desire to maintain continence. As discussed earlier in this chapter, depression can play a role in the development of functional incontinence, especially in the older adult. There are quick and easy tools that can be used in the clinical setting to screen for depression, such as the Geriatric Depression Scale [24] and the Cornell Scale for Depression in Dementia.[25] If depression is strongly suspected to be an influencing factor in the incontinence, a referral for treatment should be made in addition to initiation of a toileting program. Other factors that influence the willingness to toilet should also be assessed such as pain, fatigue, ambulatory stability, and the fear of falling. Any factors found to interfere with the individual's motivation to maintain continence must be addressed in the overall management plan; for example, the patient who avoids toileting because of pain should be referred to a pain specialist.

Mobility, Coordination, and Manual Dexterity Assessment

Functional incontinence is frequently associated with conditions that limit independent toileting. The best way to identify these factors is to observe all the behaviors associated with independent toileting. Patients should be observed as they walk to the toilet, remove clothing, perform personal hygiene, and prepare to leave the toileting area. This observation needs to be discrete in order, to preserve dignity. A focused assessment of the neurovascular and musculoskeletal functioning of the upper and lower extremities may be indicated, and positive findings should prompt referral for further evaluation and treatment. Table 6-3 summarizes factors to be included in neurovascular and musculoskeletal assessment. Assessment of balance and gait may also be helpful when identifying barriers to continence. Incontinent individuals with such problems are at high risk for falls and may limit their own mobility because of fear of falling, or independent ambulation may be restricted by well-meaning caregivers, thus creating a barrier to continence.

During toileting, the clinician should observe for other factors that affect effective toileting behaviors. It is not unusual for incontinent adults to layer clothing to maximize warmth and to contain incontinence. These clothing layers can become a barrier to continence because of the time and effort it takes to

TABLE 6-3 Elements of a Focused Assessment

Lower extremities	Hip and leg inspection for equal leg length and hip symmetry: joint deformity, fractures
	Gait: inability or limited ability to bear weight as a result of fractures, joint deformity, neuromuscular disease, deconditioning, or apraxia
	Pulses: diminished or absent, indicating vascular disease
	Pain: vascular disease and joint disease pain that limits mobility and flexibility
	Skin: changes associated with peripheral vascular disease, ulcers, and rashes
	Peripheral edema: caused by cardiovascular disease and limiting mobility because of pain, weakness, trauma
	Active range of motion : diminished by pain, joint deformity, fractures
	Sensation: decreased or absent because of neuropathies, diabetes
	Reflexes: diminished, absent, hyperactive from Parkinson's disease, cerebrovascular accident, other neuromuscular diseases
Feet	Foot and toe deformities : limited ambulation resulting from bunions, corns, hammer toes, Charcot foot, fractures
	Evidence of poorly fitting shoes limiting ambulation
	Pressure ulcers limiting ambulation
Shoulders and arms	Range of motion and strength: compromised by fracture, rotator cuff tear, joint deformity, deconditioning
Hands and wrists	Range of motion: compromised by joint deformity or pain
	Hand grasp strength: weakness caused by joint deformities, neuromuscular diseases
	Fine motor coordination: compromised by joint deformity, pain, neuropathies or apraxia

remove them. Urine containment products should be easy to remove for toileting. Highly absorbent products such as the adult brief tend to be difficult to remove quickly. Individuals with impaired manual dexterity as well as those with shoulder problems may have difficulty with clothing and product removal, which increases their risk of incontinent episodes. The clinician should also observe the toileting of dependent individuals by the caregiver. The caregiver should be observed for safe and appropriate transfer techniques including appropriate use of transfer equipment, the ability to remove and apply containment products and clothing, and the ability to provide adequate hygiene.

Environmental Assessment

Certain factors need to be considered when assessing the environment for barriers to continence. Anything that increases the time and effort required to carry out toileting should be factored into the environmental assessment. The assessment begins with a survey of the living area, whether in the home, hospital or long-term-care facility. Factors to be assessed include the following:

- What is the location of the toilet in relationship to living areas? Is the toilet close enough to allow timely access?
- Are there stairs to navigate that could create a barrier?
- Is the hallway leading to the bathroom well lit?
- In long-term care facilities, are there toilets located near nonresident care areas such as physical therapy rooms, day rooms, or activities areas? Residents in long-term care facilities may not want to participate in activities if no easily accessible toilets are nearby.
- In cramped hospital rooms, are there extra chairs or equipment blocking access to in-room bathrooms?

Assessment of functional incontinence includes an evaluation of bathrooms and toileting equipment. Clinicians should always inspect the bathroom or focus the health history to include questions about the bathroom. Are there any obstacles in the bathroom that could create a barrier? If a wheelchair or walker is needed to access a toilet, is there enough room in the bathroom to accommodate it and allow safe transfer to the toilet? Is the toilet seat at a height that is comfortable? Are there grab bars? In the presence of diminished visual acuity and/or cognitive impairment, is the bathroom clearly lit and marked? How many people use the same bathroom, and are there times when a queue forms to use this bathroom? If a bedside commode is used, is it located in a private place and is it sturdy enough to support the weight of the patient? Can the urinal be easily reached and held securely? Often, simple and relatively inexpensive environmental modifications can be made to support continence, such as providing a urinal to individuals with mobility problems or removing throw rugs or small pieces of furniture to facilitate access to the bathroom. Box 6-2 provides a sample guide for assessment of the home environment.

BOX 6-2 Guidelines for Conducting a Home Assessment

General

Firm, supportive furniture?
Edges of carpet tacked down?
Firm, supportive shoes or slippers with nonskid soles?
Low-lying furniture in walking areas?
Extension cords or telephone cords in walking areas?
Highly polished floors?
Throw (scatter) rugs or rugs and runners that tend to slide?

Bathroom

Good lighting in hallways and bathroom?
Night light near entrance to bathroom?
Grab bar by toilet?
Raised toilet seat?
Portable commode that is stable?

Stairs (if applicable)

Light switch at top and bottom?
Nonskid treads over steps or carpet attached to steps?
Handrails from top to bottom?
Objects on steps?

The Long-Term Care Challenge

Dependent individuals living in a long-term care facility are in an environment that can be challenging in terms of barriers to continence. As discussed earlier in this chapter, long-term care facilities have long been providing continence care in an environment of limited resources; yet it must be acknowledged that not all long-term care facilities have the same issues with staff turnover, inconsistent staff assignments, limited registered nurse staff, ineffective communication, and other issues. When evaluating functional incontinence in this environment, it is vital that the clinician fully evaluate all aspects of the environment for functional barriers. Many of the issues are the same as discussed previously and can be resolved on an individual basis. Special emphasis should be placed on finding out what programs are in place in the facility to support continence and evaluating their effectiveness. The clinician should evaluate how well the long-term care facility staff understands the causes of functional incontinence, how consistent staff members are in responding promptly to the needs of incontinent residents, and whether or not the facility truly supports continence care as a component of total quality care. Mueller and Cain[26] identified eight factors that can be evaluated as part of a continence quality improvement program in long-term care. These eight factors are evidence-based practice, timely and appropriate assessment, attention to environmental barriers, education, staffing, communication/documentation concerning residents' continence status, staff involvement, and evaluation/feedback regarding program effectiveness. One should not assume that a continence program is not possible because a facility has some resource issues; many times these issues can be overcome. Box 6-3 lists some of the elements that should be addressed when evaluating the effectiveness of a continence program in a long-term care facility.

MANAGEMENT OPTIONS

The major goals of treatment are to improve and to maintain continence by overcoming continence barriers and/or increasing access to a toilet or toilet substitute. Management strategies can be categorized into two major areas: (1) modification of barriers to

---

BOX 6-3   Assessment of a Continence Program in Long-Term Care

Administrative policies and procedures that support continence care
Timely evaluation of incontinence
Easily accessible toileting facilities
Staff education concerning causes and primary treatment of incontinence
Adequate staff to implement a toileting program
Involvement of staff in evaluation of continence outcomes
Adequate documentation of continence program including assessment and progress

---

continence and (2) toileting programs. In developing a management plan, the clinician must remember that there are times when the incontinent patient and/or caregivers may choose not to initiate treatment because the burden of treatment far exceeds the burden of the incontinence. It is imperative in these situations (and in fact in all situations) that the ultimate management plan reflect collaboration between the patient/caregiver and the clinician. In some cases, the most appropriate goal for treatment may be achievement of social continence via use of an appropriate containment product.

Modification of Barriers to Continence. An important component of any treatment plan for functional incontinence is the identification of barriers to continence and implementation of measures to maximize access to a toilet or toilet substitute. Table 6-4 highlights specific interventions.

Adequate Fluid Intake. A common response to urinary incontinence is to restrict fluids in an attempt to decrease the incontinence. Even if there is no intentional fluid restriction, caregivers may fail to offer fluids on a regular basis. As discussed in previous chapters, fluid restriction or inadequate fluid intake can cause increased urinary urgency and increased risk of UI. Fluid intake should be sufficient to produce pale yellow urine. Regular spacing of fluids is another important consideration. Excessive fluid intake or ingestion of large

TABLE 6-4   **Modification of Barriers to Continence**

BARRIER TO CONTINENCE	INTERVENTIONS
Immobility	Physical therapy consultation for transfer techniques, transfer aids, muscle strengthening, joint rehabilitation, gait training (Meadows, 2000)
	Appropriate assistive devices such as canes, walkers, wheelchairs, grab bars, transfer boards
	Shoes: supportive, well-fitted with nonskid soles
	Caregiver training: safe transfer techniques, use of transfer equipment such as transfer disks, transfer belts
	Use of bedside commodes, urinals
	Raised toilet seats
	Provision of access to bathroom or commode on same level as living area
	Maintenance bed at a height where feet are flat on the floor when the patient is sitting on the side
	Provision of chair cushions that are firm, chairs with arms to assist with safe standing
	Avoidance of recliners that are difficult to reposition for standing
	Avoidance of cushions or pillows that restrict easy movement out of chairs and beds
	Avoidance of restraints
Impaired manual dexterity	Physical and occupational therapy consultation
	Clothing modifications: stretch waist bands, loose fitting clothing, use of "Velcro"-type closures
	Avoidance clothing with buttons, zippers, hooks and eyes, tight or ill-fitting clothing, multilayered clothing
	Replacement bathroom door knobs with lever type handles
	Use of pull-up containment products or inserts/pads that can be easily applied and removed
	Use of perineal wipes for personal hygiene
Poor visual acuity	Adequate lighting in bathrooms and areas leading to bathrooms
	Motion-detection lighting in bathrooms
	Night lights
	Clear access to the bathroom (elimination of trash, equipment, furniture, or any other items that could impede access)
Pain	Consultation for adequate pain management
Poor motivation	Consultation for the management of depression
	Consultation for the management of fatigue, dyspnea, pain
	Positive reinforcement of desired behaviors

volumes in one sitting can also contribute to incontinence. Day-to-day distribution of fluid intake needs to be somewhat consistent because a steady pattern of fluid intake will produce a consistent pattern of urine elimination, which is critical to the success of any toileting program. To encourage appropriate fluid intake, the clinician should include in the management program a prescription for fluid intake; the prescription should specify the type and volume of fluid to be taken as well as the approximate time. The prescription should be individualized for the patient and should address his or her fluid preferences, lifestyle, and any concurrent medical conditions. For example, the fluid prescription for an individual with nocturnal polyuria would include a recommendation for decreased fluid intake in the late afternoon and evening. An effective strategy to increase compliance with the fluid prescription is to write the fluid intake prescription on the voiding diary and have the patient or caregiver record the time and amount of actual fluid intake (Fig. 6-1).

Scheduled Toileting Programs. Toileting programs have been shown to be an effective treatment strategy for functional incontinence. Scheduled toileting programs involve reminding and/or assisting the individual with functional incontinence to use the toilet, urinal, or bedpan at prescheduled times. These programs can be implemented on a fixed schedule or can be individualized based on the patient's own voiding patterns and ability to participate. *All toileting programs involve caregiver support to maintain some degree of continence.* Optimally, the goal of a toileting program is complete continence, but this may not be achievable 100% of the time because of caregiver limitations (such as high staff/resident ratios in long-term care facilities or caregiver exhaustion in a home care situation) or inconsistent compliance with toileting by cognitively impaired individuals. Inherent in the process of developing and implementing toileting programs is the assumption that other barriers to continence (as discussed earlier in the chapter) have been addressed and appropriate interventions implemented.

The environment of care can be a significant barrier to successful implementation of any toileting program, especially in the long-term care setting. Toileting programs have been shown to be effective but are frequently difficult to maintain,[19,27] and inadequate staffing serves to compound the problem and to adversely affect overall quality of care.[20,28-30] To improve chances of successful implementation, candidates for any type of toileting program should meet the following criteria: have sufficient mobility to enable safe transfer to a toilet, respond to cues sufficiently that they void somewhat consistently when toileted, and cooperate with staff efforts to toilet (at least most of the time). Residents being managed with a toileting program should be reevaluated after 1 month to determine whether they have maintained or improved continence. Program evaluation must be ongoing and progress must be documented on a monthly basis.

Time of day	Voided in toilet	Incontinent urine	Incontinent bowels	Changed pad or clothing	Fluid intake	
					Type	Amount

Fig. 6-1 Sample voiding record.

A plan of care must be developed with goals that are attainable and easily measurable, such as fewer incontinent episodes or improved skin condition (Fig. 6-2). In the long-term care environment, any type of scheduled toileting program is accounted for on the Minimum Data Set (MDS), [31] and these data are compiled by Centers for Medicare and Medicaid Services (CMS) into a monthly report called the *Quality Indicator*. The Quality Indicator report is available to the public and is also used by

---

Nursing Diagnosis: Functional Urinary Incontinence Related To:
- ☐ Imparied physical mobility
- ☐ Access to the toilet
- ☐ Impaired manual dexterity
- ☐ Altered cognition
- ☐ Other_____

Short Term Goals
- ☐ Will be wet only_____ times during waking hours through_____.
- ☐ Will experience no urinary leakage during the day through_____.
- ☐ Will show no complications of urinary incontinence such as urinary tract infection, skin breakdown, and falls, through_____.
- ☐ Will void in the toilet 50% of the time during waking hours through_____.

Plan of Approach
- ☐ Maintain bladder record.
- ☐ Avoid caffeinated beverages (coffee, tea, soda).
- ☐ Give_____ oz of fluids at_____.
- ☐ Manitain bowel record. Monitor for constipation, i.e., no BM in 2 to 3 days, abdominal bloating, abdominal discomfort, change in appetite, passage of small, hard stool, straining for BM.
- ☐ Monitor for skin breakdown daily.
- ☐ Apply moisture barrier product to_____.
- ☐ Monitor for signs and symptoms of UTI, i.e., elevated temperature (may not appear), abdominal pain, change in continence status, pain, foul urine, odor, frequency, change in mental status.
- ☐ Toileting plan (circle appropriate intervention).
  Offer: Urinal   Bedpan   Toilet   Bedside commode
  Remind resident to go to the toilet.
  Take resident to the toilet.
  Praise resident upon successful toileting.
  Scheduled times for toileting:

Upon arising	Before breakfast	After breakfast
Before lunch	After lunch	After nap
Before dinner	After dinner	Before bed
Upon request		

Take to toilet if restless, agitated, wanders, yells, picks at clothing, starts removing clothing.
- ☐ Provide containment product.
  Daytime product_____
  Nighttime product_____
- ☐ Toilet transfers: Use_____ (transfer disk, pivot turn, walker).
- ☐ Modify clothing: Elastic waist pants, avoid tight clothing, no buttons, zippers, hooks, or snaps.
- ☐ Notify continence specialist for any changes in continence status, i.e., increased incontinent episodes.

Fig. 6-2 Standardized care plan for long-term care.

the state Health Departments when evaluating a facility for annual licensure.[32] Thus, a successfully implemented and documented scheduled toileting program in long-term care is not only a first-line treatment for functional incontinence; it is also part of a facility's regulatory responsibility and a potential source of revenue.

Three commonly used scheduled toileting programs can be successfully implemented in home care and institutional settings: routine scheduled toileting, habit training, and prompted voiding.

Routine scheduled toileting. Routine scheduled toileting programs provide toileting assistance on a consistent, fixed schedule. These programs are called by many different names: timed voiding,[33] routine toileting, toilet training, habit voiding, and scheduled toileting. Terminology is often unclear in the literature, which makes it easy to confuse the various types of scheduled toileting. To be consistent with the definition used by the Minimum Data Set (MDS)[31] and to distinguish it from habit training and prompted voiding, routine scheduled toileting is the term used to describe a toileting program with a fixed schedule of assisted toileting; with routine scheduled toileting, there is no attempt to individualize the schedule to conform to normal voiding patterns and there is no attempt made to motivate the individual to remain continent. In a routine scheduled toileting program, incontinent individuals are assisted to the bathroom on a fixed, predetermined schedule, which is most often based on a routine such as every 2 to 4 hours or a schedule that is determined by the general routines of a long-term care facility such as on waking, before and after meals, and before bed. Continuation of the schedule during hours of sleep is a decision based on individual need and preferences. There is some evidence that toileting programs are not effective when continued through the night.[34] Toileting schedules can be designed to maximize sleep by identifying times when the patient normally awakens and toileting at those times.

The most appropriate candidate for routine scheduled toileting is the cognitively impaired person who is unable to identify or communicate the need to void and/or defecate or an individual who lacks the motivation to maintain independent continence but who is cooperative with toileting. In some instances, routine scheduled toileting is an appropriate treatment regimen for the cognitively intact person. A toileting routine can be designed in which a person is asked about the need to use the toilet or is taken to the toilet because he or she cannot easily communicate the need and/or independently perform all the required toileting behaviors. These individuals may be able to delay the urge to void until the scheduled time, thus creating a successful program for their functional incontinence. Routine scheduled toileting programs are used extensively in long-term care, where the goals are to reduce incontinent episodes, decrease the cost of incontinence reflected in laundry and containment products, improve quality of life, and increase social interaction.[35] Routine scheduled toileting programs are also used in the home setting for many of the same reasons.

Habit training. Habit training[36] is a scheduled toileting program based on the premise that the incontinent person will experience fewer incontinent episodes if they have timely access to a toileting facility when their bladder is full. A similar program is known as "patterned urge response training," or PURT.[37,38] The toileting schedule is designed based on the individual's usual voiding patterns.[35,39-41] Individuals who have the best potential for improvement with this type of scheduled toileting are those with moderate cognitive impairment who are cooperative with toileting.[42] Before initiating the program, caregivers should complete a modified voiding diary by toileting and/or checking the individual every 1 to 2 hours and recording whether he or she voided, was found wet, or was found dry. Data should be recorded for a minimum of 3 days and then analyzed for repeating patterns of voiding. A toileting schedule is then designed to prevent incontinence by toileting immediately before the usual voiding time as identified by the voiding diary. An alternative approach is to measure bladder volumes every 2 to 3 hours using a portable ultrasound to predict times of bladder fullness or to use an electronic device that records the times of incontinent episodes.

The initial "schedule" must be a considered a work in progress. Incontinent episodes should be tracked, and the schedule should then be modified to minimize such episodes. For example, if the toileted person is found to be wet at a scheduled toileting time (such as 10:00 AM), the schedule is adjusted to require earlier toileting (such as 9:00 AM). Adjustments in the schedule are made on an ongoing basis until an effective schedule is established. It may take a few weeks or several months to develop the most effective schedule. Caregivers should be counseled that a habit-training program takes time and may require multiple revisions of the schedule.

Management of fluid intake is also a part of habit training. The clinician should emphasize the importance of drinking all fluids as prescribed, and the caregiver must strongly encourage the cognitively impaired individual to drink all fluids offered. Fluid intake patterns should be regulated and stabilized, as described earlier in this chapter, to establish and maintain stable voiding patterns. Fig. 6-1 provides a sample form that can be used to monitor the efficacy of the toileting program as well as the adequacy of fluid intake. Toileting times can be highlighted to remind caregivers of the established schedule.

The habit training program may need further individualization when treating concurrent stress or urge-pattern UI. For example, caregivers should be taught to transfer wheelchair-bound patients with concurrent stress incontinence to the toilet as quickly as possible, to minimize time in the standing position. Similarly, caregivers for patients with concurrent urge incontinence can be taught to complete clothing manipulation (such as unbuttoning or unzipping) before taking the patient into the bathroom, where toileting cues will stimulate detrusor contractions.

The final component needed to maximize success with a habit training toileting program is adequate education and training of any caregivers taking part in the program. Box 6-4 lists essential components of an educational program for nursing assistants, home health aides and other caregivers taking part in a habit training scheduled toileting program.

Prompted voiding. Prompted voiding is a type of scheduled toileting used for individuals whose cognitive impairment is severe enough to cause

---

BOX 6-4   Toileting Programs: Caregiver Education

Risk factors for functional incontinence
 Loss of independent mobility
 Impaired manual dexterity
 Motivational issues
 Cognitive impairment
 Dementia versus delerium
 Discussion that incontinence is a treatable problem
Basic function of the bladder and bowel
Components of the continued assessment
Components of the program
 Toileting schedule: emphasis on importance of maintaining the schedule
 Fluid prescription
 Transfer techniques
 Special instructions
 Maintenance of bowel regularity
Completion of the bladder record
When to call for reevaluation of the program
 Decreased effectiveness: sudden or gradual

---

incontinence but who retain the ability to respond to simple directions and to recognize the urge to void. The goals of the program are to increase the individual's ability to respond appropriately to the urge to void, to increase self-initiated toileting, and thus to improve continence.[35,43,44] Patients with severe cognitive impairment or the inability to safely transfer to a toilet with the assistance of one person are not candidates for prompted voiding programs, nor are individuals who are not cooperative with toileting and other activities of daily living. The best candidates for prompted voiding programs are described in Box 6-5, although the best predictor of program success is a successful 3-day therapeutic trial of the program.

There are two components of a prompted voiding program, one focused on the patient and the other focused on the caregiver. The primary goal is to modify behavior and to help patients "relearn" the appropriate response to a full bladder. Caregivers learn a new approach to incontinence that involves monitoring, prompting, and praising.[36,44] Prompted voiding involves retraining the cognitively impaired individual to recognize and appropriately respond

BOX 6-5   Best Candidates for a Prompted Voiding Program

Mild to moderate cognitive impairment:
Able to recognize his or her name and common elements in the environment
Able to follow one- to two-step instructions
Able to recognize the need to void
Able to inhibit the urge to void
Able to communicate accurately the need to void
When toileted, voids at least 50% of the time
Able to transfer to a toilet with the assistance of one person
Cooperative with toileting and other activities of daily living

Data from references 34, 40, and 44.

BOX 6-6   Steps of Prompted Voiding Scheduled Toileting

1. Approach the patient at a prescheduled time.
2. Ask if the patient is wet or dry.
3. Check to verify wetness or dryness.
4. Ask the patient if he or she needs to void.
5. Take to the toilet if the answer is yes.
6. Praise if dry and/or cooperative with toileting.
7. If the patient is wet, change clothing, provide only minimal feedback other than to tell the patient that he or she is wet.
8. Inform the patient of the next toileting time
9. Encourage the patient to hold urine until the next toileting or to ask for toileting assistance.
10. Record the results on the bladder record.

From Lyons SS, Pringle Specht K: Prompted voiding protocol for individuals with urinary incontinence, *J Gerontol Nurs* 26(6):5-12, 2000.

to the urge to void. The first step in planning a prompted voiding schedule is to identify the normal voiding pattern, as described in the section on habit training. Individualizing the schedule to the patient's voiding pattern improves program success. Once a voiding pattern has been identified, the prompted voiding behavioral modification can begin. At the prescheduled times, the caregiver will approach the patient, ask whether he or she is wet or dry, check to ascertain wetness or dryness, then ask the patient whether he or she needs to void (regardless of "wet" versus "dry" status). Patients who give a negative response to questioning concerning their need to void should not be forced but gently encouraged.[43] Patients found dry and/or who use the toilet are praised. Patients found wet are changed, but minimal feedback is given other than to tell them that they are wet. Patients are told the time of the next toileting and are encouraged to hold urine until the next toileting or to ask for toileting assistance. The procedure for prompted voiding is summarized in Box 6-6.

A critical component of the program is the approach of the caregiver. By modifying the behavior of the caregiver, patients can develop a greater awareness and more appropriate response to the urge to void, and they can also receive increased positive interaction with the caregiver. Caregivers need to monitor patients for wetness and dryness on a regular schedule, prompt the patient to void, and praise them for dryness and any attempts to use the toilet. Desired behavior is reinforced with praise and positive interpersonal interaction with the caregiver. Undesired behavior, namely incontinence, is not reinforced. The patient is changed, cleaned, and informed of the wetness and the next prompting time with minimal socialization. Caregivers need to be very consistent in their adherence to the program and especially with prompting at the designated times.[35,44] In the institutional setting, a prompted voiding program requires a staff trained in its implementation and educated regarding the importance of adherence to the designated schedule; documentation of training and consistent monitoring and follow-up also contribute to success of the program.[44,45]

Prompted voiding is the most thoroughly studied of the three scheduled toileting programs described in this chapter. A growing body of research shows that prompted voiding is a successful behavioral treatment modality for individuals with moderate cognitive impairment in both institutional settings and in the home.[46] Studies of nursing home residents placed on a prompted voiding protocol have shown significant decreases in frequency of incontinence.[45,47-49] There are a few studies of homebound older adults with cognitive impairment that have also demonstrated clinically significant improvements in incontinence among individuals treated with a prompted voiding program.[43,50] In a small study of cognitively impaired adults in the home, Engberg and associates[43] found a mean 60% reduction in daytime incontinence for subjects in a prompted voiding protocol as compared with only a 37% reduction for those in the control group.

Modifying Barriers to Continence in Long-Term Care

Functional incontinence in institutional settings is caused by a complex combination of factors, some of which are directly linked to the culture of the institution. In long-term care, 46% to 56% of the residents are incontinent;[51] thus modification of the environment of care to support continence is a clinical and regulatory imperative. A continence program needs administrative commitment to improving and/or maintaining continence through resource allocation and program support. The continence clinician can help in writing a philosophy of continence care that integrates an understanding that incontinence can be treated and is not an inevitable consequence of aging and/or disability. A continence management program requires the support of the nursing home/assisted living/ hospital administrators, nursing and medical administration, and primary care providers. Continence-related policies, procedures, and clinical standards of care should become a part of everyday practice for the bedside caregivers. Procedures and standards for continence assessment and treatment should be written and easy to implement. In the long-term care environment, there should be detailed policies and procedures for continence evaluation, scheduled toileting, prompted toileting, routine bowel management, and removal of urinary catheters, as well as a plan for quality improvement.

If an outside continence consultant is assisting an institution in continence care, it is vital that the continence program as a whole belongs to the staff and the facility, not the continence consultant. It is helpful to designate a "continence champion" in the institution who can function as a key contact for all

consulting specialists and ensure that program initiatives are implemented. The optimal continence champion should be a nurse who has a commitment to continence care and a desire to gain a working knowledge of basic continence care such as skin care, containment products, behavioral management, bowel management, diet and fluid modifications, and medications. When planning continence treatment plans in the long-term care environment, the continence consultant should use a collaborative decision making model. Such a model will improve communication of and compliance with the treatment plans. Wagner and Colling[52] found that nursing assistants did not believe that they had input into the policies that affected their work, and this perception negatively influenced their compliance. Clearly, the bedside caregivers should be involved in all levels of decision making, from administrative policies to designing a plan of care for individual residents. Often the bedside caregiver has valuable insights into system-wide practice issues as well as the day-to-day care of residents. In long-term care, the interdisciplinary team that gathers to discuss resident problems and care as part of the MDS process is another valuable resource for planning and implementing care.[53]

With high staff turnover and inconsistency in staff assignments because of staffing shortages, nursing staff members in all care environments need frequent education about incontinence and its management.[19] Information about continence evaluation and management should be included as part of new employee orientation and should be repeated periodically. Information should be presented creatively, such as via flyers, newsletters, contests, walking rounds with staff to review resident status, or mini in-services; the goal is to eliminate some of the institutional barriers to continence care linked to knowledge deficits and ingrained attitudes about functional components of incontinence.

SUMMARY

Functional incontinence is directly linked to any factor that interferes with the ability to respond in a socially appropriate way to the urge to void or defecate. The first step in effective treatment is to identify barriers to toileting. Barriers to continence include cognitive impairment, lack of motivation to be continent, compromised mobility and/or manual dexterity, and factors in the living environment, whether home or an institution. Comprehensive assessment of any incontinent individual should include evaluation of factors known to contribute to functional incontinence. Primary management strategies include environmental adaptations, fluid management, and toileting programs. In the long-term care setting, effective management of functional incontinence is dependent in large part on administrative support, adequate staffing, staff education, and staff involvement in decision making.

SELF-ASSESSMENT EXERCISE

1. Define the term "functional incontinence."
2. Discuss how each factor listed below can contribute to functional incontinence.
   a. Impaired cognition
   b. Poor motivation
   c. Immobility
   d. Impaired manual dexterity
3. Explain how institutionalization such as admission to a nursing home or hospital can contribute to the development of functional incontinence.
4. Describe changes associated with normal aging that increase the risk for functional incontinence.
5. Discuss the importance of completing a cognitive evaluation before instituting a toileting program.
6. Identify the major elements of an assessment of functional incontinence that should be integrated into a comprehensive continence assessment.
7. Give an example of five different environmental modifications that can be implemented to treat functional incontinence.
8. Compare the following toileting programs including indications, implementation, and limitations:
   a. Routine scheduled toileting
   b. Habit training
   c. Prompted voiding

REFERENCES

1. Bortz WH II: A conceptual framework of frailty: a review, *J Gerontol Med Sci* 57A(5):M283-M288, 2002.
2. Chaing L, Ouslander J, Schnelle J, Reuben DB: Dually incontinent nursing home residents: clinical characteristics and treatment differences, *J Am Geriatr Soc* 48:673-676, 2000.
3. Colling JC, Owen TR, McCreedy MR: Urine volumes and voidings among incontinent nursing home residents, *Geriatr Nurs* 15:188-192, 1994.
4. Reynard J: Fluid balance therapy of nocturia in women, *Intern Urogynecol J Pelvic Floor Dysfunct* 10(1):43-48, 1999.
5. Albaugh J: Urinary dysfunction and urodynamics in the elderly, *Urol Nurs* 23(2):136-140, 2003.
6. Resnick NM: Geriatric incontinence, *Urol Clin North Am* 23(1):55-71, 1996.
7. Jirovec MM, Wells TJ: Urinary incontinence in nursing home residents with dementia: the mobility-cognition paradigm, *Appl Nurs Res* 3:112-117, 1990.
8. Schnelle JF, Leung FW: Urinary and fecal incontinence in nursing homes, *Gastroenterology* 126(1 suppl 1):S41-S47, 2004.
9. Skelly J, Flint AJ: Urinary incontinence associated with dementia, *J Am Geriatr Soc* 43:286-295, 1995.
10. National Institute on Aging: *2001-2002 Progress report on Alzheimer's disease*, NIH Pub No. 03-5333, Bethesda, Md., 2003, National Institutes of Health, US Department of Health and Human Services.
11. Dugan E, Cohen SJ, Bland DR, et al: The association of depressive symptoms and urinary incontinence among older adults, *J Am Geriatr Soc* 48:413-416, 2000.
12. Burgio KL, Locher JL, Roth DL, Goode PS: Psychological improvements associated with behavioral and drug treatment of urge incontinence in older women, *J Gerontol B Psychol Sci Soc Sci* 56(1):P46-P51, 2001.
13. Bogner HR, Gallo JJ, Sammel MD, et al: Urinary incontinence and psychological distress in community-dwelling older adults, *J Am Geriatr Soc* 50(3):489-495, 2002.
14. Heidrich SM, Wells TJ: Effects of urinary incontinence: psychological well-being and distress in older community-dwelling women, *J Gerontol Nurs* 30(5): 47-54, 2004.
15. Faison WE, Steffens DC: Prevalence and treatment of depression in the elderly, *Clin Geriatr* 9(11):46-52, 2001.
16. Tinetti M, Inouye S, Gill T, Douchette J: Shared risk factors for falls, incontinence and functional dependency, *J Am Geriatr Soc* 273:1348-1353, 1995.
17. Brown JS, Vittinghoff E, Wyman JF, et al: Urinary incontinence: does it increase risk for falls and fractures? *J Am Geriatr Soc* 48(7):721-725, 2000.
18. US Centers for Medicare and Medicaid Services: *Appropriateness of minimum nurse staffing ratios in nursing homes: phase II final report*, Cambridge, Mass., 2001, Abt associates. Retrieved 2/1/04 from: http://cms.hhs.gov/Medicaid/reports/rp1201-8.asp
19. Harke JM, Richgels K: Barriers to implementing a continence program in nursing homes, *Clin Nurs Res* 1: 158-168, 1992.

20. Lekan-Rutledge D, Palmer MH, Belyea M: In their own words: nursing assistants' perceptions of barriers to implementation of prompted voiding in long-term care, *Gerontologist* 38:370-378, 1998.

21. Maki DG, Tambyah PA: Engineering out the risk of infection with urinary catheters, *Emerg Infect Dis* 7(2): 1-6, 2001.

22. Wilde MH: Urinary catheter management for the older adult, *Clin Geriatr* 12(4):26-32, 2004.

23. Folstein MF, Folstein SE, McHugh PR: Mini-Mental State: a practical method for grading the cognitive state of patients for the clinician, *J Psychiatr Res* 12:189-198, 1975.

24. Sheikh, JI, Yessage JA: Geriatric Depression Scale: recent evidence and development of a shorter version, *Clin Gerontol* 5:165, 1986.

25. Alexopoulos GS, Abrams RC, Young RC, Shamoin CA: Cornell Scale for Depression in dementia, *Biol Psychiatry* 23(3):271-284, 1988.

26. Mueller C, Cain, H: Comprehensive management of urinary incontinence through quality improvement efforts, *Geriatr Nurs* 23(2):82-87, 2002.

27. Frantz RA, Xakellis GC, Harvey PC, Lewis AR: Implementing an incontinence management protocol in long-term care: clinical outcomes and costs, *J Gerontol Nurs* 29(8):47-53, 2003.

28. Dellenfield, ME: The relationship between nurse staffing in nursing homes and quality indicators: a literature review, *J Gerontol Nurs* 26(6):14-28, 2000.

29. Kayser-Jones J, Schell ES, Porter C, et al: Factors contributing to dehydration in nursing homes: inadequate staffing and lack of professional supervision, *J Am Geriatr Soc* 47:1187-1194, 1999.

30. Mather KF, Bakas T: Nursing assistants' perceptions of their ability to provide continence care, *Geriatr Nurs* 23(2):76-81, 2002.

31. Centers for Medicare and Medicaid Services: *Revised long-term care resident assessment instrument user's manual,* version 2.0, product number H50172, Miamisburg, Ohio, 2003, MED-PASS, Inc.

32. Kaplan MJ: A powerful new tool for nursing home consumers: the quality indicator report, *Ann Long-Term Care* 10(6):21-24, 2002.

33. Ostaszkiewicz J, Johnson L, Roe B: Timed voiding for the management of urinary incontinence in adults (Cochrane review), *Cochrane Library* 3, 2004.

34. Ouslander JG, AI-Samarrai N, Schnelle JF: Prompted voiding for nighttime incontinence in nursing homes: is it effective? *J Am Geriatr Soc* 49:706-709, 2001.

35. Palmer M: *Urinary continence assessment and promotion,* Gaithersburg, Md., 1996, Aspen, p 92.

36. Fantl JA, Newman DK, Colling J, et al: Urinary incontinence in adults: acute and chronic management, *Clinical practice guideline,* No. 2, 1996 update, AHCPR Publication No. 96-0682, Rockville, Md., 1996, US Department of Health and Human Services, Public Health Service, Agency for Health Care Policy and Research.

37. Colling J, Ouslander J, Hadley BJ, et al: The effects of patterned urge-response toileting (PURT) on urinary incontinence among nursing home residents, *J Am Geriatr Soc* 40:135-141, 1992.

38. Colling J, Owen, TR, McCreedy M, Newman D: The effects of a continence program on frail community-dwelling elderly persons, *Urol Nurs* 23(2):117-131, 2003.

39. Jirovec MM: Effect of individualized prompted toileting on incontinence in nursing home residents, *Appl Nurs Res* 4:188-191, 1991.

40. Johnson T: Nonpharmacological treatments for urinary incontinence in long-term care residents, *J Am Med Dir Assoc* 3(1 suppl):S25-S29, 2002.

41. Ostaszkiewicz J, Johnson L, Roe B: Habit retraining for the management of urinary incontinence in adults (Cochrane review), *Cochrane Library* 3, 2004.

42. Jirovec MM, Templin T: Predicting success using individualized scheduled toileting for memory-impaired elders at home, *Res Nurs Health* 24(1):1-8, 2001.

43. Engberg SJ, Organist L, Lafayette-Lucey A, McDowell BJ: Treatment of urinary incontinence among caregiver-dependent adults, *Urol Nurs* 18(2):131-136, 1998.

44. Lyons SS, Pringle Specht K: Prompted voiding protocol for individuals with urinary incontinence, *J Gerontol Nurs* 26(6):5-12, 2000.

45. Schnelle JF, Traughber B, Sowell VA, et al: Prompted voiding treatment of urinary incontinence in nursing home patients: a behavioral management approach for nursing home staff, *J Am Geriatr Soc* 37:1051-1057, 1989.

46. Eustice S, Roe B, Paterson J: Prompted voiding for the management of urinary incontinence in adults (Cochrane Review). In: *Cochrane Library* 3, 2004.

47. McCormick KA, Burgio LD, Engel BT, et al: Urinary incontinence: an augmented prompted void approach, *J Gerontol Nurs* 18(3):3-10, 1992.

48. Schnelle JF: Treatment of urinary incontinence in nursing home patients by prompted voiding, *J Am Geriatr Soc* 38:356-360, 1990.

49. Schnelle JF, Newman D, White M, et al: Maintaining continence in nursing home residents through the application of industrial quality control, *Gerontologist* 33:114-121, 1993.

50. Adkins VK, Mathews RM: Prompted voiding to reduce incontinence in community-dwelling older adults, *J Appl Behav Anal* 30:153-156, 1997.

51. Brandeis GH., Baumann MM, Hossain M, et al: The prevalence of potentially remediable urinary incontinence in frail older people: a study using the Minimum Data Set, *J Am Geriatr Soc* 45(1):179-184, 1997.

52. Wagner A, Colling J: Resistance to change: understanding the aides' point of view, *J Long-Term Care Admin* 21(2):27-30, 1993.

53. Maloney C, Cafiero M: Implementing an incontinence program in long-term care settings, *J Gerontol Nurs* 25(6):47-52, 1999.

54. Jirovec MM: Functional incontinence. In: Doughty DB, editor: *Urinary and fecal incontinence nursing management,* ed 2, Philadelphia, 2000, Mosby, pp 145-157.

Pathology and Management of Reflex Incontinence/Neurogenic Bladder

MIKEL L. GRAY

OBJECTIVES

1. Identify three consistent elements among the various definitions of reflex urinary incontinence (UI).
2. Differentiate between neurogenic detrusor overactivity and overactive bladder/detrusor instability.
3. Identify patients at risk for reflex incontinence.
4. Explain why reflex incontinence occurs only in individuals with lesions affecting the spinal cord from functional level C2 to S1.
5. Describe the Hinman syndrome and explain why children with this syndrome experience voiding dysfunction that closely mimics reflex UI.
6. Identify the two primary components of the pathophysiology of reflex UI.
7. Describe the typical pattern of urinary leakage among patients with reflex UI.
8. Define the terms "detrusor-sphincter dyssynergia" and "low bladder wall compliance" and explain the effect of each on bladder function and upper urinary tract function.
9. Explain the concept of "hostile bladder function" and implications for management of the patient with reflex UI.
10. Identify three complications associated with reflex UI that must be addressed in the management plan.
11. Outline key factors to be included in the assessment of an individual with reflex UI.
12. Explain why urodynamic evaluation should be *routinely* incorporated into the assessment of a patient with reflex UI.
13. Explain why treatment of asymptomatic bacteriuria is contraindicated in the patient with reflex UI.
14. Identify the advantages, disadvantages, and key factors to be addressed with each of the following bladder management programs: spontaneous voiding, reflex voiding with condom catheter containment, intermittent catheterization, indwelling catheter.
15. Identify the indications for anticholinergic and alpha-adrenergic antagonist drugs in management of the patient with reflex UI and the key factors to include in patient teaching and assessment relative to these medications.
16. Explain the role of bladder augmentation and continent urinary diversions in management of the patient with reflex UI.

There are several definitions for reflex urinary incontinence (UI). The International Continence Society defines reflex UI as uncontrolled urine loss occurring as a result of neurogenic disorders and caused by neurogenic detrusor overactivity; they add that the leakage occurs in the absence of any desire to urinate. The North American Nursing Diagnosis Association (NANDA) defines reflex UI as urine loss occurring at somewhat predictable intervals of time when a specific bladder volume is reached; their defining characteristics for this condition also include the absence of sensory awareness.[1-3]

Despite subtle variations in these definitions, they share key elements that provide a broad but useful definition for reflex UI. For the purposes of this text, reflex UI is defined as involuntary urine loss caused by overactive detrusor contractions and occurring with diminished or absent sensory awareness of the urge to urinate. The significance of detrusor-sphincter dyssynergia (DSD), which is typically associated with reflex UI, is also discussed.

Neurogenic detrusor overactivity is defined as the occurrence of uncontrolled bladder contractions in a patient with a neurologic lesion.[3] Among patients with reflex UI, overactive detrusor contractions may or may not produce urine loss, depending on the magnitude and duration of the contractions, and on the response of the urethral sphincter mechanism. *DSD* is the loss of coordination between the striated sphincter and the detrusor muscle; that is, the sphincter does not consistently relax when the detrusor contracts. This condition is also known as "vesicosphincter dyssynergia," and it is significant because contraction of the striated muscle components of the sphincter during bladder contraction causes a functional obstruction of the bladder outlet.

EPIDEMIOLOGY

No epidemiologic data are available for the condition of reflex UI. However, some appreciation for its prevalence can be inferred from epidemiologic data for the principal neurologic conditions associated with reflex UI: spinal cord injury, spinal cord disease, multiple sclerosis (MS), and spina bifida.

In 2004, it was estimated that 247,000 Americans were living with a spinal cord injury.[4] Estimates of the incidence of spinal cord injuries vary from 21.2 per million population to 60 per million;[5-7] approximately 85% of these injuries affect the spinal segments located above the twelfth thoracic vertebra, and these lesions commonly produce reflex UI.

Reflex UI may also occur among persons with intervertebral disk disease, spinal stenosis, and cervical spondylosis. The prevalence of these conditions is not known, but the annual incidence of surgical intervention for these problems has been estimated at 52.3 per 100,000 population. Approximately 15% of these patients will experience clinically apparent voiding dysfunction, and reflex UI may occur if the nerve pathways innervating the lower urinary tract are compressed.[8]

MS may also cause UI, and reflex UI occurs in persons with lesions of the thoracic or cervical spinal cord. The prevalence of MS in the United States is approximately 85 per 100,000 or 220,000.[9,10] The incidence of MS varies according to age and

geographic region; Hawaii's annual estimated incidence is only 8.8 cases per 100,000 population, whereas Rochester, Minnesota, has an annual incidence of approximately 173 per 100,000 population. It has been estimated that as many as 96% of individuals with MS experience voiding dysfunction, 52% to 78% experience neurogenic detrusor overactivity, and approximately 50% experience vesicosphincter dyssynergia.[11,12]

Reflex UI also occurs in certain children with spina bifida. The incidence of spina bifida is about 1 per 1000 live births.[8,13] Fortunately, emphasis on primary prevention of neural tube defects via dietary supplementation of folic acid has led to a decline of this devastating defect over the past several decades.[14] Nevertheless, spina bifida continues to account for about 25% of the voiding dysfunction seen in pediatric urology practices in the United States. Approximately 54% of newborns with myelomeningoceles will have neurogenic detrusor overactivity and vesicosphincter dyssynergia.[15] Among older children with spina bifida and neurologic deficits, 62% have neurogenic detrusor overactivity and 15% have vesicosphincter dyssynergia.[16]

In addition to neurologic lesions, a small group of children *without* neurologic disease will experience both detrusor overactivity and vesicosphincter dyssynergia that adversely affects both lower and upper urinary tract function.[17] This complex voiding dysfunction is called the nonneurogenic bladder of childhood, or the Hinman-Allen syndrome. The features of this disorder closely resemble the reflex UI associated with neurologic disease, and this disorder is therefore discussed.

ETIOLOGY

Any neurologic lesion that affects the brain or the spinal cord above the sacral micturition center can cause neurogenic detrusor overactivity; however, only those conditions affecting spinal segments C2 to S1 result in reflex UI[18-20] (Box 7-1). Neurologic disorders within or above the pons typically cause neurogenic detrusor overactivity with retention of sensory awareness and bladder-sphincter coordination; these patients are likely to experience *urge incontinence* rather than reflex UI[21] (Fig. 7-1). People do not usually survive lesions involving the medulla

BOX 7-1   Etiology of Reflex Urinary Incontinence

Traumatic disorders
Spinal cord injury
Intervertebral disk disease

Congenital disorders
Myelodysplasia
Familial hereditary spasticity
Cerebral palsy

Nontraumatic disorders
Multiple sclerosis
Acute disseminated encephalomyelitis
Arachnoiditis
Landry-Guillain-Barré syndrome
Human immunodeficiency virus infection
Transverse myelitis
Systemic lupus erythematosus

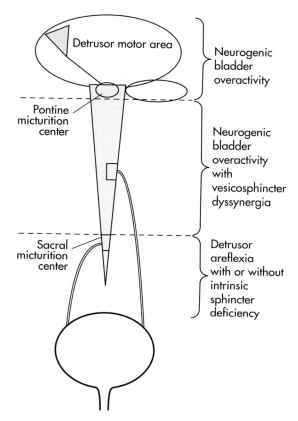

Fig. 7-1 Reflex urinary incontinence (UI) is associated with lesions that affect spinal segments C2 to S1. Lesions above C2 produce urge UI, and those below S1 produce detrusor areflexia with or without intrinsic sphincter incompetence and stress UI.

or C1 because of damage to the vital respiratory and cardiovascular centers. Lesions affecting the lower spine (below S2) or the cauda equina cause loss of bladder contractility (detrusor areflexia) and may cause intrinsic sphincter deficiency; these patients typically experience *overflow incontinence* and may also have *stress incontinence* but do not experience reflex UI. (See Chapter 2 for a review of the neurologic pathways critical to bladder function and continence.)

Spinal Cord Injuries

Spinal cord injuries represent the most common spinal lesion, and these injuries frequently result in reflex UI. The likelihood that a specific spinal injury will lead to a neuropathic bladder and reflex UI is determined by its location, its completeness, and the occurrence and severity of vascular extension. The level of a spinal cord injury can be described by the location of the affected vertebral body (the orthopedic level of injury) or by the level at which the spinal cord and nerve pathways are affected (the neurologic or functional level of injury). The orthopedic and neurologic levels are nearly identical in the high cervical region, but they do not correspond as closely in the remaining areas of the spinal column and spinal cord; therefore, it is important

to determine whether the location of a spinal cord injury is being presented by orthopedic level or by functional level. To illustrate, injuries at the *orthopedic* level of C2-T12 (or L1) are associated with *functional* injuries at the level of C2-S1[22] (Fig. 7-2). These levels of injury are associated with detrusor hyperreflexia, DSD, and reflex UI.

The effect of a specific neurologic lesion on bladder function is also influenced by the *completeness* of the injury. A complete injury produces both sensory and motor loss, whereas an incomplete injury is typically associated with loss of motor function but preservation of sensation. (In rare cases, an incomplete injury causes loss of sensation and

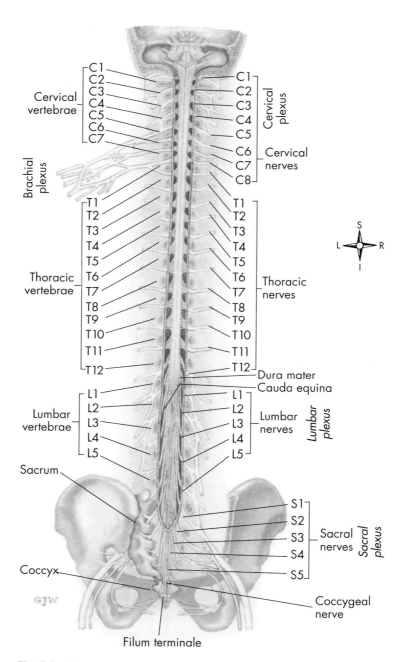

Fig. 7-2 Spine. Notice the differences in the vertebral segments, with the bony and neurologic segments in the middle and lower regions. (From Vidic B, Suarez FR: *Photographic atlas of the human body,* St Louis, 1990, Mosby).

preservation of motor function.) Approximately 46% of all spinal injuries are incomplete; this statistic may be attributable in part to the use of steroids during the early postinjury period and the resultant reduction in edema and ischemia.[22] Most patients with incomplete injuries experience reflex UI characterized by diminished awareness of bladder filling, neurogenic detrusor overactivity, and DSD; however, some patients retain bladder sensation, and a few patients with incomplete paralyzing lesions actually maintain continence.

The occurrence and severity of vascular extension comprise the third factor affecting a spinal cord injury's effect on bladder function. Vascular extension is typically caused by ischemic injury to adjacent areas of the spinal cord, and the degree of vascular extension is influenced by the mechanism of injury and the immediacy of postinjury care. Functional classification systems for spinal cord injury describe the lesion according to the highest level of neurologic involvement; however, vascular extension may cause damage to areas *below* the primary injury. This may be significant when one is considering the effect of an injury on bladder function; that is, inferior extension may account for the persistence of detrusor areflexia and intrinsic sphincter deficiency that sometimes occurs in patients with thoracic or even cervical-level injuries.

In addition to spinal cord injuries, spinal cord diseases (such as disk disease or spinal stenosis) occasionally produce compression of the spine and damage to the associated nerve pathways; if the compression is at the level of the cervical or thoracic cord, it may produce reflex UI.[23]

Nontraumatic Spinal Disorders

The most common nontraumatic spinal disorders associated with reflex UI are spina bifida and MS; additional disorders include various autoimmune disorders and polyneuropathies.

Spina bifida is an umbrella term for congenital defects characterized by failure of the vertebral bodies to close and the associated spinal cord defects.[13,24] In many cases, the defect is limited to the bony structures, but the meninges (meningocele) and the spinal cord itself (myelomeningocele) may herniate through the defect; if the spinal cord is involved,

the child typically suffers significant neurologic deficits, that is, varying degrees of motor and sensory loss and possibly disorders of the cerebrospinal drainage system (Arnold-Chiari defect). When the defect involves neurologic structures, it is termed "myelodysplasia"; this defect commonly involves multiple spinal segments, usually in the lumbar and sacral areas of the spine, although it may also involve the thoracic spine. Reflex UI is common among infants and children with myelodysplasia involving the thoracic and lumbar areas of the spine.

MS is a demyelinating disease that affects multiple levels of the central nervous system.[25] It typically strikes young adults between 16 and 50 years of age, peaking among those 23 or 24 years of age. Persons who develop MS before 40 years of age commonly experience recurring episodes of neurologic impairment followed by spontaneous remission. This pattern continues even after the disease becomes clinically overt; there are periods of spontaneous exacerbations caused by demyelination within the nervous system, followed by remission or alleviation of symptoms as remyelination occurs. However, over a period of years, the repetitive scarring of the neurons and axons causes permanent dysfunction and progressive disability. The symptoms of MS vary widely because of the wide distribution of the characteristic sclerotic plaques, but "typical" symptoms include sensory paresthesias in one or more extremities, weakness in one or more limbs, visual disturbances, and gait disturbances (or a slowly progressing weakness or spasticity of the lower extremities).

Approximately 10% of patients have voiding symptoms at the time of diagnosis, and voiding difficulties are the *only* symptom in 1% to 3% of all new cases.[25,26] The most commonly reported voiding symptoms are urinary frequency, urgency, and urge incontinence; unfortunately, this symptom pattern is *most commonly* seen in women with urge or mixed stress-urge incontinence, and therefore the patient with only voiding symptoms and no neurologic deficit may be incorrectly diagnosed. The clinician should be very thorough when assessing any young adult with apparent "urge" incontinence. If the symptoms of urge incontinence are associated with hesitancy, the recent onset of enuresis, or a urinary tract infection (UTI), the clinician should be suspicious of a neurologic deficit; these signs and symptoms indicate the possible presence of DSD, which is an ominous finding in any young adult with voiding dysfunction.

MS produces reflex UI when the lesions involve the spinal tracts that provide communication between the lower urinary tract and the modulatory areas in the spinal cord, pons, and cortex. The demyelinating plaques of MS affect the white matter of the dorsal columns of the spinal cord and especially the abundant white matter located in the cervical and thoracic areas of the cord.[27,28] The plaques affect nerve structures below the level of the pons, and they compromise both sensory and motor function; therefore, reflex UI is common in patients with MS lesions involving the spinal cord.

Multiple other diseases cause progressive degeneration of the spinal cord and the development of reflex UI; these diseases are occasionally misdiagnosed as MS.[25] For example, the human immunodeficiency virus is known to invade the central nervous system, and reflex UI sometimes occurs during the advanced stages of acquired immunodeficiency syndrome.[29] Other less common diseases that occasionally cause reflex UI include disseminated encephalomyelitis, arachnoiditis,[23] cerebellar ataxia,[30] Landry-Guillain-Barré syndrome,[31-34] and transverse myelitis. Transverse myelitis is characterized by inflammation of the spinal cord, which causes loss of motor and sensory activity below the involved segment or segments. As in spinal cord injury, the bladder dysfunction associated with transverse myelitis is affected by the location of the area of inflammation; some patients develop urinary retention, whereas others develop reflex UI.[35-38] Systemic lupus erythematosus is a well-known chronic autoimmune disorder characterized by formation of antibodies that attack the victim's own tissues and serum factors;[39] SLE is primarily known to affect the kidneys, skin, and hematologic system, but it can also affect the central nervous system, including the spine.[40] Spinal involvement produces transverse myelopathy that results in motor and sensory deficits and in reflex UI when the lesion is located above S2.[41]

Nonneurogenic Neurogenic Bladder: Hinman-Allen Syndrome

Daytime UI (characterized by frequency, urgency, and urge incontinence) and nocturia or enuresis are not uncommon among school-aged children with apparently normal neurologic function.[47] However, in as many as 20% of these children,[43] and in approximately 0.5% of all patients with urge incontinence,[44] detrusor overactivity is complicated by DSD. In most cases, this dyssynergia does not lead to serious upper tract distress, and it can usually be resolved, either by elimination of the unstable bladder contractions or by a short course of biofeedback to eliminate the dyssynergic sphincter activity. However, a few of these children develop a nonneurogenic neurogenic bladder. This syndrome, also known as the Hinman-Allen syndrome, is a functional disorder that closely mimics reflex UI.[45] It is characterized by contraction of the striated muscle of the sphincter during voiding, which produces a functional obstruction of the bladder outlet. Children with nonneurogenic neurogenic bladders have profound changes in the radiographic appearance of the urinary tract. Hydroureteronephrosis, vesicoureteral reflux, scarring of the kidneys from febrile infections, and a trabeculated bladder are common findings. Renal insufficiency may occur, and renal failure with an elevated creatinine may already be present on initial evaluation.

The cause of the nonneurogenic neurogenic bladder is not known.[17] It was originally postulated to represent an occult neurologic lesion;[46] however, more recent research has not confirmed this hypothesis.[42,47] Currently, the Hinman-Allen syndrome is attributed to persistence of the phase in toilet training when the child learns to contract the sphincter to delay voiding.[48] McGuire and Savastano have suggested that the dyssynergia associated with the Hinman-Allen syndrome may represent overutilization of "guarding behaviors" in response to unstable detrusor contractions.[49] The guarding response is the contraction of the pelvic floor and periurethral striated muscles in an attempt to prevent or minimize leakage during an unstable detrusor contraction; in children, it is often accompanied by Vincent's curtsy, that is, crossing the legs and bending the knees or placing one heel in the perineum, followed by the characteristic curtsy.[50] Bauer has studied children with nonneurogenic neurogenic bladders and their families, and he identifies several common psychogenic characteristics that may provide clues to its cause.[13] For example, he notes that many of these families include a domineering, unyielding father who is intolerant of failure; divorce and alcoholism are also common. The child's UI is frequently perceived as immature, defiant, and purposeful behavior and is commonly managed within the family by physical and mental punishment. Gray reported on a series of 10 children who had been diagnosed with Hinman syndrome; he found that 90% had abnormalities noted on the Minnesota Multiphasic Personality Inventory, and 70% had a history of sexual abuse.[51]

PATHOPHYSIOLOGY

A discussion of the pathophysiology of reflex UI must focus on two primary aspects of this condition: (1) the mechanism of leakage, and (2) the effect on upper urinary tract function. Because the potential effect of reflex UI on upper urinary tract health is so significant, the management of patients with this condition is often focused on the preservation of renal function, with little attention given to the problems caused by the urinary leakage. This section addresses each of these issues separately and also includes a discussion of the potential complications of reflex UI: UTI, renal calculi, and autonomic dysreflexia (AD). The management section focuses on the inextricable relationship of the two issues and on the effect of bladder management on continence, renal health, and quality of life.

Urinary Incontinence

The primary mechanism for leakage in reflex UI is the occurrence of overactive detrusor contractions (Fig. 7-3). These contractions occur at variable volumes, in response to bladder distension or other triggers (such as stroking the thigh or a sudden change in perineal skin temperature). In some patients, overactive detrusor contractions are well sustained with good amplitude, leading to intermittent episodes of high-volume urinary leakage;[52,53] in others, the contractions are low pressure and poorly sustained, resulting in frequent loss of small volumes of urine.[54] Because the sensation of bladder filling is diminished or absent in individuals with reflex UI, overactive detrusor contractions are associated with little or no urge to urinate. However, I have observed that many patients with little or no bladder sensation usually experience some identifiable sensation of impending micturition, however "atypical." For example, many patients with complete spinal cord injuries experience a tingling in the arms, hands, or face before micturition, whereas others report a "rushing" sensation that

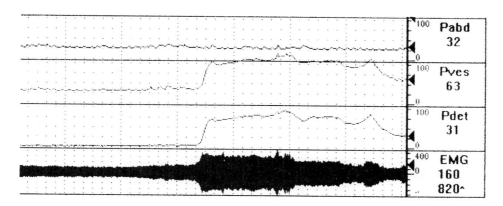

Fig. 7-3 Urodynamic tracing showing neurogenic detrusor overactivity. These contractions are elicited by a variety of stimuli and frequently occur at unpredictable intervals.

may represent a mild sympathetic discharge. Unfortunately, a literature search of the MEDLINE and CINAHL databases up to January 2004 yielded no research in this area, and it is not known whether these warnings of impending micturition can be successfully exploited in the clinical management of this complex form of incontinence.

Although neurogenic detrusor overactivity is clearly the primary cause of incontinence in patients with reflex UI, other factors may also contribute to urine loss. For example, persons with reflex UI may also experience stress UI caused by inadequate urethral sphincter resistance. This is particularly common among women who may have had preexisting stress UI before a spinal cord injury or the development of MS. Patients with lesions affecting the lower spinal segments and those with long-standing obstruction and severe trabeculation of the bladder are also at risk for low bladder wall compliance and overflow incontinence. In addition, some patients with reflex UI may develop continuous or extraurethral urinary leakage as a result of fistula development (Fig. 7-4).

Upper Urinary Tract Damage

The relationship between upper urinary tract function and reflex UI is illustrated by the history of spinal cord injury management, with particular emphasis on morbidity and mortality. During the midtwentieth century, urinary tract complications were the leading cause of death after spinal cord injury. Urosepsis and renal failure accounted for 43% of the spinal cord injury deaths reported among World War II and Korean War soldiers and veterans.[55] Fortunately, since that time, we have gained a keener appreciation and understanding of the relationship between UI and renal function. As a result, the life expectancy after a spinal cord injury has improved dramatically, and the proportion of deaths attributable to urinary tract complications has fallen to a range of 3% to 16%.[54,56]

Some individuals with reflex UI are at much greater risk for upper tract distress and compromised renal function than others; factors determining the risk for any one person include the presence of DSD, the severity of obstruction caused by this dyssynergia, and bladder wall compliance.[57] The presence of these characteristics may be said to represent "hostile bladder function," a term sometimes used to describe the potential for dysfunction in the lower urinary tract to cause distress in the upper tracts.[52,58-60]

Clearly, the effect of DSD on upper tract function is determined primarily by the severity of obstruction it produces[59] (Fig. 7-5). This severity has been evaluated and classified according to several different techniques. Chancellor and Blaivas divide DSD into three categories, based on urodynamic tracings of sphincter activity as compared with detrusor activity.[21] Type 1 DSD is characterized by an increase

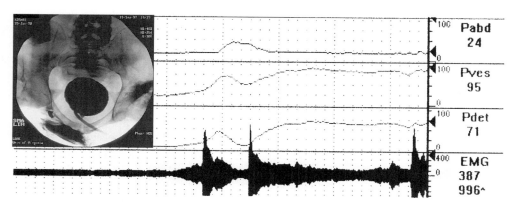

Fig. 7-4 Urethrocutaneous fistula from pressure injury in this spinal cord–injured patient produces a combination of reflex and continuous urinary incontinence.

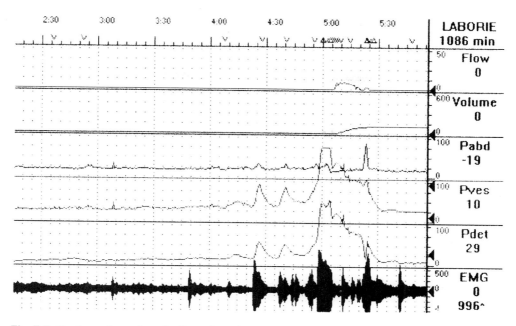

Fig. 7-5 Urodynamic tracing of reflex urinary incontinence shows high-pressure neurogenic detrusor overactivity with detrusor-sphincter dyssynergia and obstruction. (**Courtesy of** *LABORIE,* Laborie Medical Technologies, Toronto, Canada.)

in sphincter contraction that persists up to the maximum amplitude of a detrusor contraction and then abruptly subsides. Voiding occurs primarily during the phase of detrusor relaxation. It is not yet known what causes this abrupt relaxation of the sphincter followed by relaxation of the detrusor, that is, whether the striated sphincter, detrusor muscle, or both are inhibited at this point and by what mechanism. In Type 2 DSD, clonic contractions of the sphincter occur throughout the detrusor contraction, and the urinary stream is classically "intermittent." Type 3 DSD is characterized by a persistent, crescendo-decrescendo contraction of the striated sphincter that mirrors the detrusor contraction. Although clinical experience supports the observations of Blaivas and Chancellor, dyssynergia type has not been found to predict obstruction severity or risk for subsequent urologic complications.[61]

Other researchers advocate assessing obstruction severity by evaluating the detrusor pressure required to produce urine flow; that is, to overcome sphincter resistance. McGuire and colleagues[62] observed that

a high detrusor leak point pressure (LPP, the pressure required to drive urine across the urethral sphincter) increased the risk for upper tract distress. Gray and colleagues[59] measured detrusor and urethral pressures during hyperreflexic detrusor contractions in a group of spinal cord-injured male patients who were managed by reflex voiding and condom catheter containment. These investigators found that the risk for upper urinary tract distress (defined in this study as the presence of febrile UTI, vesicoureteral reflux, ureterohydronephrosis, or renal insufficiency) was directly related to the magnitude of energy required to overcome the obstructed bladder outlet.

In addition to creating obstruction to urine flow, DSD is believed to increase the risk for upper tract distress by increasing the potential for bacteriuria and UTI. Because DSD obstructs the bladder outlet, it is frequently associated with large postvoid residual urine volumes.[63,64] Residual urine in the bladder serves as a medium for bacterial growth, which may result in infection. In addition, DSD may increase the risk for UTI because it creates turbulence in the urethra; the turbulence allows urine to move from the more bacteria-laden distal portion of the urethra to the proximal portion of the urethra and bladder as it travels through the dysfunctional sphincter[65] (Fig. 7-6).

Two factors contribute to low detrusor filling pressures, which allow the ureters to overcome ureterovesical junction resistance and to fill the bladder: (1) normal detrusor tonus; and (2) normal viscoelastic properties of the bladder wall; that is, sufficient elasticity to allow the bladder to stretch and fill at low pressures.[66,67] This distensibility of the bladder wall is measured during urodynamic testing and is expressed as bladder wall compliance (see Chapter 12). Low bladder wall compliance refers to the loss of normal distensibility and results in higher intravesical filling pressures. Poor or low bladder wall compliance increases the risk of upper tract distress because the elevated intravesical filling pressures functionally obstruct the ureters and ultimately the kidneys.

Several factors associated with reflex UI may lead to low bladder wall compliance. Long-term use of an indwelling catheter is one of these factors, possibly because of the chronic infection that frequently occurs with this management approach.[68] In children with voiding dysfunction, chronic bacteriuria has been associated with increased urine levels of fibroblast growth factor; this could lead to the deposition of fibrous tissue in the bladder wall, which would be expected to reduce distensibility and thus to lower compliance.[69] In addition to the effects of infection and inflammation, prolonged bladder drainage may itself contribute to reduced compliance and thus diminish the bladder's ability to function as an effective storage vesicle.[70] Another factor that may contribute to reduced compliance in the patient with reflex UI is denervation of the lumbosacral spinal segments, as occurs in children with myelodysplasia. This denervation contributes to low bladder wall compliance because it seems to promote collagen deposition within the bladder wall, which is seen on radiographic imaging as trabeculation.[71-73] Among individuals with reflex UI, trabeculation is often seen after a prolonged period of "reflex" voiding with condom catheter containment; the reason may be that reflex voiding requires the detrusor to mount contractile pressures high enough to overcome any bladder outlet obstruction and to achieve bladder evacuation[52,54] (Fig. 7-7). Ogawa and colleagues have correlated the severity of trabeculation with the likelihood of ureterohydronephrosis (one sign of upper tract distress) in both children with myelomeningocele and adults with spinal cord injury[71,72] (Fig. 7-8).

Urinary Tract Infection

Chronic bacteriuria and symptomatic UTIs are common among patients with reflex UI.[60,74] The long-term sequelae of UTI relate to progressive damage to the renal parenchyma and ultimate renal insufficiency. The patient with DSD and bladder outlet obstruction is at particular risk for UTI because elevated residual volumes and urinary stasis increase the risk that bacteriuria will evolve from an asymptomatic to a symptomatic state.[75] Any UTI in the individual with reflex UI carries the risk of upper tract involvement, leading to pyelonephritis and bacteremia, unless *both* the infection and the voiding dysfunction are aggressively managed. The risk for pyelonephritis is increased further in the patient with low bladder wall compliance, vesicoureteral reflux, or ureterohydronephrosis. Pyelonephritis is a very significant complication from the long-term perspective because

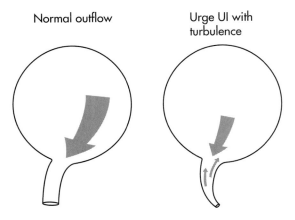

Normal outflow   Urge UI with turbulence

Fig. 7-6 Detrusor-sphincter dyssynergia produces turbulence in outflow tract that may increase the risk of subsequent urinary tract infection because urine swirls from distal to proximal segments of the urethra.

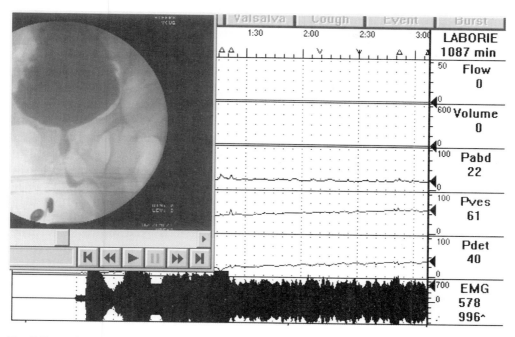

Fig. 7-7 Low bladder wall compliance and detrusor areflexia cause overflow urinary incontinence and upper urinary tract distress in this patient who has been managed by a reflex voiding program for past 13 years.

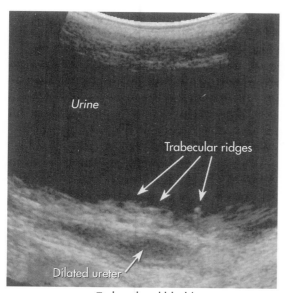

Fig. 7-8 Sonogram of the bladder in a patient with myelodysplasia and low bladder wall compliance reveals trabeculation and a dilated ureter associated with vesicoureteral reflux.

of its negative effect on the renal parenchyma; pyelonephritis may cause renal scarring, which involves the replacement of functioning nephrons with fibrotic tissue. When recurrent episodes of pyelonephritis occur, the number of scars and the volume of nonfunctioning renal parenchyma increase, ultimately leading to a poorly functioning or nonfunctioning kidney.[76] Infants and children are at greatest risk for this complication, but it also occurs among adults, especially when the infection is complicated by obstruction.[77]

In the short-term, pyelonephritis causes significant morbidity (fever, pain, and possibly nausea, vomiting, and dehydration) and can lead to bacteremia and urosepsis unless it is promptly and effectively treated.[75] Urosepsis is defined as the presence of tachypnea, tachycardia, and fever or chills in combination with hypoxemia, elevated plasma lactate concentration, or oliguria in the patient with clinical or definitive laboratory evidence of a UTI. Septic shock occurs when urosepsis results in hypotension, characterized by a sustained decrease in systolic blood pressure to 90 mm Hg or less or a drop of 40 mm Hg that lasts for at least 1 hour. Septic shock has traditionally been associated with gram-negative pathogens, but it may also occur with infections caused by gram-positive organisms.[78] Although its pathogenesis is not completely understood, the hypotension and organ failure associated with septic shock probably occur as a result of the release of bacterial endotoxins that activate humoral pathways, macrophages, and other cells involved in the inflammatory process. Septic shock constitutes a medical emergency and is associated with a mortality of 10% to 90%,[79,80] with the majority of deaths occurring within 48 hours of the onset of sepsis.[81]

Urinary Calculi

Another complication of reflex UI is urinary stone disease.[59,82] Urinary stasis and immobility, both common among patients with paralyzing spinal disorders, are known to increase the risk for urinary calculus formation. In addition, some of the pathogens commonly associated with UTI, such as the *Proteus* species and other urease-producing bacteria, predispose the individual to calculus formation. This association is explained by the finding that these bacteria can split urea to form ammonia, which raises the urinary pH as well as the concentration of ammonia; the result may be precipitation of ammonium phosphate and the formation of magnesium-ammonium phosphate stones. Urinary calculi are a significant complication for the individual with reflex UI because they create or exacerbate obstruction, increase the risk of bacteremia and sepsis, and compromise renal function.

Autonomic Dysreflexia

AD, sometimes called "autonomic hyperreflexia," is a syndrome characterized by sweating, headache, and hypertension and caused by extreme stimulation of the autonomic nervous system.[57,83] The condition is peculiar to spinal cord injury, and it primarily affects patients with functional injury levels of T6 and above, although cases of AD have been reported with injuries at T7 and T8.[84,85] It is the hypertension associated with AD that carries the greatest risk for mortality; the systolic blood pressure during an episode of dysreflexia can reach 300 mm Hg, and

the diastolic pressure can climb to 220 mm Hg.[86] Several conditions are known to precipitate episodes of AD, such as overdistension of the rectal vault or the presence of an infected pressure ulcer, but the most common stimuli for these life-threatening episodes are associated with the urinary bladder.

The relationship between the urinary bladder and AD was first observed in 1947. Specific events that may produce AD include bladder filling and overdistension; this effect is particularly pronounced during filling cystometry.[87,88] AD may also be precipitated by a hyperreflexic detrusor contraction in the presence of DSD; it is not known whether it is the presence of DSD itself, or the magnitude of detrusor stimulation produced by contraction against the obstructed outlet, that causes the episode of AD. However, it *is* known that elimination of the bladder outlet obstruction (by transurethral sphincterotomy or placement of a urethral stent) alleviates the AD, even though it does not reverse the underlying neurologic abnormality that produces the dyssynergic sphincter activity.[88-90]

ASSESSMENT

A detailed discussion of the assessment for an individual with UI is presented in Chapter 12. Nonetheless, a brief overview of the assessment for an individual with reflex UI is included in this chapter because there are some unique aspects as compared with the more prevalent types of incontinence and because of the significance of the assessment findings to the formulation of an appropriate bladder management program (Box 7-2).

History

The voiding history should emphasize the current bladder management program. Unlike persons with stress, urge, or mixed stress-urge UI, most persons with reflex UI do not manage their bladder by spontaneous voiding. In contrast, a common management approach is by intermittent catheterization (IC). In this case, it is particularly important to determine the typical frequency of catheterization and the presence of leakage between catheterizations. Some patients manage their bladders with indwelling catheters, and it is important to determine why the catheter was inserted, the length of time a catheter

BOX 7-2 **Essential Elements in the Assessment of an Individual with Reflex Urinary Incontinence**

History and review of systems

History of incontinence
Duration of UI
Current bladder management program (spontaneous voiding, reflex voiding program, intermittent
  catheterization, indwelling catheter)
Character of leakage to include factors that provoke UI

Urologic system
UTIs (febrile? obtain record of cultures if available)
Urinary calculi
Disorders of the upper tracts (hydronephrosis, vesicoureteral reflux, problems with renal function,
  renal failure)
Urologic surgery (augmentation cystoplasty, urinary diversion)

Neurologic system
Neurologic disorder associated with reflex UI (referral indicated if patient states no history of neurologic
  evaluation)
Gastrointestinal system
Bowel management program (spontaneous defecation, scheduled program, stimulation program)
Frequency and characteristics of bowel movements (to include problems with constipation, impaction, diarrhea)

Medication history
All medications currently being taken (prescription, over the counter, herbal; include medications given to
  modify bowel and bladder function)

Physical examination
General functional and neurologic examination
Focused pelvic examination
Neurologic examination of perineal sensation
Bulbocavernosus reflex and response
Anal sphincter tone and contractility
Circumvaginal muscle tone (for patient with motor control)

Laboratory studies
Urinalysis with microscopic examination
Urine culture and sensitivities for symptomatic UTI
Upper urinary tract imaging study in consultation with physician (ultrasonogram, radionuclide scan,
  intravenous pyelogram): every year or every other year for all patients managed by reflex voiding, indwelling
  catheter, or urinary diversion and at *any time that symptoms of upper tract distress occur*
Imaging study may be indicated for patients managed by spontaneous voiding, or intermittent catheterization,
  if symptoms of upper tract distress are present.

Urodynamics
During initial evaluation before selection of bladder management program
When symptoms of upper tract distress occur (such as febrile UTI, rise in serum creatinine, change in upper
  tract imaging study)
When UI patterns change and transient causes for urinary leakage or change in patterns have been excluded

UI, urinary incontinence; UTI, urinary tract infection.

has remained in place, the size of the catheter and retention balloon, the material of construction (latex, silicone, etc.), and the presence of any leakage around the catheter (bypassing) or blockage. Still other patients manage their reflex UI with spontaneous voiding and urinary containment; many men contain their leakage with a condom catheter, but women and some men use adult incontinent briefs.

The review of systems must include a careful history of the neurologic disorder leading to the reflex UI and its effect on the patient's general health and functional abilities. Adults with reflex UI and no known neurologic lesion require prompt referral to a neurologist for a thorough evaluation. The urologic history includes any history of UTI, especially febrile infections, and any urinary problem requiring hospitalization. It is helpful to query the patient about symptoms leading to suspicion of UTI. Because sensations of bladder filling are diminished or absent, dysuria and suprapubic discomfort are infrequent and unreliable indicators of infection. The appearance and odor of the urine are also unreliable indicators; cloudy urine may simply reflect phosphaturia from consumption of meat, and changes in urinary odor may be caused by the diet or the medications rather than by bacteriuria. Nonetheless, it has been my clinical experience that even patients with complete spinal cord injuries often notice changes that are indicative of UTI. Common "indicators" among this population include increased spasticity, a change in the pattern of reflex voiding, or new onset of leakage between catheterizations;[58,89,91] new-onset incontinence and changes in the pattern of reflex voiding are probably attributable to the effect of bacteriuria on detrusor contractility. Many patients with reflex UI are very well informed about their UTI history, and it is worthwhile to query the patient and to review available medical records to determine whether the patient's UTIs are caused by a *Proteus* species or another urease-producing organism. It is also important to ask the patient about any previous history of urinary calculi, because the risk of recurrent stones is about 50% in the general population,[82] and it is probably even higher among those with reflex UI and a neurologic disorder.

Physical Examination

The general examination should focus on the patient's functional status, including sensory level, mobility, and dexterity. The patient's living environment should also be assessed in terms of support for the patient's efforts to maintain continence or adequate urinary containment. The patient with reflex UI and a paralyzing neurologic condition should be assessed for seating (that is, type and design of wheelchair), assistive devices used for ambulation (if applicable), and choice of clothing. McDowell has suggested assessing the time required for an elderly person with UI to move to the bathroom and prepare for urination by removing necessary clothing and sitting on the toilet.[92] This assessment strategy is also appropriate for the individual with impaired mobility and dexterity because of a neurologic disorder. Similarly, the person who manages his or her bladder with IC should be assessed for the ability to wash his or her hands, prepare the catheter, remove or adjust clothing, and complete the catheterization procedure. If the patient relies on family members or other caregivers to assist with or perform the catheterization procedure, the assessment should include the ability of the involved individuals to perform the procedure appropriately.

In addition to routine evaluation of the genitalia and the perineal skin, a focused but thorough neurologic examination must be included in assessment of the patient with reflex UI; this should include testing for perineal sensation, bulbocavernosus reflex, and pelvic floor muscle strength.

Diagnostic Testing

A urinalysis is completed as a routine portion of any incontinence evaluation, and it is particularly important in the assessment of a patient with reflex UI because of the risk for UTI.[71] Because of this increased risk, some clinicians routinely obtain urine cultures for these patients; however, this practice has not been shown to improve patient outcomes or to be cost effective.[93] Current recommendations are to limit cultures and treatment for UTI to patients with *symptomatic* infections (that is, infections associated with fever or hematuria) and patients with reflex UI who have both bacteriuria and pyuria on microscopic examination of the urine. Treatment of asymptomatic bacteriuria is discouraged because it has not been shown to benefit patients. Instead, it may harm patients by favoring colonization with bacterial strains that are resistant to oral or parenteral antibiotics.[94,95]

Although urodynamic testing is reserved for complex or complicated cases of urge, stress, or mixed stress-urge UI, it should be routinely performed for patients with reflex UI. Urodynamic testing for the patient with reflex UI must answer two essential questions: (1) what is the mechanism underlying urinary leakage, and (2) is this bladder likely to produce upper tract distress? If you are unfamiliar with the various urodynamic studies, refer to Chapter 12 for a thorough explanation. This chapter includes only a brief review of the specific studies indicated for the patient with reflex UI.

In evaluating the mechanism or mechanisms of leakage, the examiner must be aware that the leakage may be of mixed cause. Although overactive detrusor contractions are characteristic of reflex UI, patients must also be evaluated for stress incontinence and for evidence of extraurethral UI. When evaluating for neurogenic detrusor overactivity, it is important to observe *both* the magnitude and duration of the contraction and the pressure at which urinary leakage occurs. The detrusor LPP is the detrusor pressure at which urinary leakage first occurs; an elevated detrusor LPP (particularly values greater than 80 cm H_2O) is associated with severe obstruction and upper urinary tract distress.[91] The abdominal LPP is the abdominal force required to produce urinary leakage. Any measurable abdominal LPP indicates the presence of stress UI. When assessing abdominal LPP in a patient with reflex UI, it is important to remember that many patients will be unable to perform Valsalva's maneuver effectively. Therefore, it may be necessary for the examiner to apply external pressure over the bladder to elicit stress leakage. Extraurethral UI should be suspected when urine loss is observed that is not associated with detrusor overactivity or increased abdominal pressure. However, urodynamic studies lack sensitivity in the evaluation of extraurethral UI; additional evaluation may be required if the fistula is subtle.

An evaluation of the potential of the bladder to cause upper tract distress is based on measurement of bladder wall compliance, maximum detrusor contraction pressure, the maximum urethral pressure gradient, and/or the detrusor LPP.[52,59,63,65,95] Bladder wall compliance is a measurement of the distensibility of the bladder wall during bladder filling and storage. The compliance of the bladder wall can be calculated by dividing the change in pressure that occurs during bladder filling by the corresponding change in bladder volume. Persons with normal bladder function have high bladder wall compliance (with values exceeding 30 mL/cm H_2O);[96] normal compliance allows the bladder to fill to high volumes (300 to −600 mL) while maintaining low detrusor pressures (usually less than 15 cm H_2O). Low bladder wall compliance indicates excessive detrusor pressure acting on the bladder wall, intravesical urinary contents, the bladder outlet (urethrovesical junction), and the paired inlets (ureterovesical junctions). Values of 10 mL/cm H_2O or lower are associated with a high risk for upper urinary tract distress and/or overflow UI.[97,98]

In addition to evaluating bladder wall compliance, urodynamic testing should measure urethral resistance. Four values may be used for this assessment: maximum sustained detrusor pressure during bladder filling, maximum detrusor contraction pressure, the maximum urethral pressure gradient, or the detrusor LPP. Measuring the maximum sustained detrusor pressure during bladder filling provides an alternative to calculating whole bladder wall compliance; it is measured during the filling cystometrogram, and intravesical volumes are recorded at 20, 30, and 40 cm H_2O. Maximum sustained pressures that are 20 cm H_2O or less are associated with negligible risk of upper urinary tract changes, sustained pressures of 21 to 30 cm H_2O are associated with moderate risk, and those reaching 40 cm H_2O are associated with a high risk of upper urinary tract distress. The detrusor LPP is determined by observation of the pressure level at which urinary leakage is observed during the filling cystometrogram. Values greater than 40 cm H_2O are associated with imminent risk of upper urinary tract distress when they coexist with lower bladder wall compliance, as noted previously.

When assessing the bladder's potential to produce upper tract distress, it is best to rely on multiple outcomes. A minimal assessment should include at least one variable to assess bladder filling pressures (bladder wall compliance), one to assess detrusor work during a contraction, and one to measure urethral resistance. For example, assessment of bladder wall compliance, maximum detrusor contraction pressure, and the detrusor LPP would provide a reasonable assessment of the bladder's potential to be "hostile." In addition, although this assessment is ideally completed by means of videourodynamic techniques, it can be determined by a multichannel urodynamic study and without completing the more technically challenging urethral pressure study. Table 7-1 provides the normal values for each of these variables and the values that indicate increased risk for upper tract distress.

If available, videourodynamic testing represents the best approach to evaluation of the potentially "hostile" bladder. Fluoroscopic monitoring permits evaluation of any bladder trabeculation or vesicoureteral reflux. Fluoroscopy can also be used to identify other conditions causing urethral obstruction (such as bladder neck dyssynergia or benign prostatic hypertrophy), which may complicate reflex UI and increase the likelihood of upper urinary tract distress.

Routine imaging of the urinary tract is also useful in the evaluation of upper tract distress. A baseline imaging study may be obtained during the neonatal period (in the case of myelodysplasia) or when reflex UI is first diagnosed (among persons with spinal cord injuries or nontraumatic neurologic disorders). Traditionally, an intravenous pyelogram was used to evaluate the urinary system (Fig. 7-9). However, because of the potential for patient morbidity related to the intravenous contrast, as well as the radiation exposure and the cost, an ultrasound study of the urinary system is now generally preferred[99] (Fig. 7-10).

TREATMENT

The treatment of reflex UI is based on the results of the incontinence evaluation, knowledge of the underlying neurologic disorder and its natural history, assessment of the patient's neurologic status and functional ability, and the patient's preferences. Because of the complexity of these considerations and the profound effect of the bladder management program on the lives of the patient, family, and caregivers, this decision should be made in collaboration with an interdisciplinary team, such as the rehabilitation team; at a minimum, the decision should be made in close consultation with the patient, family or significant others, primary care provider, continence care clinician, and neurologist or physiatrist. Table 7-2 provides a listing of management options and the potential for incontinence and upper tract distress with each.

Spontaneous Voiding

A few patients (17% to 20%) with spinal cord injuries or other neurologic conditions associated with reflex UI experience neurogenic detrusor overactivity and vesicosphincter dyssynergia but retain sensory awareness of bladder filling.[58] Within this small group of patients, some retain reasonable continence.

TABLE 7-1   Urodynamic Variables Used to Assess Risk for Upper Tract Distress

URODYNAMIC VARIABLE	NORMAL VALUE OR RANGE	VALUE OR RANGE INDICATING RISK FOR UPPER TRACT DISTRESS
Bladder wall compliance	Greater than 50 mL/cm H_2O	Less than 10 mL/cm H_2O
Detrusor leak point pressure	Women: less than 30 cm H_2O Men: less than 40 cm H_2O	Greater than 40 cm H_2O
Maximum urethral pressure gradient	Less than 40 cm H_2O	40 to 80 cm H_2O: significant risk Greater than 80 cm H_2O: imminent risk

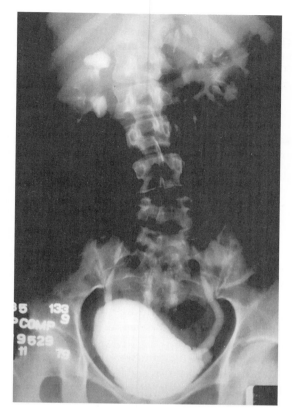

Fig. 7-9 Intravenous pyelogram in a patient with spinal cord injury shows a severely trabeculated bladder and evidence of upper urinary tract distress (in this case, ureterohydronephrosis).

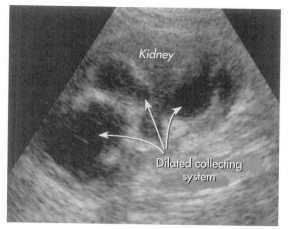

Hydronephrosis

A

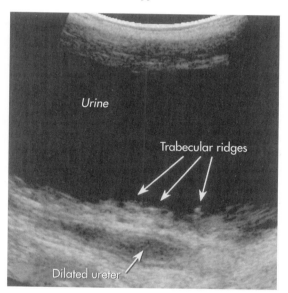

Trabeculated bladder

B

Fig. 7-10 Renal ultrasound in a patient with reflex urinary incontinence shows evidence of upper urinary tract distress. **A,** Hydronephrosis of kidney. **B,** Trabeculated bladder and dilated distal portion of ureter.

Technically, because these patients retain sensation, their UI can be classified as urge; however, their management is discussed within this chapter because they have DSD, and their neurologic condition is identical to those conditions that typically lead to reflex UI.

From the perspective of a continence nurse and from a urologic and rehabilitation viewpoint, a spontaneous voiding program is attractive. Patients who are candidates strongly prefer a spontaneous voiding program, even though they may experience some episodes of leakage, because it preserves their ability to urinate without the use of a catheter. Anson and Gray studied a group of spinal cord–injured patients who were followed for 1 to more than

TABLE 7-2 **Bladder Management Programs**

BLADDER MANAGEMENT PROGRAM	RISK OF UPPER URINARY TRACT DISTRESS	RISK OF URINARY INCONTINENCE
Spontaneous voiding	None	30%
Reflex voiding program	29% to 30%	70%*
Intermittent catheterization	7%	45%
Indwelling catheter	75%†	29%

*Urinary incontinence rate based on reported frequency of failure of condom catheter to contain urine ("wet continence").
†Risk is correlated with number of years indwelling catheter is used to manage reflex urinary incontinence.
Data from Anson C, Gray M: Secondary urologic complications of spinal injury, *Urol Nurs* 13:107-112, 1993, and Killorin WK, Gray M, Bennett JK, Green BG: Evaluative urodynamics and bladder management in predicting upper urinary tract infection in male spinal cord injury, *Paraplegia* 30:437-441, 1992.

15 years;[58] these investigators found that 30% of these patients experienced episodes of urinary leakage, but none of them developed upper tract distress. Weld and colleagues[100] evaluated renal function in a group of 308 spinal cord–injured patients who were followed for a mean of 18.7 years and found that 1.3% developed proteinuria. When records of a group of 74 spinal cord-injured patients followed for a mean of 18 years were reviewed, 44% of these patients were found to have some type of urologic complication, but none were found to have renal deterioration.[100]

The patient who is managed with a spontaneous voiding program typically perceives the urge to urinate, followed by a brief period of hesitancy. The initial desire to urinate is usually produced by an overactive detrusor contraction, and the gap between this sensation and the onset of urination can be attributed to the presence of DSD. This brief period of hesitancy is usually followed by micturition (or by urinary leakage if the patient cannot reach the toilet within a brief period of time). Because the patient is likely to have compromised mobility or dexterity caused by the underlying neurologic disorder, it is particularly important to maximize access to the toilet and to warn the patient that it will not be feasible to postpone urination for a prolonged period. Issues of mobility, dexterity, and toilet access should be addressed by a rehabilitation-oriented interdisciplinary team. The patient may benefit from referral to a physiatrist or rehabilitation nurse practitioner.

The patient should be assisted to identify and use a hand-held or bedside toilet as indicated. Anticipatory advice about the use of containment devices is indicated, particularly when the person with reflex UI is placed in an environment where toileting opportunities are limited, such as airplane travel or a sporting event. Because the volume of UI is usually significant, the patient should be advised to use a pad that is able to absorb relatively large volumes of urine. Men may be counseled to wear a condom catheter with leg bag drainage. However, these strategies should be reserved for selected situations and periods when toileting opportunities are limited, and the patient should be discouraged from relying on an absorptive pad for daily use.

The patient who retains partial control of the pelvic floor muscles may benefit from pelvic muscle reeducation with biofeedback. Tries[101] has used biofeedback techniques to improve continence among persons with neurologic disorders, including one patient with an incomplete spinal cord injury and UI associated with urgency. Because the level of residual sensation and motor control among patients with incomplete spinal cord injuries varies significantly, it follows that the decision to treat with behavioral methods would be highly selective; review of the literature revealed no large series of behavioral therapy for patients with incomplete spinal injuries and UI. Similarly, transvaginal or transrectal electrical stimulation may benefit selected patients with detrusor hyperreflexia and DSD;

however, a review of the literature revealed no relevant clinical trials.

Because most patients with reflex UI have DSD as well as neurogenic detrusor overactivity, antimuscarinic agents such as oxybutynin or tolterodine must be used with care. Given in larger dosages, these drugs may produce urinary retention, particularly if detrusor muscle contraction strength is also compromised. However, alpha-adrenergic antagonists, such as terazosin, doxazosin, alfuzosin, or tamsulosin, may be beneficial because they reduce urethral resistance; several of these agents (such as terazosin and doxazosin) also exert a mild anticholinergic effect through their actions on the central nervous system.[102] Table 7-3 provides the recommended dosage, administration, side effects, and precautions associated with administration of alpha-adrenergic blocking agents. The patient should also be taught the principles of fluid management to include avoidance of high-volume fluid intake over a short period of time and limitation of bladder irritants.

Patients managing their bladders with spontaneous voiding programs must be counseled regarding their risk for UTI. They should be taught the signs and symptoms of UTI: dysuria, suprapubic discomfort, and lower back pain. They also should be advised that a UTI is likely to produce an acute exacerbation of their UI. This information is particularly important because many patients with a UTI fail to recognize the significance of their worsening incontinence and respond by altering their fluid intake or their prescribed medication until the UTI escalates into a febrile infection.[91]

Reflex Voiding

Some patients with reflex UI may be managed by a "reflex," or "trigger," voiding program. In this program, the bladder empties by means of overactive contractions, and urinary leakage is contained by a condom catheter attached to a drainage bag. Because there is no adequate external collection device for women, the reflex voiding program is currently limited to men.

If a strict definition of continence is applied, a reflex voiding program does not provide for continence. Rather, the goal of management is to contain the urine and to maintain skin integrity. Joseph and colleagues have defined a goal of "wet continence" for the management of these patients;[103] rather than seeking to prevent urinary leakage, the nurse seeks to enable the patient to contain urine within a drainage system, to prevent soiling of clothing, and to eliminate odor. Using similar criteria to evaluate the success of a reflex voiding program in a group of 431 patients, Anson and Gray found that 70% experienced intermittent problems with urinary containment.[58]

Urinary containment relies on the successful application of a condom catheter. The selection of the condom catheter is particularly important because it represents the most likely point of containment failure. The ideal catheter should contain all urinary leakage while maintaining the integrity of the penile skin. It should fit snugly over the penile shaft but should provide sufficient distensibility to accommodate changes in penile circumference associated with erection. Many condom catheters are manufactured of latex, and these work well for many patients; however, other patients with reflex UI, especially those with myelodysplasia or allergies to latex, are unable to tolerate natural latex in contact with the skin.[104] For these patients, there are condom catheters made of alternative materials such as silicone. As discussed in Chapter 11, the condom catheter must be sized correctly to fit the penis. Various sizes are available, and most companies provide measuring guides. The clinician should consider both the length and the circumference of the catheter; the condom should generally cover most or all of the shaft of the penis and should fit snugly but not tightly. The catheter should have a reinforced end that resists twisting and kinking and that drains freely so urine does not pool.

A watertight seal is critical and may be obtained either through adhesive or by a constrictive band or balloon. Self-adhesive catheters are available and are simple for the patient or caregiver to apply; however, the patient must be monitored for any sensitivity to the adhesive. Other catheters are secured by a constrictive band or a balloon; if this type of device is used for the patient with reflex UI, it is *critical* to avoid excess pressure against the

TABLE 7-3   Alpha-Adrenergic Antagonists

AGENT	DOSAGE (APPLIES TO ALL AGENTS LISTED)	ADMINISTRATION	POTENTIAL SIDE EFFECTS (APPLIES TO ALL AGENTS LISTED)	NURSING CONSIDERATIONS
Terazosin (Hytrin)	Initial dosage, 1 mg	Titrate slowly to maximum of 5 to 10 mg HS	Orthostatic hypotension (exacerbated by dehydration)	Orthostatic hypotension can be significant. Advise the patient to take the drug at HS. arise slowly and dangle the legs briefly before getting out of bed. Missing more than two doses may cause severe orthostatic hypotension (when medications taken again); it may be necessary to retitrate the drug to a therapeutic dose.
Doxazosin (Cardura)	Initial dosage, 1 mg	Titrate slowly to maximum of 4 to 8 mg HS		
Tamsulosin (Flomax)	0.4 to 0.8 mg	Administer at HS	Drowsiness	Titration is not required; one may start patients at either 0.4 or 0.8 mg.
			Headache (uncommon) Profound fatigue (uncommon)	This is rare, but it may necessitate discontinuation of the alpha-adrenergic antagonists.
			Rhinitis	Advise the patient to avoid taking a decongestant for rhinitis. Decongestants contain an alpha-adrenergic agonist, which interferes with the intended action of the alpha-adrenergic antagonists.
Alfuzosin	10 mg	Administer 1 hour after a meal	Dizziness	No initial dose titration is needed. This is associated with reduced risk for retrograde ejaculation as compared with other agents.

HS, At hour of sleep.

penile shaft. Patients with reduced sensation are particularly vulnerable to pressure injuries, and some clinicians consider sensory compromise a contraindication to this type of external device.[105,106] One device (BioDerm, St. Petersburg, Fla.) uses ostomy technology to create a watertight seal at the level of the glans; a flower-shaped hydrocolloid adhesive wafer with a soft outflow connector is attached to the glans penis by use of heat and gentle pressure, reinforced with a hydrocolloid wafer formed into a semicircular band, and attached to a drainage bag (Fig. 7-11). This device has proved effective for many patients, although several weeks may be required before long-term adherence of a single device is consistently achieved.

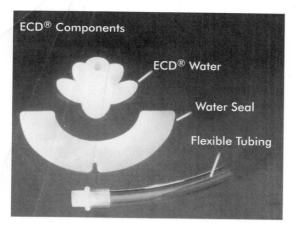

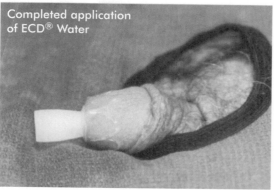

Fig. 7-11 This male containment device incorporates ostomy technology to achieve urinary containment. (Courtesy of Bioderm, Inc, St. Petersburg, Fla.)

The drainage bag must also be carefully selected. General features to consider in selecting a drainage bag are detailed in Chapter 10. For the patient with reflex UI, the drainage mechanism deserves special attention; the drain port must provide security from leakage but should allow the patient with reduced dexterity and hand strength to open and close the mechanism with a sweeping motion of the thumb or hand.

Once the external containment device and drainage system are selected, the patient or caregiver must be taught how to change the device and how to manage the system. Most patients with reflex UI being managed with condom drainage are taught to change the device daily; although some patients can "keep the condom on" for longer periods, this is generally discouraged because of the increased risk for UTI.[107,108] The importance of meticulous skin care is emphasized, as is the importance of promptly reporting any lesion on the penile skin.

Although many patients find the concept of a reflex voiding program attractive, the clinician should be aware that this management approach is associated with a significant risk of upper urinary tract distress (29% to 32%).[52,58,100] This is primarily attributable to the outlet obstruction created by DSD. Theoretically, skeletal muscle relaxants such as baclofen or diazepam could be used to reduce the activity of the striated sphincter muscle; unfortunately, the dosages required to relieve DSD are so high that the side effects and toxicities outweigh any potential therapeutic benefit.[109]

Although oral skeletal muscle relaxants have not proved beneficial in the management of DSD, intrathecal administration of baclofen has been found to relieve skeletal muscle spasticity and pain related to a variety of spinal disorders.[110] This treatment has also been found to relieve the obstruction produced by DSD in some patients; however, it carries significant risks and is therefore reserved for generalized and disabling skeletal muscle spasticity.[111-113]

In contrast to skeletal muscle relaxants, alpha-adrenergic blocking agents have proved beneficial in the management of patients with reflex UI.[114-117] Alpha-adrenergic blocking agents exert several beneficial effects: (1) they reduce the magnitude of obstruction caused by DSD, (2) they reduce urethral smooth muscle tone,[116] (3) they reduce maximum detrusor contraction pressure,[115,117] and (4) they lower residual urinary volumes and improve quality of life (as assessed by a single item on the International Prostate Symptom Score).[114] Terazosin and doxazosin must be titrated to reach optimal therapeutic dosages, whereas alfuzosin and tamsulosin require no titration. The spinal cord–injured patient with reflex UI should be evaluated for dehydration or a low serum sodium level before treatment with one of these drugs is begun; any abnormalities should be corrected before the initiation of therapy to minimize the risk for dizziness or postural hypotension. The risk for these side effects is also minimized by instructing the patient to take the drug immediately before sleep and to consult a health care provider if more than one dose is inadvertently missed.

If the patient does not respond adequately to pharmacotherapy, a sphincterotomy may be considered. The transurethral sphincterotomy has traditionally been used to treat DSD; however, this procedure has significant disadvantages. There is a significant risk of bleeding that persists for several days; in addition, although this procedure provides excellent short-term results,[118] its durability is limited, and it typically produces intrinsic sphincter deficiency that may complicate subsequent bladder management efforts. Studies indicate that significant numbers of patients develop complications such as impaired detrusor contractility or bladder neck dyssynergia, and the success rate (that is, the number of patients who are able to maintain a reflex voiding program for at least 4 years) is low.[119-121]

Because of the limitations of transurethral sphincterotomy, alternative methods of striated sphincter ablation have been explored. Rivas and colleagues used a contact neodymium:yttrium-aluminum-garnet laser to ablate the striated sphincter; they found less bleeding and excellent initial results but did not report on long-term results.[90] Other approaches include balloon dilation and the injection of botulin-A toxin, which produces prolonged muscle paralysis. Both these procedures provided excellent short-term results; however, no long-term studies are yet available, and any alternative procedure must be compared with the traditional procedure over a period of at least 4 years.[122]

Another alternative to standard sphincterotomy is the urethral stent.[123] It consists of a stainless steel circular device that is placed at the level of the membranous urethra under endoscopic guidance. (A suprapubic catheter is placed temporarily to provide urinary drainage until edema and any AD subside.) Initially, the stent is easily observed on endoscopy, but the urethral mucosa ultimately covers the stent, giving the overlying mucosa a cobblestone appearance. This procedure has been shown to reduce urethral resistance, lower detrusor contraction pressure, and improve patient satisfaction with the bladder management program.[87,123] The stent provides a viable alternative to transurethral sphincterotomy. Advantages of the urethral stent include reduced risk of bleeding, avoidance of the erectile dysfunction caused by transurethral sphincterotomy, reduced hospital stay, and the "reversible" nature of the procedure. However, bladder neck dyssynergia occurs in approximately 20% of patients and typically requires transurethral incision of the bladder neck. In addition, removal of the urethral stent is not straightforward, particularly after the device has been left in place for 1 year or longer.

Intermittent Catheterization

IC provides regular evacuation of the bladder by in-and-out catheterization. The patient is typically taught to self-catheterize using clean technique; care providers or family members may also be taught the procedure. A detailed discussion of this management technique is provided in Chapter 8; the discussion in this chapter focuses on indications for IC among patients with reflex UI and management issues specific to this patient population.

IC is effective because it provides regular, complete bladder evacuation for the patient with a neurologic disorder resulting in reflex UI. Most patients who maintain at least partial dexterity of the upper extremities are candidates for this procedure. IC as a management program may initially appear undesirable; however, it has advantages that make it an attractive option when considered carefully by the patient and caregiver. Among spinal cord–injured patients, IC ranks second only to spontaneous voiding in preservation of upper tract function; Anson and Gray found that fewer than 10% of their patients managed with IC experienced upper tract distress,[58] and Weld and associates[124] found that only 1% had proteinuria. From the patient's perspective, the benefits of IC also include reduced effect on body image (as compared with indwelling catheter or reflex voiding with condom containment, both of which require externally obvious drainage systems) and reduced risk for skin damage. The unaltered appearance of the perineum and genitalia may also promote sexual adjustment.

Despite its advantages, an IC program is associated with certain risks. In addition to the potential for upper tract distress among a small group of patients, there is an 18% risk of bladder calculi and a 9% risk of epididymitis among men.[58] The risk for bacteriuria approaches 100%; however, this statistic must be interpreted in light of the relatively low risk for symptomatic UTI, particularly when compared with patients managed with an indwelling catheter. The risk for UI among patients being managed with IC has not been adequately studied. Gray, Rayome, and Anson studied 116 patients with spinal cord injuries who were managed by IC; among this group, 45% reported perfect continence. Among the remaining 55%, more than half reported only occasional leakage (less than once per week), 10% leaked one to two times per week, and 37% leaked daily or every other day. The majority of these subjects leaked only small amounts, but 45% had sufficient volume of leakage to require a pad, containment brief, or condom catheter.[91] The prevalence of leakage between catheterizations among patients with other neurologic conditions resulting in reflex UI is not known.

Although patients may be initially hesitant to adopt IC as a bladder management program, the long-term compliance with this program is substantial. Gray, Rayome, and Anson reported a compliance rate of 95%,[91] and Chai and colleagues reported a compliance rate of 71%.[125] Harrison and Kuric accurately stated the issue of compliance as one of adjusting to the best possible solution for bladder management, as opposed to simply choosing the most convenient method; this underscores the importance of thorough and individualized education for the patient and family dealing with reflex UI and of collaborative decision–making, with the patient as an integral part of the team.[126]

Some unique issues must be addressed when an IC program is initiated for the patient with reflex UI. These patients typically have limited mobility affecting the lower and possibly the upper extremities; it is frequently advantageous to involve the occupational therapist or physical therapist in developing assistive devices and in maximizing wheelchair mobility. These strategies can prove invaluable in helping the individual to compensate for limitations in strength or dexterity. There is at least one device available to assist the female patient who has limited sight or compromised upper extremity function to locate the urethra and perform self-catheterization. This lightweight L-shaped plastic device has two "arms"; one arm is inserted into the vagina, and the other arm extends over the urethra with openings that align with the urethra and facilitate catheter insertion.[127]

If the patient is unable to perform self-catheterization even with the use of assistive devices, it may be necessary to teach one or more caregivers the procedure. Instruction of a family member or caregiver is also beneficial for the patient who is "routinely" independent with catheterization, so backup is available when needed (as during periods of illness). The patient is also taught how to direct another person through the procedure. In teaching patients and caregivers, it is important to keep the procedure simple and to emphasize a clean as opposed to sterile approach.

Medications in Conjunction with Intermittent Catheterization

IC as a single strategy is typically inadequate for management of the patient with reflex UI; overactive detrusor contractions occurring between catheterizations in response to various stimuli may cause frequent episodes of leakage. Therefore, antimuscarinic medications are commonly used to control neurogenic detrusor overactivity. Multiple anticholinergic or antimuscarinic drugs are available and appropriate for these patients; typically, these medications must be administered in significant doses, and multiple agents may be required (Table 7-4). It is usually advisable to begin with a single agent (such as oxybutynin, tolterodine, or trospium). If a second agent is needed, it is best to select one with slightly different pharmacologic properties (such as imipramine) or a different route of administration (such as adding transdermal oxybutynin to oral tolterodine or trospium).

In teaching the patient with reflex UI about the principles and specifics of his or her bladder management program, it is important to include strategies for management of recurrent leakage. Patients should be instructed to avoid significant restrictions of fluid intake unless specifically directed to do so by their health care provider. They should be taught to recognize recurrent leakage as a potential sign of UTI and should know that they should return to the clinic for urinalysis and microscopic urine examination should this develop. If the urinalysis and microscopic examination reveal UTI, the patient is treated appropriately. If the examination is negative for UTI, it may be necessary to alter the patient's antispasmodic medications or fluid intake program.

TABLE 7-4 Anticholinergic Drugs Used to Treat Reflex Urinary Incontinence

AGENT AND USUAL DOSAGE (ADULTS)	COMMON SIDE EFFECTS	NURSING CONSIDERATIONS
Immediate-release oxybutynin (Ditropan IR: 5 mg two to three times daily)	Dry mouth	This side effect can be significant and can interfere with speaking, singing, or eating.
Extended-release oxybutynin (Ditropan XL:5 to −15 mg once daily)		Encourage the patient to drink adequate amounts of fluids, chew gum, or suck on hard candy to stimulate salivation.
Extended-release tolterodine (Detrol LA: 4 mg once daily)	Intolerance to heat	Heat intolerance with flushing, fatigue, or fever when patients are exposed to heat is particularly significant for children, for the elderly, and for some individuals with a spinal cord injury or disorder that interferes with normal mechanisms for managing body temperature.
Trospium (Sanctura:20 mg twice daily)		
Transdermal oxybutynin (Oxytrol:3.9–mg/day; patch applied twice weekly)		Advise the patient of the potential for heat intolerance. Dosage may require adjustment during warmer weather.
	Blurred vision	This condition is typically limited to fine print and dissipates after the first 5 to 7 days of administration. Significant, persistent blurred vision requires adjustment of the dose or discontinuation of the anticholinergic drug.
	Confusion, altered mentation	This condition indicates drug toxicity and necessitates discontinuation or dose adjustment. Elderly patients are particularly susceptible to this side effect.
	Constipation	This may be significant, particularly for the patient with reflex urinary incontinence and limited mobility or impaired abdominal muscle tone. A change in the patient's bowel management program may be required.
	Increased intraocular pressure	This is significant for patients with narrow-angle glaucoma. It is essential to consult with an ophthalmologist before prescribing an anticholinergic medication for a patient with narrow-angle glaucoma.

If the patient with reflex UI has persistent unexplained leakage between catheterizations, repeat urodynamic evaluation may be indicated because the persistent leakage may represent a significant change in bladder function, with an associated change in risk for upper urinary tract distress.[91]

Patient education for patients managed by IC also includes nonpharmacologic measures to reduce the risk for urinary leakage between catheterizations. Appropriate measures include adequate volume fluid intake, with fluids spaced as evenly as possible, and avoidance of high volume intake over a short period of time. (The goal is to avoid overdistending the bladder between catheterizations, because bladder distension triggers detrusor overactivity and subsequent UI.) The patient is also instructed that caffeine acts as a bladder irritant and is likely to increase the risk for UI between catheterizations. Some patients who experience leakage will alter the schedule or dosage of their prescribed antimuscarinic medications or increase the frequency of catheterization.[91] However, patients should be advised *not* to alter medication dosages or schedules without consulting with their care provider, because doses in excess of recommended limits may produce adverse side effects. It may or may not be advisable to change the schedule for catheterization, and the patient should be reminded once again that unexplained leakage may represent UTI or a change in bladder function.

Reflex Voiding and Intermittent Catheterization

Some male patients with reflex UI manage their bladders with a combination of reflex voiding and IC; the combined strategy provides for complete bladder evacuation on a regular basis and also provides for containment of leakage between catheterizations. Nevertheless, this approach is associated with a relatively high risk of serious urinary complications, including UTI. One factor that increases the risk for UTI is the abundance of bacteria on the penile skin of patients managed with condom catheters.[128,129] In their study, Anson and Gray found that the combination of reflex voiding and IC was associated with more serious urinary tract complications than any other management

program, except for an indwelling catheter.[58] Therefore, this combination is recommended only when it represents the sole alternative to placement of an indwelling catheter.

Indwelling Catheter

Guidelines for insertion and management of indwelling catheters are reviewed in Chapter 10. The discussion in this chapter is therefore limited to the implications of long-term catheterization in the patient with reflex UI and management considerations unique to this population.

On initial consideration, the indwelling catheter appears to be an attractive bladder management option for the patient with reflex UI; it provides continuous urinary drainage, which prevents complications associated with high-pressure detrusor contractions and DSD, and it eliminates the necessity for chronic IC. A urethral catheter presents a barrier to sexual function, but this can be minimized by use of a suprapubic catheter. However, when viewed from a long-term perspective, an indwelling catheter presents the greatest risk for upper tract distress, significant risk for urinary leakage, and the highest rate of patient dissatisfaction (when compared with all other bladder management programs outlined in this discussion).[58] Trop and Bennett reported a 29% risk for urethral erosion leading to intrinsic sphincter deficiency and severe stress UI in patients who had indwelling catheters for prolonged periods (6 to 36 years).[130] Weld and Dmochowski[100] found evidence of urologic complications in 54% of a group of 61 patients managed by indwelling catheterization for a mean period of 18 years. In addition, Weld and associates[124] found increased incidence of proteinuria and a significantly higher mean serum creatinine in patients managed with indwelling catheters as opposed to those managed by CIC or spontaneous voiding.

Indwelling catheterization is also associated with an increased risk of bladder cancer; chronically catheterized paraplegic patients have been found to have a 2% to 10% risk of tumor development, typically squamous cell carcinoma.[131,132] This risk is attributed to chronic inflammation, but the precise mechanisms resulting in cellular mutation in these patients remain unknown.[133] The risk for cancer is greater among patients with bladder stones, which justifies annual monitoring with urine cytology, and possibly endoscopy.[134]

Despite these risks, it is unrealistic to state that an indwelling catheter should be avoided at all costs among patients with reflex UI. Short-term catheterization may be required for the treatment of pressure ulcers or for monitoring of urine output during acute illnesses. However, long-term catheterization should be used only when it represents the best management option for that patient, that is, in situations in which other strategies are not feasible. Examples of appropriate use include the terminally ill patient, the patient with altered mentation who is unable to cooperate with alternative programs, or a patient with a high cervical lesion for whom an indwelling catheter permits home management with limited assistance (as from family members who work during the day) as opposed to institutionalization.

When an indwelling catheter is selected as the best management option for an individual patient, it is important to select the catheterization site thoughtfully and then to select a catheter that best meets that patient's needs.[59] For many patients with a paralyzing neurologic disorder and reflex UI, a suprapubic cystostomy site offers significant advantages as compared with urethral catheterization. The suprapubic site eliminates the risk for urethral erosion, removes the catheter from the bacteria-laden perineum, and facilitates sexual adjustment. However, there are potential disadvantages; initial placement of the catheter requires minor surgery, and patients with stress UI may leak from the urethra despite the presence of the catheter. The decision regarding placement should be made in close consultation with the patient, urologist, and primary care provider.

Additional decisions to be made regarding an indwelling catheter include size and material of catheter, size of balloon, and type of drainage system to be used.[59] The long-term catheter should be constructed from a material that minimizes mucosal irritation and reduces the risk for latex hypersensitivity, such as an all-silicone catheter. A silver oxide–coated catheter is also now available and is reported to reduce catheter-associated bacteriuria. However, protection is transient (for about 2 weeks), and it has not been found to reduce UTI risk in the patient with a long-term indwelling catheter.[135-140] Catheter size and balloon size are important because a large catheter predisposes the individual to inflammation of the urethra and bladder base, which increases the risk of detrusor overactivity, urinary leakage, and/or UTI.[141] It is recommended that most adults use a 14- to 16-French catheter with a 5-mL balloon filled with 10 mL of fluid and that a larger catheter be used *only* if urethral erosion has already occurred and the leakage around the catheter is being caused by stress UI. If urethral erosion has not been proved, the clinician should suspect overactive detrusor contractions as the source of the leakage, and management should address the etiologic factors for the overactive contractions. The drainage system must provide adequate capacity (that is, 500 mL for leg bags and 2000 mL for bedside drainage bags) and must contain an antireflux valve to prevent the backflow of urine from the bag to the bladder.[141] The patient and caregiver must be taught the proper management of the indwelling catheter and the drainage system. Issues related to selection and management of indwelling catheters are discussed further in Chapter 10.

The patient with reflex UI and an indwelling catheter should be taught strategies for prevention of UTI and should also be taught how to recognize a symptomatic UTI. Adequate fluid intake is one of the most critical preventive measures because this helps to flush pathogens from the urinary system.[59] Another preventive measure is maintenance of a closed system whenever feasible (see Chapter10). Although antibiotic therapy is essential for the management of symptomatic UTI, suppressive antimicrobial drugs are not recommended because they increase rather than decrease the risk of symptomatic UTI with resistant organisms.[94,95] Indicators of UTI include hematuria, fever, sudden onset or exacerbation of AD or spasticity, or sudden onset of urinary leakage around the catheter (sometimes called "catheter bypassing"). Should these signs occur, a urine specimen should be promptly obtained from a newly placed catheter.

(The specimen should *never* be obtained from the drainage bag because pathogens in this urine do not represent those present in the lower urinary tract.)

MANAGEMENT OF SEQUELAE AND COMPLICATIONS

The clinician caring for individuals with reflex UI must be prepared to manage the potential complications associated with this condition, the most common of which are AD, UTI, urinary calculi, and upper tract distress.

Autonomic Dysreflexia

The primary management of AD involves identification and removal of the specific stimulus triggering the episode of sympathetic hyperreflexia. Multiple stimuli have been shown to produce AD, but distension of the bladder and detrusor hyperreflexia with DSD are the most common provocative conditions.[88,130] Other genitourinary stimuli for AD include catheterization, cystoscopy, bladder irrigation, urodynamic testing, bladder spasm in the presence of an indwelling catheter, UTI, testicular torsion, epididymitis, pressure on the testicles or glans penis, intraoperative manipulation of the renal pelvis, insertion of a vaginal speculum, electroejaculation, and sexual intercourse (in both women and men). Rectal distension is postulated to be the second most common cause of AD. Additional stimuli include rectal manipulation for bowel management, enema administration, rectal instrumentation, gastritis, gastric ulcer, ingrown nails, infection or débridement of pressure ulcers, tight clothing, and tight leg straps. In many situations, the stimulus for the episode of AD is readily apparent; in other cases, the cause of the AD is unclear, and several interventions may be required to relieve the severe hypertension and associated symptoms. When one is in doubt as to the cause, appropriate management includes positioning the patient in an upright position, evacuating the bladder, loosening any constrictive clothing, and discontinuing any instrumentation or diagnostic procedure; in addition, a 10-mg nifedipine capsule can be pierced with a needle and the fluid administered sublingually.[142] After these immediate measures to control the hypertension, additional evaluation is undertaken

to rule out bowel distension, a noxious skin lesion, or systemic infection; treatment is initiated as indicated to eliminate the stimulus for AD. In addition, patients who experience recurring episodes of AD are prescribed pharmacologic suppression, typically a long-acting alpha-adrenergic blocking agent such as terazosin,[143] titrated to a therapeutic level (2 to 5 mg) and administered routinely. It is important to understand that this drug is effective only as a suppressive agent and not as a treatment for an acute episode of AD.

Urinary Tract Infection

As has been explained, treatment of UTI should be limited to two groups: patients with symptomatic infections and patients with both pyuria and bacteriuria.[144] Because these infections are, by definition, classified as complicated UTIs, treatment should be culture specific and should last for 7 to 14 days; if there is suspicion of persistent or relapsing infection, treatment should be followed by urinalysis with microscopic exam or by repeat culture. Oral agents are preferred unless the patient has severe nausea or vomiting or urosepsis is suspected; in these cases, treatment is begun with intravenous antibiotic therapy and switched to an oral antibiotic when the patient is tolerating oral fluids and the sepsis is controlled. Ideally, the least expensive drug that is effective is ordered; daily or twice-daily dosing is also an advantage. Broad-spectrum antibiotics such as the fluoroquinolones should be reserved for UTIs that are resistant to the more common agents, to minimize the risk that the individual will develop resistant pathogens. The patient with a UTI is encouraged to drink an adequate volume of fluids, but forcing fluids is *not* recommended, because this dilutes the concentration of antibiotic in the urine.

After resolution of the acute UTI, management shifts to the prevention of future episodes. The bladder management program is evaluated and modified as indicated; for example, a febrile UTI may provide the impetus for removal of an indwelling catheter or for reevaluation of the severity of DSD and the frequency of catheter changes in the male patient previously managed with reflex voiding and condom containment. The patient's fluid intake should be reviewed and measures established as needed to reverse dehydration. The patient is instructed in the rationale for each of these measures; frequently, patients ask about prophylactic antibiotics, and the rationale for selective use of antibiotics must be explained as well.

The patient with reflex UI who develops recurring UTIs requires careful evaluation of the history of the previous infections and may need additional diagnostic studies. If a urease-producing pathogen is identified or if the same pathogen accounts for multiple infections, a KUB (kidneys, ureter, upper bladder) examination and an upper tract imaging study are justified.[82] If there is no evidence of a urinary calculus or if new-onset hydronephrosis is identified, videourodynamic evaluation is indicated to determine whether there has been an increase in the hostile potential of the bladder, which would predispose to urinary infections.

Upper Urinary Tract Distress

Upper urinary tract distress, as evidenced by febrile UTIs, renal insufficiency, dilatation of the renal pelvis or ureter, or vesicoureteral reflux, typically occurs as a result of bladder dysfunction (the organ to which the kidneys must drain). Therefore, management of the patient with reflex UI and upper tract distress is frequently directed toward the bladder, rather than the upper urinary tract. For example, a child with Hinman syndrome would appropriately be treated with pelvic muscle reeducation and biofeedback before consideration of ureteral reimplantation to correct reflux.

To reduce the potential for a hostile bladder to cause upper tract distress, treatment must reduce detrusor pressure forces; during bladder filling, these forces are reflected by the compliance of the bladder wall, and during micturition, they are evidenced by detrusor contractility or contraction pressure (see Chapter 12). Several strategies can be used to reduce detrusor forces in the bladder, thus relieving upper urinary tract distress. This discussion focuses on alterations in bladder management that are usually effective in reducing upper tract distress.

Changing the bladder management program represents a relatively straightforward and effective approach to reduction of upper tract distress. For example, a patient currently being managed by a reflex voiding program may be switched to IC, with administration of antispasmodic medications to reduce detrusor forces as well as leakage. The patient with an indwelling catheter may have the catheter removed, and a reflex voiding or IC program may then be initiated. Upper tract distress may also be relieved by measures that reduce the severity of the obstruction produced by DSD; alpha-adrenergic antagonists, sphincterotomy, and placement of a urethral stent all represent strategies for reducing urethral resistance.

Unfortunately, these measures may be inadequate when the compliance is very low (less than 10 mL/cm H_2O) and the detrusor LPP is elevated (greater than 40 cm H_2O). (See Chapter 12 for further explanations of these urodynamic findings.) Low compliance may reflect trabeculation and fibrosis within the bladder wall; these processes result in a detrusor that is refractory to antispasmodic medications (which normally reduce smooth muscle contractility). Even an IC program may be inadequate to relieve the dangerously high pressures associated with bladder filling in this situation. In this case, surgical reconstruction of the lower urinary tract is required to preserve renal function and ultimately the life of the individual.

Many surgical techniques can be used to transform a high-pressure bladder into a low-pressure reservoir. Augmentation cystoplasty is one approach;[145] in this procedure, the dome of the bladder is split, and the bladder is opened in a clam-type configuration (Fig. 7-12). A segment of bowel is then isolated from the fecal stream with its mesentery attached, detubularized, and anastomosed to the bladder[146] (Fig. 7-13). This procedure provides an excellent urinary reservoir from a urodynamic perspective; however, it is not without complications.[146] For example, because the bowel segment continues to produce mucus, ongoing mucus management is required for the majority of patients. There is also the potential for metabolic complications because of the potential for the bowel segment to absorb urinary salts (chloride and ammonium); specifically, these patients may develop a mild hyperchloremic metabolic acidosis. This can be a serious

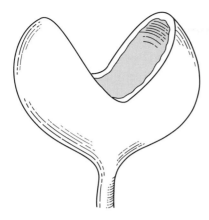

Fig. 7-12 Bladder is bivalved in preparation for augmentation.

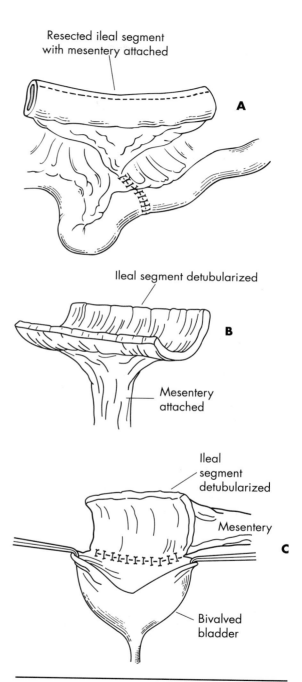

Fig. 7-13 Segment of bowel is isolated from the fecal stream, **A,** and is opened to form a U- or W-shaped configuration, **B,** that is anastomosed to the bivalved bladder. **C,** Section of stomach or an enlarged ureter may be substituted for bowel in certain patients.

problem for the patient with renal insufficiency, who is unable to compensate for this reabsorption phenomenon and who therefore requires ongoing electrolyte management. Finally, use of the terminal ileum to augment the bladder can lead to impaired absorption of vitamin B_{12}, although this deficiency does not usually become apparent for the first 1 or 2 years after surgery (because large volumes of vitamin B_{12} are typically stored in the liver). For these patients, lifelong vitamin B_{12} supplementation may be required. Gastrocystoplasty and autoaugmentation have been advocated as alternatives to augmentation enterocystoplasty, but they are no longer widely used.[147-151]

A continent urinary diversion provides another alternative to augmentation enterocystoplasty. This procedure involves the creation of a low-pressure reservoir using bowel or stomach and construction of a continent catheterizable channel between the reservoir and an abdominal stoma; the "channel" and stoma may be created from bowel, the appendix, or a ureteral segment[152] (Fig. 7-14). There are several specific approaches to creation of a continent diversion; the variations relate to the segment of bowel used, the surgical configuration of the reservoir, and the structure and surgical approach used to create the continent catheterizable channel. In construction of the reservoir, the goal should be a roughly spheric structure

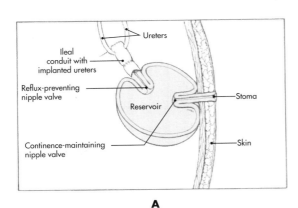

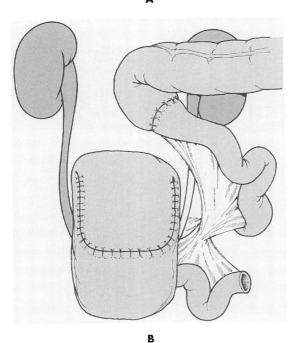

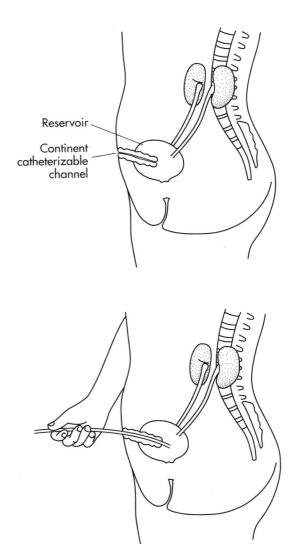

Fig. 7-14 Continent urinary diversions. **A,** Kock pouch. **B,** Indiana pouch. (**A** from Belcher A: *Cancer nursing,* Mosby's clinical nursing series, St. Louis, 1992, Mosby; **B** from Gray M: *Genitourinary disorders,* Mosby's clinical nursing series, St. Louis, 1992, Mosby.)

Fig. 7-15 The Mitrofanoff procedure uses the appendix or ureter to create a continent, catheterizable stoma.

because this configuration best reproduces the high compliance associated with the intrinsic bladder. Structures used to create the continent catheterizable channel include intussuscepted segments of bowel, the ileocecal valve, the appendix, the ureter, and even the fallopian tube[152-154] (Fig. 7-15).

Regardless of the type of surgical procedure used to create a low-pressure reservoir, the patient must be counseled regarding its effect on bladder management and life style. For many patients, augmentation cystoplasty or continent urinary diversion improves their quality of life and their satisfaction with their bladder management program,[145,155,156] in addition to preserving their life and arresting renal damage. Many patients are able to discontinue the use of anticholinergic medications and to dramatically reduce the number of catheterizations needed over a 24-hour period. In addition, the creation of a continent abdominal stoma facilitates catheterization and independence for many patients who have difficulty accessing and catheterizing the urethra while sitting in a wheelchair. The risk of urinary leakage caused by hyperreflexic contractions is eliminated or greatly reduced, as is the potential for febrile UTIs and their associated morbidity.

There are obviously many advantages to augmentation cystoplasty and continent urinary diversion in the management of reflex UI. However, the patient must realize that either of these procedures will alter their bladder management program and carries responsibilities and risks, which some patients consider to be negative. For example, all continent diversions and augmentation procedures commit the patient or caregiver to regular IC for the rest of the patient's life. In addition, some patients develop metabolic complications that require ongoing correction by medications. The patient who undergoes augmentation or continent diversion involving bowel segments may produce significant amounts of mucus and may require frequent bladder irrigations during the early postoperative period; some patients require long-term ingestion of hippuric acid or orally administered mucolytic agents to reduce mucus production. Patients whose continent urinary diversion involves resection of a significant amount of terminal ileum must be monitored for vitamin B_{12} deficiency, and many require monthly supplementation for life.

Because of these management issues, patients and caregivers must understand the care demands associated with any planned surgical intervention. Some patients may find a standard ileal conduit to be a preferable approach to protecting the upper tracts while limiting daily care demands. The continence nurse plays an important role in preoperative counseling; the goal is to clearly present the advantages, disadvantages, and management issues for each of the surgical options and to assist the patient and caregivers to select the option that is most compatible with their life style and management preferences.

SUMMARY

Reflex UI is one of the most difficult types of incontinence to manage because it involves loss of normal innervation to the bladder or the sphincter, or to both, and is typically associated with devastating injuries or illnesses that produce significant loss of sensory and motor function in addition to the disturbances in bowel and bladder function. In addition, the pathologic changes in bladder and sphincter function associated with reflex UI create a potentially "hostile" bladder that is likely to cause upper tract distress and eventual renal insufficiency. Management for any patient must be individualized and based on a comprehensive and thorough assessment; any management plan must address preservation of renal function as well as the control of urinary leakage. Major treatment options include voluntary voiding, reflex voiding with condom containment, IC, medications to reduce bladder or sphincter contractility, indwelling catheters, and surgical intervention to create a low-pressure reservoir for urine. Effective implementation of any bladder management plan requires a team approach in which the patient and caregiver or caregivers are integral members of the team; the continence nurse is also a critical member of the team and typically assumes primary responsibility for ongoing patient assessment, education, and counseling.

SELF-ASSESSMENT EXERCISE

1. Define the term "reflex incontinence," incorporating the consistent elements from the International Continence Society definition and the NANDA definition.

2. Define the terms "neurogenic detrusor overactivity" and "detrusor-sphincter dyssynergia."

3. Explain the following statement: "Reflex UI occurs only in individuals with spinal cord lesions affecting segments C2-S1; individuals with lesions above C2 typically experience urge incontinence, and those with lesions below S1 typically experience overflow incontinence."

4. Identify the two primary pathophysiologic "effects" of reflex UI and the significance of each to patient assessment and management.

5. Select an appropriate management plan for each of the following patients; briefly explain your rationale for each.

    a. 26-year-old man whose status is 3 months post spinal cord injury at T10 as a result of a motor vehicle accident. He works as a programmer analyst and is very motivated to achieve continence. He has good dexterity and mobility of upper body; he is now wheelchair bound. Urodynamic studies indicate detrusor-sphincter dyssynergia with moderately high postvoid residuals (150 to 200 mL). Compliance is normal at this time; bladder capacity on urodynamic study is 400 mL. He has no sensory awareness of bladder filling. He has had two febrile UTIs since his injury (managed with indwelling catheter for 3 weeks and subsequently with reflex voiding and condom containment).

    b. 41-year old woman with MS and reflex UI. She has had MS for 15 years and is now chair and bed bound. She is able to perform weight shifts and to get around her home with her motorized chair, and she has enough upper extremity dexterity to prepare and eat simple meals; however, she is unable to transfer from the chair to the bed or vice versa. She lives at home with her husband, who works, and her daughter, who is in school. Her bowel function is being controlled with alternate-day administration of a suppository by her husband. She has managed her bladder with IC but is now unable to reposition herself sufficiently to access the urethra; she is referred to you for modification in her bladder management program. Her urodynamic studies indicate DSD, normal compliance, capacity of 300 mL.

    c. 18-year-old man who is 4 weeks post spinal cord injury (C6-C7) incurred in motorcycle accident. He lives with girlfriend, who will help him when she is there, but she works long hours as a waitress. He has no sensory awareness of need to urinate; urodynamic studies indicate minimal DSD, normal compliance, well-sustained hyperreflexic contractions, and postvoid residual of 25 mL. He has been told about IC but states that he does *not* want to put any tubes in his penis and he does *not* want to be "tied to the clock."

6. Match the following categories of medications to the patient situations, and list key side effects to be addressed in patient teaching:
    - Anticholinergics
    - Alpha-adrenergic antagonists
    a. Patient being maintained on reflex voiding/condom containment program whose urodynamic studies indicate moderate bladder outflow obstruction secondary to DSD.
    b. Patient being maintained on IC program who frequently leaks between catheterizations because of hyperreflexic contractions.

7. Rate each of the following statements as true or false, and briefly explain your answer:
    a. _____ Prophylactic and suppressive antibiotic therapies are recommended for the patient with reflex UI because of the risk for UTI and upper tract damage.
    b. _____ AD is a potentially fatal complication for the patient with a cervical or upper thoracic spinal cord injury and can be precipitated by bladder distension.
    c. _____ Patients with UTIs caused by urease-producing bacteria are at increased risk for the formation of calculi.

8. Explain the role of bladder augmentation and continent urinary diversion in management of patients with reflex UI.

REFERENCES

1. Ackely BJ, Ladwig GB: *Nursing diagnosis handbook,* ed 6, St. Louis, 2002, Mosby.
2. Kim MJ, McFarland GK, McLane AM: *Pocket guide to nursing diagnoses,* St. Louis, 1995, Mosby.
3. Abrams P, Cardozo L, Fall M, et al: The standardization of terminology of lower urinary tract function: report from the Standardization Sub-Committee of the International Continence Society, *Neurourol Urodyn* 21: 167-178, 2002.
4. National Spinal Cord Injury Statistical Center. *Facts & figures at a glance,* August 2004, downloaded 9/15/2004, URL: http://images.main.uab.edu/spinalcord/pdffiles/factsfig.pdf.
5. Clifton GL: Spinal cord injury in the Houston-Galveston area, *Tex Med* 79:55-57, 1983.
6. Fine PT, DeVivo MJ, McEachran AB: Incidence of acute traumatic hospitalized spinal cord injury in the United States, *Am J Epidemiol* 115:475-479, 1982.
7. Griffin MR, Opitz JL, Kurland LT, et al: Traumatic spinal cord injury in Olmstead County, Minnesota, 1935-1981, *Am J Epidemiol* 121:884-895, 1985.
8. Stover SL: Epidemiology of neurogenic bladder, *Rehabil Clin North Am* 4:211-220, 1993.
9. Noonan CW, Kathman SJ, White MC: Prevalence estimates for MS in the United States and evidence of an increasing trend for women, *Neurology* 58(1):136-138, 2002.
10. Anderson DS, Ellenbery JH, Leventhal CM, et al: Revised estimate of the prevalence of multiple sclerosis in the United States, *Ann Neurol* 31:333-336, 1992.
11. Ebers GC, Sadovnick AD: The geographic distribution of multiple sclerosis: a review, *Neuroepidemiology* 12:1-5, 1993.
12. Sadovnick AD, Ebers GC: Epidemiology of multiple sclerosis: a critical overview, *Can J Neurol Sci* 20:17-29, 1993.
13. Bauer SB: Neuropathic dysfunction of the lower urinary tract. In: Walsh PC, Retik A, Vaughan ED, Wein AJ, editors: *Campbell's urology,* ed 8, Philadelphia, 2002, WB Saunders, pp 2231-2261.
14. Ray JG, Meier C, Vermeulen MJ, et al: Association of neural tube defects and folic acid food fortification in Canada, *Lancet* 360(9350):2047-2048, 2002.
15. Bauer SB: Management of the obstructed urinary tract associated with neurogenic bladder dysfunction, *Urol Clin North Am* 17(2):395-406, 1990.
16. Webster GD, El-Mahrouky A, Stone AR, Zakrzewski C: The urological evaluation and management of patients with myelodysplasia, *Br J Urol* 58:261-265, 1986.
17. Allen TD: Forty years experience with voiding dysfunction, *BJU Int* 92(suppl 1):15-22, 2003.
18. Barrington FJF: The nervous control of micturition, *Queens J Exp Physiol* 8:33, 1915.
19. Bradley WE, Teague CT: Spinal organization of micturition reflex afferents, *Exp Neurol* 22:504-516, 1968.
20. deGroat WC, Ryall W: Reflexes to the sacral parasympathetic neurones concerned with micturition in the cat, *J Physiol* (Lond) 200:87-108, 1969.
21. Chancellor MB, Blaivas JG: Detrusor-external sphincter dyssynergia, *Ciba Found Symp Neurobiol Incontinence* 151:195-205, 1990.
22. Yarkony GM: *Spinal cord injury: medical management and rehabilitation,* Gaithersburg, Md., 1994, Aspen.
23. Kennelly MJ, Rudy DC: Incontinence caused by neurologic disease. In: O'Donnell PD, editor: *Urinary incontinence,* St. Louis, 1997, Mosby.
24. Gray M: Nursing planning, intervention, and evaluation for altered urinary function. In: Broadwell Jackson D, Saunders RB, editors: *Child health nursing,* Philadelphia, 1993, JB Lippincott.
25. Paty DW, Noseworthy JG, Ebers GC: Diagnosis of multiple sclerosis. In: Paty DW, Ebers GC, editors: *Multiple sclerosis,* Philadelphia, 1998, FA Davis.
26. Bemelmans BL, Hommes OR, van Kerrebroeck PE, et al: Evidence for early lower urinary tract dysfunction in clinically silent multiple sclerosis, *J Urol* 145:1219-1224, 1991.
27. Thielen KR, Miller GM: Multiple sclerosis of the spinal cord: magnetic resonance appearance, *J Comput Assist Tomogr* 20:434-438, 1996.
28. Vita G, Fazio MC, Milone S, et al: Cardiovascular autonomic dysfunction in multiple sclerosis is likely related to brainstem lesion, *J Neurol Sci* 120:82-86, 1993.
29. Hermieu JF, Delmas V, Boccon-Gibod L: Micturition disturbances and human immunodeficiency virus infection, *J Urol* 156:157-159, 1996.
30. Leach GD, Farsaii A, Kark P, Raz S: Urodynamic manifestations of cerebellar ataxia, *J Urol* 128:348-350, 1982.
31. Bannister R: *Brain and Bannister's clinical neurology,* Oxford, UK, 1991, Oxford University Press.
32. Grbavac Z, Gilja I, Gubarev N, Bozicevic D: Neurologic and urodynamic characteristics of patients with Guillain-Barré syndrome, *Lijec Vjesn* 111:17-20, 1989.
33. Singh NK, Jaiswal AK, Misra S, Srivastava PK: Assessment of autonomic dysfunction in Guillain-Barré syndrome and its prognostic implications, *Acta Neurol Scand* 75:101-105, 1987.
34. Wheeler JS Jr, Siroky MB, Pavlakis A, Krane RJ: The urodynamic aspects of the Guillain-Barré syndrome, *J Urol* 131:917-919, 1984.
35. Berger Y, Blaivas JG, Oliver L: Urinary dysfunction in transverse myelitis, *J Urol* 144(1):103-105, 1990.
36. Hald TG, Bradley WE: *The urinary bladder: neurology and dynamics,* Baltimore, 1982, Williams & Wilkins.
37. Kandel ER, Schwartz JH: *Principles of neural science,* New York, 1981, Elsevier/North Holland.
38. Sakakibara R, Hattori T, Yasuda K, Yamanishi T: Micturition disturbance in acute transverse myelitis, *Spinal Cord* 24:481-485, 1996.
39. Miakowski C: Immunologic system. In: Thompson JM, McFarland GK, Hirsch JE, Tucker SM, editors: *Clinical nursing,* St. Louis, 1997, Mosby.
40. Hachen HJ, Chantraine A: Spinal cord involvement in systemic lupus erythematosus, *Paraplegia* 17:337-346, 1979.
41. Chan KF, Boey ML: Transverse myelopathy in SLE: clinical features and functional outcomes, *Lupus* 5: 294-299, 1996.

42. Bauer SB: The unstable bladder in childhood, *Urol Clin North Am* 7(2):321-326, 1980.

43. Webster GD, Koefoot RB Jr, Sihelnick S: Urodynamic abnormalities in neurologically normal children with micturition dysfunction, *J Urol* 132(1):74-77, 1984.

44. Jrgensen TM, Djurhuus JC, Schröder HD: Idiopathic detrusor sphincter dyssynergia in neurologically normal patients with voiding abnormalities, *Eur Urol* 8(2):107-110, 1982.

45. Hinman F Jr: Nonneurogenic neurogenic bladder (the Hinman syndrome): 15 years later, *J Urol* 136(4):769-777, 1986.

46. Mix LW: Occult neuropathic bladder, *Urology* 10(1):1-9, 1977.

47. Hinman F: Urinary tract damage in children who wet, *Pediatrics* 54(2):143-150, 1974.

48. Rudy DC, Woodside JR: Non-neurogenic neurogenic bladder: its relationship between intravesical pressure and the external sphincter EMG, *Neurourol Urodyn* 10:169-176, 1991.

49. McGuire EJ, Savastano JA: Urodynamic studies in enuresis and nonneurogenic bladder, *J Urol* 132:299-302, 1984.

50. Vincent SA: Postural control of urinary incontinence: the curtsy sign, *Lancet* 2:631, 1966.

51. Gray M: *Sphincter reeducation for pediatric voiding dysfunction complicated by dyssynergia,* Association for Continence Advice International Conference, Bournemouth, UK, April 1993.

52. Killorin WK, Gray M, Bennett JK, Green BG: Evaluative urodynamics and bladder management in predicting upper urinary tract infection in male spinal cord injury, *Paraplegia* 30:437-441, 1992.

53. Walter JS, Wheeler JS Jr, Dunn RB: Dynamic bulbocavernosus reflex: dyssynergia evaluation following spinal cord injury, *J Am Paraplegia Soc* 17(3):140-145, 1994.

54. Le CT, Price M: Survival from spinal cord injury, *J Chronic Dis* 35:487-489, 1982.

55. Hackler RH: A 24-year prospective mortality study in the spinal cord injured patient: comparison with the long term living paraplegic, *J Urol* 117:486-489, 1977.

56. DeVivo MJ, Kartus PL, Stover SL, et al: Cause of death for patients with spinal cord injuries, *Arch Intern Med* 149:1761-1766, 1989.

57. Wein AJ, van Arsdalen K, Levin RM: Pharmacologic therapy. In: Krane RJ, Siroky MB, editors: *Clinical neurourology,* Boston, 1991, Little, Brown.

58. Anson C, Gray M: Secondary urologic complications of spinal injury, *Urol Nurs* 13:107-112, 1993.

59. Gray M, Bennett JK, Green BG, Killorin WK: Urethral pressure gradient in the prediction of upper urinary tract distress following spinal cord injury, *J Am Paraplegia Soc* 14:105-106, 1991.

60. Cardenas DD, Mayo ME, Turner LR: Lower urinary changes over time in suprasacral spinal cord injury, *Paraplegia* 33:326-329, 1995.

61. Weld KJ, Graney MJ, Dmochowski RR: Differences in bladder compliance with time and associations of bladder management with compliance in spinal cord injured patients, *J Urol* 163(4):1228-33, 2000.

62. McGuire EJ, Cespedes RD, O'Connell HE: Leak point pressures, *Urol Clin North Am* 23:253-262, 1996.

63. Kieswetter H: Neurogenic bladder as a cause of urinary tract infection, *Wien Med Wochenschr* 141:560-563, 1991.

64. Petersen T, Jensen PB: Evaluation of the urinary tract in children with myelodysplasia, *Acta Neurol Scand* 75:46-51, 1987.

65. Galloway NT, Mekras JA, Helms M, Webster GD: An objective score to predict upper urinary tract deterioration in myelodysplasia, *J Urol* 145:535-537, 1991.

66. Griffiths DJ: Hydrodynamics of the bladder and urethra. In: Mundy AR, Stephenson TP, Wein AJ, editors: *Urodynamics: principles, practice, and application,* London, 1994, Churchill Livingstone.

67. Sussett JG: Cystometry. In: Krane RJ, Siroky MB, editors: *Clinical neuro-urology,* Boston, 1991, Little, Brown.

68. Stover SL: Review of forty years of rehabilitation issues in spinal cord injury, *J Spinal Cord Med* 18(3):175-182, 1995.

69. Bagli DJ, van Savage JG, Khoury AE, et al: Basic fibroblast growth factor in the urine of children with voiding pathology, *J Urol* 158:1123-1127, 1997.

70. Close CE, Carr MC, Burns MW, Mitchell ME: Lower urinary tract changes after early valve ablation in neonates and infants: is early diversion warranted? *J Urol* 157:984-988, 1997.

71. Ogawa T: Bladder deformities in patients with neurogenic bladder dysfunction, *Urol Int* 47(suppl 1):59-62, 1991.

72. Ogawa T, Yoshida T, Fujinaga T: Bladder deformity in traumatic spinal cord injury patients. *Hinyokika Kiyo* 34:1173-1178, 1988.

73. Sussett JG, Ghoneim GM: Effect of bilateral sacral decentralization in detrusor contractility and passive properties in dogs, *Neurourol Urodyn* 3:23-33, 1984.

74. Noreau L, Proulx P, Gagnog L, et al : Secondary impairments after spinal cord injury: a population based study, *Am J Phys Med Rehabil* 79(6):526-535, 2000.

75. Schaeffer AJ: Infections of the urinary tract. In: Walsh PC, Retik AB, Vaughan ED, Wein AJ, editors: *Campbell's urology,* ed 7, Philadelphia, 1998, WB Saunders.

76. Shortliffe LMD: Urinary tract infections in infants and children. In: Walsh PC, Retik AB, Vaughan D, Wein AJ, editors: *Campbell's urology,* ed 7, Philadelphia, 1998, WB Saunders.

77. Schechter H, Leonard CD, Scribner CH: Chronic pyelonephritis as a cause of renal failure in dialysis candidates: analysis of 173 patients, *JAMA* 216:514-517, 1971.

78. Glauser MP, Heumann D, Baumgartner JD, Cohen J: Pathogenesis and potential treatment for the prevention and management of septic shock: an update, *Clin Infect Dis* 18(suppl 2):S205-S216, 1994.

79. Bone RC: The pathogenesis of sepsis, *Ann Intern Med* 115:457-469, 1991.

80. Cunnion RE, Parrillo JE: Myocardial dysfunction in sepsis: recent insights, *Chest* 95:941-945, 1989.

81. Kreger BE, Craven DE, Carling PC, McCabe WR: Gram negative bacteremia III: reassessment of etiology, epidemiology, and ecology in 612 patients, *Am J Med* 68:332-343, 1980.

82. Jenkins AD: Calculus formation. In: Gillenwater JY, Grayhack JT, Howards SS, Duckett JW, editors: *Adult and pediatric urology*, St. Louis, 1996, Mosby.

83. Comarr AE, Eltorai I: Autonomic dysreflexia/hyper-reflexia, *J Spinal Cord Med* 20:345-354, 1997.

84. Comarr AE: Autonomic dysreflexia (hyperreflexia), *J Am Paraplegia Soc* 7(3):53-57, 1984.

85. Moeller BA Jr, Scheinberg D: Autonomic dysreflexia in injuries below the sixth thoracic segment, *JAMA* 224(9): 1295, 1973.

86. Guttman L, Whitteridge D: Effects of bladder distension on autonomic mechanisms after spinal cord injuries, *Brain* 70:361, 1947.

87. Joseph AC, Juma S: Autonomic dysreflexia and videourodynamics, *Urol Nurs* 14:66-77, 1994.

88. Perkash I: Autonomic dysreflexia and detrusor-sphincter dyssynergia in spinal cord injury patients, *J Spinal Cord Med* 20:365-370, 1997.

89. Abdill CK, Rivas DR, Chancellor MB: Transurethral placement of external sphincter wire mesh for neurogenic bladder, *SCI Nurs* 11:38-41, 1994.

90. Rivas DA, Chancellor MB, Staas WE, Gomella LG: Contact neodymium:yttrium-aluminum-garnet laser ablation of the external sphincter in spinal cord injured men with detrusor sphincter dyssynergia, *Urology* 45:1028-1031, 1995.

91. Gray M, Rayome R, Anson C: Incontinence and clean intermittent catheterization following spinal cord injury, *Clin Nurs Res* 4(1):6-21, 1995.

92. McDowell BJ: Basic elements of continence assessment, *Urol Nurs* 14:120-124, 1994.

93. Darouiche RO, Priebe M, Clarridge JE: Limited vs. full microbiological investigation for the management of symptomatic polymicrobial urinary tract infection in adult spinal cord injured patients, *Spinal Cord* 35: 534-539, 1997.

94. Cardenas DD, Hooton TM: Urinary tract infection in persons with spinal cord injury, *Arch Phys Med Rehabil* 76:272-280, 1995.

95. Gribble MJ, Puterman ML: Prophylaxis of UTI in persons with recent spinal cord injury: a prospective, randomized, double-blind, placebo-controlled study of trimethoprim-sulfamethoxazole, *Am J Med* 95(2):141-152, 1993.

96. Pauwels E, De Wachter S, Wyndaele JJ: Normality of bladder filling studied in symptom-free middle-aged women, *J Urol* 171(4):1567-1570, 2004.

97. Hackler RH, Hall MK, Zampieri TA: Bladder hypocompliance in the spinal cord injury population, *J Urol* 141:1390-1393, 1989.

98. Seki N, Masuda K, Tanaka M, et al: Relationship between febrile urinary tract infection and urodynamics in myelodysplastic children with vesicoureteral reflux, *Urol Int* 71(3):280-284, 2003.

99. Green BG, Foote JE, Gray M: Urologic management during acute care and rehabilitation of the spinal cord injured patient, *Phys Med Rehabil Clin North Am* 4:249-272, 1993.

100. Weld KJ, Dmochowski RR: Effect of bladder management on urological complications in spinal cord injured patients, *J Urol* 163(3):768-772, 2000.

101. Tries J: Kegel exercises enhanced by biofeedback, *J Enterostom Ther* 17:67-76, 1990.

102. Chai T, Steers WD: Neurophysiology of micturition and continence in women, *Int Urogynecol J Pelvic Floor Dysfunct* 8:85-97, 1997.

103. Joseph AC, Giroux J, Briggs DS, et al: *Clinical guidelines for bladder management in the spinal cord injured patient*, Jackson Heights, N.Y., 1998, American Association of Spinal Cord Injury Nurses.

104. Aronovitch SA, Scardillo J: Latex allergy and the WOC nurse: a review of literature, *J Wound Ostomy Continence Nurs* 25(2):93-101, 1998.

105. Bang RL: Penile edema induced by continuous condom catheter use and mimicking keloid scar, *Scand J Urol Nephrol* 28:333-335, 1994.

106. Pidde TJ, Little TW: Hydronephrosis due to improper condom catheter use, *J Am Paraplegia Soc* 17:168-170, 1994.

107. Taylor TA, Waites KB: A quantitative study of genital skin flora in male spinal cord injured outpatients, *Am J Phys Med Rehabil* 72(3):117-121, 1993.

108. Waites KB, Canupp KC, DeVivo MJ: Epidemiology and risk factors for urinary tract infection following spinal cord injury, *Arch Phys Med Rehabil* 74: 691-695, 1993.

109. Wein AJ: Neuromuscular dysfunction of the lower urinary tract and its treatment. In: Walsh PC, Retik AB, Vaughan ED, Wein AJ, editors: *Campbell's urology*, ed 7, Philadelphia, 1998, WB Saunders, pp 953-1006.

110. Loubser PG, Narayan RK, Sandin KJ et al: Continuous infusion of intrathecal baclofen: long-term effects on spasticity in spinal cord injury, *Paraplegia* 29:48-64, 1991.

111. Nanninga JB, Frost F, Penn R: Effect of intrathecal baclofen on bladder and sphincter function, *J Urol* 142:101-105, 1989.

112. Putty TK, Shapiro SA: Efficacy of dorsal longitudinal myelotomy in treating spinal spasticity: a review of 20 cases, *J Neurosurg* 75:307-401, 1991.

113. Steers WD, Meythaler JM, Haworth C, et al: Effects of acute bolus and chronic continuous intrathecal baclofen in genitourinary dysfunction due to spinal cord pathology, *J Pathol* 148:1849-1855, 1992.

114. Abrams P, Amarenco G, Bakke A, et al: European Tamsulosin Neurogenic Lower Urinary Tract Dysfunction Study Group. Tamsulosin: efficacy and safety in patients with neurogenic lower urinary tract dysfunction due to suprasacral spinal cord injury, *J Urol* 170(4):1242-1251, 2003.

115. Perkash I: Efficacy and safety of terazosin administration to improve voiding in spinal cord injury, *J Spinal Cord Med* 18:236-239, 1995.

116. Perrigot M, Delauche-Cavallier MC, Amarenco G, et al: Effect of intravenous alfuzosin on urethral pressure in patients with neurogenic bladder dysfunction: DORALI study group, *Neurourol Urodyn* 15:119-131, 1996.

117. Swierzewski SJ III, Gormley EA, Belville WD, et al: The effect of terazosin on bladder function in the spinal cord injured patient, *J Urol* 151:951-954, 1994.

118. Catz A, Luttwak ZP, Agranov E, et al: The role of external sphincterotomy for patients with a spinal cord lesion, *Spinal Cord* 35:48-52, 1997.

119. Lockhart JL, Vorstmann B, Weinstein D, Politano VA: Sphincterotomy failure in neurogenic bladder disease, *J Urol* 135:86-89, 1986.

120. Noll F, Sauerwein D, Stohrer M: Transurethral sphincterotomy in quadriplegic patients: long-term followup, *Neurourol Urodyn* 14:351-358, 1995.

121. Vapneck JM, Couillard DR, Stone AR: Is sphincterotomy the best management of the spinal cord injured bladder? *J Urol* 151:961-964, 1994.

122. Beleggia F, Beccia E, Imbriani E, et al: The use of type A botulin toxin in the treatment of detrusor-sphincter dyssynergia, *Arch Ital Urol Androl* 69(suppl 1):61-63, 1997.

123. Chancellor MB, Rivas DA, Abdill CK, et al: Management of sphincter dyssynergia using the sphincter stent prosthesis in chronically catheterized SCI men, *J Spinal Cord Med* 18:88-94, 1995.

124. Weld KJ, Wall BM, Mangold TA, et al: Influences on renal function in chronic spinal cord injured patients, *J Urol* 164(5):1490-1493, 2000.

125. Chai T, Chung AK, Belville WD, Faerber GJ: Compliance and complications of clean intermittent catheterization in the spinal cord injured patient, *Paraplegia* 33:161-163, 1995.

126. Harrison C, Kuric J: Community reintegration of SCI persons: problems and perceptions, *SCI Nurs* 6:44-47, 1989.

127. Louis DT, Joseph AC: Providing a self-catheterization prosthesis for a handicapped patient, *J Wound Ostomy Continence Nurs* 25(2):107-110, 1998.

128. Hirsh DD, Fainstein V, Musher DM: Do condom catheter collecting systems cause urinary tract infection? *JAMA* 242:340-341, 1979.

129. Johnson ET: The condom catheter: urinary tract infection and other complications, *South Med J* 76:579-582, 1983.

130. Trop CS, Bennett CJ: Autonomic dysreflexia and its urologic complications: a review, *J Urol* 146:1461-1469, 1991.

131. Hudson MA, Catalona WJ: Urothelial tumors of the bladder, upper tracts and prostate. In: Gillenwater JY, Grayhack JT, Howards SS, Duckett JW, editors: *Adult and pediatric urology,* St. Louis, 1996, Mosby.

132. Eichorn F, Thon W, Altwein JE: The risk of cancer in neuropathic bladders, *Urol Int* 39:105-109, 1984.

133. Hofseth LJ, Dunn BP, Rosin MP: Micronucleus frequencies in urothelial cells of catheterized patients with chronic bladder inflammation, *Mutat Res* 352:65-72, 1996.

134. Stonehill WH, Dmochowski RR, Patterson AL, Cox CE. Risk factors for bladder tumors in spinal cord injury patients, *J Urol* 155(4):1248-1250, 1996.

135. Cox AJ: Effect of a hydrogel coating on the surface topography of latex-based urinary catheters: an SEM study, *Biomaterials* 8:500-502, 1987.

136. Graiver D, Durall RL, Okada T: Surface morphology and friction coefficient of various types of Foley catheter, *Biomaterials* 14:465-469, 1993.

137. Johnson JR, Roberts PL, Olsen RJ, et al: Prevention of catheter-associated urinary tract infection with a silver oxide–coated urinary catheter: clinical and microbiologic correlates, *J Infect Dis* 162:1145-1150, 1990.

138. Murakami S, Igarashi T, Tanaka M, et al: Adherence of bacteria to various urethral catheters and occurrence of catheter-induced urethritis, *Hinyokika Kiyo* 39:107-111, 1993.

139. Riley DK, Classes DC, Steens LE, Burke JP: A large randomized trial of a silver impregnated urinary catheter: lack of efficacy and staphylococcal superinfection, *Am J Med* 98:349-356, 1995.

140. Talja M, Korpela A, Järvi K: Comparison of urethral reaction to full silicone, hydrogel-coated and siliconised latex catheters, *Br J Urol* 66(6):652-657, 1990.

141. Moore KN, Rayome RG: Problem solving and troubleshooting: the indwelling catheter, *J Wound Ostomy Continence Nurs* 22:242-247, 1995.

142. Thyberg M, Etzgaard P, Gylling M, Granerus G: Effect of nifedipine on cystometry induced elevation of blood pressure with a reflex urinary bladder after a high level spinal cord injury, *Paraplegia* 32:308-313, 1994.

143. Chancellor MB, Erhard MJ, Hirsch IH, Stass WE: Prospective evaluation of terazosin for the treatment of autonomic dysreflexia, *J Urol* 151:111-113, 1994.

144. Bennett JK, Bruce BG, Foote J, et al: Augmentation enterocystoplasty in the management of neurogenic bladder: a long-term study, *Neurourol Urodyn* 13:665-666, 1995.

145. McInerny PD, Mundy AR: Augmentation cystoplasty. In: Colleen S, Mansson W, editors: *Reconstructive surgery of the lower genitourinary tract in adults,* Oxford, 1995, Isis Medical Media.

146. Adams MC, Mitchell ME, Rink RC: Gastrocystoplasty: an alternative solution to the problem of urological reconstruction in the severely compromised patient, *J Urol* 140:1152-1156, 1988.

147. Gosalbez R Jr, Woodard JR, Broecker BH, Warshaw B: Metabolic complications of the use of stomach for urinary reconstruction, *J Urol* 150:710-712, 1993.

148. Gosalbez R Jr, Woodard JR, Broecker BH, et al: The use of stomach in pediatric urinary reconstruction, *J Urol* 150:438-440, 1993.

149. Muraishi O, Ogawa A, Tsuruta T, Kato H: Bladder peptic ulcer after gastrocystoplasty for radiation cystitis, *J Urol* 152:473-474, 1994.

150. Ngan JH, Lau JL, Lim ST, et al: Long-term results of antral gastrocystoplasty, *J Urol* 149:731-734, 1993.

151. Stohrer M: Bladder auto-augmentation. In: Colleen S, Mansson W, editors: *Reconstructive surgery of the lower genitourinary tract in adults,* Oxford, 1995, Isis Medical Media.

152. Davidsson T, Lindergard B, Mansson W: Long-term metabolic and nutritional effects of urinary diversion, *Urology* 46(6):804-809, 1995.

153. Mitrofanoff P: Trans-appendicular continent cystostomy in the management of the neurogenic bladder, *Chir Pediatr* 21(4):297-305, 1980.

154. Rowland RG: The plicated or tapered ileal outlet: "Indiana Pouch," *Scand J Urol Nephrol Suppl* 142:70-72, 1992.

155. Moreno JG, Chancellor MB, Karasick S, et al: Improved quality of life with continent urinary diversion in quadriplegic women with umbilical stoma, *Arch Phys Med Rehabil* 76:758-762, 1995.

156. Watanabe T, Rivas DA, Smith R, et al: The effect of urinary tract reconstruction on neurologically impaired women previously treated with an indwelling urethral catheter, *J Urol* 156:1926-1928, 1996.

Pathology and Management of Acute and Chronic Urinary Retention

KATHERINE N. MOORE

OBJECTIVES

1. Explain the difference in acute and chronic retention in terms of onset, clinical presentation, and common causes.
2. Identify the two pathologic mechanisms that may result in urinary retention.
3. Explain the effects of prolonged or severe retention on bladder function and renal function.
4. Identify common pathologic conditions that contribute to obstructed voiding in the male patient and in the female patient.
5. Define the term "lower urinary tract symptoms" and explain why this term has replaced the old term "prostatism."
6. Identify how benign prostatic hypertrophy contributes to urinary retention, and address both static and dynamic factors.
7. Describe parameters to be included in assessment of the patient with urinary retention, and identify typical assessment findings.
8. Describe behavioral strategies that may be used to enhance bladder emptying/reduce postvoid residual volume.
9. Describe guidelines for appropriate performance of clean intermittent catheterization.
10. Describe the mechanisms of action and role of each of the following in management of benign prostatic hypertrophy: alpha-adrenergic antagonists, 5-alpha-reductase inhibitors, transurethral resection of the prostate gland, minimally invasive surgical procedures for prostate resection.

*U*rinary retention is a broad term that includes any difficulty with bladder emptying; it varies in severity from incomplete emptying to total inability to void. Retention can occur in infants as a result of congenital disorders, but it is most common among men with prostatic hypertrophy, individuals with neurologic lesions, and diabetic patients with autonomic cystopathy. Retention can be classified according to onset (acute versus chronic), site of impaired emptying (upper versus lower tract), and cause (obstruction versus impaired contractility). Regardless of cause, retention is associated with increased incidence of urinary tract infection and risk for upper tract damage; thus, retention requires prompt diagnosis and prompt intervention. This chapter provides a review of types of retention, etiologic factors, pathologic effects, assessment parameters, and treatment options; in addition, pathology, assessment, and management of prostatic hypertrophy are addressed in depth, because benign prostatic hyperplasia (BPH) is one of the most common conditions associated with urinary retention.

ACUTE VERSUS CHRONIC RETENTION

Acute urinary retention is characterized by the sudden onset of inability to void and is extremely painful; as a result, these patients end up in the emergency room and are sometimes misdiagnosed as having an "acute abdomen" because of the profound pain. In patients who are unable to communicate as a result of neurologic lesions such as cerebrovascular accident, acute retention is manifest by extreme restlessness and diaphoresis. Causative factors for acute retention are typically classified as follows: (1) obstructive lesions that prevent the flow of urine, such as urethral stricture or prostate gland enlargement;

TABLE 8-1   Medications That May Contribute to Urinary Retention

TYPE OF MEDICATION	EXAMPLES
Anticholinergics, antimuscarinics, antispasmodics	Atropine, darifenacin, dicyclomine, hyoscyamine, oxybutynin, scopolamine, propantheline, tolterodine, trospium
Tricyclic antidepressants	Amitriptyline, amoxapine, clomipramine, doxepin, imipramine, nortriptyline, protriptyline, trimipramine
Other antidepressants (lower risk for retention)	Bupropion, paroxetine, sertraline, trazodone
Antipsychotics	Chlorpromazine, clozapine, perphenazine, promazine, thioridazine
Antiparkinsonian	Amantadine, bromocriptine, levodopa
Calcium-channel blockers (potential risk)	Nifedipine, verapamil
Narcotic analgesics	Morphine, meperidine
Anesthetic agents	General anesthesia, spinal/epidural anesthesia

From Gray M: Urinary retention: management in the acute care setting. Part 2, *Am J Nurs* 100:36, 2000, with permission.

(2) loss of detrusor muscle contractility caused by damage to the sensory and/or motor nerves controlling bladder function (as a result of diabetes, multiple sclerosis, and various medications); or (3) some combination of obstruction and diminished contractility.[1,2] For example, antiincontinence procedures such as vaginal slings are associated with acute transient postoperative retention, which is caused in part by the effects of anesthesia and analgesics, in part by postoperative edema and temporary nerve damage, and in part by the increased urethral resistance provided by the sling. Patients with chronic retention may inadvertently trigger an episode of acute retention by excessive alcohol intake, use of recreational drugs, or use of medications that compromise detrusor function. For example, the patient with prostatism may be placed at risk for acute retention when he is prescribed a beta blocker or a calcium-channel blocker. (Table 8-1 highlights medications that may contribute to acute retention in the "at risk" patient.)

In contrast to the dramatic onset of acute retention, chronic retention may develop over several months or even years; the most common causes are BPH and neurogenic processes such as diabetic cystopathy. Because compromised ability to empty the bladder develops gradually in these conditions, the patient may be relatively unaware of the problem.

TABLE 8-2   Lower Urinary Tract Symptoms

Voiding symptoms	Hesitancy
	Poor flow
	Straining to start flow
	Intermittent and/or prolonged stream
Storage symptoms	Frequency
	Urgency
	Nocturia

"Silent prostatism" is the historical term used to describe patients who deny lower urinary tract symptoms (LUTS), despite significant postvoid residual (PVR) urine and rising blood urea nitrogen (BUN) and creatinine levels.[3] Chronic urinary retention may be identified "incidentally" in a routine physical examination if the patient presents with LUTS such as difficulty initiating the urinary stream, a slow or "weak" stream, and feelings of incomplete emptying. Some patients complain of frequent, small-volume voids and urinary leakage during activities associated with increased abdominal pressure, but they do not realize that the underlying problem is failure to empty the bladder effectively. (See Table 8-2 for common LUTS.)

Although chronic retention causes only "low-grade" symptoms, it can produce significant damage in terms of bladder function. For example, long-term obstruction to urine flow and the subsequent bladder distension cause denervation injury and increased collagen deposits within the bladder wall; these pathologic changes produce thickening of the bladder wall, diminished sensory awareness of bladder filling, and compromised detrusor contractility. Relief of the obstruction may or may not "correct" the pathologic changes in bladder function, depending on the extent and duration of the obstruction and distension; if irreversible damage has occurred, the bladder will be large, "floppy," and unable to contract effectively. Such individuals usually require long-term management with intermittent catheterization. Alpha blockers combined with daily or twice daily catheterization may be effective for some patients with diminished voiding function. The alpha blocker helps to reduce urethral resistance, which improves bladder emptying in patients with diminished contractility; this "combination therapy" may permit the patient to manage with self-catheterization once a day, rather than four to six times a day.

ETIOLOGIC FACTORS FOR RETENTION

Retention is frequently a multifactorial condition; however, all the etiologic factors can be broadly classified as either obstructive processes or conditions that compromise detrusor contractility. This discussion therefore focuses on the two primary "groups" of etiologic factors.

Obstructive Processes

Obstructive processes include any condition or lesion that interferes with the flow of urine at any point in the urinary tract, from the calyx of the kidney to the distal urethra. Obstruction at any point causes stasis of urine above the obstruction; the urinary stasis and structural distension cause pain and infection, and untreated obstruction eventually leads to renal failure and death. Obstructive processes can be classified either by type (congenital, neoplastic, structural/functional, inflammatory, and miscellaneous)[4] or by site (upper tract versus lower tract) (Table 8-3).

TABLE 8-3   Upper and Lower Urinary Tract Causes of Obstruction

CAUSE	UPPER URINARY TRACT	LOWER URINARY TRACT
Congenital	Polycystic kidney, renal cyst, ureteropelvic junction obstruction, aberrant vessel at the ureteropelvic junction, stricture, ureterocele, ureterovesical reflux, ureteral valve, ectopic kidney, retrocaval ureter	Myelomeningocele, bladder-sphincter dyssynergia, posterior or anterior urethral valves, prune belly syndrome, meatal stenosis
Neoplastic	Wilms' tumor, renal cell carcinoma or transitional cell carcinoma of renal pelvis, multiple myeloma, carcinoma of ureter, metastatic carcinoma	Bladder tumor, invasive prostate cancer, urethral or penile carcinoma
Inflammatory	Tuberculosis, *Echinococcus* infection, schistosomiasis, abscess, ureteritis cystica, endometriosis	Acute prostatitis, paraurethral abscess
Miscellaneous	Renal calculi, trauma, aneurysm of renal artery, peripelvic cyst, sloughed papillae, retroperitoneal fibrosis, pelvic lipomatosis, radiation therapy, lymphocele, urinoma, pregnancy	Phimosis, radiation therapy, urethral obstruction from mechanical device (artificial urinary sphincter, vaginal sling, pessary), medications, neurogenic causes (diabetes, multiple sclerosis, sacral cord lesions)

Classification by Type. *Congenital* lesions include obvious and serious anomalies such as myelomeningocele as well as occult lesions of variable severity, such as posterior urethral valves or vesicoureteral reflux. Any lesion that produces significant obstruction to urinary flow places the child at risk for urinary tract infections, hydronephrosis, and permanent renal damage. *Neoplastic* lesions include Wilms' tumor, renal cell or transitional cell carcinoma, ureteral carcinoma, multiple myeloma, and metastatic lesions; these tumors represent a dual threat, in that the malignancy itself is a threat to life, and the obstruction to urine flow presents an additional threat to life and health. Common *structural* and *functional* lesions include ureteral and renal calculi, urethral strictures, BPH, pelvic organ prolapse, and even pregnancy and severe constipation. Uncommon conditions producing functional obstruction include neurologic lesions resulting in detrusor sphincter dyssynergia, such as spinal cord injury. Finally, inflammatory conditions such as endometriosis and tuberculosis are uncommon causes of urinary tract obstruction.

Classification by Site. Retention can also be classified according to site. This approach is helpful because the pathologic features and management of upper tract obstruction differ from those of lower tract obstruction.

Upper tract obstruction. Upper tract obstruction most commonly occurs at the ureteropelvic junction (UPJ),[5] in neonates and children as well as adults. In neonates, obstruction at the UPJ is typically the result of abnormal development of the UPJ during embryonic life; the UPJ begins development as a solid structure but then undergoes canalization to form a hollow channel. Incomplete canalization results in a narrow channel, abnormal resistance to urine flow, and increased vulnerability to obstructive lesions such as calculi. Obstruction at the UPJ can also be caused by aberrant blood vessels that distort the anatomy of the renal pelvis and proximal ureter,[6] by tumors, and by renal calculi. Patients with conditions producing partial UPJ obstruction are at high risk for complete obstruction from renal calculi, which are more likely to form because the increased resistance to urine flow produces varying degrees of stasis and infection, which are risk factors for calculi formation.

Untreated obstruction of the UPJ results in progressive hydronephrosis and hydroureter, atrophy of the renal parenchyma, and compromised renal function. The degree to which obstruction negatively affects renal function is affected by the severity of the obstruction (the degree to which urine flow is blocked), the duration of the obstruction, and whether or not infection occurs.

In a completely obstructed kidney, tissue damage is evident within 7 days; however, if the obstruction is relieved within 14 days following onset, return to normal or preobstructive function is probable. If complete obstruction persists for 21 days without relief, only 50% of renal function is likely to return.[7] Interestingly, the damage progresses from distal to proximal; histologic changes are first noted in the distal nephron and advance steadily to eventually involve the glomerulus. The pathologic changes include reduction in arterial flow and impaired venous drainage; the ischemia and congestion contribute significantly to the renal tissue damage. When the obstructive process is complicated by infection, the associated inflammation further intensifies the rate and severity of the pathologic process.[7]

Lower tract obstruction. Obstruction occurring at the level of the bladder neck or urethra is classified as lower tract obstruction; the most common causes of obstruction in men are pathologic conditions of the prostate,[8,9] which are discussed in detail later in this chapter, and urethral stricture. Strictures can be caused by a variety of conditions, including radiation therapy for genitourinary cancer and surgical procedures such as radical prostatectomy ; the reported incidence of stricture following radical prostatectomy is as high as 25%.[10] Additional causes of stricture include straddle injuries, pelvic fractures, and sexually transmitted diseases. The stricture gradually obstructs the urethra, causing increased pressure proximal to the obstruction; the rising pressures proximal to the lesion may cause gradual thinning of the urethral walls, formation of urethral diverticula, and "pocketing" of urine resulting in infection.[11]

In women, lower urinary tract obstruction is most commonly caused by pelvic organ prolapse and cystocele or by antiincontinence procedures (such as urethral sling procedures); rarely, obstruction is caused by urethral stricture or pelvic neoplasms. Pelvic organ prolapse causes outlet obstruction either by altering the angle of the urethrovesical junction or by directly compressing the urethra. Antiincontinence procedures cause outlet obstruction by "oversuspending" or "overcompressing" the urethra.[12,13]

An uncommon cause of outlet obstruction is "pseudodyssynergia" caused by dysfunctional voiding patterns; in this situation, the patient unconsciously contracts the pelvic floor muscles during voiding, which creates obstruction to bladder emptying ("dyssynergic" contraction of the sphincter muscles during bladder contraction).[14]

Impact of outlet obstruction. Obstruction at the level of the urethra or bladder neck has a very negative impact on bladder wall structure and function. Investigations based on Gosling's pioneering research provide convincing evidence of the following sequelae of lower urinary tract obstruction:[15] increased deposition of collagen within the bladder wall; reduced production of and response to acetylcholinesterase (which results in increased bladder contractility resulting from increased levels of acetylcholine), and changes in the function of smooth muscle cells in the bladder wall (altered intracellular communication and electrical potential).[16,17] In addition, studies indicate that obstruction causes a reorganization of the spinal micturition reflex, which results in hypertrophy of the afferent and efferent neurons, an increase in C-fiber neurons, and increased production of nerve growth fiber. These changes may explain why men with prostatic obstruction develop symptoms of overactive bladder that are not always relieved by performance of a transurethral resection of the prostate (TURP). Severe prolonged obstruction and the resulting bladder distension cause denervation, a thickened bladder wall, and loss of contractility. Once these changes have occurred, it is usually too late to "undo" the damage; relieving the obstruction does not necessarily restore normal detrusor function, and the patient may require intermittent catheterization and/or alpha-adrenergic antagonists (alpha blockers) on a long-term basis to provide effective emptying.

Effects of lower tract obstruction on upper tract. The upper tracts are normally protected against problems within the lower tract. Even when the bladder is grossly distended, the ureterovesical valves initially prevent the retrograde flow of urine (reflux). However, when distension is prolonged, the position and configuration of the ureterovesical valves are gradually distorted; the progressive distortion reduces the resistance to retrograde flow and permits urine to reflux into the ureters and kidneys. Prolonged bladder distension also causes major changes in the structure and function of the ureters; they initially hypertrophy in an attempt to overcome the resistance to urine flow, which causes them to become tortuous and elongated. Eventually, the ureters become so stretched and dilated that they lose their tone and capacity for peristalsis;[11] in addition, the tortuous and elongated ureters may become angled in a way that causes them to "self-obstruct." The end result of compromised ureteral function is back pressure on the renal pelvis and calyces. Normal renal pressures are almost zero; however, as ureteral pressures rise, pressures within the renal pelvis and calyces rise also, resulting in dilatation of the calyces and renal pelvis. The renal pelvis initially hypertrophies in an attempt to overcome the obstruction, but persistent obstruction results in total loss of tone and contractility. Table 8-4 highlights the progression of renal damage caused by persistent obstruction.[11]

Clinical Presentation. Clinical presentation varies, depending on the rate at which the obstruction develops and the "preobstruction" voiding patterns. For the patient with postprostatectomy incontinence, early obstruction (from stricture formation) produces a marked improvement in bladder control; the patient is usually pleased and typically interprets these symptoms as "progress." Over a relatively short time, however, the patient develops the classic symptoms of lower urinary tract obstruction: straining to void, progressive weakening of the urinary stream, hesitancy, intermittency, postvoid dribble, daytime frequency (voiding more often than every 2 hours), and

TABLE 8-4   **Progression of Renal Changes in Response to Obstruction**

SITE OF DAMAGE	PATHOLOGY
Calyces	Calyceal fornices become blunt and rounded, papillae become flattened and then clubbed
Renal parenchyma	Gradual atrophy from compression and ischemia as blood supply diminishes, especially in interlobular arteries
Renal tubules	Dilatation and atrophy caused by ischemia
Widespread renal effects	Progressive rise in intrapelvic pressures; when intrapelvic pressures rise to the level of glomerular filtration pressure (6 to 12 mm Hg), urine formation decreases, glomerular filtration rate and renal plasma flow are reduced, the ability to concentrate urine is lost, and the urea-creatinine concentration ratio drops (normal 1:10)

Data from Tanagho EA. Urinary obstruction and stasis. In: Tanagho EA, McAninch JW, editors: *Smith's general urology*, ed 16, New York, 2004, Lange Medical Books/McGraw-Hill, pp 175-187.

nocturia (being wakened by the urge to void more than once per night in people younger than 65 years of age and more than twice per night in people older than 65 years of age). Urgency and urge incontinence may also occur, and hematuria may be noted if the obstruction is complicated by urinary tract infection. Depending on the etiology and severity, obstructed voiding may lead to acute or chronic urinary retention. For example, postprostatectomy stricture formation can produce complete obstruction and acute retention over the course of 1 to 2 days if the patient fails to seek assistance on initial onset of voiding difficulty.[8,9]

Upper tract damage is manifest by flank pain that frequently radiates along the course of the ureter, hematuria, pyuria, fever, chills, and malaise. If the hydronephrosis is severe enough to produce uremia, the patient will also exhibit nausea, weight loss, and pallor.

Retention Caused by Compromised Detrusor Contractility

The second primary etiologic factor for urinary retention is loss of detrusor contractility. This can occur as a result of damage to the parasympathetic nerves innervating the bladder or as a result of direct damage to the detrusor muscle. Common causes of denervation damage include diabetic cystopathy, multiple sclerosis, chronic alcoholism, and sacral level cord lesions. Diabetic cystopathy is particularly common but is frequently unrecognized in the early phases, which are characterized by diminished sensory awareness of bladder filling and reduced detrusor contractility. These pathologic changes result in less frequent voiding and elevated postvoid residual volumes. The lack of sensory awareness means that the patient fails to realize that anything is wrong until severe distension has occurred; at this point, the denervation damage is complicated by further loss of contractility caused by "stretch" damage to the muscle fibers of the detrusor. To prevent permanent bladder damage, providers must monitor bladder function among individuals with diabetes, especially those with other forms of neuropathy; early indicators of diabetic cystopathy include weak or prolonged urinary stream, recurrent urinary tract infections, and elevated postvoid residual volumes.

Direct damage to the detrusor muscle is most likely to occur as a result of severe acute retention that causes overstretching of the muscle fibers; common causative factors include surgery, especially pelvic procedures, and acute neurologic lesions or processes. Risk factors for retention in surgical patients include anesthetic agents, intraoperative fluid administration, sympathetic stimulation caused by pain, sympathomimetic medications, and patient sedation; strategies to minimize the risk of significant bladder distension include reduction of intraoperative fluid volume, pain control, administration of alpha-adrenergic anatagonists, careful monitoring for evidence of distension (especially in patients who are sedated or have undergone spinal anesthesia), and prompt catheterization for patients with evidence of retention.[18] Acute neurologic lesions or processes (such as spinal cord injury, transverse myelitis, or cerebrovascular accident) may also result in acute severe retention, caused by sudden loss of both sensory awareness and bladder contractility; these patients must be closely monitored for evidence of retention, and most require short-term management with an indwelling catheter (or routine intermittent catheterization).

Failure to recognize and effectively manage acute retention causes either acute or progressive loss of detrusor contractility and a corresponding increase in bladder distension and retention of urine. As noted earlier, medications such as anticholinergics can contribute to the severity of the retention and can precipitate acute retention in the patient with compromised detrusor contractility.

ASSESSMENT OF THE PATIENT WITH KNOWN OR SUSPECTED RETENTION

Assessment of the patient with urinary incontinence or retention is described in detail in Chapter 12; the discussion in this chapter is limited to the parameters and findings most significant to the assessment of a patient with urinary retention.

History

The history should focus on the onset of voiding difficulties and any associated events (such as prostatectomy), conditions known to contribute to urinary retention (such as diabetes, multiple sclerosis, or Parkinson's disease), any history of upper tract disease, all prescription and over-the-counter medications, and the type and severity of LUTS. In assessing the impact of lower urinary tract symptoms, it is very helpful to use a validated tool such as the American Urological Association (AUA) Symptom Score (also known as the International Prostate Symptom Score) (Fig. 8-1). The nurse should also assess the patient's cognitive status, ambulatory status, and general well-being and functional ability; for patients with cognitive or functional impairment, it is critical to assess the patient's living arrangements and support system.[19-21]

Voiding Diary. As described in detail in Chapter 12, a voiding diary is extremely helpful in assessing the patient's diurnal and nocturnal voiding frequency, the frequency and severity of any urinary leakage, and the type and volume of fluid intake. (Sample voiding diaries are included in Chapter 12). The voiding diary does not accurately reflect functional bladder capacity in the patient with significant retention; determination of functional capacity in these patients requires measurement of both voided volume and PVR (the two volumes are added together).

Physical Examination

A careful physical examination is a critical element in the assessment of an individual with known or suspected urinary retention.[22] In beginning the exam, the clinician should be alert to systemic indicators of acute retention, such as diaphoresis, restlessness, and elevated heart and respiratory rates; this is particularly important when assessing patients with altered sensation or impaired ability to communicate. For example, bladder distension in the patient with a spinal cord lesion above the level of T6 can result in a life-threatening complication known as autonomic dysreflexia.[23] This condition is caused by extreme sympathetic nervous system stimulation and can be triggered by a number of conditions, including fecal impaction, pressure ulcers, bladder distension, or bladder filling during urologic procedures such as cystoscopy or urodynamics; urologic procedures are the *most* common triggering event. The most significant indicator of autonomic dysreflexia is a rapid rise in blood pressure to life-threatening levels; associated signs and symptoms include flushing, mucous membrane congestion, and blurred vision above the level of the lesion and pallor, goose bumps, increased spasticity, penile erection, and bowel and bladder spasms below the level of the lesion. The primary element of effective management is elimination of the triggering condition, such as irrigation or replacement of an obstructed urethral catheter; in addition, the patient may require a rapid-acting antihypertensive, such as sublingual nifedipine (10 mg) or glyceryl trinitrate spray.[24]

Name: _____ Date: _____	Not at all	Less than 1 time in 5	Less than half the time	About half the time	More than half the time	Almost always
Score (Scores range from 0–35, with 0 being asymptomatic and 35 indicating severe symptoms)	0	1	2	3	4	5
1. *Incomplete Emptying* Over the past month, how often have you had a sensation of not emptying your bladder after you finish urinating?						
2. *Frequency* Over the past month, how often have you had to urinate again less than 2 hours after you finished urinating?						
3. *Intermittency* Over the past month, how often have you found that you stopped and started several times when urinating?						
4. *Urgency* Over the past month, how often have you found it difficult to postpone urination?						
5. *Weak Stream* Over the past month, how often have you had a weak urinary stream?						
6. *Straining* Over the past month, how often have you had to push or strain to begin urination?						
7. *Nocturia*	None	One time	Two times	Three times	Four times	Five times

Over the past month, how many **times** did you most typically get up to urinate from the time you went to bed at night until the time you got up in the morning?

Quality of life as a result of urinary symptoms	Delighted	Pleased	Mostly satisfied	Mixed: equally satisfied and dissatisfied	Mostly dissatisfied	Unhappy	Terrible
If you were to spend the rest of your life with your urinary symptoms the way they are now, how would you feel?	0	1	2	3	4	5	6
Symptom score (0–35)							
Quality of life score (0–6)							
Total AUA score (0–41)							

Fig. 8-1 American Urological Association (AUA) Symptom Score.

Abdominal Exam. A carefully performed abdominal exam provides critical information regarding the degree of bladder distension (especially in the nonobese patient) and the presence or absence of renal tenderness, and it also provides data regarding the structure and function of major abdominal organs, such as the bowel.

The abdominal exam should be conducted with the patient in a comfortable supine position. The examiner begins by carefully inspecting the abdomen for contours and symmetry, being particularly alert to the presence of scars and visible masses. Scars alert the clinician to the potential for adhesions, which may cause discomfort perceived by the patient as pelvic, bladder, or renal pain; a visible mass in the upper quadrants may be indicative of a renal tumor or severe hydronephorosis, and a centrally located mass may indicate a distended bladder. Inspection is followed by auscultation of bowel sounds; this element of the abdominal exam is particularly relevant when assessing the patient who has recently undergone urologic surgery involving manipulation or reconstruction of the bowel. A warm stethoscope is placed on the abdominal wall, and the examiner notes the presence, frequency, and character of bowel sounds; normal findings include clicks and gurgles that occur without any definable pattern, ranging in frequency from 5 to 35 per minute. The third element of abdominal exam is percussion; all abdominal quadrants are percussed, but particular attention is paid to the suprapubic area. Normal findings are tympany over the lower quadrants (where air-filled bowel predominates) and dullness over the liver; dullness is also noted over the suprapubic area when the bladder contains more than 150 mL (approximately). The final element in the abdominal exam is palpation, which contributes to the detection of bladder distension, especially in the nonobese patient. Palpation is also used to delineate the abdominal organs and to detect subtle masses; the examiner should use the palmar surface of the fingers to palpate gently but deeply. The liver, spleen, loops of bowel, and borders of the abdominal muscles are structures that are commonly palpable; it is normal for the patient to report slight tenderness on deep palpation over the cecum, sigmoid colon, and aorta. Any palpable mass associated with muscle guarding should be evaluated in terms of size, shape, consistency, and magnitude of tenderness provoked by palpation; such findings always mandate further investigation. Following palpation of the abdominal structures, the examiner attempts to palpate the kidneys; this is realistic only in the relatively thin adult patient, and typically the right kidney is easier to palpate than the left kidney. (It is very difficult to palpate the kidneys in large, muscular, or overweight patients and in patients in pain.) One approach to palpation of the kidney is to ask the patient to assume the supine position and to inhale deeply (which elevates the flank); the examiner reaches across the patient to perform deep palpation during the inhalation. An alternate approach is to attempt to "capture" the kidney; the patient is instructed to inhale and then to exhale forcefully during deep palpation. The descending kidney can sometimes be felt between the examiner's fingers during the deep exhalation. The normal kidney is firm, nontender, and smooth, and only the lower pole is palpable; however, hydronephrosis or renal masses can distort size and cause tenderness. Even when the kidneys are nonpalpable, the examiner can assess for tenderness by placing the patient in a sitting position, placing the palm of the examining hand over the costovertebral angle, and then striking the examining hand lightly with the fist of the other hand; the patient should perceive this light blow as a dull thud, as opposed to sharp tenderness or pain.

Abdominal exam indicators of urinary retention include the following:

- Visible and palpable midline abdominal mass reflecting bladder distension. In a nonobese patient, visible and/or palpable fullness extending to the level of the umbilicus indicates bladder volume of at least 500 mL, whereas fullness/distension extending above the umbilicus is reflective of bladder volume greater than 1000 mL.
- Tenderness to suprapubic palpation. The patient with intact sensation and acute-onset retention will experience marked tenderness or discomfort in response to even light palpation; in contrast, the patient with chronic distension typically does not report pain or tenderness.

- Dullness to percussion in the suprapubic area. A full bladder produces a dull percussion note, as opposed to the tympanic sound produced by a hollow organ. However, the examiner needs to be aware that this finding is significant *only* in the nonobese patient; percussion is not a reliable indicator of bladder distension in the obese patient.

Pelvic and rectal examinations provide additional data that are contributory in selected cases of retention. For example, diminished or absent sensation in the sacral dermatomes, absence of the bulbocavernosus reflex, and absence of the anal wink are indicators of a neurologic lesion or condition involving the pelvic floor and bladder. Similarly, the patient with evidence of retention should be questioned specifically regarding bowel dysfunction (refractory constipation or incontinence) and sexual dysfunction, because the triad of bladder dysfunction, bowel dysfunction, and sexual dysfunction is highly indicative of a neurologic process or lesion. A digital rectal examination permits assessment of anal sphincter tone, presence and consistency of stool in the rectum, and (in the male) size and consistency of the prostate gland. (Digital rectal exam is discussed later in this chapter.) The pelvic examination is used to assess pelvic organ prolapse and cystocele in women, because these conditions are associated with obstructed voiding in the female patient. In assessing a trauma victim, the clinician should be alert to subtle indicators of lower urinary tract injury, such as small amounts of blood at the meatus.

Diagnostic Studies

Essential studies in the evaluation of a patient with suspected urinary retention include PVR urine measurement and urinalysis; serum BUN and creatinine are also obtained when there is any concern regarding upper tract function, such as the patient with high PVR measurements or evidence of long-standing retention. Invasive tests, such as urodynamic studies and renal scans, are typically reserved for more complex cases in which advanced diagnostic data are required to direct treatment. Table 8-5 highlights common diagnostic studies and findings.

Postvoid Residual Measurement. PVR measurement helps to confirm the diagnosis of retention and is accepted as a standard element in the assessment of a patient with LUTS or with conditions associated with retention (such as prostatic hypertrophy, pelvic organ prolapse, or neurologic lesions). PVR can be obtained either via in-and-out catheterization or via portable bladder ultrasound. To ensure accuracy, the PVR measurement must be completed within several minutes of voiding, especially in the well-hydrated or overhydrated patient; documentation should include the time and volume of voided urine as well as the time and volume of PVR measurement. Because there are individual variations in completeness of bladder emptying throughout the day or with activity, PVR measurements are ideally repeated two to three times to ensure a complete and accurate "picture" of the patient's voiding patterns and ability to empty the bladder. The exception to this guideline is an initial PVR measure exceeding 500 mL, which is always indicative of significant retention.

Guidelines for performance of PVR measurement are established and agreed on; however, the *interpretation* of PVR measurements is quite variable. At this time, there is no defined volume of PVR urine that can be used to diagnose retention or to guide practice. Although a normal PVR in a healthy individual is generally accepted as 50 mL or less, older individuals may be symptom free despite residuals of 100 mL or more.[25] Residual urine volumes greater than 50 mL usually indicate the need for further assessment; however, total bladder capacity and patient symptoms must also be taken into account. For example, the patient with a voided volume of 100 mL and a PVR of 150 mL (total bladder capacity of 250 mL) requires more active intervention than the patient with a voided volume of 450 mL and a PVR of 150 mL (total bladder capacity 600 mL), even though the PVR volumes are the same. Some men are symptom free despite relatively large PVRs, and there is consensus among members of the AUA Guideline Committee that PVR alone should not mandate treatment in men with BPH.[26] In contrast, a residual urine volume that is 25% or more of total bladder capacity is considered a mandate for intervention in children.[27]

TABLE 8-5　　**Diagnostic Studies for Patient with Urinary Retention**

STUDY	RELEVANCE AND/OR COMMON FINDINGS
Urinalysis (UA; dipstick UA or UA with microscopy)	Detects hematuria, which requires further workup; positive leukocyte esterase and nitrites (dipstick) or positive leukocytes and bacteria on microscopy indicative of infection
AUA (American Urological Association) Symptom Score (or similar symptom score)	Provides important data regarding severity of symptoms and impact on quality of life
Prostate-specific antigen (PSA)	Indicated for men with a life expectancy of more than 10 years or those in whom diagnosis of prostate cancer would change management; PSA greater than 1.5 ng/mL in symptomatic men indicative of prostate volume greater than 30 ml and suggests need for 5-alpha-reductase medications
Postvoid residual urine (PVR)	Noninvasive method of assessing bladder emptying, especially in patients with complex medical history; PVR must be interpreted within the context of other bothersome symptoms and total bladder volume
Uroflow	Helpful in assessing bladder capacity, quality of urine stream, intermittency; uroflow Qmax (maximum flow rate) less than 10 mL/sc indicative of impaired emptying; however, need pressure/flow studies to differentiate between obstruction and poor contractility (uroflow cannot differentiate)
Urodynamics (pressure/flow studies)	Gold standard for differentiating between obstruction and reduced contractility; recommended for men with suspected poor contractility who may be surgical candidates because surgery will not improve symptoms in men with impaired contractility
Cystometrogram with video (fluoroscopy)	Useful in identification of trabeculation, diverticula, and possibly tumors, stones, and enlarged intravesical prostatic lobes
Urine cytology	Indicated for selected men who present with predominantly irritative symptoms, hematuria, or risk factors for bladder cancer
Creatinine, blood urea nitrogen (BUN), hemoglobin	Urea-creatinine ratio greater than 10:1 in patients with advanced hydronephrosis; anemia possible in chronic infection
Cystoscopy/ureteroscopy	Indicated in selected patients to rule out bladder or urethral pathology
Transrectal ultrasound	Highly recommended before minimally invasive surgical procedures for prostate resection (such as transurethral needle ablation, transurethral microwave heat treatment) because prostate size is important in success of these procedures
Ultrasound	Used to evaluate bladder wall thickness, renal parenchyma, and collecting system without exposing patient to radiation (important in children and pregnant women); prone to false readings; provides evidence of hydronephrosis, pyonephrosis, bleeding, or lesions of transitional mucosa but should be interpreted cautiously if negative
Excretory urogram	Demonstrates degree of dilatation of renal pelvis, calyx, and ureters as well as the level of ureteral obstruction

Continued

TABLE 8-5 **Diagnostic Studies for Patient with Urinary Retention—cont'd**

STUDY	RELEVANCE AND/OR COMMON FINDINGS
Retrograde urogram	May show more detail than excretory urogram (must take care not to overdistend the collecting system with too much contrast)
Abdominal x-ray	Plain film of abdomen may show enlargement of renal shadows, calcification (stones), tumors, metastases to spine
CT scan	Used to evaluate degree of dilatation and parenchymal atrophy, ureteral stones, pelvic masses pressing on ureters, iliac lymph nodes compressing the ureter, retroperitoneal urine extravasation from ruptured renal fornices

Data from AUA Practice Guidelines: AUA guideline on management of benign prostatic hyperplasia, *J Urol* 170:530, 2003.

Urinalysis. Patients with retention and urinary stasis are at increased risk for urinary tract infection; therefore, the assessment of these individuals should always include urinalysis (dipstick and microscopy). Microscopy to rule out pyuria is a particularly important component of the initial assessment. If the dipstick and microscopic findings are indicative of infection, culture and sensitivity should be obtained to direct treatment. Patients with infected urine who are scheduled for urinary tract instrumentation (such as cystoscopy) should receive an intravenous aminoglycoside 30 minutes before instrumentation to prevent urosepsis. In addition to urinalysis, men who present with irritative voiding symptoms (frequency and urgency) should have urine cytology studies conducted to rule out bladder cancer.[26]

Uroflow and Urodynamic Studies. Uroflow testing is extremely beneficial in screening for problems with emptying; it may be performed separately or in conjunction with urodynamic testing. It is important to ensure that the patient has a relatively full bladder, because low voided volumes (less than 150 mL) can produce false-positive readings (that is, a flow pattern that mimics obstruction or impaired contractility). Uroflow patterns typical of compromised bladder emptying are illustrated in Figs. 8-2 and 8-3; an intermittent, "sawtooth" pattern (see Fig. 8-2), or prolonged uroflow and diminished volume of the urinary stream (see Fig. 8-3). As explained in greater detail in Chapter 12, uroflow studies can usually distinguish between normal and impaired bladder emptying, but they cannot reliably

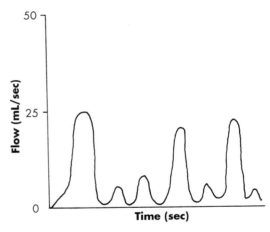

Fig. 8-2 Intermittent "sawtooth" uroflow pattern.

determine the specific etiologic factors (obstruction versus impaired contractility). (Normal uroflow patterns are illustrated in Chapter 12.)

Urodynamic testing is frequently indicated for patients with retention, because this is the only study that can accurately and reproducibly determine whether the retention is caused by obstruction, impaired contractility, or a combination of both factors. Obstruction is manifest by a poor or intermittent stream in combination with *high* detrusor pressures (greater than 40 cm H_2O), whereas impaired contractility presents as a diminished or intermittent stream in combination with *low* detrusor pressures (less than 30 cm H_2O). There is an

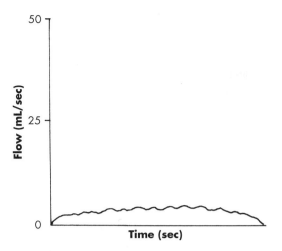

Fig. 8-3 Prolonged "poor" uroflow pattern.

argument for routinely obtaining urodynamic studies in men with BPH who are suspected of having some degree of impaired contractility, because TURP in these patients is unlikely to improve symptoms or urinary flow rate and may actually make the patient worse.[28]

Imaging Studies. Imaging studies are typically reserved for selected patients and are chosen based on the type of data needed. For example, retrograde urethrogram is commonly performed when urethral stricture is suspected, to confirm location and length of the stricture. Similarly, ultrasound can be used to assess renal and prostate size and the presence of bladder trabeculation (an indicator of prolonged obstruction). Finally, a radionucleotide scan may be done to assess renal function. Table 8-5 outlines the various diagnostic studies that may be undertaken in the evaluation of a patient with known or suspected retention.

MANAGEMENT OF THE PATIENT WITH ACUTE OR CHRONIC RETENTION

Primary management options for the patient with urinary retention include behavioral strategies, short-term (or long-term) indwelling catheterization, clean intermittent catheterization, alpha-adrenergic blocking agents, and surgical procedures to correct any obstructing lesions. The specific therapy for a given patient is determined by the particular etiologic factors and by patient/caregiver abilities and preferences. For men with retention caused by BPH, the treatment choices have changed significantly over the last decade; the development of new pharmacologic agents and noninvasive surgical procedures has reduced the number of patients treated with standard surgical procedures (such as TURP) by more than 60%.[29] The specific options now available for treatment of BPH are discussed in greater detail later in this chapter.

Behavioral Strategies

Behavioral management may be of benefit for the patient with mild retention resulting from impaired bladder contractility; this approach involves strategies such as fluid management (avoidance of diuretic fluids and even spacing of fluid intake), routine scheduled voiding to prevent increased bladder distension, and "double voiding" (voiding, waiting 1 to 2 minutes, and then attempting to void again before leaving the bathroom). Biofeedback may be beneficial for selected individuals with pseudo-detrusor-sphincter dyssynergia caused by dysfunctional voiding patterns; visual feedback of pelvic muscle activity is frequently very helpful in teaching the individual to relax the pelvic floor muscles to permit bladder emptying. However, effective use of biofeedback requires a motivated person with normal or near-normal innervation of the pelvic floor.[30]

Clean Intermittent Catheterization

Straight (in-and-out) catheterization is used in the initial assessment of a patient with known or suspected retention, and routine straight catheterization can be used to manage retention and to maintain urethral patency following stricture dilatation. In noninstitutional settings, patients are taught to perform the procedure using "clean" technique, that is, clean hands and a clean catheter as opposed to sterile gloves and a sterile catheter; studies have shown no increase in urinary tract infections when catheters are reused after being washed with soap and water.[31,32] Patients must be taught *not* to force the catheter through the urethra, because this can result in urethral tearing, creation of a "false passage," extravasation of urine, infection, and sepsis. Table 8-6 provides guidance for performance of clean intermittent catheterization.

Patients must also be taught the importance of performing catheterization on schedule (to prevent overdistension of the bladder) and the importance of maintaining adequate fluid intake. The specific schedule must be individualized for the patient. A guide for adults is that catheterization should be completed often enough to maintain catheterized volumes at approximately 500 mL. For people who void but have incomplete emptying, once-daily catheterization (such as at bedtime) may be sufficient to prevent overdistension of the bladder and to eliminate urinary stasis; for patients who do not void at all, catheterization will need to be done four to six times a day, depending on fluid intake. Urodynamic studies, which provide data regarding bladder pressure during filling and at capacity, are extremely valuable in establishing a goal for catheterized urine volumes that will prevent overdistension and vesicoureteral reflux. (For example, if urodynamic studies indicate an unacceptable rise in detrusor pressures when bladder volume exceeds 450 mL, the patient must be taught to maintain a catheterization schedule that produces catheterized volumes of less than 450 mL.) (See Chapter 12 for further discussion of urodynamic studies.)

Indwelling Catheterization

Short-term use of an indwelling catheter is commonly used to manage acute urinary retention; current recommendations include insertion of an indwelling catheter for 48 to 72 hours along with initiation of an alpha-adrenergic blocking agent. Studies indicate that as many as 42% of men presenting with acute retention will be able to void spontaneously following bladder decompression for 48 to 72 hours with an indwelling catheter; these patients can be followed and managed on alpha blockers alone.[33] Patients should be instructed to expect postobstruction diuresis resulting in large volume voids for a period of time following bladder decompression. Risk factors for *failure* to void effectively following catheter removal include the following: increased age, long-term obstruction, increased severity of LUTS, uroflow of less than 10 mL/second, large prostate gland (greater than 40 mL), more than one episode of acute retention, and the presence of comorbid conditions.[34]

A broad-spectrum antibiotic, such as a fluoroquinolone or aminoglycoside, is commonly administered before catheter insertion; this is based on the high incidence of urinary tract infection among patients in retention and the resultant high risk for urosepsis. Patients in acute retention may also benefit from the administration of systemic analgesics

TABLE 8-6 Guidelines for Performance of Clean Intermittent Catheterization

- Wash hands with soap and water.
- Lubricate the catheter as needed (usually recommended).
- Insert the catheter; drain urine into the toilet, urinal, zip-lock plastic bag, or other container.
- Withdraw the catheter slowly to allow complete urine drainage; bend or kink the catheter before final withdrawal to prevent urine drips.
- Wash the catheter and hands with soap and water, sudsing for 10 seconds; rinse and allow the catheter to air dry (such as on paper towel).
- Once dry, place the catheter in paper bag, zip-lock bag, or other convenient storage container for the next catheterization.

Tips:

Catheters can be reused many times, usually until the soap residue causes them to become opaque (about 7 to 10 days).

Catheterization intervals should be guided by patient's bladder capacity, symptoms, and fluid intake. A general guide for adults is catheterizing often enough to maintain catheterized volumes at 500 mL or less (usually every 4 to 6 hours).

e pain, promote
before catheterization, to the rhabdosphinc-
relaxation, and reduce s. Application of anes-
ter during catheter ally in men and children;
thetic gels to the ave shown that local anes-
catheter ins ective in relieving the pain
well-des'sthetic gel (lidocaine [Xylocaine]
the n these populations.[33,35] In men,
on; the urethral opening should then
osed (or the penis gently clamped) for
utes before catheter insertion to allow the
c to take effect. For men in retention,
ation should be performed with a large
Fr) catheter because larger catheters are
d easier to manipulate than smaller sizes;
rticularly important when catheterizing a
patient with prostatic enlargement.

nsertion of a catheter to relieve urinary retention
not without risk; in nonexpert hands, attempts at
catheterization can severely traumatize the urethra.
No more than three attempts should be made
to insert a catheter before urologic services are
consulted, a suprapubic catheter is inserted by an
experienced clinician, or the patient is transferred
to another center.

There is much discussion in the nursing literature about the amount of urine to drain when
inserting a catheter to decompress the bladder; many
nurses are afraid that draining large volumes of
urine may result in hematuria or vasovagal attacks.
Based on these fears, many centers have established
recommendations limiting initial drainage to
500 mL, followed by clamping of the catheter for
variable lengths of time before further decompression. In actuality, vasovagal episodes and other
adverse effects are rare; therefore, recommendations
for routine clamping of the catheter should be
replaced with cautions to assess each patient throughout the decompression procedure, to interrupt
drainage *if* adverse symptoms occur (such as sweating, pallor, or hypotension), and to resume decompression when the symptoms subside. In most cases,
the bladder can safely be emptied in one procedure.

Long-term management with an indwelling
catheter is considered to be a "last resort" treatment

option (because of multiple complications) and is
therefore limited to patients whose retention cannot
be effectively managed with surgery and/or pharmacotherapy (and who are unable to perform
intermittent catheterization). Management of the
patient with an indwelling catheter is discussed in
depth in Chapter 10

Pharmacologic Management Options

There are limited options for pharmacologic
management of urinary retention. Alpha-adrenergic
antagonists may be of benefit for patients whose
retention is caused or exacerbated by excessive
urethral tone or by prostatic hyperplasia; these agents
reduce urethral resistance by blocking sympathetic
receptors at the bladder neck. They are *most*
commonly used for patients with BPH; therefore,
they are addressed in more detail later in this chapter.
Cholinergic agents such as bethanechol are theoretically of benefit in the management of retention,
particularly when the retention is caused by impaired
contractility; however, these agents have proven
relatively ineffective in clinical practice and are
therefore not commonly used. No pharmacologic
agent can relieve upper tract obstruction; however,
these patients frequently require analgesics for pain
control and antibiotics for management of infection.

Surgical Management Options

Surgical procedures are of benefit in selected cases,
for diagnosis, primary correction of an obstructive
lesion, or to establish urinary drainage above
the point of obstruction. Cystoscopy should be
performed whenever direct visualization of the
urethra, bladder neck, or bladder is indicated;
specific situations in which cystoscopy is beneficial
include suspected urethral trauma or stricture and
signs and symptoms of bladder cancer, such as
hematuria. (Patients with hematuria should also
have urine cytology studies performed.) Surgery
can also be used to *treat* selected cases of retention;
for example, strictureplasty or dilatation may relieve
or reduce obstruction caused by urethral stricture,
surgical repair of pelvic organ prolapse and cystocele corrects any associated obstruction in women
(the alternative to surgery is use of a pessary), and
TURP or alternative prostatic ablation procedures

may be of benefit for patients with BPH. (Acute retention in men with BPH is typically treated medically, because TURP in this situation is associated with significant morbidity, that is, bleeding, pyelonephritis, and sepsis.)[36] Ureteral reimplantation is the procedure of choice for persistent vesicoureteral reflux. Finally, surgical procedures may be required to establish drainage proximal to an uncorrectable obstructive lesion; the specific procedure depends on the level of obstruction. For example, placement of a ureteral stent (or construction of a ureterostomy) may be required to maintain ureteral patency in the patient with ureteral stricture or ureteral compression, and nephrostomy tube placement may be required for the patient with uncorrectable ureteral obstruction. The goal of surgical intervention is to restore drainage promptly, because this may allow reversal of renal damage; if renal function does not improve, the kidney remains infected, and the patient is symptomatic, nephrectomy may be required.

BENIGN PROSTATIC HYPERPLASIA

BPH is a common noncancerous condition affecting nearly all aging men and a very common cause of urinary retention. The term "prostatic hyperplasia" can be defined in terms of microscopic changes in the prostatic tissue, macroscopic changes in the prostate gland, or clinical manifestations produced by the changes in the prostate gland. *Microscopically,* BPH is manifest by proliferation (hyperplasia) of the stromal and epithelial cells within the periurethral zone of the prostate gland. This cellular hyperplasia causes glandular enlargement and the typical symptoms commonly known as "prostatism," although size of the prostate, degree of urethral resistance, and severity of symptoms are not strongly correlated.[37-39] Some clinicians argue that the term "benign prostatic hyperplasia" should be used to describe histologic evidence of cellular hyperplasia and that "benign prostatic enlargement" is a more appropriate term for description of macroscopic prostatic enlargement;[38] however, BPH is the commonly used term and the one recommended by the International Consultation on BPH. The Fourth International Consultation on BPH also recommended the use of standardized terminology

to describe lower urinary tract symptoms.[40] In the past, the term "prostatism" was used to refer to symptoms associated with voiding difficulty, such as hesitancy, intermittent or weak urinary stream; however, these voiding difficulties occur in women as well as men, and to date a cause-and-effect relationship has not been established between histologic hyperplasia and voiding symptoms. Therefore, the term "lower urinary tract symptoms" has been adopted to describe symptoms of voiding difficulty and to replace the older term "prostatism."

Epidemiology

The etiology and pathogenesis of BPH are not clearly understood, and the true incidence has not yet been established. Several population studies suggest that the overall incidence is 15 per 1000 man-years and that the incidence increases from a rate of 3 per 1000 man-years in men less than 49 years of age to 38 per 1000 man-years in men aged 75 or more.[41] Indeed, as many as 50% of 60-year old men and 80% of 80-year old men suffer voiding dysfunction and LUTS related to BPH.[42] Severe LUTS have a significant impact on health and well-being,[43] and the number of men affected by this condition will continue to rise as a result of longer life expectancies.

Data regarding risk factors for BPH are inconclusive and sometimes contradictory. For example, one study of Asian men found that alcohol use and smoking appeared to reduce the risk of BPH,[44] whereas several other population surveys found these behaviors to be associated with *increased* risk. Smoking stimulates the sympathetic nervous system and theoretically may increase smooth muscle tone at the bladder neck and sphincter;[45] thus, smoking seems more likely to act as a risk factor than a protective factor. Studies supporting this hypothesis include a study conducted in the United States of African-American men in which the following factors were associated with increased risk for LUTS: history of smoking or current tobacco use, heavy alcohol consumption, history of hypertension or heart disease, and diabetes.[46] Similarly, a study of Finnish men found a higher prevalence of LUTS among those who smoked as compared with those who did not.[47] Race appears to affect the rate at which symptoms develop; African-American men develop symptoms earlier than white men, whereas Asian men develop symptoms later than white men.[44] Comorbidities associated with LUTS include neurologic disease, arthritis, and constipation or fecal impaction.[48]

Pathophysiology

Factors currently believed to be important in the development of BPH include growth factors, stromal-epithelial cell interaction (signaling), hormonal factors (production of dihydrotestosterone and relative proportion of estrogens), and nonandrogenic factors produced by the testes.[49,50] Growth factors are known to affect cell growth and cell death and are believed to function synergistically with androgens (dihydrotestosterone) to stimulate stromal cell hyperplasia. The growth factors most relevant to BPH include epidermal growth factor, keratinocyte growth factor, and basic fibroblast growth factor. A synergistic effect involving androgens and growth factors helps to explain *stromal cell hyperplasia*; however, it does not explain epithelial cell hyperplasia, because these cells are unresponsive to androgens. The mitotic response of epithelial cells is believed to be mediated by stromal-epithelial cell interactions. Although epithelial cells are unresponsive to androgenic stimulation, they are very responsive to growth factors produced by the stromal cells, and these growth factors are produced in greater quantities when the stromal cells are stimulated by androgens. Thus, androgenic stimulation may indirectly affect epithelial hyperplasia. In addition, the testes may produce a nonandrogenic substance that acts to sensitize the prostatic tissues to the effects of androgens.[50] Finally, estrogen is believed to play some type of supportive or synergistic role in the development of BPH.[44]

The typical symptoms associated with BPH (diminished urinary stream, hesitancy, intermittency, nocturia, terminal dribbling, frequency, and urgency) are thought to be caused by the gradual increase in size of the prostate gland. These symptoms may or may not be associated with significant outlet obstruction. In nonobstructed men, LUTS are thought to be caused by a complex interplay of poorly understood factors, including some degree

of urethral obstruction, impaired detrusor contractility, detrusor instability (overactive bladder), and sensory urgency.[37,51-53] Approximately two-thirds to three-fourths of patients with clinical signs of BPH are found to have some degree of obstructed voiding and urinary retention;[51] however, these patients do not necessarily progress to complete inability to void.[26] Potential predictors of complete retention include prostate size, poor uroflow, and clinical symptoms.[41] The primary risk factors for complete obstruction are increasing level of symptoms as measured by the AUA Symptom Score, the sensation of incomplete emptying, urinary frequency (urge to void every 2 hours or more often), and a weak urinary stream.[19] In North America, serious complications of BPH are rare; therefore, treatment should be guided by the patient's perceptions of symptom severity and the impact on his quality of life, as opposed to prostate size per se.

Pathology of Outlet Obstruction Secondary to Benign Prostatic Hyperplasia. As noted, BPH may or may not progress to the point of significant outlet obstruction. When outlet obstruction does occur, it is thought to develop as a result of both static (structural) and dynamic (functional) factors. The static factor is the size of the prostate gland and the degree to which it compresses the urethral lumen. Men whose prostate glands are larger than 30 mL are three times more likely to progress to obstruction than men with smaller prostates (less than 30 mL).[38] Enlargement of the median lobe of the prostate is of particular importance; median lobe hypertrophy can cause significant urethral compression even if the overall size of the prostate appears nonsignificant. This is partly because of the effect of the nonelastic prostatic capsule, which restricts the direction in which the prostate can spread.[37] Prostatic ultrasound scanning can delineate both overall gland enlargement and median lobe enlargement, and the formula obtained by ultrasound (transition zone volume/total prostatic volume) appears to accurately predict patients at high risk for acute retention.[54] The importance of median lobe enlargement (transition zone volume) and total prostate enlargement is supported by the observation that 5-alpha-reductase inhibitors reduce both transition zone volume and overall prostatic volume and also improve symptoms of voiding dysfunction.[54,55]

Dynamic factors contributing to outlet obstruction include smooth muscle tone and alpha-adrenergic receptors.[52,53] Prostatic hyperplasia appears to cause both an increased volume of smooth muscle and increased sympathetic tone, both of which contribute to increased resistance at the level of the prostatic urethra.[37,52,53,55] This has major implications for management, because pharmacologic agents can be used to increase or reduce sympathetic tone; for example, sympathomimetic agents such as pseudoephedrine increase smooth muscle tone and urethral resistance, whereas blockade of the sympathetic receptors by alpha-adrenergic antagonists produces smooth muscle relaxation and reduced resistance at the bladder neck and prostatic urethra. Clinically, the introduction of alpha-adrenergic antagonists has radically changed the management of patients with BPH, because these drugs are highly effective in improving urinary flow rates and reducing obstructive symptoms.[55] There is some controversy about the precise mechanism underlying the "dynamic obstruction" associated with increased prostatic smooth muscle tone. For example, the benefits provided by alpha-adrenergic antagonists could be explained by the reduction of resistance at the bladder neck (as opposed to the prostatic urethra) or by inhibition of various neurologic reflexes affecting vesicourethral function.[53]

Phases of prostatic obstruction. Tanagho identified two major phases in the development of outlet obstruction caused by BPH: the compensatory phase, during which the bladder wall hypertrophies in an attempt to overcome the increased urethral resistance; and the decompensation phase, during which contractility is significantly diminished and residual urine volumes rise significantly[11] (Table 8-7).

During the *compensatory* phase, the detrusor muscle gradually adapts and thickens in response to the increasing resistance caused by the prostate. Urodynamic studies during this phase demonstrate high voiding pressures and decreased compliance; voiding pressures rise to two to four times the normal values, that is, from 30 cm H_2O to as high as 120 cm H_2O.[56] The elevated intravesical pressures cause formation of cellules, small pockets that are created when segments of the bladder lining are pushed between bundles of superficial muscle fibers. If the pressures within the bladder remain high, the cellules eventually push through the entire thickness of the bladder wall to form diverticula; the diverticular sacs fail to empty effectively, thus creating pools of stagnant urine that act as a reservoir for bacterial proliferation and calculi formation. The elevated pressures within the bladder wall also promote collagen deposition and hypertrophy of the smooth muscle fibers, resulting in bladder wall trabeculation. Hypertrophy of

TABLE 8-7 **Phases of Bladder Response to Benign Prostatic Hypertrophy**

STAGE OF BLADDER RESPONSE	PATHOLOGIC CHANGES IN BLADDER
Compensatory phase	Trabeculation of bladder wall, hypertrophy of the trigone, detrusor overactivity
Decompensation phase	Changes in muscle function and loss of contractility, resulting in elevated postvoid residual urine volume, loss of bladder wall compliance resulting in elevated intravesical pressures and increased resistance at ureterovesical junction; the end result consists of ureteral dilatation, hydronephrosis, and potential for urinary tract infection, pyelonephritis, and impaired renal function

Data from Tanagho EA. Urinary obstruction and stasis. In: Tanagho EA, McAninch JW, editors: *Smith's general urology,* ed 16, New York, 2004, Lange Medical Books/McGraw-Hill, pp 175-187.

the smooth muscle fibers is particularly pronounced in the trigonal region;[15,57] this causes distortion of the ureteric orifices, which results in progressive obstruction of the ureters, reflux, and hydronephrosis. (Catheterization and bladder decompression temporarily relieve the trigonal distension and reduce distortion and obstruction of the ureteral orifices.) In addition to detrusor hypertophy, the early phases of outlet obstruction cause detrusor overactivity, as evidenced by the classic symptoms of urgency, frequency, nocturia, and possibly urge incontinence. Finally, on a microscopic level, the bladder wall is infiltrated with plasma cells, lymphocytes, and polymorphonuclear cells.

Unrelieved obstruction eventually results in bladder *decompensation*. The decompensation phase is characterized by progressive reduction in bladder contractility and ability to empty the bladder. As contractility declines, PVR volumes and the incidence of urinary tract infections rise. If treatment is not initiated, the bladder eventually becomes totally acontractile.

Assessment

Factors to be included in the assessment of any patient with known or suspected retention have been addressed earlier in this chapter. This section addresses the assessment parameters of particular relevance to the patient with BPH.

History. In obtaining patient history, the nurse must remember that LUTS and urinary retention can be caused by many factors and conditions other than BPH; even in the patient with known BPH, there may be neurologic or pharmacologic factors contributing to the degree of retention and severity of symptoms. Therefore, a complete history is always essential; this must include medical conditions, past surgical procedures, all prescription and over-the-counter medications, and a thorough discussion of urologic symptoms. Because the treatment of BPH is affected in large part by the degree of "bother" associated with LUTS, the nurse should query the patient regarding symptom onset, the degree of bother, any diagnostic procedures that have been completed in relation to the problem, and any past or current treatment. A validated tool should be used to assess symptom severity; the AUA

Symptom Score (also known as the International Prostate Symptom Score) is a validated tool that provides an objective index of symptom severity and can also contribute to the prediction of risk for urinary retention.[19,21] See Table 8-5. (The range of scores is from 0, for no symptoms, to 35, extreme symptoms; a score greater than 7 is associated with increased risk for retention.) It is also helpful to query the patient about any problems with erectile function, especially if treatment with 5-alpha-reductase inhibitors is being considered; the nurse should discuss the potential effects of these drugs on sexual function.

Physical Examination. The most critical element of the physical examination for the patient with BPH is the digital rectal exam; the prostate gland should be carefully assessed for size, shape, consistency, and masses. In addition, the clinician should note tone and contractility of the anal sphincter and the presence and consistency of stool in the rectal vault. Other factors to be assessed have been discussed earlier in this chapter and include abdominal exam and evidence of neurologic dysfunction.

Diagnostic Studies. As is true of all patients with known or suspected urinary retention, measurement of PVR urine volume and uroflowmetry provide very valuable data. Urodynamic studies should be done when there is concern regarding detrusor contractility and the patient is contemplating TURP,[58,59] and transurethral ultrasound is indicated when it is important to accurately delineate prostate size (situations in which minimally invasive procedures are being considered).

Prostate-specific antigen (PSA) is not recommended as a routine test for all men with BPH and LUTS; however, it *is* recommended for men with a life expectancy of more than 10 years and for situations in which PSA results may alter treatment.[60] For example, several trials have shown that PSA is a proxy for prostate volume and can be used to predict symptom progression and response to therapies such as 5-alpha-reductase inhibitors.[61] Men with LUTS who have a PSA greater than 1.5 ng/mL are more likely to have a prostate volume of at least 30 mL and are at higher risk for complete obstruction than men whose PSA is less than 1.5 ng/mL.[62]

Thus, men whose PSA is elevated and who are symptomatic should undergo therapy designed to reduce prostate gland volume, that is, 5-alpha-reductase inhibitors (possibly in combination with alpha-adrenergic blockers to improve voiding symptoms). Conversely, men whose PSA is less than 1.5 ng/mL are much less likely to progress to outlet obstruction; in these patients, treatment is determined by symptom severity and bother and is designed to reduce voiding difficulty, as opposed to reducing prostate volume. These patients are best managed with alpha blockers as opposed to 5-alpha-reductase inhibitors.

Risk Factors for Retention. In considering treatment options for the patient with BPH, one consideration is risk for progression to significant retention. Factors that have been identified as predictive of risk for retention include the following: age; prostate size larger than 30 mL, urinary flow rate less than 12 mL/second, AUA Symptom Score greater than 7, and PVR volumes greater than 150 mL.

Management

The introduction of new pharmacologic agents for treatment of BPH and the development of minimally invasive procedures for prostatic resection have led to significant changes in the treatment options for men with clinically significant BPH and LUTS. Men are now offered a variety of options, depending on symptom severity and potential for obstruction; these include watchful waiting, alpha-adrenergic blocking agents, 5-alpha-reductase agents, transurethral microwave heat treatment (TMT), transurethral needle ablation (TUNA), interstitial laser therapy, stent placement, TURP, and suprapubic prostatectomy. Patients who are relatively asymptomatic may be managed with "watchful waiting" as well as with reassurance and education regarding behavioral strategies (fluid management, restriction of caffeine and alcohol intake, and routine toileting).[63]

Treatment decisions should be guided by patient preference. The AUA Consensus Guidelines note that even men with moderate or severe symptoms do not necessarily require further diagnostic tests or active therapy if they are not bothered by their symptoms (and if they are relatively low risk for retention).

Management of Irritative Voiding Symptoms. As noted earlier, obstruction may produce bladder overactivity and irritative voiding symptoms (urgency, frequency, nocturia, and possibly urge incontinence), and relief of the obstruction may or may not resolve the symptoms.[16] Indeed, relief of the obstruction may actually cause worsening of any incontinence, because the "protective mechanism" provided by the obstruction has been removed. If the obstruction has not been prolonged, the symptoms may gradually resolve; in addition, numerous treatment strategies may be of benefit for these individuals, such as fluid management, restriction of caffeine intake, bladder retraining strategies, and anticholinergics (see Chapter 5).

Management of Obstructive Voiding Symptoms: Alpha-Adrenergic Blockers. As has been stated, medical management of obstructive voiding symptoms related to BPH has been revolutionized by the introduction of alpha-adrenergic antagonists (alpha blockers). (Table 8-8 outlines the currently available pharmacologic agents for treatment of obstructive voiding symptoms.) This means that many men who would formerly have required surgery can now be managed medically; it also means that patients who *do* require surgery are generally more symptomatic, with larger prostate glands, and are therefore at higher risk for complications.

Alpha-adrenergic receptors mediate catecholaminergic actions in the sympathetic nervous system, and alpha blockers bind to these receptors to "block" the effects of sympathetic neurotransmitters such as norepinephrine. At least three alpha-receptor subtypes have been identified in humans: alpha-1a, alpha-1b, and alpha-1d. In the urinary tract, the most significant alpha-receptor subtypes seem to be alpha-1a and alpha-1d, and the alpha-1d receptors have a much higher affinity for norepinephrine and epinephrine than either the alpha-1a or alpha-1b receptors[64] (Fig. 8-4). The alpha-1d receptors predominate in the detrusor and are less common in the prostatic stroma and capsule; the reverse is true of the alpha-1a receptors. Thus, blockade of these two receptor types will theoretically improve bladder contractility while reducing urethral resistance. DeGroat suggested

TABLE 8-8   **Alpha-1-Adrenergic Receptors in Lower Urinary Tract**

RECEPTOR SUBTYPE	DISTRIBUTION	EFFECTS OF RECEPTOR BLOCKADE
Alpha 1A	Prostatic stroma and capsule, bladder neck	Decreases tone in prostate and bladder neck
Alpha 1B	Prostatic epithelium, vascular smooth muscle	Relaxes blood vessels
Alpha 1D	Prostatic stroma, vascular smooth muscle	Decreases tone in prostate, relaxes blood vessels

From Kaplan SA: Use of alpha adrenergic inhibitors in treatment of benign prostatic hyperplasia and implications on sexual function, *Urology* 63(3):428-434, 2004.

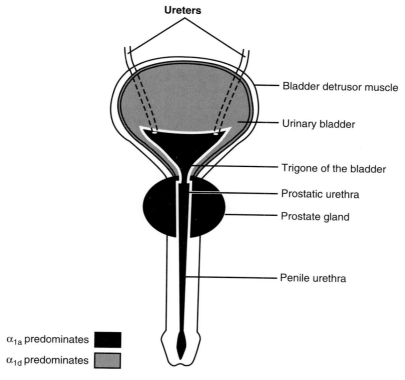

Fig. 8-4 Distribution of α_1-AR subtypes in human male urogenital system. From Roehrborn, Claus G, Schwinn, Debra A: α_1-adrenergic receptors and their inhibitors in lower urinary tract systems and benign prostatic hyperplasia, *Journal of Urology,* 2004; 171(3):1031.

that alpha-adrenergic blockers may also slightly enhance bladder contractility by a direct or indirect effect on the parasympathetic ganglia, thus further explaining their ability to improve bladder emptying.[65]

Sympathetic stimulation of the prostatic smooth muscle, which is mediated by alpha-adrenergic receptors, results in increased muscle tone (the dynamic component of outlet obstruction); the primary neurotransmitter is noradrenaline (norephinephrine). Alpha-adrenergic antagonists (terazosin, doxazosin, tamsulosin, and alfuzosin) improve voiding function by "blocking" the alpha-adrenergic receptors located in the smooth muscle of the bladder neck, proximal urethra, and prostatic stroma and capsule.[66] This blockade rapidly reverses the effects of alpha-adrenergic agonists such as ephedrine and norepinephrine.[67] A review of efficacy studies indicates that all these agents improve voiding symptoms to a similar degree,[64] and all involve once-daily dosing. However, tamsulosin and alfuzosin are associated with a lower incidence of side effects, especially postural hypotension (as compared with terazosin and doxazosin). All these agents are selective for alpha-1 receptors; however, tamsulosin is the *most* selective for the alpha-1a and alpha-1d receptor subtypes in the prostatic stroma and capsule, which may explain its reduced incidence of cardiovascular side effects. However, doxazosin and terazosin may also contribute to reduction in volume of prostatic smooth muscle through a molecular mechanism that enhances apoptosis (death) of the smooth muscle cells; this may account for the long-term benefit conferred by these particular medications.[68] Research is ongoing into the possible use of alpha antagonists to promote apoptosis in men with prostate cancer.

Men with advanced BPH and severe LUTS may not benefit from alpha-adrenergic antagonists and may require more invasive treatment. Specific indicators for more aggressive treatment include the following: prostate larger than 40 mL, severe symptoms as measured by the AUA symptom score, uroflow of less than 10 mL/second, and/or urodynamic evidence of outflow obstruction.[34]

Reduction of Prostate Size. Prostate size is the "static" element contributing to BPH-induced outlet obstruction; the degree of urethral compression is directly related to the size of the prostate as a whole and the median lobe in particular. Until the introduction of 5-alpha-reductase inhibitors, the only way to reduce the size of the prostate was surgical resection (typically TURP). However, it is well known that the prostate is an androgen-sensitive organ, and BPH can be viewed as a bulky, testosterone-dependent prostatic adenoma.[69] Thus, reduction in testosterone levels (and prostate size)

can be achieved by administration of drugs that block the effects of 5-alpha-reductase, a steroid that is necessary for the conversion of testosterone to dihydrotestosterone (a much more potent androgen). 5-alpha-reductase has two isoforms: Type I is expressed in the liver, skin, hair follicles, and the testicles; and Type 2, which is responsible for male virilization, is found in genital skin, hair follicles, and the stromal and epithelial cells of the prostate. Finasteride and dutasteride are the two 5-alpha-reductase inhibitors currently available, and both achieve reduction in prostate size and subsequent reduction in urethral obstruction.[70-72] The benefits of finasteride are well documented: reduction in size of the prostate gland, reversal of the disease process (BPH reversal), reduction in voiding symptoms, reduced episodes of urinary retention, and reduced likelihood of invasive surgery such as TURP.[49,70] Dutasteride differs from finasteride in that it is capable of inhibiting both isoforms of 5-alpha-reductase. This may result in greater inhibition of dihydrotestosterone production and therefore in more rapid clinical response; however, this has not yet been proven.[73] Clinically, to date the drugs appear comparable, although no head-to-head studies have yet been published.[74] Side effects of 5-alpha-reductase inhibitors include decreased libido, impotence, reduced volume of ejaculate, and occasional breast tenderness.[75] Fortunately, most of these side effects diminish over time.

Men who are most likely to benefit from 5-alpha-reductase inhibitors include those with prostate glands of 40 mL or more.[76,77] These drugs have been shown to control BPH-related hematuria in addition to preventing progression of the disease process; these drugs may also contribute to the prevention of prostate cancer, although further research is needed in this area.[74] Men with large-volume prostates who also have severe LUTS may benefit from dual therapy, that is, a combination of 5-alpha-reductase inhibitors (to reduce prostate volume) and alpha-adrenergic antagonists (to reduce urethral resistance); combination therapy reduces the risk of acute urinary retention more effectively than either drug alone.[66,71] (See Table 8-9 for summary of various drugs that can be used to reduce LUTS in men with BPH.)

TABLE 8-9   Medical Therapy for Lower Urinary Tract Symptoms

DRUG	ACTION	DOSE	SIDE EFFECTS
Terazosin (Hytrin)	Nonselective alpha-1 blocker; relaxes smooth muscle of bladder neck	1 mg at HS to reduce incidence and severity of side effects; gradually increase dose to 2 mg, 5 mg, 10 mg to achieve desired flow rate; 4 to 6 weeks may be required to achieve benefit	NB: All alpha-blockers should be administered cautiously in patients taking antihypertensives *Both terazosin and doxazosin: First-dose syncope; postural hypotension, fatigue, dizziness, headache, nasal stuffiness, erectile dysfunction, urinary incontinence, need to monitor blood pressure*
Doxazosin (Cardura)	Nonselective alpha-1 blocker (very similar to terazosin)	1 mg once daily; gradually increase to 2 mg, 4 mg, 8 mg to achieve benefit; each increase should be approximately 2 weeks apart	
Tamsulosin (Flomax)	Selective alpha-1 blocker (alpha-1a, 1d receptor subtypes): reduced cardiovascular side effects because of selectivity	0.4 mg once daily, increase dose to 0.8 mg after 2 weeks if necessary 10 mg once daily	Both tamsulosin and alfuzosin: absorption increased with food; take immediately following same meal each day; ejaculatory dysfunction; contraindicated in men with hepatic insufficiency; potential P450 3A4 inhibitor
Alfuzosin (Uroxatral)			
Finasteride (Proscar)	5-alpha-Reductase inhibitor: inhibits Type II isoenzyme in stromal and basal epithelial cells to prevent conversion of testosterone to dihydrotestosterone	5 mg once daily	Erectile dysfunction; decreased libido; ejaculatory dysfunction; long-term therapy required; may take 6 months to reach peak efficacy; not effective in men with small prostates
Dutasteride (Avodart)	5-alpa-Reductase inhibitor; may inhibit both Type 1 and Type 2 isoenzymes	0.5 mg	Similar side effects; dual isoenzyme inhibition should cause more rapid relief of obstructive symptoms
Phytotherapy: saw palmetto, beta-sitosterols, *Pygeum africanum*, cernitin	Actions not completely understood; believed to act as mild 5-alpha-reductase inhibitor and possibly aromatase inhibitor	Dosages and benefits vary widely depending on preparation	Advise patient that he should not take phytotherapy when using other medical therapy for obstructed voiding

Adapted from Turkoski BB, Lance BR, Bonfiglio MF: *Drug information handbook for advanced practice nursing*, ed 4, Hudson, Ohio, 2003, Lexi-Comp, p 1715, with permission.

Phytotherapy (Herbal Medications). Phytotherapy is a common form of self-treatment among men with LUTS,[78] and in Europe, nonprescription herbal agents are recommended at least as often as alpha-blocking agents or finasteride.[79] These agents are thought to "work" by inhibiting 5-alpha-reductase and possibly by inhibiting aromatase.[80] Commonly used herbal agents include saw palmetto, beta-sitosterols (Prostatic Perform), *Pygeum africanum* (pygeum bark), and cernitin (Cernilton);[81] saw palmetto is the most widely studied of these agents. Randomized controlled trials conducted to date provide the following guidance in use of herbal agents:

- Saw palmetto provides improvement in voiding symptoms with low incidence of side effects (comparable with placebo), but the clinical benefit is less than that provided by finasteride.[82]
- Beta-sitosterols improve symptoms as compared with placebo.[83]
- *Pygeum africanum* demonstrates a slight benefit over placebo.[84]
- Cernitin (rye pollen) provides a slight benefit over placebo and appears equal in effect to *Pygeum africanum*.[85]
- As compared with finasteride, saw palmetto is not effective in relieving pain or improving quality of life in men with chronic prostatitis.[86]

In the laboratory, *Opuntia* (prickly pear) cactus demonstrates 5-alpha-reductase, aromatase, and free radical properties but has not been compared with placebo.[80] Stinging nettle is associated with relief of LUTS and is associated with a decreased AUA Symptom Score; however, in the studies conducted, there was no significant difference in maximum urinary flow rate or in PVR urine.[87] In summary, the role of phytotherapeutics is not yet clearly defined, but they are frequently used; thus, the health history must always include inquiries regarding use of these agents.

Aromatase Inhibitors. Estrogen and estradiol are thought to play a role in prostate stromal growth and the resulting BPH, because the relative concentration of estrogens increases with age and the plasma levels of testosterone diminish.[88] Aromatase inhibitors block estrogen biosynthesis, which theoretically should result in reduction of prostate size. However, to date, aromatase therapy has produced no significant difference in voiding symptoms as compared with placebo; this therapy therefore remains investigational.[60]

Anticholinergics/Antimuscarinics. Anticholinergic medications bind to the muscarinic receptors and block the uptake of acetylcholine, which is released by cholinergic nerves in response to parasympathetic stimulation. These agents are the mainstay of pharmacologic therapy for overactive bladder, and it is well established that bladder outlet obstruction caused by prostatic hyperplasia often produces symptoms of overactive bladder. However, clinicians have been reluctant to prescribe anticholinergics for these patients, because a theoretic side effect is diminished bladder contractility resulting in increased PVRs or in urinary retention. Although this makes sense physiologically, a recent review of the literature suggests that men who receive either tolterodine or oxybutynin for symptoms of urgency, frequency, and nocturia do obtain symptom relief and are at no greater risk of elevated PVRs or urinary retention than men who receive placebo.[89]

Surgical Intervention: Transurethral Resection of the Prostate and Minimally Invasive Procedures

TURP is the most common approach to surgical resection of the prostate and is considered to be the gold standard in terms of treatment efficacy. Before undertaking surgical resection, it is important to determine accurately whether the patient's voiding symptoms are caused by urethral obstruction, because prostatic resection is of benefit only in these patients. LUTS in unobstructed patients are usually caused either by detrusor instability or by compromised contractility; prostatic resection does not correct detrusor instability and may actually cause worsening of the symptoms and onset of urinary incontinence,[90] and prostatic resection is of little benefit in the case of reduced contractility because it fails to address the underlying pathologic features.[59] These issues point to the value of urodynamic studies before surgical intervention, because pressure-flow data can provide the information needed to differentiate between outlet obstruction and impaired contractility; however, routine use of urodynamic testing for all patients with prostatic obstruction remains controversial.[59,91]

Risk factors for poor voiding function following TURP include the following: age more than 80 years, retention of more than 1500 mL urine, absence of detrusor instability, poor sensation, and maximal detrusor pressure lower than 28 cm H_2O.[92] These factors should be taken into consideration when considering a patient's candidacy for surgery.

Minimally Invasive Procedures. Recent advances in the field of prostate surgery include the development of minimally invasive procedures: TMT, water-induced thermotherapy, TUNA, and high-energy TMT. All these procedures use an energy source to heat the obstructing prostatic tissue, which results in coagulation tissue necrosis. Energy sources include microwave thermotherapy, water-induced thermotherapy, radiofrequency, and laser. These procedures are generally recommended for men with less severe obstructive symptoms, who have not responded to medical management with alpha blockers and/or 5-alpha-reductase inhibitors, and who do not wish to undergo more invasive surgery (or who are not candidates for more invasive procedures.)[93] Noninvasive procedures are usually attractive to patients and payors because they can usually be done in day surgery or the physician's office, and they are less costly than TURP. Outcomes vary as compared with TURP, but all appear effective in the short term.

In summary, the pathology of BPH is complex and not well understood. Of note is that pathology studies on resected prostatic tissue reveal distinct "patterns" of hyperplasia (predominantly stromal hyperplasia, predominantly glandular hyperplasia, and mixed hyperplasia),[52] which suggests distinct pathologic conditions that may affect treatment. Currently, the mechanisms believed to account for the clinical symptoms include static outlet obstruction caused by the enlarging prostate gland, dynamic outlet obstruction related to sympathetic tone in the prostate and bladder neck, and factors such as changes in sensory input and altered detrusor stability and contractility. Current treatment options include medical or surgical reduction of prostatic volume, medical inhibition of sympathetic tone, and strategies to reduce overactive bladder symptoms. It is likely that future management of patients with BPH will be based on a much clearer understanding of the specific pathologic mechanisms and a broader choice of treatment options.

SUMMARY

In this chapter, the common causes of urinary retention, defined as the inability to empty the bladder completely, have been reviewed. The most common cause of retention is in men with prostatism; retention is also common among diabetic patients and is often overlooked. Pathologic factors contributing to retention at the level of the bladder include bladder outlet obstruction, diminished bladder contractility, or a combination of both. Retention may also occur in the upper tract, as a result of obstructive lesions in the bladder, ureter, or kidney. In both cases, these may be acquired or congenital. Whatever the cause, some general principles guide assessment and treatment: maintaining renal and bladder health, preventing infections, and maintaining quality of life. Upper tract obstructions are always managed surgically. Retention caused by lower tract obstruction may be managed surgically but may also be amenable to a variety of conservative strategies such as intermittent catheterization, alpha blockers, and biofeedback. Retention caused by loss of contractility is managed by behavioral therapies (such as double voiding and timed voiding), alpha blockers, and/or catheterization. Nursing management of patients with retention is critical and involves education regarding medications (and monitoring for efficacy and for adverse effects), empathetic and thorough instruction in clean intermittent catheterization, measures to prevent or promptly manage urinary tract infections, follow-up and evaluation of the total individualized treatment plan, and ongoing attention to development and implementation of a management plan that preserves both renal health and the patient's quality of life.

SELF-ASSESSMENT EXERCISE

1. Identify the component of the storage-voiding cycle that is altered in the patient with urinary

retention and the potential effect on upper urinary tract function.

2. Describe the two pathologic processes that are known to cause or contribute to retention and identify implications for management.

3. Explain why acute retention is typically diagnosed quickly while chronic retention may go undiagnosed for prolonged periods of time.

4. Identify strategies to reduce the risk of acute urinary retention in the postoperative patient.

5. Define the term "lower urinary tract symptoms" and explain why this term has replaced the term "prostatism."

6. Outline typical assessment findings for the patient in acute urinary retention and the patient with chronic urinary retention.

7. Explain how urodynamic studies help to differentiate retention caused by outlet obstruction from retention caused by impaired contractility.

8. Explain the role of static and dynamic factors in the development of BPH and outlet obstruction.

9. Explain why surgical reduction of the prostate gland may *not* result in clinical improvement for the patient with BPH and explain the rationale for use of medical therapies such as finasteride or alpha-adrenergic antagonists in the management of these patients.

10. Explain the role of each of the following in management of the patient with urinary retention:

    • Behavioral therapies
    • Clean intermittent catheterization
    • Indwelling catheterization
    • Alpha-adrenergic antagonists
    • Surgical removal of obstructing lesion or tissue

11. Outline key factors to be included in a teaching plan for a patient with a sacral cord lesion who is being taught to manage her chronic retention with clean intermittent catheterization. (She is ambulatory with braces.)

REFERENCES

1. McNeill SA: The role of alpha-blockers in the management of acute urinary retention caused by benign prostatic obstruction, *Eur Urol* 45:325, 2004.
2. Gray M: Urinary retention: management in the acute care setting. Part 1, *Am J Nurs* 100:40, 2000.
3. Finestone AJ, Rosenthal RS: Silent prostatism, *Geriatrics* 26:89, 1971.
4. Gulmi FA, Felsen D, Vaughan ED Jr: Pathophysiology of urinary tract obstruction. In: Walsh PC, Retik AB, Vaughan ED Jr, editors: *Campbell's urology*, ed 8. Philadelphia, 2002, WB Saunders, pp 411-462.
5. Koff SA, Mutabagani KH: Anomalies of the kidney. In: Gillenwater JY, Grayhack JT, Howards SS, et al, editors: *Adult and pediatric urology*, ed 4, vol 3, Philadelphia, 2002, Lippincott Williams & Wilkins, pp 2129-2154.
6. Joseph DV: Vesicoureteral reflux. In: Gearhart JP, editor: *Pediatric urology*, Totowa, N.J., 2003, Humana Press, pp 51-82.
7. Gillenwater JY: Hydronephrosis. In: Gillenwater JY, Grayhack JT, Howards SS, et al, editors: *Adult and pediatric urology*, vol 1, Philadelphia, 2002, Lippincott Williams & Wilkins, pp 879-905.
8. Murray K, Massey A, Feneley RC: Acute urinary retention: a urodynamic assessment, *Br J Urol* 56:468, 1984.
9. Roehrborn CG, Bruskewitz R, Nickel GC, et al: Urinary retention in patients with BPH treated with finasteride or placebo over 4 years: characterization of patients and ultimate outcomes, *Eur Urol* 37:528, 2000.
10. Kostakopoulos A, Argiropoulos V, Protogerou V, et al: Vesicourethral anastomotic strictures after radical retropubic prostatectomy: the experience of a single institution, *Urol Int* 72:17, 2004.
11. Tanagho EA. Urinary obstruction and stasis. In: Tanagho EA, McAninch JW, editors: *Smith's general urology*, ed 16, New York, 2004, Lange Medical Books/McGraw-Hill, pp 175-187.
12. Cross, Cespedes R, English S, McGuire E: Transvaginal urethrolysis for urethral obstruction after anti-incontinence surgery, *J Urol* 159:1199-1201, 1998.
13. Stevenson K: Voiding dysfunction in women, *Curr Opin Obstet Gynecol* 8:343-346, 1996.
14. Kaplan S, Santarosa R, D'Alisera P, et al: Pseudodyssynergia (contraction of the external sphincter during voiding) misdiagnosed as chronic nonbacterial prostatitis and the role of biofeedback as a therapeutic option, *J Urol* 157:2234-2237, 1997.
15. Gosling JA, Gilpin SA, Dixon JS, et al: Decrease in the autonomic innervation of human detrusor muscle in outflow obstruction, *J Urol* 136:501, 1986.
16. Christ GJ, Venkateswarlu K, Day NS, et al: Intercellular communication and bladder function, *Adv Exp Med Biol* 539:239, 2003.
17. Koelbl H, Mostwin J, Boiteux JP, et al: Pathophysiology. In: Abrams PH, Cardozo L, Khoury S, et al: *Incontinence: Second International Consultation on Incontinence*, ed 2, Plymbridge, UK, 2001, Health Publications, pp 203-241.

18. Zaheer S, Reilly, Pemberton J, Ilstrap D: Urinary retention after operations for benign anorectal disease, *Dis Colon Rectum* 41:696-704, 1998.

19. Meigs JB, Barry MJ, Giovannucci E, et al: Incidence rates and risk factors for acute urinary retention: the Health Professionals Followup Study, *J Urol* 162:376, 1999.

20. Bhargava S, Canda AE, Chapple CR: A rational approach to benign prostatic hyperplasia evaluation: recent advances, *Curr Opin Urol* 14:1, 2004.

21. Barry MJ, Fowler FJ Jr, O'Leary MP, et al: The American Urological Association Symptom Index for benign prostatic hyperplasia, *J Urol* 148:1549, 1992.

22. Gray M: Assessment. In: Gray M, editor: *Genitourinary disorders*, St. Louis, 1992, Mosby–Year Book, pp 20-31.

23. Blackmer J: Rehabilitation medicine: autonomic dysreflexia, *Can Med Assoc J* 169:931, 2003.

24. Shergill IS, Arya M, Hamid R, et al: The importance of autonomic dysreflexia to the urologist, *BJU Int* 93:923, 2004.

25. Mold JW: Pharmacotherapy of urinary incontinence, *Am Fam Physician* 54:673, 1996.

26. AUA Practice Guidelines: AUA guideline on management of benign prostatic hyperplasia, *J Urol* 170:530, 2003.

27. Gray M: Urinary retention: management in the acute care setting. Part 2, *Am J Nurs* 100:36, 2000.

28. Thomas AW, Cannon A, Bartlett E, et al: The natural history of lower urinary tract dysfunction in men: the influence of detrusor underactivity on the outcome after transurethral resection of the prostate with a minimum 10-year urodynamic followup, *BJU Int* 93:745, 2004.

29. Borth CS, Beiko DT, Nickel JC: Impact of medical therapy on transurethral resection of the prostate: a decade of change, *Urology* 57:1082, 2001.

30. McKenna LS, McKenna PH: Modern management of nonneurogenic pediatric incontinence, *J Wound Ostomy Contin Nurs* 31:351-356, 2004.

31. Moore KN, Kelm M, Sinclair O, et al: Bacteriuria in intermittent catheterization users: the effect of sterile versus clean reused catheters, *Rehabil Nurs* 18: 306, 1993.

32. Schlager TA, Clark M, Anderson S: Effect of a single-use sterile catheter for each void on the frequency of bacteriuria in children with neurogenic bladder on intermittent catheterization bladder emptying, *Pediatrics* 108: E71, 2001.

33. Gerard LL, Cooper CS, Duethman KS, et al: Effectiveness of lidocaine lubricant for discomfort during pediatric urethral catheterization, *J Urol* 170:564, 2003.

34. de la Rosette JJ, Kortmann BB, Rossi C, et al: Long term risk of retreatment of patients using alpha-blockers for lower urinary tract symptoms, *J Urol* 167:1734, 2002.

35. Siderias J, Guadio F, Singer AJ: Comparison of topical anesthetics and lubricants prior to urethral catheterization in males: a randomized controlled trial, *Acad Emerg Med* 11:703, 2004.

36. Pickard R, Emberton M, Neal DE: The management of men with acute urinary retention, *Br J Urol* 81:712, 1998.

37. Shapiro E, Lepor H: Pathophysiology of clinical benign prostatic hyperplasia, *Urol Clin North Am* 22:285, 1995.

38. Girman CJ: Natural history and epidemiology of benign prostatic hyperplasia: relationship among urologic measures, *Urology* 51:8, 1998.

39. Guess HA: Benign prostatic hyperplasia: antecedents and natural history, *Epidemiol Rev* 14:131, 1992.

40. Denis L, McConnell O, Yoshida S, et al: Recommendations of the International Scientific Committee. In: Denis L, Griffiths K, Khoury S, et al, editors: *Fourth Inter-National Consultation on Benign Prostatic Hyperplasia (BPH)*, Plymbridge, UK, 1998, Health Publications, pp 669-684.

41. Naderi N, Mochtar CA, de la Rosette JJ: Real life practice in the management of benign prostatic hyperplasia, *Curr Opin Urol* 14:41, 2004.

42. Verhamme KM, Dieleman JP, Bleumink GS, et al: Incidence and prevalence of lower urinary tract symptoms suggestive of benign prostatic hyperplasia in primary care: the Triumph Project, *Eur Urol* 42:323, 2002.

43. Koskimaki J, Hakama M, Huhtala H, et al: Is reduced quality of life in men with lower urinary tract symptoms due to concomitant diseases? *Eur Urol* 40:661, 2001.

44. Kang D, Andriole GL, Van de Vooren RC, et al: Risk behaviors and benign prostatic hyperplasia, *BJU Int* 93:1241, 2004.

45. Haass M, Kubler W: Nicotine and sympathetic neurotransmission, *Cardiovasc Drugs Ther* 10:657, 1997.

46. Joseph MA, Harlow SD, Wei JT, et al: Risk factors for lower urinary tract symptoms in a population-based sample of African-American men, *Am J Epidemiol* 157:906, 2003.

47. Koskimaki J, Hakama M, Huhtala H, et al: Association of smoking with lower urinary tract symptoms, *J Urol* 159:1580, 1998.

48. Koskomaki J, Hakama M, Huhtala H, et al: Association of non-urological diseases with lower urinary tract symptoms, *Scand J Urol Nephrol* 35:377, 2001.

49. Foley CL, Bott SR, Shergill IS, et al: An update on the use of 5-alpha reductase inhibitors, *Drugs Today* 40:213, 2004.

50. Lee C, Kozlowski JM, Grayhack JT: Etiology of benign prostatic hyperplasia, *Urol Clin North Am* 22:237, 1995.

51. Blaivas JG: Obstructive uropathy in the male, *Urol Clin North Am* 23:373, 1996.

52. Bosch J, Kranse R, Van Mastrigt R, et al: Reasons for the weak correlation between prostate volume and urethral resistance parameters in patients with prostatism, *J Urol* 153:689, 1995.

53. Elbadawi A. Voiding dysfunction in benign prostatic hyperplasia: trends, controversies, and recent revelations: II. Pathology and pathophysiology, *Urology* 51:73, 1998.

54. Kurita Y, Masuda H, Terada H, et al: Transition zone index as a risk factor for acute urinary retention in benign prostatic hyperplasia, *Urology* 51:595, 1998.

55. Nickel C: Long-term implications of medical therapy on benign prostatic hyperplasia end points, *Urology* 51:50, 1998.

56. Roehrborn CG: Etiology, pathophysiology, epidemiology, and natural history of BPH. In: Walsh PC, Retik AB, Vaughan ED Jr, et al, editors: *Campbell's urology*, ed 8, vol 2, Philadelphia, 2002, WB Saunders, pp 1297-1336.

57. Levin RM, Monson FC, Haugaard N, et al: Genetic and cellular characteristics of bladder outlet obstruction, *Urol Clin North Am* 22:263, 1995.

58. Comiter CV, Sullivan MP, Schacterle RS, et al: Urodynamic risk factors for renal dysfunction in men with obstructive and nonobstructive voiding dysfunction, *J Urol* 158:181, 1997.

59. Javle P, Penkins SA, West C, et al: Quantification of voiding dysfunction in patients awaiting transurethral prostatectomy, *J Urol* 156:1014, 1996.

60. Lepro H, Lowe FC: Evaluation and nonsurgical management of benign prostatic hyperplasia. In: Walsh PC, Retik AB, Vaughan ED Jr, et al, editors: *Campbell's urology*, ed 8, vol 2, Philadelphia, 2002, WB Saunders, pp 1337-1378.

61. Roehrborn CG, Boyle P, Bergner D, et al: Serum prostate-specific antigen and prostate volume predict long-term changes in symptoms and flow rate: results of a four-year, randomized trial comparing finasteride versus placebo (PLESS Study Group), *Urology* 54:662-669, 1999.

62. Bartsch G, Fitzpatrick JM, Schalken JA, et al: Consensus statement: the role of prostate-specific antigen in managing the patient with benign prostatic hyperplasia, *BJU Int* 93:27, 2004.

63. Brown CT, van der Meulen J, Mundy AR, et al: Defining the components of a self-management program for men with uncomplicated lower urinary tract symptoms: a consensus approach, *Eur Urol* 46:254, 2004.

64. Roehrborn CG, Schwinn DA: Alpha 1 adrenergic receptors and their inhibitors in lower urinary tract symptoms and benign prostatic hyperplasia, *J Urol* 171:1029, 2004.

65. DeGroat WC: Anatomy and physiology of the lower urinary tract, *Urol Clin North Am* 20:383, 1993.

66. Kaplan SA: Use of alpha-adrenergic inhibitors in treatment of benign prostatic hyperplasia and implications on sexual function, *Urology* 63(3):428-434, 2004.

67. Mycek MJ, Harvey RA, Champe PC: *Pharmacology*, ed 2, Philadelphia, 2000, Lippincott Williams & Wilkins, p 514.

68. Kyprianou N: Doxazosin and terazosin suppress prostate growth by inducing apoptosis: clinical significance, *J Urol* 169:1520, 2003.

69. Kortmann BB, Floratos DL, Kiemeney LA, et al: Urodynamic effects of alpha-adrenoreceptor blockers: a review of clinical trials, *Urology* 62:1, 2003.

70. Roehrborn CG, Bruskewitz R, Nickel JC, et al: Sustained decrease in incidence of acute urinary retention and surgery with finasteride for 6 years in men with benign prostatic hyperplasia, *J Urol* 171:1194, 2004.

71. McConnell JD, Bruskewitz R, Walsh P, et al: The effect of finasteride on the risk of acute urinary retention and the need for surgical treatment among men with benign prostatic hyperplasia, *N Engl J Med* 338:557, 1998.

72. Roehrborn CG, Boyle P, Nickel JC, et al: Efficacy and safety of a dual inhibitor of 5-alpha-reductase types 1 and 2 (dutasteride) in men with benign prostatic hyperplasia, *Urology* 60:434, 2002.

73. Clark RV, Hermann DJ, Cunningham GR, et al: Marked suppression of dihydro-testosterone in men with benign prostatic hyperplasia by dutasteride, a dual 5-alpha reductase inhibitor, *J Clin Endocrinol Metab* 89:2179, 2004.

74. Foley Cl, Kirby RS: 5-alpha reductase inhibitors: what's new? *Curr Opin Urol* 13:31, 2003.

75. Turkoski BB, Lance BR, Bonfiglio MF: *Drug information handbook for advanced practice nursing*, ed 4, Hudson, Ohio, 2003, Lexi-Comp, p 1715.

76. Boyle P, Gould AI, Roehrborn CG: Prostate volume predicts outcome of treatment of benign prostatic hyperplasia with finasteride: meta analysis of randomized clinical trials, *Urology* 48:398, 1996.

77. Nickel CJ: Long-term implications of medical therapy on benign prostatic hyperplasia end points, *Urology* 51:50, 1998.

78. Barqawi A, Gamito E, O'Donnell C, et al: Herbal and vitamin supplement use in a prostate cancer screening population, *Urology* 63:288, 2004.

79. Chow RD: Benign prostatic hyperplasia: patient evaluation of obstructive symptoms, *Geriatrics* 56:33, 2001.

80. Jonas A, Rosenblat G, Krapf D, et al: Cactus flower extracts may prove beneficial in benign prostatic hyperplasia due to inhibition of 5 alpha reductase activity, aroma-tase activity, and lipid peroxidation, *Urol Res* 26:265, 1998.

81. Lowe FC, Fagelman E: Phytotherapy in the treatment of benign prostatic hyperplasia, *Curr Opin Urol* 12:15, 2002.

82. Wilt T, Ishani A, MacDonald R: *Serenoa repens for benign prostatic hyperplasia (Cochrane Review)*, *Cochrane Library*, Chichester, UK, 2004, John Wiley and Sons.

83. Wilt T, Ishani A, MacDonald R, et al: *Beta-sitosterols for benign prostatic hyper-plasia (Cochrane Review)*, *Cochrane Library*, Chichester, UK, 2004, John Wiley and Sons.

84. Wilt T, Ishani A, MacDonald R, et al: *Pygeum africanum for benign prostatic hyperplasia (Cochrane Review)*, *Cochrane Library*, Chichester, UK, 2004, John Wiley and Sons.

85. Wilt T, MacDonald R, Ishani A, et al: *Cernilton for benign prostatic hyperplasia (Cochrane Review)*, *Cochrane Library*, Chichester, UK, 2004, John Wiley and Sons.

86. Kaplan SA, Volpe MA, Te AE: A prospective, 1-year trial using saw palmetto versus finasteride in the treatment of category III prostatitis/chronic pelvic pain syndrome, *J Urol* 171:284, 2004.

87. Schneider T, Rubben H: Extract of stinging nettle root extract (Bazoton-uno) in long term treatment of benign prostatic syndrome (BPS): results of a random-ized, double-blind, placebo-controlled multicenter study after 12 months, *Urologe* 43:302, 2004.

88. Sciarra F, Toscano V: Role of estrogens in human benign prostatic hyperplasia, *Arch Androl* 44:213, 2000.

89. Reynard JM: Does anticholinergic medication have a role for men with lower urinary tract symptoms/benign prostatic hyperplasia either alone or in combination with other agents? *Curr Opin Urol* 14:13, 2004.

90. Nitti VW, Adler H, Combs AJ: The role of urodynamics in the evaluation of voiding dysfunction in men after cerebrovascular accident, *J Urol* 155:263, 1996.

91. Comiter CV, Sullivan MP, Schacterle RS, et al: Prediction of prostatic obstruction with a combination of isometric detrusor contraction pressure and maximum urinary flow rate, *Urology* 48:723, 1996.

92. Djavan B, Madersbacher S, Klingler C, et al: Urodynamic assessment of patients with acute urinary retention: is treatment failure after prostatectomy predictable? *J Urol* 158:1829, 1997.

93. Larson TR: Rationale and assessment of minimally invasive approaches to benign prostatic hyperplasia therapy, *Urology* 59:12, 2002.

Pathology and Management of Postprostatectomy Incontinence

JOANNE P. ROBINSON

OBJECTIVES

1. Describe the pathophysiology and risk factors for each of the following:
   - Postprostatectomy stress incontinence
   - Postprostatectomy urge incontinence
2. Explain why the prevalence rates for postprostatectomy incontinence (PPI) vary widely from study to study.
3. Explain the influence of physiologic, psychologic, and situational factors on the patient's experience related to PPI.
4. Identify the impact of each of the following on the risk for PPI: age, postoperative urethral length, uncertainty regarding prognosis, poor self-esteem and diminished cognitive control, social support system, and availability of professional education and support.
5. Identify key factors to be included in nursing assessment of the individual with PPI.
6. Describe the role of pelvic floor muscle exercises and fluid management in treatment of patients with PPI.
7. Identify medications that may be of benefit to patients with postprostatectomy stress incontinence and postprostatectomy urge incontinence.
8. Identify indications for surgical intervention in the patient with PPI and types of procedures that may be effective.

Prostate cancer is the most commonly diagnosed cancer in American men and the second leading cause of male cancer deaths in the United States. It is estimated that 232,000 new cases of prostate cancer will occur in the United States during 2005, and the disease will claim 30,350 lives.[1] Fortunately, with improved methods of detection and heightened public awareness, most prostate cancers today are diagnosed in the local or regional stages.

Radical prostatectomy is considered the gold standard for treatment of early-stage prostate cancer in otherwise healthy men with localized disease.[2] More than 25,000 radical prostatectomies are performed each year on Medicare patients alone.[3] This procedure provides high 10-year disease-specific survival rates;[4] however, the procedure is also associated with significant risk for urinary incontinence (UI) and erectile dysfunction (ED). UI occurs in many men for several weeks or months following surgery, and it persists permanently in up to 35%.[5] Among those who fail to regain continence, research suggests that quality of life is significantly impaired and UI is more distressing than ED.[6-9]

This chapter describes the scope of the problem of postprostatectomy incontinence (PPI) in the context of radical prostatectomy and examines clinical presentation, pathophysiology, and what is known about risk factors. Guidelines for assessment and management of PPI are also presented.

SCOPE OF THE PROBLEM

The age-adjusted rate for radical prostatectomy increased almost sixfold between 1984 and 1990,[10] and it continues to climb as men pursue early detection, cure, and survival of prostate cancer.[11,12] Despite continued refinements in surgical technique, however, radical prostatectomy carries a significant risk of PPI caused by urethral sphincter incompetence, detrusor dysfunction, or both.

Prevalence rates of PPI range from 3% to 87%,[13-23] varying with the definition of PPI, source of data, timing and method of data collection, and surgical approach. In the largest study,[22] patients who had undergone radical prostatectomy were randomly selected from population-based cancer registries in six geographic regions of the United States and were surveyed at 6, 12, and 24 months after diagnosis. Surgery for all subjects ($n = 1291$) occurred within 6 months of diagnosis. At 24 months from diagnosis, 1.6% still reported no bladder control, 6.8% reported frequent leakage, and 40.2% percent reported occasional leakage. Moreover, research suggests that even in the most experienced hands at major treatment centers, at least 8% of patients experience some degree of PPI following radical prostatectomy.[2]

Negative effects of PPI on health-related quality of life are well documented.[6-8,13,24-30] In the account of his journey through diagnosis and treatment of prostate cancer, author Michael Korda[31] reflected poignantly on the implications of PPI:

> It meant that there wasn't a moment, day or night, that you weren't *conscious* of your urine, weren't thinking about it, weren't concerned that you were leaking it, or dripping it, or that other people could smell it on you, no matter how much you washed... and sprayed Lysol everywhere around you... From being Topic Z, way down at the bottom of anybody's list of daily concerns, it had leapt right up there to Topic B or C, if you took cancer as A, by a long shot, and included impotence on the list.

PATHOPHYSIOLOGY AND CLINICAL PRESENTATION

Removal of the prostate gland may be accomplished through either an abdominal or a perineal approach. The abdominal or retropubic approach is employed most often and is frequently preferred since this approach provides the potential for "sparing" of nerve bundles important to continence and erectile function. The perineal approach is usually limited to situations in which shorter surgical time and minimal blood loss are priorities, because the nerve bundles cannot be spared with this procedure.

Whether performed retropubically or perineally, radical prostatectomy involves removal of the prostate gland, seminal vesicles, affected nerve bundles, pelvic lymph nodes as indicated, and surrounding tissue as necessary to obtain clean surgical margins. The prostatic urethra, which contains voluntary sphincter muscle that prevents urine flow when contracted, is inevitably removed with the prostate gland. The bladder neck, which contains involuntary sphincter muscle that contracts as the bladder fills, is preserved if possible and is anastomosed to the remaining distal urethra.[32]

Following radical prostatectomy, stress, urge, or mixed UI can occur. Stress UI involves urine loss with coughing, sneezing, laughing, or other physical activities that cause pressure within the abdomen to rise.[33] Stress UI results from damage to the rhabdosphincter, a specialized striated muscle that extends from the verumontanum, where ejaculatory and prostatic ducts open into the urethra, to the bulbar urethra[34] (Fig. 9-1). After radical prostatectomy, continence depends mostly on integrity of the rhabdosphincter because the prostate gland, prostatic urethra, and possibly the bladder neck are surgically removed.[35,36] Incompetence of the rhabdosphincter is considered the primary cause of PPI.[37,38] Factors that increase the risk for SI include the following: scarring or atrophy resulting in reduced mobility of the rhabdosphincter, ischemic injury to the rhabdosphincter during surgery, injury to the pudendal nerve, and shortening of the urethra to less than 2.5 cm (the hypothesized critical functional length).[35,37]

Urge UI involves urine loss associated with a precipitous urge to void.[33] Following radical prostatectomy, urge UI is caused by detrusor instability, poor detrusor compliance, or both. Detrusor dysfunction is considered a secondary cause of PPI and can be caused by a variety of factors: bladder denervation during the surgical procedure, surgical alteration of bladder wall configuration, fibrosis, infection, aging, and age-associated comorbidities such as Parkinson's disease or cerebrovascular accident.[35,37,38] Detrusor instability and urge incontinence may also result from persistence of high-pressure bladder contractions; preoperatively, these high-pressure contractions help to override the increased urethral resistance created by prostatic tumor and prostate gland enlargement. Once the prostate gland is removed, persistence of these high-pressure contractions can cause overactive bladder

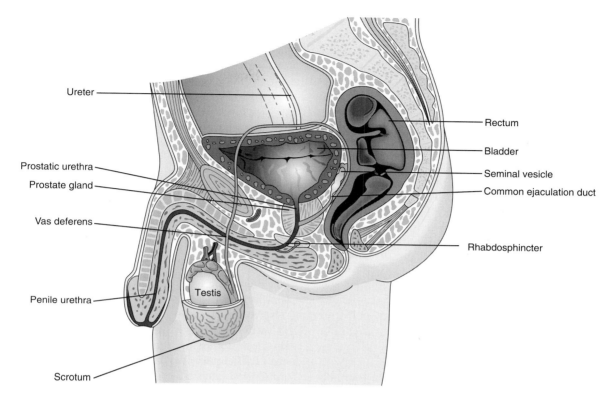

Fig. 9-1 Anatomy of the lower urinary tract in the male. Note location of the rhabdosphincter just inferior to the prostate gland. (Modified from Copstead LC, Banasik JL: *Pathophysiology,* ed 3, St. Louis, 2005, Saunders.)

and urge UI.[38,39] In addition, prolonged preoperative efforts to overcome bladder outlet obstruction may cause hypertrophy and connective tissue infiltration of the detrusor muscle, thus producing postoperative urge UI related to poor detrusor compliance.[35]

Mixed UI is a combination of stress and urge UI[33] caused by both damage to the rhabdosphincter and detrusor instability.[37] In one large study, the majority of patients referred for PPI treatment 1 year or more following radical prostatectomy had urodynamically demonstrated mixed UI rather than isolated stress or urge UI.[40]

RISK FACTORS
Theoretic Perspective

Risk factors for PPI can be understood within the context of the Theory of Unpleasant Symptoms.[41,42] This theory posits that physiologic, psychologic, and situational factors interact to influence the symptom experience. Physiologic factors are defined as somatic contributors to the expression of the target symptom. Psychologic factors refer to mental state and mood. Situational factors include aspects of the social and physical environment that can affect the experience and reporting of the symptom. The theory further depicts the symptom experience as a composite of four separable but related dimensions: timing, intensity, quality, and distress.

Together, these dimensions influence the individual's symptom experience and performance. Timing refers to the duration and frequency of the symptom's occurrence. Intensity refers to the severity, strength, or amount of symptom experienced. Quality is generally specific to a given symptom and refers to how the symptom is manifested and experienced (such as stress, urge, or mixed UI). Distress refers to the degree of bother associated with the symptom. Finally, performance refers to functional and cognitive activities that are affected by the symptom experience, including physical activity, activities of daily living, social activities and interaction, role performance, concentration, thinking, and problem solving. Based on the Theory of Unpleasant Symptoms, the physiologic, psychologic, and situational factors that influence the timing, intensity, quality, and distress of PPI are reviewed.

Physiologic Factors

Physiologic factors have been examined primarily for their influence on the timing of PPI. Surgical alterations of the lower urinary tract during radical prostatectomy have received the most attention.

Evidence from several studies suggests that urinary continence following radical prostatectomy is essentially a function of the extent to which the maximum possible urethral length is preserved. In all but one study reviewed,[43] surgical procedures designed to preserve maximum possible urethral length were associated with reduced incidence of PPI and diminished prevalence of persistent PPI.[44-50] Two studies found that surgical techniques designed to preserve urethral length were also associated with a significant reduction in the duration of transient PPI.[43,46]

Despite much investigation, it remains unclear whether nerve-sparing surgery or preservation of the bladder neck influences the duration of transient PPI or prevalence of persistent PPI following radical prostatectomy. Evidence that supports preservation of one or both neurovascular bundles as effective in minimizing persistent PPI[44,47,51-54]

and in reducing transient PPI duration[47] is refuted by contradictory findings from equally impressive studies.[2,23,49,55-59] Similarly, there is evidence that preservation of the bladder neck during radical prostatectomy may reduce the duration of transient PPI,[46,60] but it may[44,61] or may not[46,56,60] affect the prevalence of persistent PPI.

The merits of perineal and retropubic approaches to radical prostatectomy are beginning to be compared relative to their impact on PPI, but findings are contradictory. Bishoff and colleagues[15] found significantly lower rates of persistent PPI among patients who experienced the perineal approach to prostatectomy, although this group suffered significantly greater rates of postoperative fecal incontinence than those who underwent the retropubic approach. In contrast, Gray and colleagues[17] found no clinically significant differences between the two approaches in terms of the prevalence or intensity (severity) of persistent PPI.

Various preoperative physiologic factors have also been studied for their influence on the timing of PPI. There is evidence that the incidence of PPI and the prevalence of persistent PPI increase after age 65 years;[2,10,22,46,52,54,58,62,63] however, age may[49,57] or may not[46,55,59,64,65] influence the duration of transient PPI. The influence of age on UI-related distress has been studied in men with lower urinary tract symptoms and prostate conditions; these findings are also inconclusive.[66,67-69] There is, however, some evidence that preoperative micturition disorders[18,54,70] and preoperative prostate specific antigen (PSA) values of greater than 10 ng/mL[56] are predictive of greater risk for persistent PPI. Several other studies suggest that prostate weight has no influence on duration of transient PPI,[49,55,57,59] and tumor characteristics do not affect the incidence of PPI, the prevalence of persistent PPI, or the duration of transient PPI.[2,48-49,55-57,59,70] Some studies suggest that prior prostate surgery has no effect on transient PPI duration;[49,55,57,59] however, the prevalence of persistent PPI may[54,71,72] or may not [46,73-76] be influenced by previous surgery on the prostate gland.

Likewise, several complications of radical prostatectomy have been investigated for their influence on the timing of PPI. Schatzl and colleagues[77] found that urine extravasation at the anastomosis 18 days after radical prostatectomy did not affect PPI prevalence at either 3 months or 6 months following surgery. Similarly, Davidson and colleagues[78] found that urine loss during the initial 24 hours following catheter removal was not predictive of duration of transient PPI. The presence of an anastomotic stricture was associated with greater prevalence of persistent PPI and transient PPI duration in one study;[46] however, anastomotic strictures did not contribute to the prevalence of persistent PPI in other investigations.[17,56]

Psychologic Factors

There is evidence from research on patients with a variety of symptoms that the mental states of anxiety and depression contribute to the timing, intensity, distress, and quality of symptoms in general.[41] A literature search revealed no studies reporting the effects of anxiety and depression on the timing of PPI following radical prostatectomy. However, several studies were identified that addressed the influence of psychologic factors on the level of distress experienced by patients who had undergone radical prostatectomy. These findings are relevant because distress level may affect performance of self-care measures that promote recovery of bladder control and avoidance of persistent PPI.

At 1 year or more following radical prostatectomy, Herr[27] found that patients who expressed uncertainty about the curative effects of surgery were more upset by the presence of urinary problems than those who expressed confidence in cure. Qualitative research by Paterson[79] suggests that patients who have undergone prostatectomy and who are able to develop "a new sense of self that is accepting of their leaking body" can overcome the stigma associated with PPI. Similarly, in women, greater self-esteem is associated with lower levels of UI-related distress.[80] Mastery over the management of UI is also associated with reduced depression and improved quality of life in women,[80] and it was found to be critical to emotional recovery from radical prostatectomy in a qualitative descriptive study of couples' experiences of PPI and ED.[81] These findings are consistent with a large body of

research suggesting that gaining cognitive and behavioral control over threatening situations enhances psychologic well-being.[82]

Situational Factors

Aspects of the social and physical environment that have been examined for their influence on the experience of PPI include demographic factors, professional education and support, cancer treatments, and social support.

Income, marital status, race, and education are beginning to be explored relative to their influence on the duration of transient PPI and prevalence of persistent PPI. There is preliminary evidence that income affects neither the prevalence of persistent PPI[18] nor the duration of transient PPI[64] following radical prostatectomy. However, Litwin and colleagues[64] found that marital status and race were independent predictors of recovery of baseline urinary function 1 year after radical prostatectomy, with recovery occurring to a greater extent among married and white men than among their unmarried and nonwhite counterparts. After controlling for age and income, an inverse relationship between education and recovery of urinary function was also observed, such that those with more education recovered to a lesser extent than their less educated counterparts. Education did not, however, influence the prevalence of persistent PPI in a study by Heathcote and colleagues.[18]

Existing evidence suggests that ongoing professional education and support are crucial in minimizing distress associated with PPI. Participants in a qualitative study by Maliski and colleagues[81] described advanced practice clinicians (who provided a standardized home care intervention) as invaluable sources of information, instruction, support, and affirmation during the process of gaining control over urinary function and dysfunction. Participants who were not exposed to the intervention reported dealing with PPI by "trial and error" and expressed more uncertainty about recovery of bladder control. Findings from a qualitative study by Moore and Estey[83] suggest that neither the information nor professional support needs of patients are routinely met, resulting in much concern, worry, and uncertainty about PPI and other surgical sequelae. Participants in this study indicated that they were unable to process the detailed teaching offered preoperatively because they were overwhelmed by the cancer diagnosis, which interfered with comprehension and retention of the information. Similarly, participants in a study by Herr[27] indicated that continuing education during the postoperative period would help them to cope with the distress related to PPI.

Cancer treatments have also been examined for their influence on the timing of PPI. There is some evidence that preoperative endocrine therapy is predictive of greater prevalence of persistent PPI, probably because fibrosis around the prostatic apex following endocrine therapy complicates surgical dissection.[56] In contrast, although postoperative adjuvant radiation therapy was associated with greater prevalence of persistent PPI in an early study,[84] more recent investigations negate its influence on either the incidence of PPI or prevalence of persistent PPI.[56,85,86] Finally, experts assume that the skill and experience of the surgeon performing radical prostatectomy influence both the incidence of PPI and the prevalence of persistent PPI.[54,87,88] Indeed, several studies suggest that continence outcomes associated with surgery performed outside major treatment centers are less favorable.[74]

The influence of social support on the experience of PPI has been described by Maliski and colleagues[81] in their qualitative study of couples' mastery of PPI and ED. Wives encouraged pelvic floor muscle exercise (PFME), modeled PFME, routinized PFME, stocked continence supplies, praised accomplishments, and provided reassurance, which patients considered essential to the process of gaining control over urinary function and dysfunction. Patients also talked with friends and used prostate cancer Internet sites and chat rooms to network with other patients who had undergone radical prostatectomy, with whom they compared progress and exchanged tips for hastening recovery of continence. No other studies of the influence of social support on UI in either men or women were found in the literature. Social support needs of prostate cancer patients are, however, well documented in research literature.[89-92] There is also good empiric evidence that social support interventions have beneficial effects for patients with prostate cancer.[93-98]

Summary

There has been great interest in determining physiologic risk factors for both transient and persistent PPI, to inform surgical practice. Findings from several studies suggest that when efforts are made to preserve maximal urethral length during radical prostatectomy, the incidence of PPI, the duration of transient PPI, and the prevalence of persistent PPI decline. There is also evidence that older age is associated with a higher incidence of PPI and prevalence of persistent PPI. Findings are less clear, however, concerning other potential physiologic risk factors such as surgical approach, preoperative genitourinary status, and untoward surgical sequelae.

Several studies suggest that psychologic factors, including uncertainty about prognosis, self-esteem, and cognitive control, influence the distress dimension of PPI in patients who have undergone radical prostatectomy and also affect the performance of self-care measures that promote recovery of bladder control.

Findings regarding the influence of demographic factors and adjuvant cancer treatments on PPI-related distress and recovery of bladder control following radical prostatectomy are either inconsistent or lack replication. Existing research does, however, indicate that ongoing professional education and support are crucial in minimizing PPI-related distress, and social support from wives, friends, and other patients is essential to the process of gaining control over urinary function and dysfunction.

ASSESSMENT

A focused history and physical exam are the basis for treatment of patients with PPI. The Theory of Unpleasant Symptoms[41,42] can be used to guide the assessment process.

History

First, a detailed description of each dimension of the PPI symptom experience should be elicited from the patient. Relative to the dimension of *timing*, information about the onset, duration, and frequency of PPI should be gathered. The *intensity* or volume of PPI episodes should also be ascertained from the patient's perspective. It is usually helpful to supplement patient interviews concerning the timing and intensity of PPI with information obtained from a 3-day bladder diary, designed to capture the frequency and pattern of voiding, leakage episodes, and fluid intake, and a 24-hour pad test, which yields objective data on the amount of leakage.[99] To explore the *quality* of the PPI symptom experience, explicit questions should be asked about associated symptoms, including urgency, frequency, nocturia, dysuria, hesitancy, and feelings of incomplete emptying. Patients should also be asked about precipitants of leakage such as sneezing, coughing, lifting, physical exertion, and ingestion of caffeinated beverages or other bladder irritants. The degree of *distress* or bother associated with PPI is another essential component of the discussion.

To guide therapeutic management and to shape realistic treatment goals, information concerning risk factors for PPI and quality of life issues should be collected.[32,100] Medical and surgical history should be reviewed with particular attention to preoperative UI, neurologic symptoms, urethral stricture, and pelvic radiation. Current medications, fluid and fiber intake, bowel habits, and exposure to bladder irritants should also be determined, as should past and present strategies used to treat or manage leakage. Stress level, self-esteem, and social support should be appraised because they can affect performance of self-care measures that promote recovery of bladder control. Finally, functional and cognitive activities that are affected by PPI should be discussed, and the patient's expectations of treatment should be noted.

Physical Examination

The focused physical exam involves evaluation of the patient's neurologic status, abdomen, perineum, and rectum. Neurologic evaluation includes gross assessment for problems with cognition, gait, balance, and manual dexterity. The abdomen should be evaluated for signs of bladder tenderness and distension. Skin of the genitalia and perineum should be examined for signs of irritation, infection, and breakdown.

Perineal and perianal sensation, internal anal sphincter tone, strength of external anal sphincter contraction, and presence of a fecal impaction should also be assessed. Performance of a cough stress test for direct observation of urine loss is recommended, as is a urinalysis to screen for urinary tract infection. Finally, if urinary retention is suspected, postvoid residual volume should be measured by bladder ultrasound.[32,100]

MANAGEMENT

Every patient with PPI deserves education to address the uncertainty inherent in the PPI symptom experience. Based on the Theory of Uncertainty in Illness,[101] patients should be helped to form a cognitive schema for PPI, which includes an understanding of the pattern and meaning of their PPI symptoms, familiarity with the circumstances of their leakage episodes and how these episodes are best prevented and/or managed, and a realistic appreciation of the expected course of PPI in their own situation. Individualized patient teaching should also include resources for additional information and support, including the National Association for Continence (*www.nafc.org*) and Simon Foundation (*www.simonfoundation.org*) for information on continence treatment, products, and services, and *Us Too!* (*www.ustoo.com*) and the American Cancer Society (*www.cancer.org*) for prostate cancer education and support.[32] Beyond this, behavioral, pharmacologic, surgical, and supportive interventions are available for patients with PPI. Patient education and interventions should always be individualized based on specific assessment findings.

Behavioral Interventions

PFME training and diet modification should comprise the first line of treatment for patients with PPI.[33] PFME training involves building the strength and endurance of the pubococcygeus, puborectalis, and ileococcygeus segments of the levator ani muscle. The levator ani supports pelvic organs like a sling and, when contracted, helps to maintain close apposition of the mucosal folds of the urethra to prevent urine leakage. Contraction of the levator ani muscles also triggers an inhibitory spinal cord reflex that reduces bladder sensitivity and suppresses involuntary bladder contractions.[32,102,103]

The patient should first be taught to identify and contract the levator ani without recruiting adjacent abdominal, buttock, and thigh muscles. Biofeedback is often used as an instructional aid and tool for evaluating progress. Electrical or electromagnetic stimulation of the levator ani is also sometimes used to teach muscle isolation or to supplement active PFME. Once the patient has mastered muscle isolation, he is taught to work up to a contraction of 10 seconds' duration, followed by a relaxation period of 10 seconds. Between 15 and 20 repetitions are typically prescribed three times daily in sitting, standing, and lying positions to condition the pelvic floor. Ongoing performance of PFME is usually recommended to maintain improvements in muscle function and bladder control.[32,100] See Chapter 4 for more information.

Optimal timing for instruction in PFMEs has yet to be determined. Findings from one pilot study suggest that the frequency and volume of urinary leakage improve to a greater extent when PFME training is conducted preoperatively (as compared with training conducted during the early postoperative period); however, these findings are based on a very small sample size ($n = 16$), and the authors acknowledge the need for repeated studies with larger samples.[104] Preoperative PFME training may be overwhelming to patients who have recently been diagnosed with prostate cancer and who are focused primarily on "getting rid of the cancer" as well as the numerous tests required during the preoperative period.[105] This may explain why seven of eight previous studies on PFME for patients who had undergone radical prostatectomy employed postoperative PFME training.[29,106-111] Four of these studies demonstrated reduced frequency and volume of urinary leakage in patients who underwent PFME training postoperatively.[108-111]

Techniques to inhibit stress and urge UI can be taught when sufficient strength and control of the pelvic floor are developed. To prevent stress UI, patients should be taught to contract the levator ani muscle before and during activities that increase intraabdominal pressure, such as coughing, sneezing, or rising from a chair. To prevent urge UI, patients should be instructed to refrain from voiding in the presence of urgency. To suppress urgency, patients can be taught to engage in a combination of 5 to 10 quick flicks or flutters of the levator ani, deep breathing, and mental distraction. Bladder training can also be introduced to patients with urge UI when comfort with urge suppression is achieved. (Bladder training is described in greater depth in Chapter 5.) An intervoiding interval of 3 to 4 hours is generally the goal.[32,100]

Modification of diet and fluid intake is integral to the success of any continence promotion program, particularly if the patient presents with urge or mixed UI. An intake of at least 1.5 to 2 liters of fluid per day should be encouraged to maintain dilute urine, which helps to minimize bladder spasms and the resultant urgency. Consumption of whole grain foods and five servings of fruits and vegetables each day should be promoted to prevent constipation, because a full rectum can crowd the bladder and contribute to bladder spasms and urgency. Finally, patients should be instructed to limit or avoid consumption of foods, beverages, and other products that can be irritating to the bladder. Caffeine is the substance with the strongest evidence base as a bladder irritant; however, anecdotal reports suggest that numerous substances may act as bladder irritants for selected individuals. The list of possible irritants includes alcohol, tobacco, carbonated beverages with or without caffeine, decaffeinated coffee or tea, milk and milk products, citrus fruits and juices, tomatoes and tomato-based products, spicy foods, sugar, honey, chocolate, corn syrup, and artificial sweetener.[32,100,112]

Pharmacologic Interventions

Medications that adversely affect bladder control, such as diuretics, sedatives, narcotic analgesics, and alpha-adrenergic blocking agents, should be reduced or eliminated if possible. Selected drugs can also be added to the therapeutic regimen to augment behavioral interventions when stress and urge UI symptoms are intractable.

For urge UI symptoms, drugs with anticholinergic properties are often helpful in reducing bladder spasms. Most commonly prescribed are the antispasmodics oxybutynin (Ditropan), hyoscyamine (Levsin), and tolterodine tartrate (Detrol). Less often used are calcium-channel blockers, such as nifedipine (Procardia), which are also thought to have a depressant effect on the bladder. For stress UI symptoms, alpha-adrenergic agonists, particularly pseudoephedrine (Sudafed) and phenylpropanolamine (Entex), are sometimes prescribed to strengthen bladder neck contractions (so long as the patient has no contraindications to use of adrenergic agonist agents). Recent research into the physiology of sphincter innervation indicates that both serotonin and norephinephrine are significant neurotransmitters; based on this research, a combined serotonin norepinephrine uptake inhibitor has been evaluated for treatment of stress incontinence.[113,114] Clinical trials have shown impressive improvement, and the drug (duloxetine) may obtain approval by the Food and Drug Administration (FDA) for use in the United States. If FDA approval is obtained, this drug is expected to become the primary pharmacologic agent for treatment of stress incontinence.[113,114] For mixed UI symptoms, the tricyclic antidepressant, imipramine (Tofranil), may be helpful as it exerts antispasmodic effects on the bladder and also stimulates contractions of the bladder neck. Of course, the introduction of any medication must be coupled with thorough patient education about the drug and careful monitoring for adverse effects.[100,115]

Surgical Interventions

Surgical interventions are reserved for patients with PPI that persists beyond 6 to 12 months following radical prostatectomy and for whom behavioral and pharmacologic interventions have not provided sufficient improvement. All these procedures target stress UI symptoms.

Injection of the bladder neck with bulking material, typically collagen, is performed to enhance sphincter competence and is considered the first-line surgical intervention. The procedure can be performed on an outpatient basis and has a low rate of complications; however, repeated injections may be necessary, and long-term outcomes are disappointing. Bladder neck suspension or suburethral sling procedures are designed to reduce leakage by lifting and compressing the urethra so the bladder neck remains in its proper anatomic position and urethral resistance is maintained

when intraabdominal pressure rises. Finally, implantation of an artificial urinary sphincter (AUS) is a last resort for PPI that is refractory to other surgical interventions. Essentially, the AUS is a three-part device consisting of a pump that is situated in the scrotum, an inflatable cuff that is wrapped around the urethra, and a reservoir that is implanted beneath the skin (Fig. 9-2). As long as the cuff is filled, continence is maintained; patients are taught to use the pump mechanism to deflate the cuff when they are ready to void. (Reinflation of the cuff occurs automatically within a few minutes.) Satisfactory continence has been reported by many men following AUS implantation; however, surgical revision is required for many patients as a result of infection, erosion, and atrophy.[100]

Supportive Interventions

Every patient with PPI should be helped to select and obtain products to contain urine leakage and to protect the skin. Use of the resource guide to continence products and services published annually by the National Association for Continence (*www.nafc.org*) will greatly facilitate this process. In the presence of leakage, twice-daily cleansing of

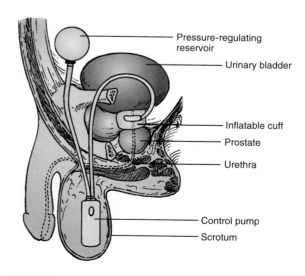

Fig. 9-2 The artificial sphincter. The three elements include an inflatable cuff positioned around the urethra, a reservoir placed in the abdomen, and a pump implanted in the scrotum.

the skin and the use of moisturizers, emollients, and waterproof barrier ointments are recommended. An extensive array of absorbent products is available, including pads for light loss (6 to 10 oz), guards for moderate loss (10 to 14 oz), undergarments for moderate to heavy loss (14 to 17 oz), and briefs for heavy loss (more than 17 oz).[116] Drip collectors, which can be purchased or homemade, are absorbent pouches that pocket the penis and best serve patients with mild to moderate stress UI symptoms. Condom catheters should be reserved for patients with heavy urine loss and demand attention to proper fit and correct application. Finally, penile clamps are available, but they should be used judiciously on selected occasions, given the hazards of penile ischemia and necrosis associated with prolonged wearing time. Clamps should be applied with the minimum pressure necessary to prevent leakage and should be released every 3 hours.[32, 100]

SUMMARY

Cases of postprostatectomy UI are escalating as growing numbers of men with localized prostate cancer choose radical prostatectomy to maximize survival. Despite continued refinements in surgical technique, radical prostatectomy carries significant risk of stress, urge, or mixed UI, which persists permanently in up to 35% of patients. This distressing outcome occurs within the context of a cancer diagnosis and affects patients who are recovering from major surgery, thus creating considerable potential for diminished quality of life.

PPI is caused by incompetence of the rhabdosphincter and/or detrusor dysfunction, and it can present as stress, urge, or mixed UI. From the perspective of the Theory of Unpleasant Symptoms, physiologic, psychologic, and situational risk factors interact to influence the timing, intensity, quality, and distress associated with PPI. Research suggests that older age and suboptimal postoperative urethral length increase the incidence and duration of PPI. There is also some evidence that uncertainty about prognosis, loss of self-esteem, and diminished cognitive control increase the distress dimension of PPI. Research findings also indicate that ongoing professional education and support are crucial in minimizing PPI-related distress in patients who undergo radical prostatectomy, and social support is essential to the process of gaining control over urinary function and dysfunction.

Assessment of the patient with PPI should include: (1) a detailed description of the timing, intensity, quality, and distress from the patient's perspective; (2) collection of information concerning risk factors and quality of life issues; (3) gross evaluation of the patient's neurologic status and focused physical examination of the abdomen, perineum, and rectum; and (4) urinalysis, cough stress test, and bladder ultrasound as appropriate.

Management of PPI is based on assessment findings and involves education and support to address the uncertainty inherent in the PPI symptom experience, as well as behavioral, pharmacologic, surgical, and supportive interventions as indicated. Behavioral interventions should be the first line of treatment and include PFME training, stress and urge inhibition techniques, bladder training, and modification of diet and fluid intake. Pharmacologic interventions include reduction or elimination of medications that adversely affect bladder control and the addition of selected drugs to augment behavioral interventions when stress and urge UI symptoms are intractable. Surgical interventions are available to target stress UI symptoms, but they should be reserved for patients with PPI that persists beyond the sixth postoperative month and who have not been helped by behavioral or pharmacologic interventions. For these patients, urethral bulking injections, bladder neck suspension surgery, and AUS implantation can be effective. Supportive interventions consist of a wide variety of absorbent products as well as drip collectors, condom catheters, and penile clamps that can be used to contain urine leakage and protect the skin.

SELF-ASSESSMENT EXERCISE

1. Radical prostatectomy is associated with which of the following?
   a. Stress incontinence
   b. Urge incontinence
   c. Reflex incontinence

d. Both stress and urge incontinence

2. Which of the following is thought to be most critical to maintenance of continence after prostatectomy?

   a. Preservation of the bladder neck

   b. Use of "nerve-sparing" surgical technique

   c. Postoperative urethral length greater than 2.5 cm

   d. Patient age less than 65 years

3. Explain the role of each of the following in postprostatectomy bladder function and continence:

   • Rhabdosphincter

   • High-pressure bladder contractions

4. Outline parameters to be included in assessment of the patient with PPI.

5. Describe behavioral therapy for the patient with PPI, to include fluid modifications and pelvic floor muscle exercises.

6. Identify indications and mechanisms of action for each of the following:

   • Anticholinergic agent such as tolterodine

   • Serotonin norepinephrine uptake inhibitor such as duloxetine

7. Explain indications and advantages/disadvantages of each of the following:

   • Urethral bulking procedure

   • Suburethral sling procedure

   • AUS

REFERENCES

1. Jemal A, Murray T, Ward E, et al: Cancer statistics, 2005. CA: *Cancer J Clin* 55(1):10-30, 2005.
2. Catalona WJ, Ramos CG, Carvalhal GF: Contemporary results of anatomic radical prostatectomy, *CA Cancer J Clin* 49:282-296, 1999.
3. Yao S, Lu-Yao G: Population-based study of relationships between hospital volume of prostatectomies, patient outcomes, and length of hospital stay, *J Natl Cancer Inst* 91:1950-1956, 1999.
4. Gerber GS, Thisted RA, Scardino PT, et al: Results of radical prostatectomy in men with clinically localized prostate cancer, *JAMA* 276:615-619, 1996.
5. National Comprehensive Cancer Network: *Prostate cancer: treatment guidelines for patients, version III,* October 2001, Available from: URL: http://www. nccn.org/patient_gls/english/_prostate/index.htm
6. Fowler FJ, Barry MJ, Lu-Yao G, et al: Effect of radical prostatectomy for prostate cancer on patient quality of life: results from a Medicare survey, *Urology* 45:1007-1015, 1995.
7. Litwin MS, Hays RD, Fink A, et al: Quality-of-life outcomes in men treated for localized prostate cancer, *JAMA* 273:129-135, 1995.
8. Shrader-Bogen CL, Kjellberg JL, McPherson CP, et al: Quality of life and treatment outcomes: prostate carcinoma patients' perspectives after prostatectomy or radiation therapy, *Cancer* 79:1977-1986, 1997.
9. Mazur DJ, Merz JF: Older patients' willingness to trade off urologic adverse outcomes for a better chance at five-year survival in the clinical setting of prostate cancer, *J Am Geriatr Soc* 43:979-984, 1995.
10. Talcott JA, Rieker P, Clark JA, et al: Patient-reported symptoms after primary therapy for early prostate cancer: results of a prospective cohort study, *J Clin Oncol* 16:275-283, 1998.
11. Palmer MH: Postprostatectomy incontinence: the magnitude of the problem, *J Wound Ostomy Continence Nurs* 27:129-137, 2000.
12. Walsh PC: Surgery and the reduction of mortality from prostate cancer, *N Engl J Med* 347:839-840, 2002.
13. Jonler M, Madsen F, Rhodes P, et al: A prospective study of quantification of urinary incontinence and quality of life in patients undergoing radical retropubic prostatectomy, *Urology* 48:433-440, 1996.
14. Bates T, Wright M, Gillat D: Prevalence and impact of incontinence and impotence following total prostatectomy assessed anonymously by the ICS-Male Questionnaire, *Eur Urol* 33:165-169, 1998.
15. Bishoff JT, Motley G, Optenberg SA, et al: Incidence of fecal and urinary incontinence following radical perineal and retropubic prostatectomy in a national population, *J Urol* 160:454-458, 1998.
16. Goluboff ET, Saidi JA, Mazer S, et al: Urinary continence after radical prostatectomy: the Columbia experience, *J Urol* 159:1276-1280, 1998.
17. Gray M, Petroni D, Theodorescu D: Urinary function after radical prostatectomy: a comparison of the retropubic and perineal approaches, *Urology* 53:881-891, 1999.
18. Heathcote P, Mactaggart P, Boston R, et al: Health-related quality of life in Australian men remaining disease-free after radical prostatectomy, *Med J Austr* 168:483-486, 1998.
19. Jonler M, Messing E, Rhodes P, et al: Sequelae of radical prostatectomy, *Br J Urol* 74:352-358, 1994.
20. Ojdeby G, Claezon A, Brekkan E, et al: Urinary incontinence and sexual impotence after radical prostatectomy, *Scand J Urol Nephrol* 30:473-477, 1996.
21. Poon M, Ruckle H, Barnshad R, et al: Radical retropubic prostatectomy: bladder neck preservation versus reconstruction, *J Urol* 163:194-200, 2000.
22. Stanford JL, Feng Z, Hamilton AS, et al: Urinary and sexual function after radical prostatectomy for clinically

localized prostate cancer: the prostate cancer outcomes study, *JAMA* 283:354-360, 2000.

23. Talcott JA, Rieker P, Propert KJ, et al: Patient-reported impotence and incontinence after nerve-sparing radical prostatectomy, *J Natl Cancer Inst* 89:1117-1123, 1997.

24. Braslis KG, Santa-Cruz C, Brickman AL, et al: Quality of life 12 months after radical prostatectomy, *Br J Urol* 75:48-53, 1995.

25. Fleshner N, Herschorn S: The artificial urinary sphincter for post-radical prostatectomy incontinence: impact on urinary symptoms and quality of life, *J Urol* 155:1260-1264, 1996.

26. Haab F, Trockman BA, Zimmern PE, et al: Quality of life and continence assessment of the artificial urinary sphincter in men with minimum 3.5 years of follow-up, *J Urol* 158:435-439, 1997.

27. Herr HW: Quality of life of incontinent men after radical prostatectomy, *J Urol* 151:652-654, 1994.

28. Kornblith AB, Herr HW, Ofman US, et al: Quality of life of patients with prostate cancer and their spouses, *Cancer* 73:2791-2802, 1994.

29. Moore KN, Griffiths D, Hughton A: Urinary incontinence after radical prostatectomy: a randomized controlled trial comparing pelvic muscle exercises with or without electrical stimulation, *BJU Int* 1999;83:57-65, 1999.

30. Yarbro CH, Ferrans CE: Quality of life of patients with prostate cancer treated with surgery or radiation therapy, *Oncol Nurs Forum* 25:685-693, 1998.

31. Korda M: *Man to man: surviving prostate cancer,* New York, 1996, Vintage Books, p 177.

32. Moorhouse DL, Robinson JP, Bradway C, et al: Behavioral treatments for post-prostatectomy incontinence, *Ostomy Wound Manage* 47(12):30-42, 2001.

33. Fantl JA, Newman DK, Colling J, et al: *Urinary incontinence in adults: acute and chronic management,* Clinical Practice Guideline No. 2, 1996 update, Rockville, Md., 1996, US Department of Health and Human Services, Public Health Service, Agency for Health Care Policy and Research; 1996.

34. Elbadawi A: Functional anatomy of the organs of micturition, *Urol Clin North Am* 23:177-210, 1996.

35. Haab F, Yamaguchi R, Leach GE: Post-prostatectomy incontinence, *Urol Clin North Am* 23:447-457, 1996.

36. Raz S: Pathophysiology of male incontinence, *Urol Clin North Am* 5:295-304, 1978.

37. Diokno AC: Post prostatectomy urinary incontinence, *Ostomy Wound Manage* 44:54-60, 1998.

38. Desautel MG, Kapoor R, Badlani GH: Sphincteric incontinence: the primary cause of post-prostatectomy incontinence in patients with prostate cancer, *Neurourol Urodyn* 16:153-160, 1997.

39. Joseph AC: Male pelvic anatomy/post-prostatectomy incontinence, *Urol Nurs* 21:25-27, 2001.

40. Leach GE, Trockman B, Wong A, et al: Post-prostatectomy incontinence: urodynamic findings and treatment outcomes, *J Urol* 155:1256-1259, 1996.

41. Lenz ER, Pugh LC, Milligan RA, et al: The middle-range theory of unpleasant symptoms: an update, *ANS Adv Nurs Sci* 19:14-27, 1997.

42. Lenz ER, Suppe F, Gift AG, et al: Collaborative development of middle-range nursing theories: toward a theory of unpleasant symptoms, *ANS Adv Nurs Sci* 17:1-13, 1995.

43. Poore RE, McCullough DL, Jarow JP: Puboprostatic ligament sparing improves urinary continence after radical retropubic prostatectomy, *Urology* 51:67-72, 1998.

44. Gaker D, Gaker L, Stewart J, et al: Radical prostatectomy with preservation of urinary continence, *J Urol* 156:445-449, 1996.

45. Hammerer P, Schuler J, Gonnermann D, et al: Urodynamic parameters before and after radical prostatectomy, *J Urol* 149:235, 1993.

46. Kaye KW, Creed KE, Wilson GJ, et al: Urinary continence after radical retropubic prostatectomy: analysis and synthesis of contributing factors: a unified concept, *Br J Urol* 80:444-451, 1997.

47. O'Donnell PD, Finan BF: Continence following nerve-sparing radical prostatectomy, *J Urol* 149:235, 1989.

48. Presti JC, Schmidt RA, Narayan PA, et al: Pathophysiology of urinary incontinence after radical prostatectomy, *J Urol* 143:975-978, 1990.

49. Ramon J, Leandri P, Rossignol G, et al: Urinary continence following radical retropubic prostatectomy, *Br J Urol* 71:47-51, 1993.

50. Veenema RJ, Gursel EO, Lattimer JK: Radical retropubic prostatectomy for cancer: a 20-year experience, *J Urol* 117:330-331, 1977.

51. Catalona WJ, Biggs S: Nerve-sparing radical prostatectomy: evaluation of results after 250 patients, *J Urol* 143:538-544, 1990.

52. Eastham JA, Kattan MW, Rogers E, et al: Risk factors for urinary incontinence after radical prostatectomy, *J Urol* 156:1707-1713, 1996.

53. Fowler JE, Mouli K, Clayton M, et al: Early experience with the Walsh technique of radical retropubic prostatectomy, *Urology* 3:242-246, 1987.

54. Van Kampen M, De Weerdt W, Van Poppel H, et al: Prediction of urinary continence following radical prostatectomy, *Urol Int* 60:80-84, 1998.

55. Catalona WJ, Basler JW: Return of erections and urinary continence following nerve sparing radical retropubic prostatectomy, *J Urol* 150:905-907, 1993.

56. Egawa S, Minei S, Iwamura M, et al: Urinary continence following radical prostatectomy, *Jpn J Clin Oncol* 27:71-75, 1997.

57. Klein EA: Early continence after radical prostatectomy, *J Urol* 148:92-95, 1992.

58. Rossignol G, Leandri P, Ramon J, et al: Radical prostatectomy in the management of stage-A carcinoma of the prostate, *Eur Urol* 20:179-183, 1991.

59. Steiner MS, Morton RA, Walsh PC: Impact of anatomical radical prostatectomy on urinary continence, *J Urol* 145:512-515, 1991.

60. Lowe B: Comparison of bladder neck preservation to bladder neck resection in maintaining postprostatectomy urinary continence, *Urology* 48:889-893, 1996.

61. Seaman EK, Benson MC: Improved continence with tubularized bladder neck reconstruction following radical retropubic prostatectomy, *Urology* 47:532-535, 1996.

62. Griffiths TRL, Neal DE: Localized prostate cancer: early intervention or expectant therapy? *J R Soc Med* 90: 665-669, 1997.

63. Licht MR, Klein EA, Tuason L, et al: Impact of bladder neck preservation during radical prostatectomy on continence and cancer control, *Urology* 44:883-887, 1994.

64. Litwin MS, McGuigan KA, Shpall AI, et al: Recovery of health related quality of life in the year after radical prostatectomy: early experience, *J Urol* 161:515-519, 1999.

65. Walsh PC, Quinlan DM, Morton RA, et al: Radical retropubic prostatectomy: improved anastamosis and urinary continence, *Urol Clin North Am* 17:679-684, 1990.

66. Hunskaar S, Sandvik H: One hundred and fifty men with urinary incontinence, *Scand J Prim Health Care* 11:193-196, 1993.

67. Dugan E, Cohen SJ, Robinson D, et al: The quality of life of older adults with urinary incontinence: determining generic and condition-specific predictors, *Qual Life Res* 7:337-344, 1998.

68. Hunter DJW, McKee M, Black NA, et al: Health status and quality of life of British men with lower urinary tract symptoms: results from the SF-36, *Urology* 45:962-971, 1995.

69. Naughton MJ, Wyman JF: Quality of life in geriatric patients with lower urinary tract dysfunction, *Am J Med Sci* 314:219-227, 1997.

70. Aboseif SR, Konety B, Schmidt RA, et al: Preoperative urodynamic evaluation: does it predict the degree of urinary continence after radical prostatectomy? *Urol Int* 53:68-73, 1994.

71. Elder JS, Gibbons RP, Correa RJ, et al: Morbidity of radical perineal prostatectomy following transurethral resection of the prostate, *J Urol* 132:55-57, 1984.

72. Scardino PT, Cantini M, Wheeler T: Radical prostatectomy: assessment of morbidity and pathological findings [abstract], *J Urol* 137:192A, 1987.

73. Bandhauer K, Senn E: Radical retropubic prostatectomy after transurethral prostatic resection, *Eur Urol* 15: 180-181, 1988.

74. Bass RB, Barrett DM: Radical retropubic prostatectomy after transurethral prostatic resection, *J Urol* 124:495-497, 1980.

75. Donnellan SM, Duncan HJ, MacGregor RJ, et al: Prospective assessment of incontinence after radical retropubic prostatectomy: objective and subjective analysis, *Urology* 1997;49:225-230, 1997.

76. Lindner A, de Kernion JB, Smith RB, et al: Risk of urinary continence following radical prostatectomy, *J Urol* 129:1007-1008, 1983.

77. Schatzl G, Madersbacher S, Hofbauer J, et al: The impact of urinary extravasation after radical retropubic prostatectomy on urinary incontinence and anastomotic strictures, *Eur Urol* 36:187-190, 1999.

78. Davidson PJT, van den Ouden D, Schroeder FH: Radical prostatectomy: prospective assessment of mortality and morbidity, *Eur Urol* 29:168-173, 1996.

79. Paterson J: Stigma associated with postprostatectomy urinary incontinence, *J Wound Ostomy Continence Nurs* 27:168-173, 2000.

80. Chiverton PA, Wells TJ, Brink CA, et al: Psychological factors associated with urinary incontinence, *Clin Nurse Spec* 10:229-233, 1996.

81. Maliski SL, Heilemann MV, McCorkle R: Mastery of postprostatectomy incontinence and impotence: his work, her work, our work, *Oncol Nurs Forum* 28:985-992, 2001.

82. Brockopp DY, Hayko D, Davenport W, et al: Personal control and the needs for hope and information among adults diagnosed with cancer, *Cancer Nurs* 12:112-116, 1989.

83. Moore KN, Estey A: The early post-operative concerns of men after radical prostatectomy, *J Adv Nurs* 29:1121-1129, 1999.

84. Barrett DM, Furlow WL: Radical prostatectomy incontinence and the AS791 artificial urinary sphincter, *J Urol* 129:528-530, 1983.

85. Green N, Treible D, Wallack H: Prostate cancer: post-irradiation incontinence, *J Urol* 144: 307-309, 1990.

86. Van Cangh PJ, Richard F, Lorge F, et al: Adjuvant radiation therapy does not cause urinary incontinence after radical prostatectomy: results of a prospective randomized study, *J Urol* 159:164-166, 1998.

87. Feneley MR, Walsh PC: Incontinence after radical prostatectomy, *Lancet* 353:2091-2092, 1999.

88. Paulson DF: Editorial comment, *J Urol* 145:515, 1991.

89. Boudioni M, McPherson K, Moynihan C, et al: Do men with prostate or colorectal cancer seek different information and support from women with cancer? *Br J Cancer* 85:641-648, 2001.

90. Gray RE, Fitch M, Phillips C, et al: To tell or not to tell: patterns of disclosure among men with prostate cancer, *Psychooncology* 9:273-282, 2000.

91. Fitch MI, Gray R, Franssen E, et al: Men's perspectives on the impact of prostate cancer: implications for oncology nurses, *Onc Nurs Forum* 27:1255-1263, 2000.

92. Jakobsson L, Hallberg IR, Loven L: Experiences of daily life and life quality in men with prostate cancer: an exploratory study. Part I, *Eur J Cancer* Care 6(2):108-116, 1997.

93. Adamsen L, Midtgaard Rasmussen J, Sonderby Pederson L: 'Brothers in arms': how men with cancer experience a sense of comradeship through group intervention which combines physical activity with information relay, *J Clin Nurs* 10:528-537, 2001.

94. Coreil J, Behal R: Man to Man prostate cancer support groups, *Cancer Pract* 7(3):122-129, 1999.

95. Shrock D, Palmer RF, Taylor B: Effects of a psychosocial intervention on survival among patients with stage I breast and prostate cancer: a matched case-control study, *Altern Ther Health Med* 5(3):49-55, 1999.

96. Hellbom M, Brandberg Y, Glimelius B, et al: Individual psychological support for cancer patients: utilisation

and patient satisfaction, *Patient Educ Couns* 34(3): 247-256, 1998.

97. Gray RE, Fitch M, Davis C, et al: Interviews with men with prostate cancer about their self-help group experience, *J Palliat Care* 13(1):15-21, 1997.

98. Gregoire I, Kalogeropoulos D, Corcos J: The effectiveness of a professionally led support group for men with prostate cancer, *Urol Nurs* 17(2):58-66, 1997.

99. Groutz A, Blaivas JG, Chaikin DC, et al: Noninvasive outcome measures of urinary incontinence and lower urinary tract symptoms: a multicenter study of micturition diary and pad tests, *J Urol* 164:698-701, 2000.

100. Robinson JP: Managing urinary incontinence following radical prostatectomy, *J Wound Ostomy Continence Nurs* 27:138-145, 2000.

101. Mishel MH: Uncertainty in illness, *Image J Nurs Sch* 20(4):225-232, 1988.

102. Bo K, Berghmans LCM: Nonpharmacologic treatments for overactive bladder: pelvic floor exercises, *Urology* 55(suppl 5A):7-11, 2000.

103. Stein M, Discippio W, Davia M, et al: Biofeedback for the treatment of stress and urge incontinence, *J Urol* 153:641-643, 1995.

104. Sueppel C, Kreder K, See W: Improved continence outcomes with preoperative pelvic floor muscle strengthening exercises, *Urol Nurs* 21:201-210, 2001.

105. Maliski S, Heilemann MSV, McCorkle R: From "death sentence" to "good cancer": couples' transformation of a prostate cancer diagnosis, *Nurs Res* 51:391-397, 2002.

106. Franke JJ, Gilbert WB, Grier J, et al: Early post-prostatectomy biofeedback, *J Urol* 163:191-193, 2000.

107. Opsomer RJ, Castille Y, Abi Aad AS, et al: Urinary incontinence after radical prostatectomy: is profes-sional pelvic floor training necessary? [abstract] *Neurourol Urodyn* 13:382-384, 1994.

108. Burgio KL, Stutzman RE, Engel BT: Behavioral training for post-prostatectomy urinary incontinence, *J Urol* 141:303-306, 1989.

109. Meaglia JP, Joseph AC, Chang M, et al: Post-prostatectomy urinary incontinence: response to behavioral training, *J Urol* 144:674-676, 1990.

110. Jackson J, Emerson L, Johnston B, et al: Biofeedback: a noninvasive treatment for incontinence after radical prostatectomy, *Urol Nurs* 16:50-54, 1996.

111. Van Kampen M, DeWeerdt W, Van Poppel H, et al: Effect of pelvic floor re-education on duration and degree of incontinence after radical prostatectomy: a randomized controlled trial, *Lancet* 355:98-102, 2000.

112. National Association for Continence: *Frequently asked questions*, 2004, Available from: URL: http://www.nafc.org/about._incontinence/faqs/faq2.htm

113. Fraser MO, Chancellor MB: Neural control of the urethra and development of pharmacotherapy for stress urinary incontinence, *Br J Urol* 91(8):743-748, 2003.

114. Thor KB: Serotonin and norepinephrine involvement in efferent pathways to the urethral rhabdosphincter: implications for treating stress urinary incontinence, *Urology* 62(4 suppl 1):3-9, 2003.

115. Ebersole P, Hess P, Luggen AS: *Toward healthy aging: human needs and nursing response*, ed 6, St. Louis, 2004, Mosby.

116. Newman D, Dzurinko M: *The urinary incontinence sourcebook*, ed 2, Los Angeles, 1999, Lowell House.

CHAPTER 10

Current Concepts in Catheter Management

JOANN MERCER SMITH

OBJECTIVES

1. List four situations in which long-term use of an indwelling catheter is appropriate.
2. Name two benefits of suprapubic catheter placement and explain why suprapubic catheterization may be better for certain patients.
3. Define "closed urinary system" and explain how to maintain a closed system in a patient with an indwelling catheter.
4. Identify catheter and balloon characteristics that reduce the risk of catheter-related complications.
5. Name three points of bacterial entry into a catheter and drainage system and appropriate nursing actions to minimize or delay bacterial growth/contamination.
6. Describe strategies for prevention or management of the following catheter-related complications:
   - Catheter-associated urinary tract infection (CAUTI)
   - Bladder spasms and leakage
   - Catheter encrustation and obstruction
7. Outline key patient assessment criteria for identification of CAUTI in a patient with an indwelling catheter, and describe the procedure for obtaining a urine specimen for culture and sensitivity from a patient with an indwelling catheter.
8. Outline a teaching plan for a patient with an indwelling catheter. Include insertion site care (suprapubic or urethral), maintenance of a closed system, catheter securement, selection, use and care of the drainage system, signs and symptoms of CAUTI, and appropriate response.
9. Explain the process whereby the use of large catheters and overfilling or underfilling catheter balloons lead to urinary leakage around the catheter.
10. Compare and contrast suprapubic and urethral catheters, including indications, contraindications, advantages, disadvantages, and key nursing management strategies.
11. Identify guidelines for effective use of external male catheters and compression devices.
12. Describe three options available for patients who wish to resume sexual activity after catheter insertion and specific suggestions a nurse should give when teaching the patient and partner these techniques.

Individuals with intractable urinary incontinence and/or persistent urinary retention present major management challenges. The goals of care include effective bladder emptying and effective containment of urine; management options include clean intermittent catheterization, use of indwelling catheters, and use of external devices (for patients with incontinence but no retention). This chapter provides guidelines for the management of patients with indwelling urinary catheters and external urinary collection devices.

INDWELLING CATHETERS

The indwelling catheter, also known as the "Foley" catheter, is one of the most commonly used medical devices in hospitals, long-term care facilities, and the home. Indwelling catheters may be placed for a variety of reasons: to keep patients dry and prevent skin maceration (and for the convenience of hospital staff or caregivers), to decompress the bladder during and after surgery, or to provide for accurate monitoring of urine output. Although catheters can provide many benefits, they are also the primary risk factor for nosocomial urinary tract infection (NUTI), which is the number 1 hospital-acquired infection in the United States.[1] Complications associated with indwelling catheters lead to increased health care costs, patient discomfort, morbidity, and even death.[1-3] Pain and discomfort caused by catheters can be significant issues; studies indicate that patients view their catheters as uncomfortable, painful, and embarrassing.[2-4] Catheters also restrict activities of daily living, act as a physical restraint, and limit the patient's ability to function freely and with dignity.[2]

Despite general recognition that indwelling catheters lead to many complications, they continue to be widely used, even when other options are available. In addition, physicians sometimes forget that hospitalized patients have catheters, and these "forgotten" catheters remain in place until a catheter-related complication occurs or the patient is discharged. Once a patient is sent home with a catheter, it may remain in place, unquestioned by the nurse or caregiver, who focus on catheter maintenance as opposed to removal.

Once a catheter is placed, ongoing decision making and management typically are left to the nurse. Studies have shown that catheter care routines vary widely and frequently are not evidence based.[4-6] Although some common catheter management practices are well supported in the medical literature, others are based on nursing habits or institutional traditions.[7] The goal throughout health care today is evidence-based practice, and the care of patients with indwelling catheters should be guided by this principle. The first questions a nurse should ask when encountering a patient with an indwelling catheter are these: "Why is this catheter being used?" "What are the plans for removal?" "What other options are available for management of incontinence in this patient?"

Indications for Use

The first step in preventing catheter-related complications is to limit indwelling catheter use to patients for whom they are the only option or the best option. Short-term catheter use (less than 30 days) is indicated for a variety of reasons, including management of acute urinary retention, intraoperative and postoperative bladder decompression, and monitoring of urinary output in acutely ill patients.[1,8] Short-term catheter use is usually well tolerated, although UTI is a significant issue. In contrast, long-term catheter use (more than 30 days) can be associated with multiple complications including infection, bladder spasms, urethral erosion, hematuria, stones, epididymitis, urethritis, periurethral abscess, accidental removal, pain, fistula formation, obstruction secondary to encrustation, and leakage.[1,9] Long-term catheterization has also been associated with inflammatory and proliferative lesions of the bladder, including transitional cell and squamous cell carcinomas.[10,11] For these reasons, indwelling catheters are generally considered a last-resort option for management of urinary incontinence. The Centers for Disease Control and Prevention (CDC) and the Agency for Health Care Policy and Research (AHCPR) identify four situations in which long-term use of indwelling catheters is appropriate: (1) urinary retention that cannot otherwise be managed, (2) management of terminally ill or severely ill patients, (3) management of patients with stage 3 or stage 4 pressure ulcers on the trunk or pelvis until the ulcer is healed, and (4) management of urinary incontinence in the homebound patient who is incapable of self-toileting and whose caregiver is unable to manage the incontinence effectively with toileting, containment devices, or absorptive products.[9,12] Neither the CDC nor the AHCPR advocates use of long-term indwelling catheters as a primary approach to the management of urinary incontinence.

Catheter Selection

Although catheters should not be considered first-line therapy, they do represent the *best* management option for selected patients; in these cases, appropriate catheter selection, meticulous nursing care, and comprehensive patient education are paramount.

In selecting the best catheter for an individual patient, the clinician must consider both the primary (base) material and the coating. There are two types of base materials, latex and silicone, and a variety of coatings: hydrogel, silicone elastomer, and antimicrobial substances. Teflon, which was once a commonly used coating, is no longer available in the United States. Coatings are designed to provide a smooth, slippery surface that reduces friction, protects against irritation of the urethral mucosa, and resists encrustation; coatings also prevent direct contact with latex (when the catheter is latex based). Antimicrobial coatings also delay or prevent catheter-associated urinary tract infections (CAUTIs).

The best catheter is soft, smooth, and hydrophilic; these properties serve to minimize urethral irritation and trauma, and to resist encrustation and bacterial attachment. In addition, short-tipped catheters (length from balloon to tip) are better because they provide optimum drainage and are less likely to cause bladder irritation. Finally, the nurse must consider any patient preferences; patients who have been managed with indwelling catheters may have strong preferences and beliefs regarding the catheter that "works best" for them.

Latex Catheters. Latex catheters are soft, flexible, comfortable and inexpensive; they continue to be one of the best catheter choices available. Red rubber latex catheters are radiopaque because of the addition of barium, which also makes them firmer; therefore, they are less likely to kink and are frequently used for patients with enlarged prostates. However, the clinician must rule out latex sensitivity before placing a latex-based catheter. Latex sensitivity most commonly occurs in medical personnel, rubber industry workers, or patients with repeated exposure, such as children with spina bifida.[13] In addition, individuals with a history of atopy or allergies to bananas, avocado, kiwi, or chestnuts may cross-react to latex; therefore, a thorough history is necessary to identify patients who are at risk.[13] Strict latex precautions, including use of latex-free catheter kits and drainage systems, should be followed with patients known to be latex sensitive and for patients with repeated exposure, who are at risk for latex sensitivity. Latex reactions from indwelling catheters can range from severe anaphylaxis with respiratory distress and generalized urticaria, to redness and swelling of the urinary meatus, meatal discharge, complaints of bladder pain, or localized urticaria involving the skin in contact with the catheter.

Complete latex-free kits with latex-free catheters, drainage bags, and gloves are available and should be used if there is any question of latex sensitivity. Since 1998, the United States Food and Drug Administration has required that medical devices containing latex be identified by including a warning statement on the label. Nurses should check labeling carefully when selecting a catheter for a latex-sensitive patient and should be aware that "latex-free" labeling is not required (so latex-free products can be identified by the absence of a label indicating latex, as opposed to a label stating that the product is latex free). Some facilities are now removing all latex products and going latex free.

Although latex sensitivity can be an issue for some patients, the actual prevalence of latex allergy in the general population is low (approximately 1%).[14] In addition, quality catheter manufacturers use a leaching process that removes latex proteins and processing chemicals that could lead to a reaction. This means that latex-based catheters are safe for most patients.

Silicone Catheters. Silicone catheters are available uncoated, hydrogel coated, and antimicrobial coated. Currently, only 100% silicone catheters are considered "safe" for patients with latex sensitivity. The term "Silastic" is sometimes used interchangeably with "silicone", but Silastic (C.R. Bard, Covington, Ga.) catheters are actually a brand-name green latex catheter, compounded with a silicone coating that is nonstick. These catheters are not latex free and should not be used on latex-sensitive patients.

Silicone catheters have the advantage of thinner walls, which provide larger internal lumens per external diameter, and they are less likely to collapse during aspiration. The larger internal lumen results in greater flow, which is advantageous for patients with blood clots, mucus, or sediment in their urine. Silicone catheters also resist encrustation, and the larger internal lumen delays time until blockage.[15,16] Some studies suggest that silicone is more biocompatible with urethral tissues than latex, which may lead to reduced incidence of urethritis and possibly reduced incidence of urethral stricture.[17] However, studies of catheters used for more than 6 weeks in animals showed no difference between silicone and latex catheters in terms of inflammatory changes.[17]

A disadvantage of silicone catheters is the permeability of the balloons, which results in loss of fluid over time.[18] Therefore, when silicone catheters are used, the balloon should be checked at least every 2 weeks and fluid added as needed. Another disadvantage of silicone catheters is the tendency of the balloon to form creases or cuffs when deflated, which can lead to painful and difficult catheter removal.[19,20] Finally, silicone is much firmer than latex, and patients may complain that silicone catheters cause more discomfort than the softer latex catheters.

Silicone Elastomer–Coated Catheters. Silicone elastomer-coated catheters are sometimes confused with 100% silicone catheters; these catheters are actually latex catheters coated inside and out with silicone. The difference between silicone-coated and 100% silicone catheters is worth noting for two reasons: (1) patients who are latex sensitive should be managed with 100% silicone catheters, and (2) patients who are not latex sensitive may prefer silicone-coated catheters to all-silicone catheters because these catheters combine the strength and flexibility of latex with the durability and reduced encrustation typical of all-silicone catheters. Silicone elastomer is not considered a permanent coating and will wear off over time.

Hydrogel-Coated Catheters. Hydrogel-coated catheters are soft and highly biocompatible. The hydrophilic coating absorbs fluid to form a soft, hydrated cushion around the catheter; the coating is slippery when wet, which results in easier insertion and less potential for urethral irritation and trauma. In addition to promoting patient comfort, hydrophilic coatings may resist encrustation as compared with coatings that are hydrophobic (that is, coatings that repel fluid). The coating is considered permanent for the life of the catheter.

Antimicrobial-Coated Catheters. New advances in catheter coating technology have led to the development of antimicrobial coatings; the purpose of these coatings is to reduce the incidence of CAUTIs and NUTIs. The first antimicrobial catheter was a silver oxide–coated catheter released in the 1980s. Silver has been used for many years in medicine and is known to be an effective antimicrobial at low concentrations, with a low incidence of bacterial resistance. However, the silver oxide catheter was removed from the market after a large randomized trial failed to demonstrate efficacy in the prevention of catheter-associated bacteriuria.[21] The silver oxide coating was reported to rub off, which caused loss of bactericidal efficacy and also discolored the meatal and perineal tissue. The second attempt at a silver coated–catheter involved use of a thin layer of silver alloy combined with hydrogel (Bardex IC, C.R. Bard Inc., Covington, GA.) applied either to latex or latex-free catheters; the silver coating was designed to reduce bacterial attachment, colonization, and migration, and thereby to decrease or prevent NUTIs and CAUTIs. The silver hydrogel coating is permanent and nonstaining, and multiple studies have shown it to be effective in reducing CAUTI without causing bacterial resistance.[1,12,22-24] One randomized double blind study of 850 catheterized patients demonstrated that use of these catheters provided a 26% reduction in CAUTI in patients managed with indwelling catheters for up to 20 days; the greatest benefit was in prevention of infections caused by gram-positive organisms (*enterococci, staphylococci,* and *Candida).*[1] The silver hydrogel coating was not found to offer protection against CAUTIs caused by gram-negative organisms, which typically gain access intraluminally.[1] Although numerous randomized studies support the effectiveness of silver hydrogel catheters in reduction of NUTIs, these studies have all focused on short-term use of indwelling catheters; these catheters have *not* yet been studied in patients with long-term indwelling catheters. However, patients who are immunocompromised and patients with recurrent CAUTIs may benefit from a trial of these catheters.

Another antiinfective catheter is the all-silicone controlled-release nitrofurazone-coated catheter (RELEASE-NR, Rochester Medical, Stewartville, MN.). This catheter is designed as a drug delivery system; when inserted into the fluid environment of the urinary tract, the coating delivers the chemosynthetic compound nitrofurazone to the tissues lining the urethra. Although antibiotic resistance is a growing concern within the medical community, nitrofurazone has been used for many years as a systemic agent with very little resistance. Furthermore, the catheter provides localized delivery of the antiinfective, which reduces the need to systemically treat CAUTIs. Nitrofurazone is broadly active against many gram-positive and gram-negative bacteria. In vitro, this catheter has also been shown to have a high level of activity against many types of multidrug resistant bacteria that are associated with NUTIs including methicillin-resistant *Staphylococcus aureus* (MRSA).[25] One investigator-masked trial of 344 catheterized patients demonstrated a decrease in CAUTIs for up to 7 days; after 7 days, the catheter did not appear to provide protection. In addition, the catheter failed to reduce the incidence of infections caused by *Candida* or *Enterococcus*.[1,26]

Catheter Size. When determining catheter size, the clinician must consider both diameter and length. The diameter of indwelling catheters is measured by the French scale, with 1 Fr equal to 0.33 mm. Balloon-tipped catheters come in even sizes 6 to 10 Fr (12 inches in length) for children and 12 to 30 Fr (16 to 17 inches in length) for adults. The "female-length" balloon-tipped catheter (C. R. Bard, Covington, Ga.) is typically 8 inches in length; these catheters are appropriate for small women, but they may not be long enough for tall or obese women.

When selecting a catheter, the prevailing guideline is to use the smallest diameter that will provide good drainage, typically 14 to 18 Fr (adult) unless the patient has blood clots or sediment that frequently occlude the lumen. "Small"-diameter catheters are preferred because the goal is to minimize the distortion of the normal urethral contours. The urethra normally has a flattened noodle-like shape, and the urethra usually conforms to the shape of the catheter as a result of its normal elasticity. Large catheters (catheters larger than 18 Fr) cause distortion of the urethra and also cause significant intraurethral friction. Long-term use of large catheters can lead to erosion of the urethral mucosa, stricture formation, and predisposition to UTIs. In addition, larger catheters are uncomfortable for the patient, and they impair paraurethral gland function. The urethra is lined with paraurethral glands, which produce a mucoid substance that protects against ascending bacteria. Normally, this mucus is flushed away with urination; however, in catheterized patients, the mucus drains by gravity and peristaltic action. (The mucus may appear as a stain on the patient's underwear or a dark, dried "crust" outside the urethra or on the catheter surface.[27]) Large catheters obstruct the paraurethral glands, leading to glandular distension and congestion and accumulation of the normal secretions. These accumulated secretions, in addition to the urethral trauma also associated with large catheters, predispose the patient to UTI and to potential sequelae such as abscess and stricture formation.[28,29] In managing a patient who has a large catheter (larger than 18 Fr) in place, the catheter should be downsized with each catheter change until the catheter is in an acceptable size range. Long-term use of a large catheter in a woman may cause permanent loss of urethral elasticity; in this case, downsizing leads to persistent leakage and possibly to spontaneous dislodgement of the catheter.[30] In this situation, a larger catheter may be required to manage the damaged urethral outlet.

Balloon Size and Balloon Inflation. The size of the balloon is another very important consideration in indwelling catheter selection. Confusion exists among nurses regarding selection and filling of catheter balloons, and 5-mL and 30-mL balloons are frequently used interchangeably. Caregivers need to realize that the purpose of the balloon is to hold the catheter in the bladder, not to occlude the urethra or prevent leakage. For routine use, the clinician should select a 1.5- or 3-mL balloon for pediatric patients and a 5-mL balloon for adult patients and should fill the balloon per manufacturers' directions.

Fig. 10-1 illustrates the difference in a 16-Fr catheter with a 5-mL balloon and a 16-Fr catheter with a 30-mL balloon. When filled, the 30-mL balloon weighs approximately 48.2 g; these balloons are designed to provide short-term postprostatectomy hemostasis by applying pressure to the surgical site. However, these balloons should generally *not* be used for routine or long-term use. Use of a 30-mL balloon (or the addition of extra fluid to a 5-mL balloon) in an attempt to "stop leakage" or "to keep the patient from pulling the catheter out" actually has the opposite effect; the large balloon

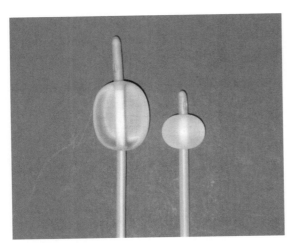

Fig. 10-1 Comparison of 16-Fr catheters with 30- and 5-mL balloons. Note the size of the balloons and the balloon to drainage eye length. The 30-mL balloons were designed for postprostatectomy hemostasis. The drainage eyes of a 30-mL ballooned catheter sit high in the bladder and lead to stasis of urine; the extra weight can damage the bladder neck. (**Courtesy of Dawn Smith-Popielski.**)

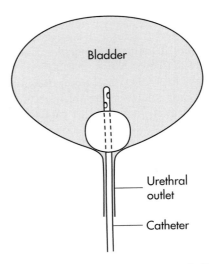

Fig. 10-2 Indwelling catheter with a 30-mL balloon illustrating proximal displacement of the drainage eyes, leading to increased residual urine volume.

acts as a major irritant to the bladder, thus provoking the bladder spasms that cause the leakage and increasing the patient's discomfort and awareness of the catheter.[28,31-33] In addition, long-term use of a large balloon can damage the bladder neck, resulting in inability to retain the catheter.[27] When teaching caregivers about the negative effects of large balloons, it may be helpful to fill a 30-mL balloon with water so caregivers can appreciate the weight that such a balloon places against the bladder neck. Large balloons also sit high in the bladder and displace the drainage eyes proximally, resulting in urinary stasis, residual urine, and the potential for bacterial overgrowth[28,29] (Fig. 10-2).

Much confusion exists about the proper volume to be used for balloon inflation. Because balloons are labeled "5 mL," some clinicians may assume that they only hold 5 mL of fluid and fear breaking the balloon by adding extra fluid. The term "5-mL balloon" is actually a misnomer because these balloons can hold much more fluid without breaking. (In the United Kingdom, the same balloons are

labeled 10 mL). The guiding principle is to follow the manufacturer's instructions. Catheter manufacturers test their balloons to determine the amount of fluid required to obtain symmetric inflation. Underinflation or overinflation can result in an asymmetric balloon, which can deflect the catheter tip to one side (Fig. 10-3). This deflection can cause occlusion of the drainage eyes, irritation of the bladder wall, and bladder spasms. In general, a 5-mL balloon requires about 10 mL of fluid for symmetrical inflation. Manufacturers recommend that sterile water be used to fill catheter balloons as opposed to normal saline or air; saline can lead to crystal formation in the inflation lumen, which can lead to difficulty deflating the balloon, and inflation with air will cause the balloon to float in the bladder.[34] Silicone balloons lose fluid over time as fluid diffuses out into the urine; therefore, the fluid levels in silicone balloons should be checked at least every 2 weeks and fluid added as needed.[4]

Special note. Patients with long-term catheters are at significant risk for bladder calculi that can puncture the retention balloon. Patients who experience repetitive, spontaneous balloon deflation should be evaluated by a urologist for the presence of bladder calculi.

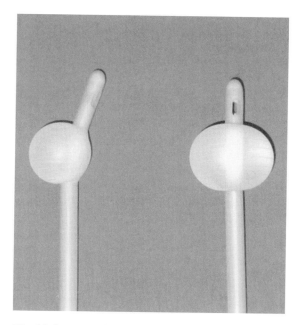

Fig. 10-3 A 5-mL balloon filled with 10 mL of fluid. Proper balloon inflation leads to a symmetric balloon that sits evenly in the bladder. Underinflated balloons can lead to tip deflection that can tip the balloon to the side, irritate the bladder, or occlude drainage eyes. (Courtesy of Dawn Smith-Popielski.)

Guidelines for Catheter Insertion

Guidelines for catheter insertion are outlined in Table 10-1. Placement of an indwelling catheter should be accomplished by techniques that prevent or minimize urethral trauma and bacterial contamination. Copious lubrication should be used to minimize trauma to urethral tissue and any discomfort to the patient. Strict aseptic technique should be followed to prevent bacterial contamination because periurethral contamination at the time of catheter insertion is an important risk factor for CAUTI. The meatus and surrounding area should be cleansed with either 10% povidone-iodine or 1% to 2% aqueous chlorhexidine solution;[12] in addition, perineal cleansing with soap and water or a perineal cleanser is recommended *before* the sterile preparation to further reduce the potential for introduction of bacteria into the bladder.[1,12]

Hand Washing. Thorough hand washing is considered to be the single most important action.[35] Patients and caregivers alike should be taught to wash their hands with antibacterial soap or alcohol-based hand cleaners before and after catheter insertion or manipulation of the drainage system.

Balloon Pretesting. Pretesting of catheter balloons is commonly recommended as a way to prevent insertion of a catheter with a defective balloon. However, balloons are now pretested during the manufacturing process, and some catheter manufacturers no longer recommend pretesting. Although pretesting latex catheter balloons does not usually cause a problem, pretesting is not recommended for silicone catheter balloons. This is because the balloon does not return to its original shape after inflation, and the enlarged balloon area can form a cuff or crease that can traumatize the urethra during catheter insertion.

Documentation. Documentation should include type of catheter inserted, French size, balloon size, amount of fluid used for inflation, ease of insertion, and any problems (resistance to insertion, bleeding, pain) encountered with catheter insertion. Additionally, the amount and description of urine returned and the patient's response to the procedure should be documented.

Female Catheterization. Proper positioning and good lighting facilitate visualization of the female meatus and increase the potential for successful insertion, without contamination or trauma. Ideally, the patient should be positioned on her back with her knees bent and legs apart; use of the sidelying position (as recommended in some nursing procedure manuals) may introduce fecal bacteria into the bladder and should be avoided unless the patient has limited mobility or restricted range of motion or the urethra cannot be otherwise visualized. The female urethra is only 1.5 to 2.0 inches in length; therefore, it is only necessary to lubricate and insert 2 to 3 inches of the catheter. Identification of the female urethra may be difficult in obese women, and in older women the urethra may be prolapsed into the upper vaginal wall. In patients with urethral prolapse, the catheter can be inserted by placing a sterile gloved finger into the vagina and sliding the

TABLE 10-1   Guidelines for Catheter Insertion

GENERAL PROCEDURAL STEPS AND GUIDELINES	MALE CATHETER INSERTION	FEMALE CATHETER INSERTION
Select a closed-system catheter kit with a 14- or 16-Fr catheter and a 5-mL balloon.	Rule out a history of strictures or previous genitourinary surgery. Refer to the urologist if known insertion difficulties occur.	Position the female patient on her back with legs bent and apart; avoid catheter insertion from the rear; identify the urethra before beginning sterile preparation.
Position patient for urethral exposure: cleanse perineal area and rinse well.	Inject 2% lidocaine jelly into the urethra, occlude the tip of the urethra with the finger to prevent leakage, and wait 2 to 5 minutes for anesthetic effect, or push the catheter through a large "mound" of lubricant applied to the end of the penis.	Use the nondominant hand to open the labia; maintain the sterility of the dominant hand throughout the procedure.
Set up sterile tray; don sterile gloves.		
Use rayon balls or swabs soaked in antimicrobial solution to prepare the urethra.		The urethra may be prolapsed into the vagina: to insert catheter place a gloved finger into the vagina and insert the catheter along the tip of the finger, directing the catheter cephalad into the urethra.
Avoid pretesting catheter balloons (especially silicone) unless recommended by manufacturer.	Choose a Coude-tipped catheter for older men or if prostatic enlargement is suspected; insert Coude-tipped catheters with the tip up in 12 o'clock position throughout insertion.	
Insert catheter	Have the patient breathe deeply or bear down if resistance is felt; do not force against resistance.	Lubricate and insert only 2 to 3 inches of catheter.
Confirm urine return then fill the balloon per the manufacturer's directions.	Insert the catheter almost to the bifurcation.	
Lubricant in drainage eyes may delay urine return, and gentle aspiration using safe sampling port may be necessary.	Gently pull the catheter to seat the balloon at the bladder neck.	If the catheter is inadvertently placed into the vagina, leave it as a landmark and obtain a sterile catheter for insertion into the urethra.
Secure the catheter post insertion.	Retract the foreskin for cleansing and catheter insertion in uncircumcised male patients and reposition the foreskin over the head of the penis after insertion.	
Tip	Secure the catheter to the upper thigh or the lower abdomen; position the penis with a slight upward curve to decrease pressure at the penile-scrotal junction.	
A larger catheter or balloon may be used in selected situations but should not be routinely used.		

catheter along the top of the finger, directing it cephalad and into the urethra.[30] If the catheter is inadvertently placed into the vagina, it should be left temporarily as a landmark and a new sterile catheter kit obtained for insertion into the bladder.

Male Catheterization. Male catheterization can be particularly difficult because of the greater urethral length and the prostatic curve. Difficult catheter insertion can be caused by inadequate lubrication, a urethral stricture, inability to thread the catheter through the S-shaped bulbar urethra, or excessive resistance at the bulbomembranous urethra, with tightening of the external sphincter.[30,34] It is helpful to obtain a medical history before attempting to insert the catheter, to identify patients who may have difficult insertions (that is, patients with a history of urethral strictures, prostatic enlargement, or prostate surgery). In uncircumcised patients, the foreskin is retracted to clean the penis and for catheter insertion; the foreskin is then repositioned over the head of the penis after insertion. Particular caution should be used when inserting a catheter into an uncircumcised patient with severe penile and scrotal edema because it may be very difficult to reposition the foreskin once the catheter has been inserted. Patients with severe edema are also at greater risk for penile erosion.

Inadequate lubrication can cause urethral trauma and pain and can also result in inability to pass the catheter through the prostatic urethra. Common nursing practices such as squirting lubricant on the end of the catheter or dragging the end of the catheter through lubricant are not usually sufficient for male catheterization, and applying lubricant to the entire insertion length can make the catheter very slippery and difficult to handle. One effective technique is to apply a very large mound of lubricant to the tip of the penis; the catheter is lubricated along the entire insertion length as it enters the penis, but the remainder of the catheter stays dry. Another approach is to inject 10 mL of water-soluble lubricant directly into the male urethra; this is the technique used by urologists, and it effectively distends the urethra and places the lubricant high in the urethra, where it is needed.[34,36] This technique is not typically taught in nursing schools, so nurses may be hesitant to inject the lubricant into the urethra.

Many experts recommend the use of lidocaine jelly 2% injected directly into the urethra to reduce discomfort and prevent urethral spasm.[34] The lidocaine syringe tip is inserted into the urethra, and the anesthetic jelly is injected; catheter insertion should then be delayed for 2 to 5 minutes for the anesthetic to take effect.[34,36] (Placing a gloved finger over the tip of the penis prevents the lidocaine from leaking out during the waiting period.) If resistance is met during catheter insertion, the patient can be instructed to perform deep-breathing exercises to relax the sphincter, at which point the catheter is passed. The catheter should be advanced almost to the bifurcation to avoid inflation of the balloon in the urethra,[28,29] and placement should be confirmed by urine return before the balloon is inflated. Lubricating jelly in the drainage eyes may delay urine return; in this case, gentle aspiration of urine (through the drainage bag safe sampling port) can be used to confirm placement.

Forcing a catheter during insertion should be strictly avoided, because this can lead to the formation of a false passage, where the catheter is pushed into tissues alongside the urethra. This is a serious condition that can lead to urethral strictures, bleeding, and infection, and may require surgical intervention. Strategies that promote successful catheterization in male patients include use of a Coude-tipped catheter, copious lubrication, and insertion with slow steady pressure.[30,34] Coude catheters, as seen in Fig. 10-4, have a firm curved tip designed to negotiate the male prostatic curve, and are helpful for patients with prostate gland enlargement. Coude catheters are inserted with the tip pointed upward (toward the patient's umbilicus) in the 12 o'clock position and are passed using steady gentle pressure.[30] An arrow or raised indicator on the catheter shaft indicates the position of the tip during insertion. If a Coude catheter cannot be inserted in accordance with these guidelines, the patient should be referred to a urologist.

Securement Recommendations and Drainage Bag Selection

Catheter Securement. After insertion, all urinary catheters should be secured. Unsecured catheters can lead to bleeding, trauma, pressure sores, penile

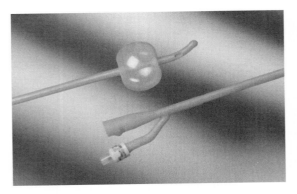

Fig. 10-4 Coude catheters facilitate negotiation of the prostatic urethra. The tip is inserted upward in the 12 o'clock position throughout insertion. A raised indicator on the funnel indicates the direction of the tip. (Courtesy of C.R. Bard, Inc., Covington, Ga.)

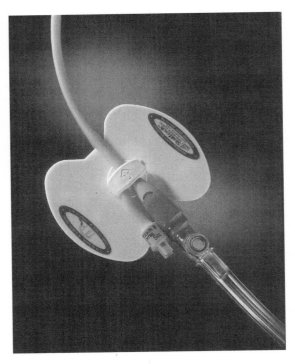

Fig. 10-5 StatLock Foley Securement Device. (Courtesy of StatLock Foley, Venetec International, Inc., San Diego, CA)

erosion, and bladder spasms from pressure and traction[37] (see Plate 2). Securement devices stabilize the catheter and prevent tension and drag, thus reducing friction and trauma within the urethra and the bladder.[28,29,32] It is recommended that the catheter be secured to the thigh for women and to the upper thigh or lower abdomen for men. The lower abdominal or upper thigh position in men gently curves the penis up and to the side and decreases the potential for pressure necrosis and urethral erosion at the penile-scrotal junction.[30,32,34] Ambulatory men may find abdominal securement difficult; these patients can be instructed to secure the catheter to the upper thigh in the daytime and to change the position to the lower abdomen for sleep. Many securement devices are available including adhesive and nonadhesive tube stabilization devices, leg straps with Velcro fasteners, and catheter-specific anchors. Use of an anchoring device should be a standard of care for the patient with an indwelling catheter. A new catheter-specific anchor (StatLock Foley, Venetec International, Inc., San Diego, CA; Fig. 10-5) offers advantages that include a reclosable locking mechanism that swivels as the patient moves and an adhesive comfort pad that can be left in place for up to 1 week without altering skin integrity.[37] Whatever product is selected, nurses should instruct patients and caregivers in the proper use and removal of the securement device.

Drainage Bag Selection. In selecting a drainage system, the clinician should consider the patient's vision, dexterity, and mobility in addition to aesthetic issues.[28,38] The goal is to select a system that is easy for the patient or caregiver to manage and that minimizes any embarrassment or psychological discomfort associated with use of an indwelling catheter. Critical components of an acceptable drainage system include the following: an antireflux chamber or device, a large reservoir (at least 2000 mL for sleep), a stable hangar mechanism, a drainage tube clamp that is easy for the patient or caregiver to operate, and an anchoring strap that is comfortable and easy to use. Antireflux devices or chambers prevent retrograde urine flow once the urine drains into the bag, and this helps to reduce the incidence of CAUTI. Some drainage bags also have antimicrobial tubes located in the drainage spout; these provide a microbicidal barrier that further inhibits the retrograde migration of pathogens.

The Belly Bag (Rusch, Inc., Duluth, Ga.) has 1000 mL urine capacity, fastens around the waist, and is designed to be worn on the abdomen over the bladder. This drainage bag is easily concealed under clothing and can be used day and night; however, drainage depends on normal bladder pressures to push the urine "uphill" from the bladder into the bag. The physician should be consulted before use of this drainage bag to make sure that the patient's bladder pressures are sufficient.

Many patients prefer leg bags because they are easy to conceal under clothing. Leg bags have an antireflux device that prevents urine from refluxing into the drainage tubing, but they use gravity to drain and work best when attached to the lower leg. Leg bags are available in a variety of designs and capacities, and have various types of leg straps. Some leg bags contain "baffles" (seams that create equal compartments) to ensure even distribution of the urine and to promote conformity of the bag to the leg. Drainage spigots are available in push-pull, twist and pull, or removable cap forms. One disadvantage of leg bags is their reduced capacity; they have insufficient capacity for nighttime use (although many patients use them for nighttime drainage). Some patients use leg bags during the day and switch to bedside bags at night; however, this involves breaking the closed system, which should be avoided because of the increased risk for CAUTI. Instead, patients should be taught to maintain a closed connection between the leg bag and the catheter, and to attach the leg bag spout to the night drainage bag tubing. Another potential problem with leg bags is that many are unvented, which can create a vacuum lock and impaired drainage, especially when the patient is lying down. An unvented bag can also cause discomfort when the bag is drained. In an unvented leg bag, air lock can be prevented by leaving a small amount of urine in the bottom of the bag when emptying; air lock can be *alleviated* by opening the spigot and pulling the sides of the bag apart to pull air into the bag.

Nurses should be knowledgeable about the available products and should assist patients to find the products that best fit their needs; nurses should also be aware that patients may have strong preferences regarding the type of bag or outlet device that works best for them. For example, patients with disabilities or limited mobility may require a special type of outlet device, and the nurse should assist the patient to find the one that works best for them.

Routine Care

Routine care protocols for patients with indwelling catheters are designed to reduce the incidence of catheter-related complications, such as infection and damage to the bladder neck. Key elements include positioning of the drainage bag and drainage tubing to prevent retrograde flow of urine, measures to maintain a closed system, measures to reduce contamination of the outlet spout, catheter stabilization, and adequate fluid intake.

Position of Drainage Bag and Tubing. It is important to maintain the drainage bag and tubing below the level of the patient's bladder to prevent reflux of urine from the drainage tubing into the bladder; in addition, the tubing should be maintained in a "straight line" without kinks or loops to promote unobstructed urine flow.[12] (Hanging the drainage bag on the end of the bed makes it easier to avoid loops and kinks in the tubing.) All staff members should be taught to strictly avoid placement of drainage bags on patients' abdomens or between their legs during transport. Devices that promote appropriate positioning of the drainage bag and tubing include stainless steel drainage bag holders (available from medical supply companies); patients can also be taught to use a chair, new plastic trashcan, or tub to hang the bag properly. When teaching patients and caregivers how to manage catheters and drainage bags, the following points must be emphasized:

- Keep drainage bags off the floor.
- Position the drainage bag below the bladder at all times; keep the drainage tubing straight and "unkinked," and do not allow loops of tubing to fall below the level of the drainage bag.
- Empty the drainage bag when one-half to two-thirds full, to avoid traction on the catheter from the weight of the drainage bag.
- When emptying the drainage bag, do not allow the drainage spout to contact the collection container or the floor.

- Disinfect urine collection containers after use, and provide each patient with his or her own drainage container.

Fluid Intake. Many strategies can be used to reduce the incidence of CAUTI; one of the most important is provision of adequate fluid intake, which promotes a constant antegrade flow of urine that opposes retrograde migration of bacteria. In addition, adequate fluid intake helps to maintain dilute and typically acidic urine, which acts to inhibit bacterial growth. Increased fluid intake has also been shown to delay time until blockage in patients with catheter encrustation.[39] Patients with indwelling catheters should be encouraged to limit intake of caffeinated fluids, because caffeine is a bladder irritant and can lead to bladder spasms. The use of carbonated beverages should also be discouraged because these beverages are thought to promote alkaline urine.

Site Care/Perineal Care. At one time, scheduled meatal care was considered effective and necessary after catheter insertion; however, studies have not demonstrated that meatal care with soap, water, povidone-iodine, or antibacterial ointments or creams decreases the incidence of CAUTI.[12] Although routine perineal care *is* recommended, catheter manipulation should be avoided, because this is thought to contribute to bacterial migration into the bladder around the catheter-meatal junction.[1,12] Patients who are ambulatory can still shower, but they should be instructed to cleanse the perineal area gently, to minimize catheter manipulation, and to keep the drainage bag lower than the bladder and off the floor. Application of petrolatum-based creams or ointments around the meatus can degrade latex catheters and should be avoided.

Catheter Change Intervals. There is no evidence to support routine monthly catheter changes; rather, nurses should monitor patients closely for signs of blockage or encrustation and should change the catheter based on specific patient needs.[9,12] The frequency of catheter change should be increased for the patient who consistently develops encrustation and obstruction before the next scheduled change. Data indicate that 96% of all unplanned catheter changes can be attributed to the following three factors: inadvertent dislodgement or removal

by the patient (41%), leakage (31%), and encrustation (24%).[28] Patients who are disoriented or confused should be observed closely, and every effort should be made to reduce any catheter-related discomfort, because this can lead to removal of the catheter with the balloon inflated (and resultant trauma to the urethra and bladder).

Closed Catheter Systems. Closed systems are catheter kits that contain a catheter that is pre-connected to the drainage bag, and sealed at the catheter-drainage bag junction. Maintenance of a closed drainage system has been found to be a key element in prevention of CAUTI;[1] studies have shown that bacteriuria occurs within 4 days when open systems are used, as compared with 30 days when a closed system is used.[1,36] Disconnection of the catheter from the drainage tube invites bacterial invasion; thus catheter irrigations and drainage bag changes are more likely to cause UTI than to prevent it. However, maintenance of a closed system can be very difficult for home care patients, who frequently switch from standard drainage bags at night to leg bags in the day. These frequent breaks in the system greatly increase the risk of CAUTI. Currently, there are no leg bag systems designed to hold the urine volume produced during sleep. However, nurses can attach a sterile leg bag to the catheter at the time of catheter insertion and use extension tubing or an adapter to attach the standard drainage bag to the leg bag at bedtime. The standard drainage bag can be removed and cleaned each morning. In light of the importance of maintenance of a closed system, further product development is needed in this area.

Catheter Irrigation. Catheter irrigation is not recommended unless obstruction with clots or mucus is anticipated; breaking the catheter-drainage bag connection (closed system) is a major contributor to bacterial entry into the system.[12,41] Closed continuous irrigation with a three-way catheter may be necessary for patients with repeated obstructions caused by blood clots, mucus, or sediment.[12] The CDC recommends that catheter irrigations be limited to management of acute obstruction and performed using aseptic technique with sterile saline and a sterile syringe; however, some home care agencies have a policy for cleaning and reuse of irrigation supplies. Catheter irrigation solutions should be instilled by gravity or with gentle pressure. Vigorous irrigation and aspiration with an irrigating syringe should be avoided as this can result in damage to the bladder mucosa.

Use of Safe Sampling Port. Drainage bags designed with "safe sampling" ports allow the nurse to obtain urine specimens while maintaining a closed system; the CDC recommends that urine specimens be obtained directly through these ports using aseptic technique.[12] To collect a specimen, the drainage tubing is occluded below the port temporarily, thus allowing the urine to collect in the tubing. The port is swabbed with alcohol, and the urine is withdrawn following manufacturer's instructions, using a needle, blunt cannula, or Luer lock/Luer slip syringe. (Needleless systems with Luer lock or Luer slip syringes prevent needlestick injuries when obtaining specimens.) Urine for culture and sensitivity should only be obtained from a newly inserted catheter and drainage bag to avoid culturing the system (catheter and drainage bag) rather than the urine.[30,41] If large volumes of urine are needed (for example, a 24-hour urine collection), a new drainage bag can be attached to collect the specimen.

Guidelines for Cleansing and Reusing Equipment

Over the past few years, there has been a shift from sterile to clean technique in the home care setting; cleaning and reusing catheter drainage bags and irrigation equipment are now common in home care. Cleaning of medical products can be an added burden for patients or caregivers who may be confused regarding cleaning procedures. Cleaning procedures should therefore be individualized, taking into consideration patient and caregiver needs and their ability to follow the procedures. Cleaning solutions designed for urinary equipment are available from medical suppliers or pharmacies, but common household products such as bleach or vinegar are less expensive and readily available. Recommended solutions for cleaning urine drainage bags or irrigation equipment include: one part vinegar to three parts water (1:3), or 1 oz bleach (sodium hypochlorite 5.25%) to 10 oz water (1:10).[42,43] Vinegar solutions are safer for elderly

patients or caregivers and for individuals with limited mobility or dexterity, for whom spills could be an issue. Vinegar has been used safely in the home for many years; it effectively decrystalizes sediment that may build up, and it changes the pH balance, which inhibits bacterial growth.[4]

Bleach solutions have excellent antimicrobial activity, but they lose strength quickly and must be mixed daily.[4,42,44] If bleach is used, patients must be taught proper handling including measures to prevent inhalation or contact with the skin, eyes, or clothing. A study by Dille and Kirchhoff demonstrated that daily decontamination of drainage bags with a 1:10 bleach solution was effective in reducing colony-forming units (CFUs) to a negligible number; specifically, they found growth rates of zero to 100 CFUs for 100% of the cultures from bedside drainage bags and 95.6% of the cultures from leg bags they tested.[42] The drainage bags were used for 4 weeks; none of the cleaned bags leaked, and only two of the 54 bags exhibited separation of the air vent. In addition to reducing bacterial count, the bleach solution also prevented odor in the drainage bags.

Box 10-1 outlines cleaning and decontamination procedures using both bleach and vinegar solutions. If bleach is used, the patient or caregiver should be instructed to use only regular household bleach (5.25% sodium hypochlorite solution) rather than the newer, more concentrated bleach. Whichever solution is used, caregivers should be taught to instill the cleaning solution down the tubing and into the bag, taking care to avoid wetting the air vent located at the top of the drainage bag.

Complications: Causes and Prevention Strategies

A major element of care for the patient with an indwelling catheter is complication prevention; common complications include UTI, bladder spasms and leakage, and encrustation. This section focuses on nursing measures for prevention and management of these complications.

Catheter-Associated Urinary Tract Infection. Of the complications associated with indwelling catheters, the most common and most serious is CAUTI; prevention and management of these

BOX 10-1   Guidelines for Cleansing Reusable Equipment

Vinegar Water Solution 1:3

Supplies:
A large (at least 1 gallon) clean bucket or basin
1 quart white vinegar mixed with 3 quarts tap
water
Turkey baster, catheter tipped syringe, or funnel

Procedure:
1. Empty all urine from the system.
2. Wash hands.
3. Flush system with water. Use a turkey baster, syringe, or funnel or hold tubing under faucet.
4. Drain water from drainage spout and close spout.
5. Fill the bag half full with vinegar solution (using the baster, syringe, or funnel).
6. Close the tubing cap, and allow the solution to dwell for 30 minutes.
7. Release air from the bag or put in more solution, making sure that the inside surfaces that touch urine are cleansed by the solution.
8. Drain the vinegar solution and rinse the entire system with tap water and drain again.
9. Use the baster or syringe to instill air in the system.
10. Hang the system to dry with all caps and the drainage spout open.
11. After drying, store in a covered container.

Bleach Solution 1:10

Supplies:
Tap water
Protective gloves
Irrigating bottle
15 mL (1 Tbsp) liquid bleach (must be regular
bleach 5.25% sodium hypochlorite) mixed
with 150 mL (5 oz) water

Procedure:
1. Wash hands and don protective gloves.
2. Place 150 mL (5 oz) tap water in an irrigating bottle and add 15 mL (1 Tbsp) bleach (5.25%); invert the bottle to mix well.
3. Empty all urine from the drainage bag.
4. Fill the drainage bag and all extension tubing from the top of the tubing with 200 mL of cold tap water; agitate for 10 seconds; empty through spout.
5. Repeat this step.
6. Instill 1 oz or more of the premixed bleach/water solution into the bag with the irrigating bottle. Agitate for at least 30 seconds. Make sure the bleach touches all inner surfaces of the bag.
7. Empty the bag and hang to air dry, do not rinse.
Note: Use only liquid bleach containing 5.25% sodium hypochlorite. Bleach solution must be made fresh daily.

Data from Dille C and Kirchhoff K. Increasing the wearing time of vinyl urinary drainage bags with bleach. *Rehabil Nurs* 18(5):292-295, 1993 and National Association for Continence Care and Cleansing Reusable Catheters and Accessories. NAFC, Charleston, SC (1999).

infections are *the most important aspects of nursing management.*

Impact and significance. CAUTI is the most frequently reported complication of urinary catheterization; more than 40% of all nosocomial infections are catheter associated.[1] More than 1 million patients in hospitals and extended care facilities acquire a CAUTI each year, and studies suggest that CAUTIs are associated with substantially increased death rates; in addition, CAUTIs have been identified as a leading source of nosocomial antibiotic-resistant pathogens.[1,45] Although not all CAUTIs can be prevented, it is believed that proper catheter management could significantly reduce the incidence of these infections.[12] The CDC

guideline for prevention of CAUTI (Box 10-2) addresses preventive measures for patients with short-term urinary catheters; however, patients with long-term indwelling catheters may have different needs.[12] Some experts now recommend the routine use of antimicrobial-coated catheters to reduce rates of infection and costs associated with NUTI.[1,24]

Risk factors. Risk factors for catheter-related infection include: prolonged catheterization (longer than 6 days), female gender, catheter insertion outside the operating room, ureteral stents, azotemia, other active infections, diabetes, malnutrition, renal insufficiency, monitoring of urine output, and placement of the drainage bag above the bladder or allowing loops of drainage tubing to drop below the level

BOX 10-2 Centers for Disease Control Prevention Guidelines for Prevention of Catheter-Associated Urinary Tract Infections Summary of Major Recommendations

Category I. Strongly Recommended for Adoption*

Educate personnel in correct techniques of catheter insertion and care.
Catheterize only when necessary.
Emphasize hand washing.
Insert catheter using aseptic technique and sterile equipment.
Secure catheter properly.
Maintain closed sterile drainage.
Obtain urine samples aseptically.
Maintain unobstructed urine flow.

Category II. Moderately Recommended for Adoption

Periodically reeducate personnel in catheter care.
Use smallest suitable-bore catheter.
Avoid irrigation unless needed to prevent or relieve obstruction.
Refrain from daily meatal care with either of the regimens discussed in text.
Do not change catheters at arbitrary fixed intervals.

Category III. Weakly Recommended for Adoption

Consider alternative techniques of urinary drainage before using an indwelling urethral catheter.
Replace the collecting system when sterile closed drainage has been violated.
Spatially separate infected and uninfected patients with indwelling catheters.
Avoid routine bacteriologic monitoring.

*Refer to complete CDC *Guideline for prevention of catheter-associated urinary tract infections. (Centers for Disease Control and Prevention, Atlanta, GA, 1981.)*

of the collection bag.[1] Other contributing factors are contamination during insertion, fecal incontinence (contamination by *Escherichia coli* in women), and interruption of the closed catheter system.[1] The incidence of bacteriuria is directly related to the duration of catheterization; the rate at which bacteriuria develops is approximately 3% to 10% per day.[1,24] Once the urine is colonized with bacteria, 10% to 25 % of patients will develop symptoms of CAUTI, and about 3% will develop systemic bacteremia.[1] The most important and potentially modifiable risk factor is prolonged catheterization (longer than 6 days); it is critical to note that *all patients are colonized* by the thirtieth day of catheterization.[1]

Causes. All patients with long-term indwelling catheters will develop bacteriuria, for the following reasons:

1. The catheter is a foreign body to which bacteria can adhere.

2. There is loss of the normal defensive mechanism associated with voiding, which flushes bacteria from the urethra.

3. The catheter-drainage bag system provides three routes of bacterial entry into the bladder: the catheter-meatal junction, catheter-drainage tubing connection, and the drainage bag outlet device[45,46] (Fig. 10-6). Current prevention and management strategies for CAUTI focus on these three routes of entry:

- Catheter-meatal junction: Bacteria can enter the bladder at the time of catheter insertion as a result of periurethral contamination or later because of capillary action.[1,12] Periurethral bacterial colonization has been found to be an important risk factor in both men and women; however, extraluminal migration at the catheter-meatal junction is thought to occur more frequently in women, because of the short

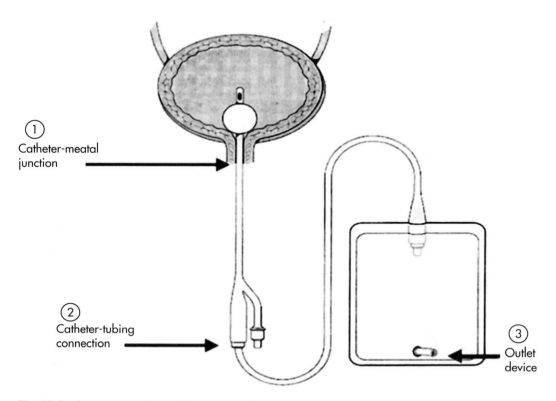

Fig. 10-6 Three routes of bacterial entry for catheter-associated infection: (1) catheter-meatal junction, (2) catheter-tubing connection, (3) outlet device. **(Courtesy of C.R. Bard, Inc., Covington, Ga.)**

female urethra.[1,47] To reduce the risk of bacterial introduction at the time of catheter insertion, the perineal area should be thoroughly washed with soap and water before the sterile catheterization procedure is begun. In practice, this is not routinely done unless the patient has fecal incontinence, but inclusion of this step could help to reduce the incidence of CAUTI. Once the catheter has been inserted, it should be manipulated as little as possible because manipulation is thought to promote bacterial migration at the catheter-meatal junction.[1] (This underscores the importance of catheter stabilization, which helps to reduce traction and manipulation of the catheter at the meatal junction.)

- Catheter-drainage tubing connection: Choosing a closed catheter system and maintenance of the

closed drainage system can reduce the overall risk of CAUTI by 25% for up to 2 weeks of catheterization.[1] The safe sampling port should be used for obtaining urine specimens and routine catheter irrigation should be avoided. Catheters and drainage bags should be changed at the same time and a new closed system provided.

- Drainage bag outlet device: Studies have shown that retrograde migration of bacteria from the urine drainage bag outlet tube is a major source of bacterial contamination.[1] Bacteria enter through the drainage spigot and advance in a retrograde fashion into the drainage bag and up the drainage bag tubing. The collection tubing and bag should always remain below the level of the patient's bladder, and the drainage tubing should always be above the level of the collection bag. Allowing the drainage tubing to drop below the drainage bag is associated with a significant increase in the risk for CAUTI; in one large prospective study, this was the only catheter care violation associated with a significantly increased risk of CAUTI.[1]

Role of biofilms. Much of the recent research on indwelling catheters has focused on the role of biofilms in the development of CAUTI, NUTI, antibiotic resistance, and catheter encrustation. Biofilms are of particular concern in the medical community because they can develop on any indwelling device, including intravenous catheters, needleless connectors, endotracheal tubes, pacemakers, mechanical heart valves, and urinary catheters, and they are highly resistant to traditional antimicrobial treatment.[16,48] The biofilm matrix can interact with and neutralize antibiotics, and biofilms are 1000-fold more resistant than "planktonic" or "free-swimming" forms of bacteria.[16,48] Device-related factors that favor biofilm formation include hydrophobic materials such as uncoated latex and silicone, materials that are rough or textured, and placement within a fluid environment, such as blood or urine.[16,48] Furthermore, urine provides a layer of proteinaceous material that may change the chemical properties of the surface of the catheter and promote biofilm growth.[48]

Biofilm formation has important implications for the pathogenesis, treatment, and prevention of catheter-related infections (and catheter encrustation). Biofilms develop when bacteria adhere to and multiply on catheter surfaces, forming mushroom-like colonies that are protected by a thick polysaccharide matrix.[16,48] Bacterial migration is triggered by chemical signals called "quorum sensing;"[16] the bacteria may originate from the hands of health care workers, cross-contamination from other patients, or from the patient's own colonic or perineal flora.[1,24] Once the bacteria attach, they multiply quickly, swarm over the extraluminal (and/ or intraluminal) surfaces of the catheter, and advance in a retrograde fashion.[1,48] Studies suggest that microorganisms most frequently gain access to the bladder extraluminally, especially in women, because of the shorter urethral length and proximity of the urethra

to the rectum.[1] (Intraluminal contamination usually occurs as a result of retrograde reflux of contaminated urine from the drainage system; infections caused by intraluminal contamination may not be associated with biofilm growth.[1]) The bacteria, most commonly *E. coli* and *Klebsiella,* enter the bladder by adhering to the multiple layers of biofilm.[16,29,31,32] Because the bacteria are protected by the biofilm, they cannot be eliminated by a simple change of the drainage bag or irrigation of the catheter.

While the role of bacterial biofilms in the development of CAUTIs is not completely understood, catheters with antimicrobial coatings have been found to significantly reduce the risk of CAUTI, presumably by inhibiting bacterial growth and adherence.[1] All traditional catheter materials are subject to biofilm development; however, catheter coatings that are very smooth and hydrophilic (such as hydrogel coatings) may delay biofilm formation.[15,16,48]

Nursing measures to prevent or delay colonization include choosing catheters that are made of smooth, hydrophilic materials, maintenance of a closed system, use of aseptic technique for emptying the drainage bag, and maintenance of the drainage spout in a position that limits contamination (that is, fastened securely into the "spigot holder" as opposed to dragging along the floor). Use of catheters with antimicrobial coatings may also be of benefit. Drainage bags should be kept lower than the patient's bladder with the tubing above the base of the bag.[1] Cross-contamination should be prevented by providing each patient with his or her own urine drainage container, which should be washed and decontaminated after each use.

Diagnosis. Urine is normally sterile; it passes from the kidneys and bladder free of microorganisms. Bacteriuria is the presence of microorganisms in the urine, regardless of the source. Normally voided urine contains low levels of bacteria acquired during passage through the urethra and perineal area; "normal" bacterial levels in voided specimens are fewer than 10,000 CFUs of bacteria per milliliter of urine (CFU/mL). The term "significant bacteriuria" is characterized by bacterial multiplication and the presence of at least 100,000 CFU/mL of urine. Bacteriuria can be categorized as either asymptomatic or symptomatic. Asymptomatic bacteriuria produces no symptoms and is considered a normal state for individuals with indwelling catheters; therefore, routine cultures or antibiotics are not indicated. Prophylactic antibiotic therapy is not recommended as it leads to antimicrobial resistance. In addition, research indicates that strategies aimed at reducing or eliminating bacteriuria (that is, bladder irrigations, antibiotic ointments, and antibiotic solutions) are ineffective and, therefore, contraindicated for routine catheter management.[45,46,49] Indications for treatment of asymptomatic bacteriuria are controversial; most clinicians agree that children less than 2 to 3 years of age should be treated, and some authors also recommend treating patients with diabetes, pregnant women, immunosuppressed individuals, and individuals known to have *Proteus* in their urine.[45,46]

Symptomatic bacteriuria is defined as a positive urine culture in a patient who has signs and symptoms indicative of bacterial invasion of the urinary tract. Common signs and symptoms of infection in a patient with an indwelling catheter include bladder spasms and leakage, suprapubic pain or discomfort, a burning sensation in the bladder, malodorous cloudy urine, malaise, chills and fever, anorexia, or flank pain.

Diagnosis of UTI in the patient with a long-term indwelling catheter can be difficult because these patients do not always present with clear clinical symptoms of UTI;[50] for example, altered mental status (with or without fever) may be the only indicator of UTI in an elderly patient.[31] Whenever CAUTI is suspected, the existing catheter should be removed and a new catheter inserted. A specimen for culture and sensitivity should then be obtained via the new system; specimens obtained via a newly inserted catheter reflect bacterial counts in the urine itself, whereas specimens obtained from the existing catheter may reflect residual organisms within the catheter.[30,41,45,46] A broad-spectrum antibiotic may be initiated pending the culture results. Urine cultures obtained from the safe sampling port that show colony counts of more than 10^{2-3} CFU/mL are considered to be significant and indicative of CAUTI, because these colony counts rise to 10^5 CFU/mL within 24 to 48 hours. Infections in patients with long-term indwelling catheters are frequently polymicrobial and bacterial species may change every few weeks; this underscores the importance of obtaining the specimen from a newly placed catheter. Microorganisms commonly associated with CAUTI include *E. coli, Pseudomonas aeruginosa, Candida albicans, Klebsiella* spp, *Proteus* spp, *Providencia, Enterobacteriaceae, Morganella,* and enterococci.[8,12,51] Treatment of CAUTI is based on factors such as culture and sensitivity results, clinical symptoms, and comorbid conditions. As noted earlier, the catheter should be changed when a CAUTI is suspected; in addition to providing an accurate culture and sensitivity, this intervention hastens clinical improvement, reduces febrile days, and decreases the rate of relapse.[8,52] Specific guidelines for initiation of treatment for CAUTI are outlined in Table 10-2.[52,53]

Leakage Around the Catheter. No other catheter management issue causes more unnecessary catheter changes than leakage around the catheter (also known as "bypassing"). Leakage around the catheter is thought to affect as many as 25% to 65% of patients with indwelling catheters.[54]

TABLE 10-2 **Criteria for Treatment of Urinary Tract Infection in Catheterized Patients**

SOCIETY FOR HEALTHCARE EPIDEMIOLOGY OF AMERICA (SHEA) CONSENSUS PANEL	ASSOCIATION FOR PRACTITIONERS IN INFECTION CONTROL (APIC)
One or more signs or symptoms: Fever higher than 37.9°C or new costovertebral tenderness Rigors Delirium	Two signs or symptoms: Fever greater than 38°C or chills New flank or suprapubic pain Changes in urine character Alteration in mental status or function

From Smith J: Indwelling catheter management: from habit-based to evidence-based practice, *Ostomy/Wound Manage* 49(12):34-45, 2003.

TABLE 10-3   **Troubleshooting Guidelines for Catheter Leakage**

PROBLEM	CAUSE	SOLUTION/PREVENTION
Kinked catheter tubing or drainage tubing	Patient lying on tubing; Tubing twisted Unsecured catheter	Teach the patient to check tubing, especially after changing positions or clothing. Secure the catheter with catheter-specific securement device. Teach the patient to position drainage tubing over the thigh, not under the thigh.
Constipation or fecal impaction	Occlusion of lumen Pressure on bladder leading to spasm	Check for fecal impaction and remove. Increase fluids, fruits, and vegetables in the diet. Instruct the patient and caregiver in a bowel program.
Bladder spasms	Forceful involuntary bladder contraction; common in patients with neurologic or spinal cord injuries Underinflated or overinflated balloons (can deflect tip to one side) Large balloons (stretch and irritate bladder)	Remove known bladder irritants from the diet (alcohol, caffeine). Decrease French size of the catheter (recommended size 14 to 18 Fr for adults). Inflate the balloon per the manufacturer's instructions. Do not overinflate or underinflate catheter balloons. Use a 5-mL balloon inflated with 10 mL sterile water. Secure the catheter: thigh or lower abdomen for male patients. Antispasmodic medications can be used. Hang the drainage bag properly. Empty the drainage bag when half to two-thirds full. Rule out bladder calculi and infection.
Infection	Three entry sites for bacteria: catheter-meatal junction, catheter-drainage bag junction, drainage bag outlet port Infection causes bladder irritation and spasm May be asymptomatic	Follow CDC Guidelines including: Hand washing or alcohol hand wash before any intervention. Use strict aseptic technique; wash the perineum before sterile preparation for catheter insertion. Maintain a closed system. Monitor patients for signs of infection: APIC or SHEA guidelines. Position the drainage bag lower than the bladder at all times. Do not allow tubing to fall below the level of the drainage bag. Secure the catheter appropriately. Use an individual urine collection device for each patient. Avoid manipulation of the catheter and drainage system. Obtain urine for culture and sensitivity from a new sterile catheter.
Luminal occlusion	Blood clots, sediment or mucus	Irrigate the catheter with 60 mL sterile saline using sterile technique. Consider a three-way catheter with continuous irrigation if the problem is ongoing. Increase French size of the catheter; do not increase the size of the balloon. Consider a 100% silicone catheter (larger internal lumen). Encourage increased fluids.

Continued

TABLE 10-3 Troubleshooting Guidelines for Catheter Leakage—cont'd

PROBLEM	CAUSE	SOLUTION/PREVENTION
Encrustation with luminal occlusion	Colonization with urease-producing bacteria; pH increases causing minerals to precipitate from urine and attach to catheter surface; result is blockage	Inspect the catheter for encrustation. Increase fluids. Monitor the time until usual blockage; change the catheter before usual blockage. Keep extra catheter kits available. Monitor spinal cord-injured patients closely; autonomic dysreflexia can occur. Consider acidic bladder washouts if blockage occurs in less than 7 to 14 days (Renacidin, less than 50 mL, instilled by gravity twice).
Urethral dilation: unable to retain catheter, leakage with no other causes	Usually female patients Large catheters and balloons Traction on catheter Unsecured catheters	Use the smallest French size that provides good drainage (that is, 14 to 16 Fr). Select 5-mL balloons. Never use 30-mL balloons or overinflate or underinflate balloons. Refer to the urologist for other options. Secure the catheter to the thigh and avoid traction.

Adapted from Smith J: Indwelling catheter management: from habit-based to evidence-based practice, *Ostomy/Wound Manage* 49(12):34-45, 2003.

Although leakage around the catheter is less serious than a UTI, it is very frustrating for patients and caregivers.

The two most common reasons for urinary leakage are catheter obstruction and bladder spasms. Luminal occlusion can be caused by kinked tubing or catheter encrustation; bladder spasms are typically the result of infection, fecal impaction or constipation, or bladder overactivity caused by a large catheter or large balloon. Leakage can also be caused by loss of urethral elasticity and conformability (in the female) or by development of a small fibrotic bladder with very limited capacity, which is a potential complication of long-term catheterization and the associated bacteriuria.[54-56]

The nurse must focus first on identifying the cause of the leakage; interventions can then be tailored to the cause of the problem. Table 10-3 outlines common causes of leakage and nursing management strategies. For example, the catheter should be irrigated or changed if the catheter lumen is occluded by blood clots, sediment, mucus, or crystals. Irrigation with normal saline can remove clots or debris, but saline is ineffective in dissolving occlusions caused by catheter encrustations; in this situation, the catheter must be changed.[40] If sediment or blood clots are causing frequent occlusion, placement of a larger catheter and routine catheter irrigations may be necessary.

Management of bladder spasms. Bladder spasms are involuntary contractions of the bladder and are common in patients with urinary catheters, spinal cord injuries, and conditions resulting in neurologic deficits.[30,54] Bladder spasms may be caused by various factors including infection, concentrated urine, a large catheter or large balloon that irritates the bladder, failure to stabilize the catheter with resultant "drag" on the bladder neck, and pressure against the bladder caused by fecal impaction. Known bladder irritants such as caffeine and alcohol should be avoided in patients with a history of bladder spasms. Additionally, large catheters and balloons should be avoided to prevent pressure on the sensitive trigone area. Symmetrical balloon inflation, catheter securement, and adequate fluid intake all help to reduce the risk for bladder spasms and resultant leakage. Several studies have shown a direct correlation among increased bladder spasms, leakage, and infection; urine culture and sensitivity testing are therefore indicated if a patient experiences leakage and other causes of leakage are excluded.[55]

One common cause of leakage is stool in the rectal vault or colon, which leads to bladder spasms and leakage by occluding the catheter lumen or compressing the bladder. In a study by Ziemann and colleagues, 81% of all patients with leakage had constipation or fecal impaction.[56] This finding underscores the importance of bowel management programs designed to prevent, or promptly correct, constipation. Patients with urinary catheters frequently have other medical problems that may lead to constipation. Bowel movements should be monitored for frequency and consistency, and a bowel program should be instituted as needed to prevent constipation and fecal impaction. Patients with urinary leakage should also have a digital rectal exam to rule out fecal impaction, although impactions can be high in the colon and not felt on digital exam.

Bladder spasms can be strong enough to push the catheter out of the urethra with the balloon inflated. The most critical intervention for the patient with bladder spasms is elimination of the triggering condition, such as treatment of infection, downsizing of a large catheter, or elimination of constipation. If bladder spasms are severe, the clinician may also consult the physician regarding possible short-term use of antispasmodic or anticholinergic drugs; however, the benefits of reduced leakage must be balanced against the potential adverse effects of these drugs.

Leakage from dilated urethra. Over time, large-diameter catheters can stretch the urethra, which results in leakage and/or the inability to retain the catheter. Urethral dilatation is particularly common in women with long-term urethral catheters.[30] Urethral dilatation should be suspected in a patient with a history of large catheters or large balloons who experiences persistent leakage with no apparent cause. These patients should be referred to a urologist and evaluated for other management options.

Leakage from obstruction and catheter encrustation. Catheter encrustation is a significant problem for up to 50% of patients with long-term catheters and can lead to frequent catheter changes, unplanned nursing visits (in home care), or costly emergency room visits.[40] It is important for nurses to understand the process of encrustation and to develop a proactive plan of care to keep the catheter open and draining. Catheter encrustation is a complex process in which crystalloid and colloid substances adhere to the catheter surface and block the drainage eyes, resulting in decreased urine flow and blockage of the drainage lumen. The primary cause of encrustation is infection of the urinary tract by *Proteus mirabilis* or other urease-producing bacteria (such as *S. aureus, Pseudomonas aeruginosa,* or *Klebsiella* species).[16] The normally acid urine becomes more alkaline as these bacteria multiply and urease raises the urinary pH (greater than 7); the alkaline environment promotes precipitation of calcium and magnesium phosphate, and these substances then adhere to the catheter's inner and outer surfaces, forming a crystalline biofilm.[16] (This precipitate is also known as struvite crystals.) *P. mirabilis* is the organism that is most effective at producing crystalline biofilms, and currently all available catheters are susceptible to biofilm formation and encrustation.[16] Biofilms form initially in the area of the catheter drainage eyes; the crystalline material accumulates around the bacterial cells as the biofilm develops (Fig. 10-7). Studies have shown that saline irrigations, antibiotics, and antiseptic solutions are ineffective in eradicating crystalline biofilms that lead to encrustation; therefore, treating the patient with antibiotics will not result in less encrustation.[40,57]

Encrustation may not be visible on the exterior of the blocked catheter; when encrustation is suspected, the nurse can cut the catheter 1 to 2 cm below the drainage eyes to observe the crystalline deposits that have formed in the inner lumen. Forms of encrustation can range from sandlike granules to an eggshell-shaped crust that either prevents catheter removal or fractures during catheter removal. These fragments act as a nidus for stone formation if they are left in the bladder.

Patients can be classified either as "blockers" or "nonblockers." Nonblockers are patients who will never develop catheter encrustation, whereas

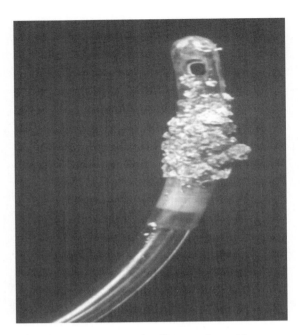

Fig. 10-7 Encrustation of a silicone catheter. Heavy deposits of encrustation on an all-silicone catheter balloon. The drainage eyes appear open, but the internal catheter lumen is blocked. Fragments of encrustation left in the bladder act as a nidus for stone formation. (Courtesy of Dr. Roger Feneley, Bristol, United Kingdom.)

"blockers" are patients who consistently and repeatedly develop encrustations resulting in decreased urine flow.[15,40] Once a patient has been identified as a blocker, it is important to monitor catheter

function closely and to modify the catheter change schedule with the goal of changing the catheter *before* it blocks. Routine administration of vitamin C (to acidify the urine) or of cranberry juice or pills (to reduce bacterial adherence) has been shown to be effective in preventing UTIs in noncatheterized patients, but it has not been shown to delay or decrease infection, encrustation, or blockage in patients with indwelling catheters.[26,58] However, a recent study suggests that increasing fluid intake significantly decreases time until blockage.[39] In addition, studies have shown that acidic solutions instilled into the bladder can dissolve encrustations, although further studies are needed regarding optimal volume and frequency and the effects on bladder mucosa.[40] In patients with frequent blockage resulting from encrustations, a prescription citric acid bladder irrigant solution (Renacidin Guardian Laboratories, Hauppauge, NY) may be instilled into the bladder to dissolve encrustations. Current recommendations for nursing management of encrustation and blockage are listed in Box 10-3.

Catheter Removal

Patients with indwelling catheters should be frequently reevaluated for possible catheter removal; the clinician must carefully consider the reasons for the indwelling catheter and possible alternatives to management. For example, a catheter placed for management of a full-thickness pressure ulcer should

---

BOX 10-3   Guidelines for Management of Catheter Encrustation and Blockage

- Inspect and palpate the catheter for signs of encrustation with each change (or cut the catheter 1 to 2 cm below the drainage eyes to visualize encrustation).
- Schedule catheter changes based on blockage history (that is, usual time to blockage).
- Schedule the catheter change the week before the catheter normally blocks.
- Increase fluid intake and attempt to acidify the urine; this is controversial, but it may be of benefit with some patients.
- Keep extra catheter kits available; when possible, teach the caregiver or patient how to change the catheter in the event of blockage.
- Ensure prompt replacement of the catheter if blockage occurs; if the patient and caregiver are unable to remove and replace the catheter at home, they should be instructed to call the nurse or physician or go to the emergency room.
- Perform two sequential bladder washouts with less than 50-mL acidic bladder irrigant solution instilled by gravity no more than every other day.[40]

be discontinued when the ulcer is healed; the patient should then be placed on an alternative bladder management program. Whenever the decision is made to discontinue an indwelling catheter, it is critical to carry out preremoval data collection, patient preparation, and patient and caregiver education to maximize the potential for successful transition to a controlled voiding program.

Evaluation and Transition. It is recommended that urine output be recorded every 6 to 8 hours for at least 2 days to establish the patient's usual pattern of urine elimination.[30,33] It is important to identify and eliminate any reversible factors that could negatively affect a successful transition to spontaneous voiding; that is, factors that contribute to urinary retention or urinary incontinence. Factors that can contribute to urinary retention are fecal impaction, anticholinergic medications, calcium-channel blockers, and alpha-adrenergic agonists;[30,33] contributing factors for urinary incontinence include altered mental status, depression, atrophic vaginitis, and UTI.[30,33] All these conditions must be eliminated or controlled before removing the catheter. It is also important to remove the catheter at a time that permits accurate recording of urine output and allows for postvoiding recatheterization if necessary. Intermittent clamping and releasing of the catheter before removal have not been shown to affect bladder function positively and are not recommended.[28,30,33] Finally, the clinician must educate the patient or caregiver regarding the plan for bladder management *before* removal of the catheter.

The bladder is normally able to resume its usual cycle of filling and emptying; however, it is essential to evaluate postvoid residual volumes (PVRs) to monitor the completeness of bladder emptying. This may be accomplished by straight catheterization or a portable bladder ultrasonogram. The measurement should be obtained as soon as possible (ideally within 5 minutes) after the patient has voided.

Patients who are able to void effectively, as evidenced by a residual urine volume of less than 100 mL, should have a repeat PVR measurement at 1 to 2 weeks after catheter removal.[30,33] An immediate PVR measurement is indicated for any patient who develops signs or symptoms of retention, such as frequency, small voided volumes, or the sensation of incomplete emptying.[30,33] The patient who is able to void but who demonstrates urge-pattern incontinence should be placed on an appropriate program that includes fluid management and bladder retraining strategies.

The patient who is unable to void requires repeat catheterization (or at least an ultrasound determination of bladder volume) at an established point in time after catheter removal.[30,32,33] In this situation, some clinicians recommend catheterizing the patient 4 to 6 hours after catheter removal.[28,29,30] Ideally, the time for catheterization is based on the "preremoval" data regarding patterns of urine elimination and a preset "limit" of 600 to 800 mL.[30,33] Patients with "borderline" PVR volumes (that is, 100 to 400 mL) should be carefully followed for voided versus residual volumes. Catheterization is indicated for any patient who complains of or demonstrates discomfort and is unable to void and for the patient who is able to void but who has a high PVR (more than 400 mL).[30,33] There are two options for patients who are unable to effectively void after catheter removal: establishment of a clean intermittent catheterization program and reinsertion of an indwelling catheter.

An optional assessment measure immediately after catheter removal is the performance of a bedside cystometrogram; this study provides very valuable data regarding the bladder's filling capacity and stability, the patient's sensory awareness of bladder filling, and the patient's ability to empty the bladder effectively. A cystometrogram should not be performed if a UTI is suspected.

Technique for Catheter Removal. Traditionally, nurses have been taught to aspirate fluid from catheter balloons for balloon deflation. More recent studies have demonstrated that aspiration may result in collapse of the inflation lumen, formation of creases, ridges or cuffing at the balloon area, and an increased diameter of the balloon area on deflation.[19,20] Enlargement of the balloon area can result in difficult removal and urethral trauma. As noted earlier, this "cuffing" effect is seen more frequently with silicone catheters. One major catheter manufacturer is now recommending that the fluid be allowed to return by gravity into the syringe, not by aspiration. Because of the small diameter of the inflation lumen, it may take 30 to 45 seconds for all of the fluid to return. Box 10-4 outlines recommended catheter removal guidelines. Manufacturers' instructions for removal should be followed. If aspiration is used, it should be very gentle.

Management of nondeflating catheter balloons. Failure of a Foley catheter balloon to deflate may be caused by several factors: collapse of the inflation lumen by forceful syringe aspiration of the fluid; a malfunctioning catheter valve; internal or external clamping, crushing or kinking of the inflation channel; luminal obstruction by crystals (if saline is used to inflate the balloon); or encrustation on or within the balloon.[59-62] Forcible removal of an inflated catheter balloon may lead to bleeding, retention of balloon fragments, and injury to the prostate or urethra with resulting formation of urethral strictures.[62] Therefore, every attempt should be made to deflate the catheter balloon using the least invasive technique.

When removing a catheter, the nurse can minimize the risk for nondeflation by following the guidelines in Box 10-4. Before attempting to deflate the balloon, the nurse should make sure the balloon is not in traction at the bladder neck; the balloon may be pulled into the bladder neck from traction on the catheter, in which case it is necessary to push the catheter slightly inward toward the bladder to disengage it from the bladder neck. The nurse should then attach either a Luer lock or a Luer slip syringe into the catheter valve and should allow the fluid to return without aspiration. It is important to avoid application of excessive pressure when attaching the syringe because this may damage the inflation valve. The fluid usually returns within 30 to 45 seconds when this technique is used. If the fluid does not return, the clinician should reposition the patient and should try to inject 3 to 5 mL of sterile water gently into the inflation valve. This maneuver usually dislodges any debris lying against the valve and/or opens a stuck valve. After the fluid is injected, the empty syringe should be reattached to the

---

BOX 10-4   Guidelines for Catheter Removal

1. Select syringe recommended by manufacturer: Luer lock or Luer tip.
2. Loosen the plunger by moving it up and down in the syringe barrel.
3. Withdraw the plunger 0.5 mL from the end of the syringe.
4. Attach the syringe to the valve:
    a. Luer lock: insert and twist to lock.
    b. Luer tip: seat firmly and do not twist or force.
5. Allow water to come back by gravity.
6. DO NOT ASPIRATE ON THE PLUNGER.
7. DO NOT CUT OFF INFLATION PORT.
8. Allow at least 30 seconds for the balloon to deflate.

If the water does not return:
1. Reposition the patient.
2. Ensure that the catheter is not in traction (balloon compressed at bladder neck).
3. Check to see if urine is flowing freely in tubing.
4. Attempt to add 5 mL fluid to balloon.
5. Attach the empty syringe to the inflation port and wait 5 to 30 minutes.
6. Apply very gentle aspiration (forceful aspiration can collapse inflation lumen).
7. Cut inflation port valve (if valve has already been cut use a blunt cannula to inject 5 mL fluid into balloon).
8. Follow protocol regarding further options and notify the physician.

Adapted from CountItDown (Foley Catheter Deflation, C.R. Bard, Inc., Covington, Ga.)

deflation port with the plunger positioned 0.5 mL from the end of the syringe. It may take as long as 30 minutes for the fluid to return; in some cases, the fluid drips very slowly into the syringe, and the nurse finds that the catheter has fallen out when he or she returns. If these maneuvers prove unsuccessful, the inflation valve can be cut off. If the problem is a defective valve, the fluid will run out and the balloon will deflate. If the valve has already been removed, the nurse can attempt to inject 5 mL of fluid into the side port with a syringe attached to a blunt-tipped cannula or angiocath. If these measures are ineffective and the balloon is still inflated (or if the fluid drains out of the balloon but the catheter resists removal), a urologist should be called. Urethral catheters should never be forcibly removed against resistance. There could be several reasons that the catheter will not come out; these include accidental suturing of the catheter during a surgical procedure, heavy encrustation of the catheter with mineral deposits, an enlarged prostate, or scar tissue formation after a surgical procedure such as prostatectomy.

The urologist will either inject mineral oil or pass a lubricated wire up the inflation port to open the inflation channel. Some urologists prefer the lubricated wire technique, because mineral oil inflation may produce balloon fragments that are left in the bladder and that necessitate cystoscopy.[62]

With the mineral oil technique, the bladder is filled with at least 200 mL of fluid followed by an injection of 10 to 15 mL of mineral oil (a rubber solvent) into the inflation lumen to dissolve the balloon; this technique works only with latex catheters, because silicone is not dissolved by mineral oil. (Other solutions such as ether, chloroform, and acetone are no longer commonly used because, although they dissolve the latex balloon, the chemicals escape into the bladder and can cause chemical cystitis and bladder contractures.)[61,63] The latex balloon will start to dissolve in about 15 minutes. Disadvantages to this technique include the potential for bladder irritation from the mineral oil, and the risk that balloon fragments may be left in the bladder.[61,62]

An alternate method is to pass a well-lubricated 3- or 4-Fr ureteral catheter set, a 0.028-inch ureteral stylet, a No. 26 orthopedic wire suture, or a 22-gauge central venous catheter over a guidewire; the intent is to open the inflation lumen, not to puncture the balloon.[59-63] Once the inflation channel is opened, the water drains out beside the wire.

If these less invasive techniques do not work, the urologist may deflate the balloon with a transurethral or transvaginal balloon puncture (in women) or a transrectal or transperitoneal puncture (in men). Alternately, the urologist may puncture the catheter balloon through a cystoscope passed alongside the catheter.

Nursing measures that reduce the risk of creating a nondeflating catheter balloon include use of water to inflate catheter balloons, filling the balloon with the recommended amount of fluid, use of passive deflation techniques (that is, avoidance of aspiration and avoidance of negative pressure on the catheter valve), and pushing the catheter in slightly before attempting catheter removal (to ensure that the balloon is not "caught" at the bladder neck).

Special note. It is increasingly common for indwelling catheters to be placed in women in active labor. This practice is contraindicated unless a cesarean section is to be performed, in which case the catheter should be placed immediately before the procedure. With each uterine contraction, the balloon is pushed with great force against the bladder neck, and, as the baby's head descends, the pressure can compress the inflation lumen; this prevents removal of fluid from the balloon. In addition to a nondeflating balloon, the repetitive thrust of the balloon against the bladder neck can cause bladder neck trauma and urethral injury.

Suprapubic Catheters

Suprapubic catheters (SPCs) are urinary catheters that are inserted via a cystotomy, an incision through the abdominal wall into the bladder. Although nurses encounter patients with SPCs, there has been little research, and few clinical articles are available regarding the management of patients with SPCs. An understanding of the insertion procedure and function of these catheters permits nurses to develop a comprehensive plan of care for these patients.

Indications. SPCs are indicated on a short-term basis for patients undergoing urethral, gynecologic, or pelvic surgery, to relieve urinary retention caused by prostatic hypertrophy or urethral stricture, and for patients with trauma or tumors that would prevent catheter insertion through the urethra.[30,64] In patients with restricted hip mobility or arthritis, it may be impossible to insert a urethral catheter, and an SPC may be indicated. SPCs may also be used for patients who require long-term catheterization as an alternative to urethral catheters.

Advantages and Disadvantages. Although SPCs are thought to have advantages such as lower infection rates, increased patient acceptance, and ease of self-care, they are not without problems.[8,64,65] Studies comparing SPCs with urethral catheters have produced mixed results and similar long-term complication rates.[9] SPCs are contraindicated in patients with intrinsic sphincter deficiency or chronically unstable bladders, known carcinoma of the bladder, and hematuria of unknown origin.[9,64]

SPCs enter the body though the lower abdominal wall, and some studies suggest lower rates of bacteriuria among patients with SPCs as compared with patients with urethral catheters. One advantage of SPC placement is that a voiding trial can be attempted before catheter removal; this is very helpful with postsurgical patients because patients do not have to undergo repeated catheterization if they are unable to void. Voiding trials are conducted by clamping the catheter until urine accumulates in the bladder, at which time the patient is encouraged to void. If the patient is not able to urinate, the catheter is unclamped to allow urine drainage from the bladder, and another voiding trial is attempted at a later time. SPCs also eliminate the risk of urethral trauma, necrosis, or catheter-induced urethritis.[9] Patients with hypercontractile neuropathic bladders can expel a catheter with the balloon inflated, which leads to urethral trauma; suprapubic placement prevents this complication. Suprapubic catheterization is also advantageous for wheelchair-bound patients because it provides easier access to the entry site for cleaning and catheter changes, does not interfere with sexual function, and prevents pressure-related tissue damage caused by lying on the catheter or drainage tubing.[64] Suprapubic placement may *not* be the best choice for obese patients

because the catheter may become trapped between folds of skin.[64]

The primary problems associated with SPC use are mechanical problems such as catheter dislodgement, obstruction, or failed insertion.[9] Other complications, such as UTI, bladder spasms, leakage around the catheter, and difficult removal, are not uncommon.[19,20,65] Furthermore, leakage from the urethra can occur, especially in women; this may require a surgical procedure to suture the urethra closed (Feneley procedure). In addition, although patients with SPCs have lower infection rates, they also experience a significant increase in bladder stone formation.[66,67] Finally, health care providers may lack knowledge and expertise in the management of SPCs.[9]

Placement Procedure. Initial SPC placement typically involves percutaneous placement of a standard indwelling urinary catheter into the bladder (punch cystotomy). This involves a surgical procedure and is usually performed by a urologist in an outpatient surgical center; the procedure may be performed under either local or general anesthesia. A cystoscope is used to visualize the inner bladder wall, and the bladder is distended with fluid. The bladder is then punctured percutaneously with a trocar/stylet above the suprapubic bone, and a standard balloon-tipped catheter or a Pezzer or Malecot catheter is inserted.[30] Some physicians may perform an open surgical cystotomy during a surgical procedure; however, open surgical cystotomies create larger stomas, take longer to heal, and may leak more than the percutaneous or punch cystotomy.[30] Pezzer and Malecot catheters are drainage catheters that have a mushroom or winged head instead of a balloon and are placed over a stylet that straightens out the mushroom or winged area. Once the Pezzer or Malecot catheter is inserted, the stylet is removed, and the mushroom or wings pop into position, thus securing the device in the bladder. Initially, SPCs may be sutured to the skin with several non-absorbable sutures until the stoma tract heals. The catheter should be left in place until the stoma tract is well established.[30,64] Nursing care of a patient with a new SPC is the same as with any new surgical wound. The area is cleaned with an antimicrobial solution or saline, and split gauze or other dressing is applied until the tract heals. The patient should be monitored for pain, urinary output, bleeding, signs of infection, or changes in vital signs that could indicate bowel perforation or misplacement of the catheter.

Changing a Suprapubic Catheter. Once the stoma tract has healed, a standard indwelling catheter is used to replace the SPC; this is usually about 4 weeks after placement. Removal and replacement of Pezzer and Malecot catheters involves the use of a stylet; therefore, physicians usually change these catheters, unless the nurse or caregiver has had special training. It is important to have all supplies at the bedside and to work quickly because the stoma tract can close rapidly. Before beginning the procedure, the clinician should observe the angle of the catheter as it leaves the abdomen and the length of catheter protruding from the abdominal surface. To determine proper catheter insertion depth, the clinician should gently pull the catheter to seat the balloon on the anterior bladder wall. A nontoxic marker or a piece of tape can be used to mark the old catheter at skin level; this provides guidance on depth of insertion for the new catheter. Using this depth marking as a guide helps to ensure that the new catheter enters the bladder and that the balloon is inflated in the bladder, rather than the abdominal cavity or urethra.

SPCs, unlike urethral catheters, can be difficult to remove; a gentle pull may be necessary to remove the catheter from the stoma tract. This can be especially pronounced with all-silicone catheters, because the deflated balloon does not return to its original shape and may develop a cuffed enlargement at the balloon area.[19,20] Nurses may be fearful that the catheter is "stuck" and may be hesitant to use the necessary force to remove the catheter. Lidocaine jelly or lubricating jelly inserted down the tract alongside the catheter can help ease removal.[64] It is also helpful to rotate the catheter in the stoma tract 360 degrees before removal, to ensure that the catheter is not adhered to surrounding tissue. In patients with known difficult removal, it is helpful to have the patient relax and breathe deeply during removal. In some cases a muscle relaxant may be necessary to relax the patient and the bladder before attempting to remove the catheter, or the

catheter may need to be replaced by a urologist. To minimize cuffing of the balloon, it is important to deflate the catheter balloon slowly by attaching an empty syringe and allowing the water to return without aspiration (see Box 10-4). Once the old catheter is removed, the clinician should quickly change to sterile gloves, clean the stoma with antimicrobial solution using aseptic technique, lubricate the catheter to the depth marked on the catheter (plus 1 to 2 inches), and insert the new catheter into the stoma tract. A delay of only a few minutes can result in partial closure of the tract.[64] The balloon should be inflated according to the manufacturer's directions, and the catheter should be secured to the abdomen. If urine does not immediately return, having the patient cough or bear down can help to initiate urine flow.

Care of the Patient with a Suprapubic Catheter. Care of the patient with an SPC is very similar to care of a patient with a urethral catheter, with special considerations. Maintaining a closed catheter system, strict hand washing, and keeping the drainage bag lower than the bladder are important to prevent CAUTIs. Two important aspects of management of the patient with an SPC are catheter securement and catheter removal. Unsecured catheters lead to enlargement of the stoma tract, leakage, and the need for larger-diameter catheters; it is not unusual to see a patient with a 24-Fr or larger SPC. Balloon-tipped catheters do not come larger than 30 Fr; hence patients with very large stoma tracts may have to use a Pezzer or Malecot catheter to prevent leakage around the site. (Pezzer and Malecot catheters are available in sizes 10 to 40 French.) However, use of larger catheters is problematic because they can irritate the bladder and lead to further leakage. Thus, the goal is to prevent enlargement of the stomal tract by stabilizing and supporting the catheter in position on the abdominal wall; stabilization also helps to prevent kinking of the tube and blockage of urine flow.[64] Vertical tube holders (such as Vertical Tube Attachment Device, VTAD, Hollister Inc., Libertyville, Ill.) secure catheters up to 40 Fr at a right angle that prevents kinking; these devices also protect the peritubular area with a hydrocolloid disk. Because clothing can sometimes "kink" an SPC, patients should be taught to check catheter positioning and urine flow after clothing changes.

For a new SPC, a split gauze or other dressing can be used to absorb secretions until the surgical site heals; after the tract is established a dressing is unnecessary and can lead to bacterial colonization.[68] Patients should be instructed to avoid the use of creams and ointments around the catheter, because petrolatum-based products can degrade latex catheters and may lead to yeast infection or maceration. Secretions around the stoma site can be removed during routine bathing or with plain water; there is no research to support the use of peroxide or other solutions for stomal cleaning. Skin barrier wipes can be applied after washing and drying the peristomal area, to protect the area from secretions or leakage.

Persistent weeping may occur, usually caused by patches of hypergranulation tissue; this is most effectively managed by cauterization with silver nitrate sticks to reduce or eliminate the hypertrophic tissue.[68] Another challenge with SPCs is removal. As noted earlier, "cuffing" of the catheter balloon on deflation can result in difficult removal, tissue trauma, and bleeding; this is most likely to occur with silicone catheters.[19] Nurses can minimize balloon cuffing by selecting a latex catheter (if the patient is not latex sensitive) and by avoiding aspiration when deflating the catheter balloon. Allowing the fluid to return by gravity allows a small amount of water to stay in the balloon, which minimizes wrinkling and cuffing. Development of bladder stones is another significant complication, and patients should be encouraged to have a yearly cystoscopy to check for stone formation and to provide for stone removal.

The Spinal Cord–Injured Patient

When managing incontinence in spinal cord–injured patients, the focus is on ensuring low bladder pressures (to avoid renal damage) and preventing UTIs. Management options include clean intermittent catheterization, indwelling catheters, use of external catheters (for men), pharmacologic treatment, augmentation cystoplasty, and urinary diversion. For some patients, an indwelling catheter may be the *best* choice, and SPCs may be preferable to urethral catheters for selected patients (such as wheelchair-bound patients who have difficulty managing an indwelling urethral catheter). Patients who are unable to empty their drainage bags without assistance may need an extra large capacity (4000-mL) drainage system.

Patients with loss of sensation cannot tell when they are lying on the catheter or drainage tubing; as a result, they can develop urethral or scrotal erosion or pressure sores around the meatus or legs. To prevent these ulcers, patients should be taught to position the tubing over their leg and to change the catheter's position throughout the day, just as they change their body position, to prevent pressure-related damage. Patients should be instructed to inspect all areas in contact with the catheter daily for redness, discoloration, or other signs of pressure.

Catheter encrustation or inadvertent blockage of the catheter lumen in spinal cord-injured patients can lead to a distended bladder, which can cause autonomic dysreflexia (AD) or hyperreflexia. This condition is considered a medical emergency; the patient must receive care quickly. Patients with lesions above T9 can develop dangerously high blood pressures in response to a noxious stimulus below the level of the injury.[69-71] Stimuli such as bladder distension, UTI, a full bowel, a new pressure sore, or sexual activity can cause AD. The signs and symptoms of AD include severe headache, facial flushing, sweating above the level of injury, postnasal drip, and anxiety.[69-72] Extremely high blood pressure can develop in patients whose pressure is usually normal and can lead to stroke, coma, seizure or even death.[69-72] The treatment of AD focuses on safely lowering the blood pressure and removing the initial noxious stimulus. The patient and family members should be taught the signs and symptoms of AD and should be instructed to check the catheter and tubing following clothing changes and to monitor the catheter closely for signs of blockage. Caregivers and patients should also be taught the signs and symptoms of CAUTI and should know to seek medical attention at the first sign of infection. Bowel function should also be closely monitored, because fecal impaction can be a primary causative factor for AD and can also contribute to AD by exerting pressure against the catheter tubing (which blocks urine flow and contributes to bladder distension.). Extra catheter kits should be left in the home for emergency use, and the patient and caregivers should be taught to change the catheter (if they are able to do so). If catheter encrustation is a problem, the patient or caregiver can be taught to monitor the time until blockage and to remove and replace the catheter the week before it would usually block. Scheduled acidic bladder washouts may be needed to prevent repeated encrustations that result in blockage.

Studies indicate that patients with spinal cord injuries who have long-term indwelling catheters are also at increased risk for bladder malignancy. It is thought that chronic mucosal irritation from the catheter itself and from repeated CAUTIs leads to inflammatory and proliferative pathologic cell changes.[10,11] In one study, 20% to 25% of spinal cord–injured patients with long-term catheters had evidence of premalignant lesions on bladder biopsy.[10] In addition, spinal cord-injured patients with SPCs have higher rates of bladder stone formation.[66,67] These findings underscore the importance of yearly cystoscopic examination by a urologist to check for bladder stones and changes in bladder tissues.

Patient Adaptation Issues

In addition to physical complications, long-term catheterization also affects emotional well-being and sexuality and can require significant financial resources. Research is limited regarding how patients respond and adapt to long-term indwelling catheters. A study by Wilde found that, despite the negative aspects of using the device, most patients viewed the catheter in a balanced way, minimizing the negative and emphasizing the positive.[38] This study found that, over time, patients with catheters became accepting of the catheter and stated that it made their lives easier and was a better alternative than incontinence. These patients came to accept the catheter as part of themselves, but they felt embarrassed and wanted to hide the catheter and drainage bag. Wilde also found that these patients were keenly aware of their own bodies and developed increased awareness of bladder and catheter function. Some patients learned to accommodate for sensory changes resulting from disease or injury and to recognize changes in urine flow through

the catheter.[38] Understanding the ways in which indwelling catheters affect patients' lives can assist nurses in sensitive decision making about care and can help nurses to become better patient advocates.[4,38] Nursing measures for patients with long-term catheters should include the following:

1. Teaching the patient/caregiver to manage the catheter and drainage system independently, including techniques for cleaning and disinfecting equipment, maintaining a closed system, emptying and positioning drainage systems to minimize contamination, changing catheters (if appropriate), securing the catheter, and hand washing before and after catheter-related care

2. Assisting the patient or caregiver to find appropriate products (that is, maintaining a list of local retailers or mail order suppliers and providing guidance in relation to product procurement and reimbursement)

3. Assisting the patient or caregiver to develop strategies for concealing the catheter and drainage device under clothing

4. Listening to and considering patients' insights about the catheter and their bodies

5. Introducing the subject of sex proactively and providing basic information and specific suggestions (see the next section)

6. Teaching the patient or caregiver signs and symptoms of catheter-related complications such as CAUTI and catheter blockage and developing a plan of care for patients with bladder spasms, leakage, or encrustation (see the earlier section on complications)

Sexuality

Wearing an indwelling catheter can severely interfere with a person's self-esteem and dignity, and it is natural for the catheterized patient to have anxieties about whether his or her partner finds him or her sexually attractive. There is little research related to the effects of catheter use on sexuality and intercourse, and nurses and physicians are frequently hesitant to broach the subject. It is a common misconception that the presence of an indwelling catheter prevents sexual intercourse, and the patient and partner may feel that sex is no longer a viable option unless they are given appropriate information.[49,66] There are many unanswered questions regarding strategies for remaining sexually active with an indwelling catheter and little information to guide patients though the process of resuming a fulfilling sex life. The nurse can provide basic counseling and information using the PLISSIT intervention model for sexual counseling.[49,73] This model incorporates four levels of sexual counseling; each level requires increasing knowledge and teaching/counseling skills.[74] PLISSIT is an acronym that identifies the following four levels of intervention:

P: Obtaining Permission from the patient to initiate discussion of sexual issues and giving the patient Permission to ask questions regarding sexual issues

LI: Providing Limited Information regarding sexual function with an indwelling catheter, specifically the fact that an indwelling catheter does not preclude sexual activity and sexual intercourse

SS: Giving Specific Suggestions for safely managing the catheter during sexual activity

IT: Referring the patient with complex issues regarding sexuality for Intensive Therapy[74]

The nurse who lacks advanced preparation in sexual counseling can meet the needs of patients and their partners on the first three levels. Teaching within the first three levels of the PLISSIT model can be accomplished though active listening, use of communication strategies that promote free discussion of feelings, demonstration of acceptance, permission to discuss sexual issues, provision of basic information, and assistance with problem solving.[38,39,74] Nurses can reduce the anxiety related to this issue by introducing the subject of sexuality proactively.[38] In assisting patients and their partners, the nurse needs to be knowledgeable regarding options for engaging in sexual activity with a catheter and also needs to be comfortable discussing sexual issues without embarrassment.[49] Initial assessment should include questions regarding whether the patient and partner desire to have sex, what concerns or questions they have about fulfilling their sexual needs, and specific information requested from the nurse.[49] Although some patients need referral for intensive therapy, many do not. Patients and their partners need someone to whom they can express their feelings and worries who can offer understanding and support and who can provide accurate, basic information.

There are several options for patients with indwelling catheters who desire to be sexually active. SPC placement promotes unhindered sexual freedom; patients who are frequently sexually active may prefer an SPC and should be encouraged to discuss this with their clinician. Another option is to teach the patient or caregiver to remove the catheter before sexual activity and to replace it with a new sterile catheter after intercourse. Other patients may prefer to leave the catheter in place during intercourse, but they must understand that there is an increased risk of bladder neck or urethral trauma; this is especially true for patients with paralysis or diminished sensation. If the catheter is to be left in place, it is critical that patients be instructed regarding appropriate techniques. For example, patients should be taught to avoid positions that would increase traction on the catheter and bladder neck, such as the man-on-top (so-called "missionary") position; a side-lying position is preferred because it minimizes traction on the catheter and pressure on the bladder neck. Men are usually taught to fold the catheter back alongside the penis, secure it with a condom, and apply copious amounts of water-soluble lubricant over the penis and condom to minimize friction.[38,75] (Oil-based lubricants should be avoided because they degrade latex catheters.) Women can be taught to tape the catheter to the abdomen or thigh so the catheter is out of the way.[38] The drainage bag should be emptied and positioned out of the way or removed completely and a catheter plug inserted. During intercourse, care should be taken to ensure that the catheter and drainage bag lumens are not occluded and that the catheter is not being held in traction. It may take time for the patient and partner to find what works best for them as a couple. The nurse can help in the adjustment process by giving permission to ask questions, providing information and suggestions as needed, teaching necessary skills (such as catheter removal and insertion or insertion of a catheter plug), and providing referrals to counselors or sex therapists when indicated.

Purple Urine Bag Syndrome

Purple urine bag syndrome (PUBS) or indigo urine bag syndrome is a condition in which the urine drainage bag develops purple or blue-purple discoloration. This can occur hours or days after catheterization; the longer the drainage bag is used, the deeper the color becomes.[76] Over time, the urinary catheter may also show purple discoloration. (Purple discoloration can occur with urinary stoma pouches as well.) The phenomenon is also associated with very strong urinary odor, especially in warmer temperatures.[76]

This phenomenon was first reported in 1978, and the first explanation regarding possible cause came in 1988, when Dealler and colleagues demonstrated that compounds produced by *Providencia stuartii* and *Klebsiella pneumoniae* (that is, phosphatase and sulfatase) converted urine indican into indigo and indirubin.[77] The purple in urinary drainage bags was found to be a mixture of indirubin dissolved in the plastic bag and indigo deposited on its surface.[77] More recent studies have identified a higher prevalence of PUBS in women with alkaline urine, chronic constipation leading to bacterial overgrowth in the colon, and high urine bacterial counts.[78,79] In one study, patients with PUBS had significantly higher urine bacterial counts (by 1 to 2 logs), but a causative relationship between PUBS and specific bacterial species was not found.[78] Another study demonstrated significantly lower serum levels of the amino acids valine and tryptophan in patients with PUB, possibly related to decreased colonic motility with resulting bacterial overgrowth.[79]

PUBS can be disturbing to the patient or caregiver, but there is no evidence that it is harmful; patients are frequently asymptomatic and show no obvious signs of UTI. Possible interventions include urine culture and sensitivity (with specimen obtained from a newly placed catheter), antibiotic treatment if indicated, measures to acidify the urine, and establishment of a bowel program to eliminate constipation and the resulting bacterial overgrowth.

Other conditions that can result in discoloration of urine or drainage bags include high levels of uric acid and various drug and dietary metabolites. High levels of uric acid can produce a red-pink precipitate in the drainage bag; although uric acid tends to be yellow, the presence of blood (red) and/or amorphous urates (pink) gives the precipitate its red-pink color. These patients frequently have acidic urine (less than 6 pH) and are at increased risk for uric acid stone formation; management involves treatment of the underlying metabolic disorder, maintenance of dilute urine, and possibly measures to keep the urine alkaline. Drug metabolites, amino acids, bacteria, and dyes (that is methylene blue) may also discolor drainage bags or catheters, depending on the patient's individual body chemistry. Anecdotally, patients taking certain antidepressives (that is sertraline hydrochloride) have reported a dark green discoloration of the external portion of their latex catheters.

EXTERNAL DEVICES FOR MANAGEMENT OF INTRACTABLE INCONTINENCE

In general, external devices are preferable to indwelling catheters for patients who have intractable incontinence but no retention or reflux. External devices should be carefully selected after a thorough assessment of the patient's needs and desires. The clinician should remember that the best device for a patient is the one that the patient thinks works best. Over time, patients may have to try different types of products before finding a product that fits their needs. In assisting the patient with device selection, the clinician must consider the pattern and volume of urine loss, the patient's or caregiver's sensory and cognitive status, visual acuity, mobility and dexterity, motivation, and concerns. Any selected device should effectively contain the urine, be easily concealed beneath clothing, and be easy for the patient or caregiver to use.

Devices for Men

External devices for men can be divided into two general categories: urethral compression devices and external catheters.

Male External Catheters. Male external catheters (MECs) are indicated for men with urinary incontinence who are able to empty their bladders effectively. These devices, also known as "Texas" catheters, were initially made by cutting a hole in the tip of a condom and attaching a drainage bag. Traditional condom type MECs are rolled onto the penis and secured with adhesive or nonadhesive straps. They are available in a variety of styles, both latex and latex free (silicone). Patients with spina bifida or latex allergy should always be managed with a latex-free device. One advantage of the nonlatex MECs is their transparency, which allows the patient to check placement and to assess skin status while the MEC is in place.

The most commonly used MECs are the single-use devices. The self-adhesive MEC has a thin coating of adhesive inside the sheath and is rolled onto the penis and pressed into place. Nonadhesive MECs come with a double-sided adhesive strip that is wrapped around the penis; the sheath is then rolled over the adhesive strip and pressed into place. In selecting a device with a double-sided adhesive strip, the clinician must consider whether or not the patient still has erectile function; patients who retain erectile function need an adhesive strip that can stretch and that has memory (the capacity to return to original size and shape). MECs with double-sided adhesive strips come with either adhesive-coated foam strips or with adhesive skin barrier strips. The foam strips lack elasticity and should be avoided with patients who retain erectile function. Barrier strips have the ability to stretch and have variable degrees of memory; they generally work well for patients with erectile function. Companies that make MECs with adhesive barrier strips include Coloplast (Marietta, Ga.) and C.R. Bard (Covington, Ga.).

A less commonly used form of MEC is the nonadhesive reusable type; these devices involve an external catheter secured by an external strap or foam ring or by an inflatable internal ring. This type of MEC is useful for patients who need only intermittent containment and for patients who are unable to tolerate adhesives or adhesive-barrier strips. Nonadhesive systems are best for individuals with intact cognition and intact sensation. The user must be instructed to apply the strap without tension or to avoid excessive inflation of the internal ring to prevent ischemic damage to the soft tissue of the penis.

A common problem encountered with use of MECs is adherence, especially in men with penile retraction. There is now an external device

designed specifically for these patients, the BioDerm ECD (BioDerm, Inc., Largo, FL). This device includes a thin hydrocolloid adhesive wafer attached to an outlet tube; the adhesive wafer is designed to adhere directly to the glans (Fig. 10-8). To apply the BioDerm ECD, the outlet tube opening is positioned over the urethral opening, and the "petals" of the hydrocolloid adhesive are sealed to the glans of the penis. A hydrocolloid seal is then applied over the adhesive "petals" (for additional security), and the drainage tube is attached to the outlet tube. The BioDerm tube holder (sold separately) stabilizes

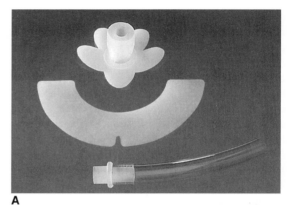

A

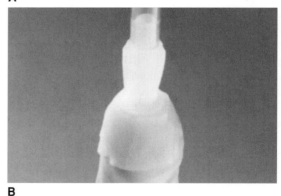

B

Fig. 10-8 BioDerm External Continence Device. **A,** Three-piece system consists of a hydrocolloid wafer and strip and drainage tube. **B,** This male external catheter adheres to the tip of penis with hydrocolloid "petals." The design directs urine into the drainage tube away from skin; the drainage tube can be removed to allow for intermittent catheterization. (Courtesy of Boderm Inc., Largo, FL)

the tubing on the inner thigh. This device has several advantages over a condom-type catheter: the design directs urine directly into the tubing, which prevents urine reflux onto the penis; one size fits most men, including men with a small or retracted penis; and the drainage tube can be disconnected, to allow for clean intermittent catheterization or urination, without removing the wafer. (This device is also a good choice for men who retain erectile function.) The wear time for new users is between 6 and 8 hours; wear times increase to 1 – 2 days after three or four applications. The ECD is changed when the adhesive wafer and wafer seal become white or opaque. The device is removed by loosening with a warm wet cloth and rolling the wafer off. This device is more expensive than standard MECs; the cost is comparable to absorbent briefs. (However, the device is very cost effective for men who are unable to maintain a seal with a standard MEC, and it provides much better clinical outcomes than absorbent briefs, that is, reduced risk of skin breakdown and UTI.)

The following guidelines should be utilized to ensure optimal results with MECs:

1. Select an MEC with a nonkinking junction between the catheter tip and the drainage tubing; this "antitwist" feature prevents obstruction to urinary flow and subsequent urinary leakage.

2. Size the catheter appropriately; measuring guides are available from most MEC manufacturers and are designed so the penile diameter can be discreetly measured at the base.

3. Ensure a dry skin surface free of hair. Moisture in the bathroom can affect the adhesive seal; if the bathroom is steamy, the patient should wait until the steam clears or move to a room where the air is not so moist. Patients should be instructed to clip hairs on the penis and any pubic hair that could become caught in the catheter as it is rolled to the base of the penis. If pubic hair is an issue, a paper towel "barrier" can be used to keep the hair out of the way while the condom is rolled into place; the patient is taught to cut a hole in the paper towel the diameter of the penis and to place the penis through the hole in the paper towel. The MEC is then rolled onto the penis, and the paper towel is torn away.

4. Consider use of a skin sealant to protect the penile skin from adhesive damage. Adhesive strips that wrap around the penis adhere well, but they may leave an adhesive film that can be difficult or painful to remove. Application of a skin sealant (skin "prep") plasticizes the skin, protects the delicate penile tissue from urine that refluxes into the condom, and prevents skin stripping when the adhesive is removed. (Many manufacturers provide a skin sealant with each MEC and adhesive strip.)

5. Ensure that the catheter is placed correctly with sufficient "clearance" of the glans. The patient should be instructed to position the rolled condom catheter over the tip of the penis with enough space so the head of the penis does not rub against the tip of the MEC.

6. When using adhesive coated sheaths, teach the patient or caregiver to unroll the MEC slowly while pressing the condom against the skin. When the MEC is completely unrolled, the patient or caregiver should grip the penis all around for 10 to 15 seconds to be sure that any wrinkles are sealed together and to eliminate air bubbles. (Excessive wrinkles in the sheath indicate that the catheter is too large.) If the condom catheter does not fully unroll (because the sheath is longer than the penile shaft), the patient or caregiver should carefully clip the remaining roll in several places (or cut the residual rim away completely) to prevent pressure sores or compression at the base of the penis.

Wear time for an external catheter varies from 24 to 72 hours depending on the product design, patient tolerance, and manufacturer's directions for use. In general, the MEC should be changed every 24 hours and the penile skin inspected for signs of skin irritation or pressure necrosis. The MEC may be changed less frequently if the device has an extended wear feature or the patient has demonstrated the ability to tolerate longer wear times without skin breakdown.[80] The patient and caregiver should be instructed in how to apply the MEC and should demonstrate correct technique for application. Men who are uncircumcised should be instructed to keep the foreskin in its normal position (down over the head of the penis) when applying the external catheter.[80] An extension tube is usually added to the MEC, and then a leg or overnight bag is attached to the extension tube; this practice allows the drainage device to be positioned on the lower leg around the calf or ankle. Whenever possible, it is helpful to give the patient several different samples to try; manufacturers are usually willing to send samples to doctors and nurses to pass on to patients. This allows the patient to experiment and to find the best product for his situation without incurring unnecessary expense.

Complications related to MECs include superficial skin damage related to maceration, monilial infections, or epidermal "stripping" from adhesives, full-thickness ischemic damage related to improper sizing or application technique, and UTI.[80] Nursing measures for patients using these devices include assisting with product selection and sizing, teaching the patient or caregiver how to apply the device, teaching skin care measures to prevent skin breakdown under the MEC, and instructing the patient or caregiver in proper cleaning and disinfection of drainage systems. In addition, the patient and caregiver should be taught to notify their health care provider of any complications, such as skin breakdown, rash, swelling of the genitals, or signs and symptoms of UTI (urinary urgency or frequency, fever, cloudy or malodorous urine, or flank pain).[80]

Penile Clamps and Cuffs. Urethral compression devices obstruct the flow of urine by mechanically compressing the soft tissue of the penis and the urethra. Active male patients may prefer the penile clamp to MECs because a drainage device is not needed and the device can be removed easily for voiding and then reapplied. Compression devices include penile clamps and inflatable compression cuffs (Fig. 10-9, *A*). The penile clamp is a plastic or metallic device lined with foam that is closed around the penis. The Cunningham Clamp (C.R. Bard, Covington, GA.) and the Geezer Klip (Gyrx LLC, Jacksonville, FL.) are two types of penile clamps. These devices have V-shaped notches or indentations that are designed to be aligned with the urethra; this ensures maximum compression force in the area of the urethra. The inflatable compression cuff (Fig. 10-9, *B*) is a soft band that is wrapped around the penis and secured with a

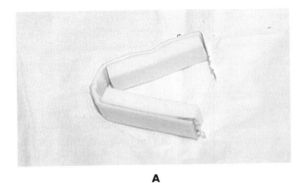

A

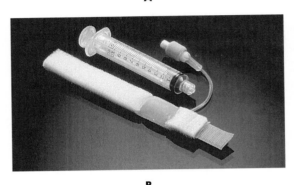

B

Fig. 10-9 Penile compression devices. **A,** Penile clamp. **B,** Penile cuff.

Velcro fastener; the band incorporates a small bladder that is positioned along the ventral aspect of the penis and then inflated with air to partially compress the urethra.

The newest compression device, known as the Freedom Valve (FreedomValve.com, Las Vegas, NV), was designed by a patient who suffered from postprostatectomy incontinence (Fig. 10-10). This U-shaped plastic device fits high on the penis near the body and has a plunger type design for urethral compression. The device opens on the side, and the base of the penis is placed into the U-shaped center, a small amount of petrolatum is placed on the plunger, and the plunger is pushed down onto the penile tissues. One advantage is that the design stops urine flow while minimizing compression of the main penile artery and vein. Another advantage is that there is no foam or similar material to wear out, and the manufacturer provides a lifetime warranty. Finally, the shape of the device supports

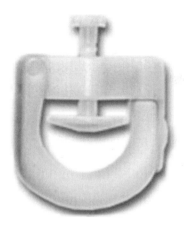

Fig. 10-10 Freedom Valve Penile Compression Device. The U-shaped design opens to fit around the base of the penis. The plunger is lubricated with petrolatum and is engaged to compress penile tissue. (Courtesy of FreedomValve.com, Las Vegas, Nev.)

concealment under clothing because it is positioned at the base of the penis. One disadvantage is that it could be dislodged in a man with a large abdomen.

Compression devices could potentially cause ischemic damage to the penis if used incorrectly; therefore, their use should be limited to individuals who have intact cognition, normal sensation, and the manual dexterity to apply the device correctly. The patient must also have the visual acuity to correctly align the notch or indentation with the urethra (as opposed to tightening the device until urine leakage stops). Ideally, a trained individual should fit the device, to ensure that the patient has the correct size, and should also assess the patient's ability to apply and remove the device as directed. The patient should be instructed to remove the device at least every 3 hours and as needed for voiding; in addition, patients are taught to remove the device immediately if they experience pain or if discoloration or excoriation of the penis is observed. Compression devices should not be used during sleep and must be removed during an erection; because nocturnal erections are normal, it is particularly important for patients with intact erectile function to avoid use of the device during sleeping hours. Some patients find that using the compression device in the daytime and absorptive

products or an MEC at night works well. Patients should be instructed in the potential complications associated with these devices and must be followed closely to assure appropriate use. These devices are most appropriate for men who have postprostatectomy stress incontinence and who meet the criteria described previously.

Female Urethral Inserts

External devices for women are limited and can be difficult to use. Despite attempts since ancient times to develop a watertight, nonirritating, and comfortable device that fits women of different body types and with different activity levels, no such device is currently available.[81] External pouches are available for short-term use (for example, for 24-hour urine collection); however, these devices are not feasible for long-term management. Many women find absorptive products easy to obtain and use, although these products can be expensive and odor can be an issue. Urethral inserts (FemSoft, Rochester Medical, Stewartville, Minn.) are tiny, tampon-like single-use devices designed to occlude the bladder neck and temporarily prevent urine leakage from stress incontinence. The narrow silicone tube is enclosed in a soft, thin, mineral oil–filled sleeve that forms a balloon at the tip. At the opposite end, the sterile tube and sleeve form an external retainer. FemSoft is inserted into the urethra with a disposable plastic applicator; as the tip of the device is advanced to the bladder, the oil flows back into the balloon, creating a seal at the neck of the bladder that prevents urine leakage. FemSoft is removed and discarded when the patient wants to urinate; a new device must then be inserted. Typically, these devices are used on an as-needed basis, such as during exercise class or other incontinence-producing activity. The patient must be cognitively intact with sufficient dexterity to insert and remove the device for urination. The patient should be instructed in signs and symptoms of complications such as UTI or urethritis.

SUMMARY

In summary, patients in retention or patients with reflux may require management with an indwelling catheter, and many patients with intractable incontinence require either an indwelling catheter or an external collecting device. All these devices are associated with significant complication rates, particularly the indwelling catheter; therefore, it is essential for the nurse managing these patients to be knowledgeable regarding their use, to assist patients or caregivers with device selection, and to educate patients and caregivers thoroughly regarding measures to prevent or minimize complications.

SELF-ASSESSMENT EXERCISE

1. Explain why indwelling catheters are considered a "last resort" for management of the patient with voiding dysfunction or urinary incontinence.

2. For each of the following patients, indicate whether or not an indwelling catheter is an appropriate option and explain your answer.
   - Elderly woman in long-term care facility with frequent episodes of incontinence related to midstage Alzheimer's disease
   - Male patient at home being cared for by his frail wife, who has difficulty changing absorptive products and who is unable to take him to the toilet
   - Paraplegic woman who is unable to position herself for self-catheterization and whose husband works from 7 AM to 5 PM
   - Patient with a pressure ulcer on the trunk and frequent episodes of urinary incontinence

3. Identify advantages and disadvantages of silicone, latex, and Silastic catheters and the implications for catheter selection.

4. Explain the following statement: The incidence of CAUTI increases with the duration of catheter use, but catheters with antimicrobial coatings are recommended primarily for patients requiring short-term catheterization in the acute care setting.

5. Outline current guidelines for catheter size and balloon size and explain the rationale.

6. Rate the following statement as True or False and explain your answer.
   Thirty-milliliter balloons are most appropriate for patients who require long-term

catheterization, especially those who experience leakage around smaller balloons.

7. Outline strategies to facilitate catheter insertion in each of the following situations:
   - Morbidly obese woman in whom the urethra cannot be visualized in the supine position
   - Male patient with an enlarged prostate
   - Female patient in whom the urethra has prolapsed into the vagina

8. Which of the following statements regarding stabilization of indwelling catheters in men is *correct*?
   a. The catheter should be secured to the lower abdomen
   b. The catheter should be stabilized to the inner thigh
   c. The catheter should be stabilized to the outer thigh
   d. The catheter should not be stabilized because this may cause undue traction on the bladder neck

9. List at least four guidelines for positioning and emptying a bedside drainage bag that should be utilized to reduce the risk of NUTIs.

10. Indicate which of the following measures *has* been found to reduce the incidence of CAUTI and should therefore be incorporated into routine care.
    - Maintain adequate fluid intake.
    - Keep urine alkaline if possible.
    - Provide thorough meatal care with an antibacterial soap and ointment twice daily and as needed.
    - Change indwelling catheters monthly; change drainage bags every 2 weeks.

11. List the three most common reasons for unplanned catheter changes.

12. Janice is a 26-year-old paraplegic woman with an indwelling catheter; she connects to a leg bag during the day (for work) and then changes to a bedside drainage bag at night. What suggestion should you make to Janice to reduce her risk for CAUTI?

13. Identify the three routes of bacterial entry into the bladder of a catheterized patient and

identify implications for prevention of infection.

14. Explain the significance of biofilms in development of CAUTI and identify measures to reduce biofilm formation.

15. Explain the following statement: Asymptomatic bacteriuria is a normal state for patients with indwelling catheters; therefore, routine cultures or antibiotics are not indicated.

16. Define the term "symptomatic bacteriuria" and outline appropriate management.

17. List at least four factors *other than* luminal occlusion that could cause leakage around the catheter ("bypassing"), and identify implications for management.

18. The most common cause of encrustation is:
    a. Concentrated urine with elevated calcium levels
    b. Infection with urease-producing bacteria
    c. Alkaline urine
    d. Prolonged catheterization (longer than 6 months)

19. Explain the term "blocker" and explain how the care plan should be modified for the patient who has been identified as a "blocker."

20. Rate the following statement as True or False: "Intermittent clamping and releasing of the catheter enhances the potential for normal bladder function after catheter removal."

21. Which of the following represents the best *initial* approach to removal of an indwelling catheter that resists balloon deflation?
    a. Inject water into the balloon port to dislodge debris; repeat attempts to aspirate the fluid using firm negative pressure.
    b. Cut off the inflation valve to allow the fluid to drain.
    c. Advance catheter into the bladder slightly; attach the syringe to the balloon port and allow the fluid to drain by gravity.
    d. Instill mineral oil into the balloon port to dissolve the balloon.

22. Identify at least one advantage and one disadvantage of SPCs as compared with urethral catheters.

23. Identify two complications associated with indwelling catheters that are unique or more common in the spinal cord–injured population.

24. Identify options for the patient with an indwelling catheter who wishes to engage in sexual intercourse.

25. Jack S. is a 66-year-old man with an indwelling catheter secondary to multiple sclerosis. He calls to report that his drainage bag is "turning purple." Which of the following represents the *best* response?
    a. Question him regarding any signs and symptoms of UTI and any problems with constipation; reassure him that this is not harmful.
    b. Notify the physician immediately.
    c. Instruct Jack to come to the clinic immediately for a metabolic panel; tell him he will probably need medication to alkalinize his urine.
    d. Tell Jack this is probably caused by some of the medications he is taking but is not likely to be harmful.

26. An MEC is *contraindicated* as a method of management for which of the following patients?
    a. 82-year-old man with functional incontinence secondary to advanced dementia
    b. 26-year-old paraplegic man with moderately severe bladder-sphincter dyssynergia
    c. 72-year-old man with severe stress incontinence following radical prostatectomy
    d. 28-year-old man with severe urge incontinence following traumatic brain injury

27. Identify one option for the male patient who is unable to wear an MEC because of penile retraction.

REFERENCES

1. Maki DG, Tambyah PA: Engineering out the risk of infection with urinary catheters, *Emerg Infect Dis* 7(2): 342-347, 2001.
2. Saint S, Lipsky BA, Goold SD: Indwelling urinary catheter: a one-point restraint? *Ann Intern Med* 137(2):125-127, 2002.

3. Jain P, Parada JP, David A, Smith LG: Overuse of the indwelling urinary tract catheter in hospitalized medical patients, *Arch Intern Med* 155(13):1425-1429, 1995.

4. Wilde M: Long-term indwelling urinary catheter care: conceptualizing the research base, *J Adv Nurs* 25(6):1252-1261, 1997.

5. Dobson C, Naidu S, Johnson M: Nurses' perceptions of urinary catheter selection and management, *Urol Nurs* 16:140-144, 1996.

6. Evans E: Indwelling catheter care: dispelling the misconceptions, *Geriatr Nurs* 20(2):85-89, 1999.

7. Smith J: Indwelling catheter management: from habit-based to evidence-based practice, *Ostomy Wound Manage* 49(12):34-45, 2003.

8. Cravens DD, Zweig S: Urinary catheter management, *Am Fam Physician* 61(2):369-376, 2000.

9. Fantl JA, Newman DK, Colling J. et al: Urinary incontinence in adults: acute and chronic management, *Clinical Practice Guidelines*, No. 2, Publication No.96-0682. Rockville, Md., 1996 Update, United States Department of Health and Human Services, Public Services Agency for Health Care Policy and Research.

10. Delnay KM, Stonehill WH, Goldman H, et al: Bladder histological changes associated with chronic indwelling urinary catheters, *J Urol* 161(4):1106-1108, 1999.

11. West DA, et al: Role of chronic catheterization in the development of bladder cancer in patients with spinal cord injury, *Urology* 53(2):292-297, 1999.

12. Wong ES, Hooten TM: Guideline for prevention of catheter-associated urinary tract infection, *Centers for Disease Control and Prevention*, 1981 [serial online]. Available at: *http://www.cdc.gov/ncidod/hip/GUIDE/uritract.htmnece*. Accessed September 8, 2003.

13. Vila L, Sanchez G, Ano M, et al: Risk factors for latex sensitization among health care workers, *J Invest Allergol Clin Immunol* 9(6):356-360, 1990.

14. Liss GM, Sussman GL: Latex sensitization: occupational versus general prevalence rates, *Am J Ind Med* 35(2):196-200, 1999.

15. Kunin CM, Chin QF, Chambers S: Formation of encrustations on indwelling urinary catheters in the elderly: a comparison of different types of catheter materials in "blocker" and "nonblocker," *J Urol* 138(4):899-902, 1987.

16. Stickler DJ: Bacterial biofilms and encrustations of urethral catheters, *Biofouling* 9(4):293-305, 1996.

17. Tullock AGS, Ferguson AF: Catheter-induced urethritis: a comparison between latex and silicone catheters in a prospective clinical trial, *Br J Urol* 57(3):325-328, 1985.

18. Studder UE, Bishop ML, Zingg EJ: How to fill silicone catheter balloons, *Urology* 22(3):300-302, 1983.

19. Parkin J, Scanlan J, Woolley M, et al. Urinary catheter "deflation cuff" formation: clinical audit and quantitative in vitro analysis, *Br J Urology* 90(7):666-671, 2002.

20. Robinson J: Deflation of a Foley catheter balloon, *Nurs Stand* 17(27):33-38, 2003.

21. Riley DK, Classen DC, Stevens LE, Burke JP: A large randomized clinical trial of a silver-impregnated urinary catheter: lack of efficacy and staphylococcal superinfection, *Am J Med* 98(4):349-356, 1995.

22. Karchmer TB, Giannetta ET, Muto CA, Strain BA, Farr BM, et al: A randomized crossover study of silver-coated urinary catheters in hospitalized patients, *Arch Intern Med* 160:3294-3297, 2000.

23. Saint S, Veenstra DL, Sullivan SD, et al: The potential clinical and economic benefits of silver alloy urinary catheters in preventing urinary tract infection, *Arch Intern Med* 160(17):2670-2675, 2000.

24. Salgado CD, Karchmer TB, Farr BM: Prevention of catheter-associated urinary tract infections. In: Wenzel RP, editor: *Prevention and control of nosocomial infections*, ed 4, Philadelphia, 2003, Lippincott Williams & Wilkins, pp 297-311.

25. Johnson JR et al: Activities of a nitrofurazone-containing urinary catheter and a silver hydrogel catheter against multidrug-resistant bacteria characteristic of catheter-associated urinary tract infection, *Antimicrob Agents Chemother* 43(12):2990-2995, 1999.

26. Maki DG, Knasinski V, Halvorson KT, et al: A prospective, randomized, investigator-blinded trial of a novel nitrofurazone-impregnated urinary catheter, *Infect Control Hosp Epidemiol* 18(suppl):50, 1997.

27. Robinson J: Urethral catheter selection, *Nurs Stand* 15(25):39-42, 2001.

28. Jeter KJ, Faller N, Norton C: *Nursing for continence*, Philadelphia, 1990, WB Saunders.

29. Newman D, Blackwood N: Application and perspectives on the use of indwelling catheters. Lecture presented at the National Multispecialty Conference on Urinary Incontinence, Kissimmee, Fla., 1999.

30. Carter HB: Instrumentation and endoscopy. In: Walsh PC, Retik AB, Vaughan ED Jr, editors: *Campbell's urology*, ed 8. Philadelphia, 2002, WB Saunders.

31. Brechtelsbauer D: Care with an indwelling urinary catheter, *Postgrad Med* 92(1):127-132, 1992.

32. Fiers S: Indwelling catheters and devices: avoiding the problems, *Urol Nurs* 14:141-144, 1994.

33. Resnick N: Geriatric incontinence, *Urol Clin North Am* 23(1):55-77, 1996.

34. Cancio LC, Sabanegh ES JR, Thompson IM: Managing the Foley catheter, *Am Fam Physician* 48(5):829-836, 1993.

35. Chinnes L, Dillion A, Fauerbach L: *HomeCareHandbook ofInfection Control.*, 2002, Association of Professionals in Infection Control and Epidemiology (APIC), Washington, DC.

36. Gerard L, Sueppel C: Lubrication technique for male catheterization, *Urol Nurs* 17(4):156-158, 1997.

37. Hanchett M: Techniques for stabilizing urinary catheters, *Am J Nurs* 102(3):44-48, 2002.

38. Wilde M. with commentary by Cameron B: Meanings and practical knowledge of people with long-term urinary catheters, *J Wound Ostomy Continence Nurs* 30(1):33-43, 2003.

39. Morris NS, Stickler DJ. Does drinking cranberry juice produce urine inhibitory to the development of crystalline, catheter-blocking *Proteus mirabilis* biofilms? *BJU Int* 88(3):192-197, 2001.

40. Getliffe KA: Managing recurrent urinary catheter blockage: problems, promises and practicalities, *Wound Ostomy Continence* 30(3):146-151, 2003.

41. Newman DK: Managing indwelling urethral catheters, *Ostomy Wound Manage* 44(12):26-35, 1998.

42. Dille C, Kirchhoff K: Increasing the wearing time of vinyl urinary drainage bags with bleach, *Rehabil Nurs* 18(5):292-295, 1993.

43. Hewitt J, Wells J: *Reusable catheters and accessories care and cleansing,* a publication of the National Association for Continence, 1999. Web site *http://www.nafc.org*

44. Rutala WA, Barbee SL, Aquiar NC, et al: Antimicrobial activity of home disinfectants and natural products against potential human pathogens, *Infect Control Hosp Epidemiol* 21(1):33-38, 2000.

45. Stamm WE: Catheter-associated urinary tract infections: epidemiology, pathogenesis, and prevention, *Am J Med* 91(3B):65S-71S, 1991.

46. Rubin L, Berger SA, Zodda FN Jr, Gruenwald R: Effect of catheter replacement on bacterial counts in urine aspirated from indwelling catheters, *J Infect Dis* 142(2):291, 1980.

47. Daifuku R., Stamm WE: Association of rectal urethral colonization with urinary tract infection in patients with indwelling catheters, *JAMA* 252(15):2028-2030, 1984.

48. Donlan RM: Biofilms and device-associated infections, *Emerg Infect Dis* 7(2):277-281, 2002.

49. Wilson RE: The nurse's role in sexual counseling, *Ostomy Wound Manage* 41(1):72-78, 1995.

50. Tambyah PA, Maki DG: Catheter-associated urinary tract infection is rarely symptomatic: a prospective study of 1,497 catheterized patients, *Arch Intern Med* 160(5):678-682, 2000.

51. Warren JW: Catheter-associated urinary tract infections, *Int J Antimicrob Agents* 17(4):299-303, 2001.

52. Gammack JK: Use and management of chronic urinary catheters in long-term care: much controversy, little consensus, *J Am Med Dir Assoc* 3(3):162-168, 2002.

53. McGeer A, Campbell B, Emori TG, et al: Definitions of infection for surveillance in long-term care facilities, *Am J Infect Control* 19(1):1-7, 1991.

54. Switters DM: Assessing leakage from around the urethral catheter, *Urol Nurs* 9(3):8-10, 1989.

55. Bhatia NN, Bergman A: Cystometry: unstable bladder and urinary tract infection (abstract), *Br J Urol* 58(2):134-137, 1986.

56. Ziemann LK, Lastauskas NM, Ambrosini G: Incidence of leakage from indwelling urinary catheters in homebound patient, *Home Healthcare Nurse* 2(5):22-26, 1984.

57. Stickler DJ, Hewitt P: Activity of antiseptics against biofilms of mixed bacterial species growing on silicone surfaces, *Eur J Clin Microbiol Infect Dis* 10:416-421, 1991.

58. Jepson R, Mihaljevic L, Craig J: Cranberries for preventing urinary tract infections, *Cochrane Database Syst Rev* 2 CD001321, 2004.

59. Birch S, Dewbury K: Technical report: a simple non-invasive method for deflating blocked Foley balloon, *Clin Radiol* 5(2):136, 1996.

60. Daneshmand S, Youssefzadeh D, Skinner EL: Review of techniques to remove a Foley catheter when the balloon does not deflate, *Urology* 59(1):127-129, 2002.

61. Khan SA, Landes F, Paola AS, Ferraratto L: Emergency management of the nondeflating Foley catheter balloon, *Am J Emerg Med* 9(3):260-263, 1991.

62. Reigle M, Sandcock DS, Resnick MI: When a Foley won't deflate, *Contemp Urol* 1996 (April).

63. Shapiro AJ, Soderdahl D, Stack R, North JH Jr.: Managing the nondeflating urethral catheter, *J Am Board Fam Pract* 13:116-119, 2000.

64. Getliffe KA: Suprapubic catheterization, *Prim Health Care* 12(6): 25-26, 2002.

65. Addison R, Mould C: Risk assessment in suprapubic catheterization, *Nurs Stand* 14(36):43-46, 2002.

66. Mitsui T, Minami K, Furuno T, et al: Is suprapubic cystostomy an optimal urinary management in high quadriplegics? A comparative study of suprapubic cystostomy and clean intermittent catheterization, *Eur Urol* 38(4):434-438, 2000.

67. Nomura S, Ishido T, Teranishi J, Makiyama K: Long-term analysis of supra-pubic cystostomy drainage in patients with neurogenic bladders, *Urol Int* 65(4):185-189, 2000.

68. Evans A, Feneley R: A study of current nursing management of long-term supra-pubic catheters, *Br J Commun Nurs* 5(5):240-245, 2000.

69. Blackmer J: Rehabilitation medicine: 1. Autonomic dysreflexia, *Can Med Assoc J* 169(9):931-935, 2003.

70. Consortium for Spinal Cord Medicine: *Acute management of autonomic dysreflexia: individuals with spinal cord injury presenting to healthcare facilities (clinical practice guideline),* ed 2, Washington, D.C., 2001, The Consortium, Paralyzed Veterans of America.

71. Helkowski WM, Ditunno JF Jr, Boninger M: Autonomic dysreflexia: incidence in persons with neurologically complete and incomplete tetraplegia, *J Spinal Cord Med* 26(3):244-247, 2003.

72. Bennett C: Urgent urological management of the paraplegic/quadriplegic patient, *Urol Nurs* 23(6):436-437, 2003.

73. McInnes RA, Chronic illness and sexuality, *Med J Aust* 179(3):263-266, 2003.

74. Annon JS: The PLISSIT model: a proposed conceptual scheme for the behavioral treatment of sexual problems, *J Sex Ther* 2:1-15, 1976.

75. Sackett C: Genitourinry conditions and sexuality. In: Fogel CI, Lauver D, editors: *Sexual health promotion,* Philadelphia, 1989, WB Saunders, pp 407-435.

76. Robinson J: Purple urine bag syndrome: a harmless but alarming problem, *Br J Commun Nurs* 8(6):263-266, 2003.

77. Dealler SF, Hawkey P, Millar R: Enzymatic degradation of urinary indoxyl sulfate by *Providencia stuartii* and *Klebsiella pneumoniae* causes the purple urine bag syndrome, *J Clin Microbiol* 26(10):2152-2156, 1988.

78. Mantani N, Ochiai H, Imanishi N, et al: A case-control study of purple urine bag syndrome in geriatric wards (abstract), *J Infect Chemother* 9(1):53-57, 2003.
79. Nakayama T, Kanmatsuse K, Serum levels of amino acid in patients with purple urine bag syndrome (abstract), *Nippon Jinzo Gakkai Shi* 39(5);470-473, 1997.
80 Wound, Ostomy, and Continence Nurses Society: *External catheters: clinical fact sheet,* Glenview, Ill. Accessed online at *www.wocn* April 2004.
81. Pieper B, Cleland V, Johnson D, O'Reilly JL: Inventing urine continence devices for women, *Image J Nurs* 21(4):205-209, 1989.

ADDITIONAL REFERENCES

Ahern DG, Grace DT, Jennings MJ, Borazjani RN, Boles KJ, Rose LJ, Simmons RB, Ahanotu EN: Effects of hydrogel/silver coatings on in vitro adhesion to catheters of bacteria associated with urinary tract infection, *Curr Microbiol* 41:120-125, 2000.
Burke JP, Jacobson JA, Garibaldi RA, Conti MT, Alling DW: Evaluation of daily meatal care with poly-antibiotic ointment in prevention of urinary catheter-associated bacteriuria, *J Urol* 129:331-334, 1983.
Classen DC, Larsen RA, Burke JP, Alling DW, Stevens LE: Daily meatal care for prevention of catheter-associated bacteriuria: results using frequent applications of polyantibiotic cream, *Infect Control Hosp Epidemiol* 12:157-162, 1991.
Food and Drug Administration, Department of Health and Human Services: Natural rubber-containing medical devices: user labeling, *Fed Reg* 62(189):51021-51030, 1997.
Kohler-Ockmore J, Feneley RC: Long-term catheterization of the bladder: prevalence and morbidity, *Br J Urol* 77:347-351, 1996.
Kunin CM, Chin QF, et al: The association between the use of urinary catheters and morbidity and mortality among elderly patients in nursing homes, *Am J Epidemiol* 135:291-301, 1992.
Tambyah PA, Maki DG: The relationship between pyuria and infection in patients with indwelling urinary catheters: a prospective study of 761 patients, *Arch Intern Med* 160:673-677, 2000.
Thees K., Dreblow L: Trial of voiding: what's the verdict? *Urol Nurs* 19:20-22, 1999.
Weber EM, McDowell BJ. et al: Protocol for indwelling bladder catheter removal in the homebound older adult, *Home Healthcare Nurse* 16(9):603-609, 1998.

CHAPTER 11

Management of Urinary Incontinence: Skin Care, Containment Devices, Catheters, Absorptive Products

DEBORAH LEKAN-RUTLEDGE

OBJECTIVES

1. Describe normal skin integrity and identify risk factors for perineal skin breakdown in the incontinent patient.
2. Describe the role of skin care products, absorbent products, and urine containment devices in the management of intractable incontinence.
3. Explain the significance of transepidermal water loss in assessment of the skin's barrier function.
4. Describe the significance, signs, symptoms, and management for each of the following:
   - Irritant dermatitis
   - Perineal yeast infection
   - Estrogen deficiency
5. Describe guidelines for appropriate selection and use of skin care products designed for cleansing and protection of the perineal skin.
6. Describe the role of the following skin care products in the management of incontinence: perineal cleansers, moisturizers, moisture barriers, powders, liquid barrier films.
7. Describe male and female portable urine containment devices (urinals).
8. Identify guidelines for effective use of external male catheters.
9. Describe indications for long-term use of indwelling catheters.
10. Identify common indwelling urinary catheter-related complications and their management: urinary tract infection, bladder spasms and leakage, and catheter encrustation and obstruction.
11. Identify attributes of the urinary catheter that may reduce the risk of catheter-related complications.
12. Describe the attributes of disposable and reusable absorbent products.
13. Identify features and indications for use for each of the following types of absorbent products: shields or guards, pant and pad systems, adult briefs, and underpads.

The treatment of urinary incontinence (UI) has advanced markedly over the past decade. Although continence care for many years focused almost exclusively on containment and skin care, recent advances have changed this focus; behavioral, pharmacologic, and surgical therapies now offer people with UI a myriad of treatment options for the restoration of continence, and this has become the focus of care for the majority of individuals with UI. Factors previously considered to be relative contraindications to a restorative approach are now being reevaluated. For example, the magnitude of UI should no longer be considered a deterrent to treatment because marked improvement can be achieved even in those with severe UI. Similarly, frail elderly patients can frequently benefit from interventions designed to promote social continence and prevent excess disability,[1] although frailty and physical and cognitive disabilities present challenges that require more directed and thoughtful intervention from clinicians and caregivers. The ultimate goals for any

UI management plan are to improve the quality of life for the patient and caregiver and to prevent or minimize incontinence-related complications.[2] Key elements of restorative care are discussed in depth in other chapters in this text: identification and management of reversible factors, modification of contributing factors, and treatment designed to correct or compensate for the specific pathologic factors causing the incontinence. Establishment of an appropriate plan requires a comprehensive and accurate assessment; the data obtained are used to identify the causative and contributing factors that must be addressed in the treatment plan and also to inform the treatment plan in terms of patient and caregiver goals and priorities. Synchronous administration of treatment approaches such as toileting regimens and management approaches such as absorbent products and bedside equipment holds promise for markedly improving the health and well-being of incontinent individuals; because UI is frequently multifactorial in origin, and because the causative factors include both physiologic[3] and behavioral factors, it is all the more important that any management program be multimodal.

Although the primary focus for incontinence management has fortunately shifted from containment to correction, containment devices and skin care still play a role in effective management of many individuals with UI. For example, management of urine loss with absorbent products, containment devices, and skin care is often needed as adjunctive therapy during the initial phases of treatment and until treatment effects occur. In the following situations, absorptive products, containment devices, and skin care are the primary focus of management: individuals in whom UI is intractable; that is, in whom the causative factors cannot be corrected; situations in which treatment is unlikely to be recommended or of benefit; or situations in which the individual is unable or unwilling to pursue treatment because of cognitive, psychological, or social barriers. However, it is important to discourage the indiscriminate use of these options as a substitute for proper assessment, diagnosis and consideration of appropriate treatment options. This chapter provides guidelines for the appropriate utilization of containment devices, absorptive products, and skin care products in the management of UI. Judicious use of these technologies can foster dignity, quality of life, and social continence in individuals with UI.

SKIN CARE
General Concepts

Prevention and treatment of perineal skin breakdown are important considerations in the management of patients with frequent or chronic exposure to urine or stool. Irritants, friction, and occlusion all contribute to the development of various skin disorders, including candidiasis, dermatitis, and skin breakdown in the perineal region. Factors identified as increasing the risk for perineal skin breakdown among incontinent individuals include the following: number of incontinent episodes, fecal incontinence, poor skin condition, pain, poor oxygenation, fever, and mobility problems.[4] Age may also be a risk factor, because there is evidence that the barrier function of the skin is diminished in the elderly.[5] This is partly the result of thinning of the epidermis in older individuals; with aging, the capacity for epidermal proliferation is decreased, so more time is needed for epidermal cells to migrate to the skin surface. This prolonged epidermal cell turnover time results in thinning of the top layer of corneocytes and increased potential for fluid loss. Another factor that increases the potential for skin damage in the elderly is reduced production of skin oils (sebum); normally, these oils fill the gaps between the epidermal cells, thus contributing to maintenance of an intact epidermal barrier. The loss of these skin oils creates gaps in the epidermal barrier that allow irritants and pathogens to penetrate the skin surface; in addition, the decreased sebum production permits increased evaporative loss of fluid from the skin, which is seen clinically as drying of the skin surface. Dry skin, or xerosis, affects as many as 59% to 85% of people over the age of 64 years and contributes to itching and scratching, which further increase vulnerability to dermal complications.

Incontinence obviously poses a significant threat to the elderly, particularly incontinence that is high volume and high frequency. In one study, the incidence and prevalence of nine common perineal skin disorders were measured prospectively over a 60-day period;[6] this study found that frail elders in long-term care experienced a high incidence of skin disorders. All subjects were noted to have at least one skin disorder during the observation period. The most commonly observed skin condition was blanchable erythema, which occurred in 94% of the subjects, predominantly in the areas of skin adjacent to the urethra and anus. Forty-six percent of residents developed macular rashes, and 19.4% developed papular rashes. Twenty-one percent developed either nonblanchable erythema or partial-thickness skin loss, stage 1 ulcers, and stage 2 ulcers, respectively. The incidence of other skin disorders in this study population included scaling (14.3%), maceration (10.7%), and pressure ulcers (15.5%).[6]

The relationship between incontinence and pressure ulcers remains unclear. "True" pressure ulcers are usually full-thickness lesions caused by prolonged compression of the tissues over bony prominences; the early clinical indicators for these ulcers typically include blanchable or nonblanchable erythema. (In this study, Schnelle and colleagues found that immobility and blanchable erythema were jointly predictive of nonblanchable erythema and increased risk for pressure ulcer development.[6]) In contrast, incontinence is more likely to damage the epidermal and dermal layers, resulting in partial-thickness skin lesions. Incontinence is a common finding among individuals with pressure ulcers, possibly because both pressure ulcers and incontinence are more common among individuals who are inactive and immobile. However, incontinence may also render the skin and underlying tissues more susceptible to injury from pressure.

Further research is needed to determine the prevalence of dermatologic disorders in noninstitutionalized adult and frail elderly populations with incontinence. There is very little information regarding perineal dermatitis in these populations.

Characteristics of the Skin Barrier

To understand the effect of incontinence on the skin and to evaluate and utilize the many hygienic and protective skin products on the market appropriately, it is necessary to understand the structure and characteristics of the skin. The outermost layer of the epidermis is the stratum corneum; this layer provides a critical barrier to invasion by microorganisms and other foreign substances and also serves to retain moisture, thus maintaining the skin's hydration. The stratum corneum is 70% protein, 15% lipids, and 15% water, with a structure that has been described as "brick and mortar."[7] The protein component is the corneocyte; these cells are held in a dense matrix with a variety of lipids (that is, ceramides, free fatty acids, and cholesterol). The lipids are critical to the barrier function of the stratum corneum; they are formed by structures known as "lamellar bodies," which are located in the underlying layers of the epidermis. Water content is another important factor in the skin's ability to function as a barrier. The amount of water is affected by age, various pathologic conditions, environmental humidity, and the use of moisturizers. Cells shrink and change shape when the water content is reduced to less than 10%; this renders the stratum corneum subject to invasion. Overhydration is also damaging; when the water content of the skin exceeds 30% to 40%, the skin's permeability increases, and its ability to function as a barrier is reduced.

The integrity of the skin barrier is promoted by the continual replacement of the stratum corneum; old cells are sloughed (a process known as "desquamation") and replaced by new cells. The rate of epidermal reproduction is increased by skin damage; any disruption of the stratum corneum stimulates a rapid increase in the rate of cell regeneration, lipid synthesis, and skin repair. However, the process of desquamation and replacement may actually create defects in the barrier, which then create the potential for skin damage. Contact with allergens or irritating substances during this process may result in enhanced absorption.

The integrity of the skin barrier is commonly measured by transepidermal water loss (TEWL), which reflects the rate at which water evaporates from the stratum corneum. TEWL is affected by many factors, including skin condition, disease states, age, and environmental humidity. Because TEWL is considered a critical indicator of the barrier's integrity, it is frequently used as a parameter when the health of the skin is studied. When the TEWL increases (that is, when the barrier is impaired), lipid synthesis is stimulated to restore or maintain barrier integrity.[8]

Factors Affecting Barrier Integrity

The healthy stratum corneum has a low pH (4.3 to 5.9)[9] and possesses significant protective buffering capacity; the low pH is frequently referred to as the "acid mantle" of the skin and is thought to be hostile to overgrowth of pathogens. Higher pH levels are correlated with increased TEWL, indicating reduced barrier function. Berg reported high pH as an important factor in the development of diaper dermatitis, but a complete understanding of the effect of skin pH remains elusive.[10]

Microorganisms may also affect the skin's barrier function. Normal skin flora include *Staphylococcus aureus*, frequently found in the perineum, diphtheroids including *Corynebacterium,* and some gram-negative bacilli. *Candida* is not commonly found on the skin of the perineum; however, it is a resident of the gastrointestinal tract and as a result is often deposited on the skin when the individual is incontinent of liquid stools. Factors that affect the skin flora include humidity levels, skin lipid levels, skin condition and the rate of desquamation, and microbial characteristics such as antagonism and adherence.

An increase in skin temperature or hydration also produces increased permeability and reduced barrier function, which may permit the penetration of microorganisms and irritants through the stratum corneum.[11]

Mechanisms of Damage

The stratum corneum can be damaged or altered in numerous ways. As noted earlier, water alone can serve as an irritant. When the water content of the skin exceeds a range of 30% to 40%, there is an increase in TEWL, signifying increased permeability and a reduction in barrier function.[7,12,13] Prolonged contact with water triggers an inflammatory response in the skin, evidenced by erythema. The presence of inflammation, in turn, increases the potential for diffusion of other irritants through the stratum corneum. Overhydration also reduces the skin's resistance to friction. The drag of wet skin against linens or garments during position changes may produce sufficient friction to injure the epidermis. Friction injuries may also result from the rubbing together of two moist skin surfaces. In addition, the plastic and cloth underpads commonly used to manage incontinence trap heat and perspiration, thus creating an environment even more conducive to skin damage. It has long been believed that urine damages skin because of its ammonia content; however, it is now generally accepted that urine causes skin damage primarily through the application of moisture.[14]

Fecal enzymes have been shown to cause epidermal damage in adults as well as children.[15] These enzymes are rendered more active and, as a result, more irritating with an increase in pH.[15,16] Consequently, it is generally accepted that a mixture of urine and feces produces an irritant with greater potential to cause skin damage. Thus, any patient who is incontinent of urine may be additionally vulnerable during diarrheal episodes, when liquid stool with residual enzymes is discharged onto the skin at frequent intervals. It is clear then that patients with chronic diarrhea are at risk for skin damage; this includes patients receiving high-dose or long-term antibiotic therapy, patients with enteropathy related to acquired immunodeficiency syndrome, and patients with short-gut syndrome. In addition to the risk of exposure to liquid stool, these patients often have mobility problems that interfere with independent toileting.

Containment garments, used to maintain hygiene and dignity, unfortunately increase the risk of skin damage by creating an occlusive environment that traps heat and moisture. Conversely, containment garments may help to separate urine (the source of "moisture-related" damage) and to sequester it into the absorbent material, thus preventing the mixing of stool and urine.

Another mechanism of incontinence-related skin damage is microbial invasion. Microbial adherence is enhanced in the presence of dermatitis, and many organisms flourish in an occlusive environment, especially if heat and moisture are also present. For example, *Candida albicans* rarely affects intact skin in an otherwise healthy individual.[17] However, as an opportunistic pathogen, it thrives on skin that has been rendered more permeable by moisture or damaged by irritants.

Pathophysiology of Perineal Dermatitis. Incontinence causes perineal dermatitis through two simultaneous mechanisms: exposure of the skin to irritants and pathogens and damage to the epidermis/compromise of the epidermal barrier resulting from inappropriate use of absorptive products and repetitive traumatic cleansing. Exposure to irritants and pathogens is unlikely to cause damage so long as the epidermal barrier remains intact; when the barrier is damaged, these substances are allowed to penetrate the skin, thereby triggering the pathologic processes that ultimately result in perineal skin infections and skin damage.

Prolonged exposure of the perineal skin to urine or stool (or to diaphoresis) results in overgrowth of bacteria; this is further enhanced by an occlusive environment.[18] In addition, pooled urine causes a shift in the pH of the skin to an alkaline level (approximately 7.1), which may further contribute to overgrowth of bacterial and fungal organisms.[18] Patients receiving prolonged antibiotic therapy may develop alterations in intestinal flora that result in overgrowth of opportunistic pathogens such as *Clostridium difficile;* this organism produces a particularly virulent toxin that results in profuse watery stools of a highly corrosive nature that tremendously increase the risk for skin breakdown via enzymatic damage.

Clinicians using absorptive products for management of incontinence must be aware that these products can increase the risk for perineal dermatitis by significantly compromising the epidermal barrier. Two factors known to affect the barrier function of the skin adversely are overhydration and elevated skin temperature; both these conditions are created when occlusive absorptive products are closed around the patient, resulting in trapping of heat and moisture.[18] Absorptive products should therefore be left open when possible (such as, at night) to avoid creation of an occlusive environment; nonocclusive (breathable) absorptive products should be used for individuals in whom this is not feasible.[18,19] Another factor contributing to perineal dermatitis in the incontinent individual is repetitive cleansing; the friction associated with cleansing "strips" layers of skin cells, thus accelerating the rate of epidermal cell removal, and the agents used for cleansing remove the skin lipids that act as "mortar" between the skin cells. The combined loss of epidermal cells and epidermal lipids can create significant defects in the barrier that permit penetration of the skin by irritants and pathogens. (As noted earlier, elderly persons are at particular risk because aging is associated with thinning of the epidermis and reduced production of skin lipids.) Finally, the "acid mantle" of the skin can be disrupted by exposure to alkaline urine and stool and by repetitive cleansing, which removes the acidic lipids; loss of the normal acidity at the skin surface creates an environment favorable to pathogens. The multiple pathogens and irritants associated with pooled urine or stool can then easily invade the damaged epidermis, triggering inflammatory changes. As noted, fecal incontinence is particularly damaging, because stool contains multiple pathogens and intestinal enzymes that can be activated in the alkaline environment associated with combined urinary and fecal incontinence.[18,20-23]

Compromised mobility can increase an individual's risk for perineal dermatitis by interfering with his or her ability to toilet independently or regularly enough to keep the skin clean and dry, or the ability to cleanse the perineal skin effectively after toileting. Cognitive impairment may create a similar risk, in that patients with cognitive deficits may be unaware of the need to use the toilet or to carry out perineal hygiene. Inadequate toileting and hygiene are significant risk factors for skin breakdown in the incontinent patient. Fig. 11-1 provides a schematic overview of the mechanisms by which incontinence causes skin damage.

In caring for individuals with incontinence, the clinician should be alert to comorbidities that adversely affect the ability to heal should breakdown occur. These include conditions that compromise oxygenation, perfusion, or nutrition, such as edema, hypoxia, and malnutrition.

Specific Types of Incontinence-Related Skin Damage

Types of skin damage commonly seen in the incontinent population are irritant dermatitis, yeast dermatitis, and partial-thickness skin loss caused by the combination of maceration (overhydration) and friction (Table 11-1). These are discussed in detail.

Incontinence Dermatitis

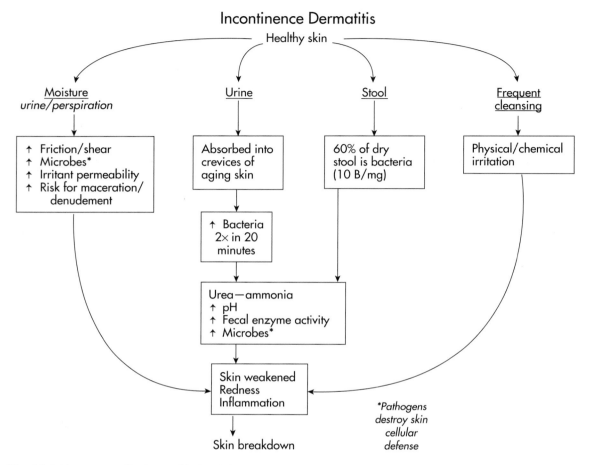

Fig. 11-1 Factors contributing to skin breakdown in incontinent patient. B/mg, billion per milligram. (Reprinted with permission from Sheila Howes-Trammel, FNP-C, MSN, CWOCN.)

Atypical lesions (such as erythrasma and herpes simplex) are addressed briefly.

Irritant Contact Dermatitis. Exposure of the skin to urine or feces may induce changes that are reflective of an irritant contact dermatitis. Irritant dermatitis refers to an inflammatory process caused by direct damage to the water-protein-lipid matrix of the skin (such as exposure to cold dry air or prolonged contact with moisture). In contrast, allergic contact dermatitis results from a hypersensitivity reaction to an antigen (such as poison ivy or a specific ingredient in a skin care product). Early signs of irritant dermatitis include erythema and edema;

as additional damage is sustained, vesicles may develop. Failure to remove the irritant will result in progressive inflammation evidenced by blistering, erosion (patchy loss of the epidermis), and weeping. Eventually, the area will exhibit signs of a chemical "burn," with intense erythema, epidermal destruction, pronounced edema, and pain (see Plate 3). The area of involvement usually corresponds to the area of exposure, although body folds may be spared, especially in younger individuals with good skin turgor. Mild inflammation produces itching and burning, whereas severe inflammation and epidermal loss results in exposure of the dermis and of

TABLE II-I   **Types of Perineal Skin Damage and Treatment**

TYPE OF DAMAGE	ETIOLOGY	TREATMENT
Irritant dermatitis	The cause is primary damage to the epidermal cells, such as occurs with prolonged exposure to urine. The injury to the skin cells triggers an inflammatory response, which is manifest initially by erythema and mild edema; if the process is not interrupted, the inflammation becomes more severe, and the patient develops blistering, erosion of the epidermis, and weeping.	Irritant dermatitis from urine or feces is best managed with a moisture barrier paste. These products combine a moisture barrier ointment such as zinc oxide with an absorptive powder to adhere to moist skin, absorb moisture, and provide a waterproof barrier against external moisture and contaminants. Because these products are designed to resist washing and removal, caregivers must be taught to use perineal cleansers and gentle technique for removal.
Yeast dermatitis	This develops when *Candida albicans* organisms adhere to and penetrate the compromised epidermis. Characteristic skin changes include a maculopapular rash that is confluent in the center with distinct "satellite" lesions at the periphery. The involved area is usually reddened, pruritic, and tender.	Yeast dermatitis requires treatment with an antifungal agent such as miconazole or nystatin; many nonprescription moisture barrier products now offer an antifungal formulation that is appropriate for patients with yeast dermatitis. Alternatively, an antifungal powder or cream can be applied to the affected area and then covered with a moisture barrier product.
Friction damage	This occurs when macerated skin is exposed to external "rubbing" forces, as may occur with cleansing or with patient movement against absorptive garments or the bed linens. The superficial skin loss is characterized by shallow, painful lesions that are moist and red. Friction damage involves the skin surfaces in contact with the bed or chair, that is, the buttock area including the ischial tuberosities and sacrum. Skin-to-skin friction can occur between the thighs and in the creases of the upper thigh and perineum in obese individuals.	Friction damage and abrasion are best managed by minimizing frictional forces and by covering the affected area with a protective absorptive dressing, such as a hydrocolloid wafer or a moisture barrier paste.

From Lekan-Rutledge D, Doughty D, Moore K, Wooldridge L: Promoting social continence: products and devices in the management of urinary incontinence, *Urol Nurs* (23)6:416–428, 458, 2004.

nerve endings. Pain management is therefore an essential element to be addressed in product selection and treatment of the patient with extensive epidermal damage.

Perineal Candidiasis ("Yeast Dermatitis"). Perineal yeast infections are common among individuals with incontinence; they are often misdiagnosed as irritant dermatitis and are therefore left untreated. As noted, *C. albicans* is an opportunistic organism that readily invades damaged skin. It produces an enzyme (akeratinase) that stimulates an intense inflammatory response, which further damages the stratum corneum. The organism thrives in a warm and moist environment, and this feature contributes to the prevalence of this condition among individuals with incontinence and among obese individuals with skin folds. It is also more common among individuals with diabetes or other conditions resulting in compromised immune function. A *Candida* infection produces a characteristic rash; that is, an area of confluent erythema that is more intense in the center and may lack a distinct (or "advancing") border. Typically, pinpoint satellite lesions are visible at the periphery; these lesions usually develop as tiny vesicles, but they frequently present clinically as macules because they have been "unroofed" by friction from garments or bed linens (see Plate 4). Moist or dry scaling may also be observed. The infection commonly involves the perineum but may extend into the groin and thigh folds. Hyperpigmentation of the area (that is, a dark, ruddy red or purple hue) is common in long-term infections that are left untreated and may be mistaken by an inexperienced clinician for a pressure ulcer, especially when observed over the coccyx or sacrum. "Yeast" rashes are typically diagnosed and treated empirically (that is, based on clinical observation); however, a skin scraping may be stained with potassium hydroxide (KOH) and viewed under the microscope for a definitive diagnosis.

Effective treatment of *Candida* infections requires an appropriate antifungal agent, specifically one with activity against yeast organisms. The standard of care for *Candida* infections is nystatin; however, this agent requires a prescription and is costly. Alternatively, there are many over-the-counter (OTC) products; these vary in terms of active agent (such as miconazole or clotrimazole) and concentration, as well as formulation (powder, cream, or ointment). The appropriate formulation is determined by the severity of the infection, the condition of the skin, and the contours of the affected area. Powders are useful in skin folds because they help to absorb moisture; they may also be applied to areas of weepy, peeling epidermis before the application of a protective ointment. Creams are most useful on intact or minimally damaged skin because they provide additional moisture. Ointments are useful over eroded areas and in areas where powder may not adhere reliably. Ointments also provide the benefit of a moisture barrier. The choice of an OTC versus prescription agent as initial therapy should be determined by the severity of the infection and the patient's overall health status. All patients treated with OTC agents should be carefully evaluated for their response to treatment. In women, it is common for the vagina to become contaminated with *Candida* organisms, particularly when diarrhea is present; therefore, vaginal treatment should be considered.

Partial-Thickness Skin Loss Resulting from Maceration and Friction. As noted, overhydration of the skin is common among incontinent individuals, especially those managed with occlusive absorptive products; this overhydration reduces the skin's tensile strength and increases its vulnerability to mechanical trauma. Thus, the incontinent individual is at continual risk for epidermal loss resulting from aggressive perineal cleansing or from friction exerted by the absorptive products or by bed linen. This is most commonly manifest as large areas of superficial skin loss corresponding to the areas in contact with the bed linen (see Plate 5). However, this type of skin loss may also occur as isolated "patches;" this is most commonly seen in patients with fecal incontinence in whom zinc oxide preparations are being used for skin protection and is caused by aggressive removal of the protective ointment via "scrubbing" or "picking." Intertrigo is the term sometimes used to refer to partial-thickness skin loss that occurs on opposing skin surfaces as a result of friction and maceration. Common sites for intertrigo include skin folds in the groin and the skin between the buttocks; clinical presentation includes erythema, superficial linear erosions at the base of the fold (as within the gluteal cleft), or circular erosions between the buttocks. Intertrigo is particularly common in diabetic patients and obese individuals, especially those with impaired mobility (see Plate 6).

Pruritus ani is a less common condition that is sometimes incorrectly assessed as irritant dermatitis. It is characterized by intense perianal itching and chronic scratching, which result in perianal inflammation and skin damage (see Plate 7). Poor perineal hygiene, heat, and psychologic factors are currently thought to be causative factors.

One condition that may be incorrectly attributed to incontinence is atrophic changes in the urethral and vaginal tissues of postmenopausal women. The vaginal mucosa in these women appears dry, pale, and nonrugated, and the urethral meatus may be abnormally prominent and cherry red; in addition, the patient may complain of itching, irritation, or a sense of uncomfortable "dryness." This condition is most appropriately treated with topical estrogen, as discussed elsewhere in this text.

Atypical Skin Problems in Incontinent Individuals

The presence of other dermatologic problems must be considered in the patient with perineal skin damage who fails to respond to conventional topical therapy. Some of the more common but atypical problems that may be seen include miliaria, erythrasma, perineal psoriasis, and herpes simplex.

Miliaria is caused by obstruction of the sweat glands and overhydration of the stratum corneum; it may mimic candidiasis. It occurs as a rash with tiny discrete lesions and is pruritic; however, it lacks the confluent areas of erythema and the scaling that are characteristic of *Candida* infections. Treatment primarily involves use of nonocclusive absorptive products and a nonocclusive moisture barrier (such as dimethicone), to provide protection against maceration while avoiding occlusion of the sweat glands.

Erythrasma is another skin infection that may be mistaken for candidiasis. It is caused by a bacterium of the *Corynebacterium* family and shares some of the same predisposing factors as *Candida*

infections, that is, obesity, heat, and damaged skin. The rash is typically distributed along the inner thighs but may also be found along the gluteal cleft; in men, the area around the scrotum may be involved as well. This infection does not produce the satellite lesions and scaling that are typical of candidal infections, and it is diagnosed by the use of fluorescence rather than culture or a KOH stain (see Plate 8). Treatment usually involves antibiotic agents. The clinician should be aware that erythrasma is sometimes mistaken for tinea cruris. Tinea cruris is a fungal infection that typically occurs in men, is localized to the groin, and requires treatment with an antifungal agent as opposed to an antibiotic. A dermatology referral is indicated for any patient in whom the diagnosis is unclear.

Perineal psoriasis is an uncommon problem that may sometimes be mistaken for irritant dermatitis or candidiasis; however, it can be distinguished by its silvery color, distinct margins, lack of satellite lesions, and absence of pruritus (see Plate 9). Dermatologic management is typically required for these patients.

Perianal herpes (either simplex or zoster) is another potential cause for perineal skin breakdown. The typical presentation of herpes simplex is a cluster of small (less than 1 cm) vesicles on a red base. However, in the patient who is relatively immobile, the vesicles may be "unroofed" by friction before an accurate assessment can be done and may therefore be unrecognized. The lesions of herpes zoster localize along a dermatome, most commonly the perianal dermatome (along the anal verge) or along the buttock. Discrete vesicles or ulcerations in the perineal area should always raise suspicion of herpetic infection, particularly when the patient is immunocompromised. Additional "clues" to herpetic infection include pain and irregular distribution or unusual grouping or presentation of lesions (Plate 10). Diagnosis involves viral culture or Tzanck smear, which the clinician obtains by scraping the lesions with a scalpel and then applying the "scraped" material to a preserved slide for microscopic evaluation. However, it is frequently difficult to obtain a definitive diagnosis for herpetic lesions, especially when the lesions have dried and no fluid is retrievable (so a viral culture cannot be done).

The conventional approach to management of herpetic lesions has been to keep them dry; however, this is not practical for perianal herpes in an incontinent patient. Most clinicians apply occlusive protective ointments over the lesions to protect them from further irritation and from superinfection and to reduce pain by occluding the nerve endings; in addition, systemic antiviral agents are typically prescribed.[24]

In evaluating and managing the patient with perineal dermatitis, the clinician should remember that the patient may develop allergic contact dermatitis to any of the products used for protection or treatment of the perineal skin, particularly if the skin is damaged. Because the clinical presentation may be indistinguishable from that of nonallergic irritant dermatitis, allergic dermatitis obviously complicates both assessment and intervention. Therefore, the clinician should be conservative in the use of topical products and should be familiar with each product's ingredients and any common sensitizers.

Prevention and Management of Skin Damage

In managing the individual with severe diarrhea or intractable incontinence, the primary goal must always be prevention of skin breakdown. This is particularly important for the patient with intractable incontinence, because it is difficult to create an environment for skin repair when there is constant or repeated exposure to urine or feces; skin damage may therefore produce a vicious cycle of damage and inflammation that results in cumulative injury.[25] In addition, damaged skin is more likely to mount an allergic response to topical products used to treat the injury.

Care of perineal skin in the incontinent patient should be based on the following goals: (1) promoting the health of the epidermis; that is, maintaining an intact epidermal barrier; (2) eliminating or minimizing exposure to irritants; (3) treating infection, if present; and (4) creating an environment for healing damaged skin, if present.

Maintaining an Intact Barrier. The Agency for Health Care Policy and Research (AHCPR) Pressure Ulcer Prediction and Prevention Guidelines include several recommendations designed to maintain the integrity of intact skin; factors addressed include bathing technique and frequency, water temperature, cleansing solution, and topical product use.[26] Key elements of preventive care are maintenance of the normal lipid and water content of the skin (prevention of dry skin), and prevention of epidermal "stripping." Specific strategies to keep the epidermis healthy include the following:

- Use gentle techniques for cleansing; avoid rubbing and scrubbing the skin, because this causes epidermal stripping.
- Avoid products and bathing rituals that increase the loss of skin lipids and adversely affect skin pH; avoid use of soaps, harsh cleansers, and solvents, and use warm (not hot) water. Neutral pH skin care cleansers with emollients are suggested. Skin care rituals such as daily bathing, the use of basins for bathing, the use of soapy, hot water, and vigorous scrubbing of the skin "do more harm than good" and should be abandoned.[27] Basins that are used for bathing are a significant source for bacterial contamination and should be avoided if at all possible; the availability of disposable soft bathing cloths impregnated with pH-balanced no-rinse cleansers and emollients render soap and water and bath basins obsolete. Another factor that must be considered in regard to bathing is transmission of bacteria from the patient to the caregiver; caregivers must be aware that use of gloves does not provide complete protection, and gloves can become a reservoir for bacterial organisms. Careful attention to hand hygiene, such as, use of antimicrobial cleansers, helps to prevent transmission of organisms during bathing and is important both for the patient and for the caregiver.[28,29]

Studies performed in the long-term care setting provide evidence that the implementation of skin care protocols involving use of perineal cleansers (body washes) and moisturizer-moisture barrier products (skin protectants) can significantly reduce the incidence of skin disorders including perineal dermatitis, breakdown, and pressure ulcers.[30,31] These data indicate that simplified protocols and appropriate products can maintain or even improve skin condition, promote staff adherence, and provide cost savings (by reducing the time for delivery of the skin care protocol).[31]

The cornerstones of effective skin care are gentle and physiologic approaches to perineal cleansing and the use of moisturizers and moisture barriers to maintain the lipid content of the skin and to provide a barrier against irritants and pathogens. The most commonly used protective products include creams, ointments, liquid films, and powders. Unfortunately, there are few published clinical trials related to the management of perineal dermatitis in the adult population;[32-34] therefore, the selection of a particular product or regimen is based primarily on theoretic principles and clinical experience, as opposed to scientific evidence.

Many of the topical products used for the prevention and management of perineal dermatitis are prepared according to recipes and techniques commonly accepted in the pharmaceutical and cosmetic industries; as such, they share properties with cosmetic formulations. The clinician must carefully review the list of ingredients to determine indications and contraindications to use.

Safety testing is part of good manufacturing practices, and data should be available from the manufacturer. Labeling must conform to Food and Drug Administration (FDA) guidelines with active ingredients (if present) identified. Ingredients are generally listed in descending order of percentage in the product. Inactive ingredients may or may not be listed. For more complete information, the clinician should request the MSDS (material safety data sheet) from the manufacturer. This sheet includes a complete listing of all ingredients as well as safety precautions. In general, products that have dermal or ocular warnings should be used cautiously or not at all for patients with fragile or sensitive skin.[22]

Accurate interpretation of product information presents a challenge; clinicians are often at a loss to understand the purpose and implications of a bewildering array of chemical ingredients used in formulations. The FDA recognizes thousands of ingredients as safe; hundreds are commonly used in skin care products. The purpose, safety, and efficacy of any individual ingredient are determined by its chemical composition, its concentration in the formulation, and its role in combination with other ingredients. It is beyond the scope of this text to present a comprehensive discussion of formulation chemistry; however, Table 11-2 provides a partial list of common ingredients and their functions. Some basic questions that should be asked by the clinician when evaluating a product include the following: (1) Is the intended use or indication consistent with the patient's skin care needs? (2) Are the ingredients disclosed on the label? (3) Are the manufacturer's claims for the product consistent with the ingredients? (4) Are the claims supported by clinical data? (5) Are safety testing data available? (6) Is the product compatible with the characteristics of normal skin; that is, is it pH balanced, is it supportive of normal skin flora, and does it allow normal skin function such as desquamation? (7) If an antimicrobial component is present, is it FDA approved?

Dyes, fragrances, and preservatives are known to be irritants. Their presence in a formulation is not an absolute contraindication to product use but requires the clinician to evaluate use carefully, particularly in patients with allergies. Hypoallergenic formulations that are free of fragrances, dyes, and preservatives or that contain minimal preservatives may be beneficial for patients with severe allergic or atopic disease. Product selection is also affected by attributes such as ease of application or, more importantly, ease of removal, fragrance, ability to control odor, cost, and proven or perceived effectiveness. Unfortunately, the lack of a strong scientific base for product selection and utilization contributes to the lack of standardization and the continued use of a multitude of products and practices, including the hazardous practice of compounding products by hand at the bedside.

Guidelines for Appropriate Use of Topical Products

Topical products are broadly classified as cleansers, moisturizers, moisture barriers, and powders. The indications and guidelines for appropriate use of each of these categories is briefly reviewed.

Cleansers. Irritants such as stool and urine should be removed from the perineum as promptly and gently as possible to prevent skin damage. Perineal cleansers are liquid solutions or emulsions designed to remove effluent and bacteria. They commonly

TABLE 11-2 **Ingredients and their Functions in Skin Care Products: Partial List**

FUNCTIONS OF INGREDIENTS	EXAMPLES OF INGREDIENTS
Antimicrobials* (FDA-approved active ingredients used in over-the-counter antimicrobial drug products that kill microorganisms)	Alcohol, benzalkonium chloride, benzethonium chloride, hydrogen peroxide, Poloxamer 188, phenol, povidone-iodine complex, methylbenzethonium chloride
Humectants (skin-conditioning agents that draw water into the stratum corneum)	Glycerin, urea, propylene glycol
Surfactants-emulsifiers† (agents that lower surface tension between liquids or a liquid and a solid)	Sodium laurel sulfate, polyethylene glycol (many); Poloxamer (many); propylene glycol (many)
Emulsion stabilizers (assist in formation and stabilization of emulsions)	Polyethylene glycol (many), cetyl alcohol, stearyl alcohol, cholesterol
pH adjusters (control pH of finished product)	Sodium citrate, sodium bicarbonate, citric acid
Chelating agents (complex substances with metal ions that prevent adverse changes in the stability or appearance of formulations)	EDTA (many), citric acid
Preservatives (prevent or retard microbial growth and protect products from spoiling)	Chloroxylenol (PCMX); triclosan; methyl, propyl, and butyl parabens; imidazolidinyl urea; diazolidinyl urea
Skin protectants‡ (FDA-approved ingredients for use in over-the-counter drugs)	Allantoin, calamine, dimethicone, glycerin, lanolin, mineral oil, petrolatum, zinc oxide
Solvent (liquid used to dissolve components of formulation)	Water; alcohol; methyl, ethyl, and isopropyl alcohols; polyethylene glycol (many); propylene glycol; specially denatured (SD) alcohol (many)

FDA, Food and Drug Administration.
*Refer to "Topical antimicrobial drug products for over-the-counter human use: tentative final monograph for first aid antiseptic drug products," *Federal Register* 56:33644, July 22, 1991.
†Other surfactant categories include cleansing agents and foam boosters.
‡A product labeled as a skin protectant must include one or more of the 21 FDA-approved ingredients in a quantity as designated. Refer to "Skin protectant drugs: products for over-the-counter human use," *Federal Register* 59:28767, June 3, 1994.

contain water and a surfactant (surface active agent), which helps to loosen soil from the skin. This eliminates the need for aggressive cleansing with washcloths, which should generally be avoided because they can cause significant frictional forces and mechanical skin damage. Cleansers frequently contain antimicrobials; these agents are added to limit bacterial growth and to reduce odor. Dyes and fragrances may be added to make the product esthetically pleasing, but these substances can increase the potential for adverse skin reactions, such as allergic contact dermatitis. The pH of the cleanser should be compatible with skin pH (within the range

of 4 to 7).[22] The cleanser should also leave minimal residue and should be nonirritating. Most bar soaps have an alkaline pH and leave substantial residue, both of which can compromise the barrier function of the skin. Cleansers that are formulated as "no-rinse" preparations are generally recommended because of the following advantages: reduced time required for bathing/cleansing; elimination of irritating residues; and the avoidance of water, which can cause drying of the skin by removing skin lipids.

Moisturizers. Moisturizers are an essential element of skin care for the incontinent individual, because these agents replace lost lipids and thus contribute to an intact epidermal barrier. Moisturizers are often formulated as creams and include one or more of the following skin conditioning ingredients: emollients, which soften the skin and improve its texture; humectants, which draw water into the stratum corneum; and occlusive agents, which prevent evaporation of water from the stratum corneum.

Moisture Barriers. The terms "moisture barrier," "skin barrier," and "skin protectant" are used interchangeably to describe formulations such as ointments, pastes, and creams that protect the skin from irritants and moisture. Petrolatum, dimethicone, and zinc oxide are ingredients commonly used in these products. The quality of petrolatum varies according to its source and manufacturing process. Refined white petrolatum is desirable for skin care preparations. Dimethicone (a silicone product) provides a water-repellant barrier that is nonocclusive and compatible with normal function of the stratum corneum. It has been used since the early 1960s for the prevention of diaper dermatitis. Zinc oxide also provides moisture protection and has limited absorbent and antifungal properties as well. Although it is believed that moisture barriers create an environment for healing, the effect of these products on the repair process is not really known. Occlusion is known to interfere with normal skin function and has been reported to delay healing of superficial injuries; however, Welzel and colleagues[35] were unable to detect any significant delay in repair as evidenced by TEWL. This is an area in which further study is needed.

Ointments are thick, anhydrous semisolids that are occlusive. Many ointments used in perineal care have a petrolatum base, which is believed to reduce TEWL and possibly to enhance hydration of the epidermal barrier. Barrier pastes are formed by mixture of an ointment with a fine powder. Addition of an ingredient such as methylcellulose or karaya results in an extremely thick material that has an absorbent and drying effect when applied to weeping skin. Pastes provide an effective barrier to irritants and moisture. These same properties make them more difficult to remove than conventional ointments, and inappropriate removal techniques may actually cause additional skin damage.

Caregivers should follow the manufacturer's guidelines for application and removal; the latter typically involves use of a liquid cleanser that contains surfactants. Paste products are most often used to protect or treat skin that is frequently exposed to liquid stool because these products are more resistant to cleansing and enzymatic breakdown.

Creams (water-in-oil or oil-in-water emulsions) can also be formulated as barrier products. They vary greatly in texture. Occlusive creams may exhibit the physical properties of an ointment or even a paste. Concerns associated with occluding the stratum cornuem and potentially interfering with normal skin function and healing have prompted manufacturers to develop nonocclusive (breathable) barrier creams. The appearance and texture of these formulations may resemble those of moisturizers, but they differ in that they provide a barrier to moisture and irritants. A moisture barrier product may be labeled as an OTC *skin-protectant* drug if it includes one or more of several FDA-approved active ingredients within a specified range (see Table 11-2). Such ingredients must be noted on the product label.

Liquid Barrier Films. These products, sometimes known as skin "sealants," are composed of polymers and a solvent; the solvent evaporates (after application to the skin), and the polymers dry to form a protective film. Although these products are commonly used for skin protection, one drawback to their use is the alcohol contained in most brands of films. Products containing alcohol have the potential to cause skin irritation, even when the stratum corneum is intact. Skin irritation is *more* likely to occur if the film is not allowed to dry (that is, the solvent is not allowed to evaporate) before an occlusive product such as an ointment is applied. (Occlusion enhances the potential for penetration into the stratum corneum.) In addition, alcohol-containing products cause discomfort or even pain when applied to damaged skin and are cytotoxic. Therefore, liquid barrier films that contain alcohol have no place in the management of damaged skin. Alcohol-free liquid barriers are available and may be used in this situation.

Powders. Powders are formulated to absorb moisture upon application; by reducing moisture, powders reduce the frictional forces that are present.

In clinical practice, powders may help to reduce moisture and friction wherever opposing skin surfaces meet, such as the gluteal or inguinal folds and along the inner thighs. However, the clinician must select the specific powder carefully. Cornstarch has been a favorite "home remedy" for control of moisture and friction; however, its use is now discouraged because it may act as an irritant and an allergen.[36]

Guidelines for Skin Care

An algorithm for prevention and management of perineal dermatitis is presented in Fig. 11-2.

Preventive Skin Care. A preventive skin care program for an individual with intact skin but frequent exposure to urine and/or stool involves three elements: cleansing, moisturizing, and protecting. Traditionally, this has involved three steps and three products. The first step involves gentle cleansing with a pH-balanced no-rinse cleanser that contains minimal or no additives. The second step involves application of a moisturizer (to replace lipids and contribute to an intact barrier); this element is particularly critical when the perineal skin is dry and chapped. The third step is application of a moisture barrier cream or ointment to create a barrier to stool and urine and thereby to reduce the potential for skin damage. Recently developed alternatives to this three-step procedure (cleanse, moisturize, protect) are products designed to reduce the care to two steps or one step. Two-step protocols involve cleansing followed by application of a moisturizer-moisture barrier cream that provides both emollients and a moisture barrier/skin protectant. One-step products involve use of a disposable cleansing wipe that is impregnated with emollients and moisture barriers; with this approach, the patient or caregiver is able to

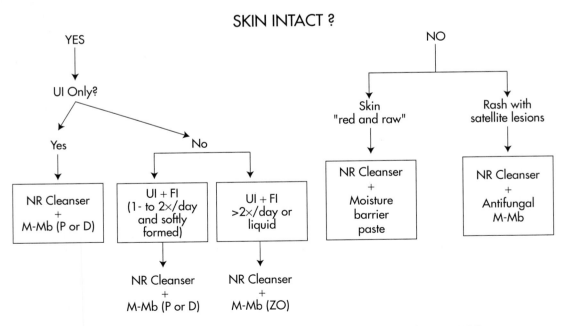

Fig. 11-2 Algorithm for prevention and management of perineal dermatitis. D, dimethicone; M-Mb, moisturizer/moisture barrier combination; Mb, moisture barrier; NRC, no-rinse perineal cleanser; P, petrolatum; ZO, zinc oxide. (From Lekan-Rutledge D and Collin J, 2003, Urinary incontinence in the frail elderly. *Am J of Nursing* Supplement: 36–46.)

cleanse, moisturize, and protect all at the same time. The advantages of two-step and one-step products are increased efficiency and increased adherence to the care protocol in busy care settings; these advantages translate into better clinical outcomes and more cost-effective care.

An alternative to the use of a moisture barrier cream or ointment is the use of an alcohol-free plasticizing film barrier.[37] These films provide effective protection against urine and against intermittent contact with feces. The patient or caregiver should be instructed to cleanse and dry the skin before applying the barrier film and to allow the liquid to dry completely before applying a second layer. Films are not typically used in combination with creams or ointments and in some cases may be incompatible.

Individuals exposed to liquid stool or to stool mixed with urine require aggressive preventive skin care. Prompt removal of soiled pads and garments is essential, followed by gentle cleansing to remove the irritants and the bacteria. Protection with moisture barrier creams or ointments is required, and many clinicians find that products containing zinc oxide or dimethicone provide more effective protection than products containing only petrolatum. It is critical to instruct the patient or caregiver in the appropriate application and removal of the selected products, especially when zinc oxide products are used.

The presence of mild erythema indicates an inflammatory response and is indicative of developing dermatitis; in this case, application of a barrier ointment or cream or an alcohol-free barrier film provides protection against the offending substance and is usually sufficient intervention (along with measures to minimize the incontinence or the duration of skin exposure to urine and stool).

Management of Perineal Dermatitis with Epidermal Loss. The patient with perineal erosion or ulceration is usually best managed with a skin barrier paste to absorb drainage and to provide an effective barrier against irritants. In this situation, a thick coating of the protective paste or ointment is applied to the involved area, and caregivers must be carefully instructed regarding appropriate cleansing and reapplication. (Cleansing should be designed to remove only the soiled layer of paste, using mineral oil or a perineal cleanser and *gentle* technique, followed by reapplication of the protective paste or ointment.) If there are large areas of epidermal loss associated with weeping, intermittent application of aluminum acetate (Burow's solution) compresses may be used. This solution is an astringent that causes protein precipitation and also has a drying and soothing effect; the compresses are typically applied three times daily. Although these compresses provide temporary comfort, they do not provide a barrier against the irritants; therefore, application of the compresses must be followed by application of a protective paste or ointment. Wound dressings such as hydrocolloids or transparent film dressings are usually ineffective for the management of incontinence-induced perineal ulceration because of problems with excessive moisture, frequent soiling, and irregular contours.

Management of Yeast Dermatitis. As noted earlier, yeast dermatitis is a fairly common type of perineal dermatitis among incontinent individuals. There are two different approaches to treatment of yeast dermatitis in the individual who also requires protection from urine and stool. One approach is to apply an antifungal powder or cream (such as nystatin) followed by a moisture barrier cream or ointment; alternatively, the clinician may select a moisture barrier product that contains an antifungal agent such as miconazole.

The use of topical antimicrobials is usually not indicated unless there is clinical or laboratory evidence of infection. Most topical products contain preservatives to prevent spoilage over time and to preserve the product's integrity. These preservatives should not be confused with an active antimicrobial agent intended to inhibit or kill bacteria on the skin.

Topical corticosteroids may be prescribed on a short-term basis to mitigate the symptoms of inflammation; however, the clinician must bear in mind that these agents may actually interfere with reepithelialization. Steroids are not indicated for long-term use because they can induce thinning of the epidermis, which renders it more susceptible to breakdown.

DEVICES FOR MANAGING INTRACTABLE INCONTINENCE

Containment devices represent an alternative to absorbent products that may provide better outcomes for selected patients; however, the device must be selected carefully based on a thorough assessment of the patterns of incontinence and the patient's needs. In addition to assessing the pattern and volume of urine loss, the clinician must consider sensory status, cognitive status, visual acuity, mobility, dexterity, motivation, and concerns of the patient or caregiver, including aesthetic issues. Ideally, the equipment must effectively contain the urine or stool and must be easy and comfortable for the patient or caregiver to use.

External Devices for Men

External devices for men can be divided into two general categories, urethral compression devices and external catheters. Urethral compression devices obstruct the flow of urine by mechanically compressing the soft tissue of the penis and the tissue surrounding the urethra, the corpus spongiosum. There are two types of devices, a penile clamp and an inflatable compression cuff (see Fig. 10-9). Penile clamps include plastic and metallic devices lined with foam that are closed around the penis and a device constructed of foam with a soft foam bolster that is positioned against the urethra; all provide urethral compression that reduces or eliminates leakage. The inflatable compression cuff is a soft band that is wrapped around the penis and secured with a Velcro fastener; the band incorporates a small bladder that is positioned along the ventral aspect of the penis and is then inflated with air to partially compress the urethra. These devices are not commonly used because of their potential for ischemic damage to the penis if they are used incorrectly. Therefore, their use is limited to individuals who are cognitively intact, with normal sensation and the manual dexterity to apply and remove the device every 3 hours and as needed for voiding. Patients must be carefully instructed in the potential complications associated with these devices and must be followed closely to ensure appropriate utilization. These devices are most appropriate for men who have postprostatectomy stress UI and who meet the criteria described earlier.

External, or condom, catheters are very frequently used for the management of urinary leakage in men. External catheters are a good choice for men with intractable incontinence who have no problems with urinary retention, such as men with normal bladder function but severe functional disabilities resulting in incontinence.[38] External catheters are usually effective in controlling urine elimination and are associated with a lower incidence of bacteriuria as compared with indwelling catheters, and a reduced incidence of perineal dermatitis and skin breakdown as compared with absorptive products. In addition, an external catheter may be more acceptable to the male patient than absorbent products. However, these products *can* result in local penile irritation, so it is critical to select and apply them appropriately. To reduce the risk of bacteriuria and skin complications, external catheters may be used for short periods of time when social continence is most desired. For some men, this may be during daytime hours when they are socially active. For others, external urethral catheters are used only at night to minimize sleep disruption.

External urinary devices were traditionally manufactured of latex rubber; however, the recognition of latex sensitivity and allergy spurred the production of external catheters from nonlatex materials, usually silicone. The various designs for external catheters are outlined in Box 11-1. The types most commonly used are the self-adhesive sheath and the nonadhesive sheath used with a double-sided adhesive strip. To apply the nonadhesive sheath, the adhesive strip is wrapped around the penis, and the nonadhesive sheath is then rolled over the adhesive strip and is pressed into place. There is also a nonadhesive reusable device that is useful for patients who need only intermittent containment and those who are unable to tolerate adhesives; with this device, correct application is essential to prevent ischemic damage to the soft tissue of the penis.

There are several guidelines to be followed for optimal results with external catheters. The first is to select a catheter with a nonkinking junction

BOX 11-1 Categories and Features of External Collection Devices for Men

Single-Use Condom Catheters
Self-adhesive
Available in latex and synthetic materials
Internal surface of sheath coated with adhesive; catheter rolled on and gently pressed into place
Double-sided adhesive strip and nonadhesive sheath
Adhesive strips available with foam base or skin barrier base; barrier strips have stretch and memory, so good for patient with erectile function
Adhesive strip wraps around penis; nonadhesive catheter rolled over strip
Nonadhesive catheter sheaths available in latex and synthetic materials

Reusable Condom Catheters
Nonadhesive sheath with Velcro strap fastener
Catheter rolled into place over penis and then secured with Velcro closure strap
Inappropriate for patient with sensory impairment because of potential for necrosis if strap fastened too tightly around penis
Nonadhesive sheath with inflatable inner ring
Catheter rolled into place over penis; syringe used to inflate internal ring
Inappropriate for patient with sensory impairment because of potential for necrosis if ring overinflated

Male "Urinal"
Nonadhesive device; consists of athletic support garment with integral condom type of collection device
Reusable

between the catheter tip and the drainage tubing; this "antitwist" feature prevents obstruction to urinary flow (and subsequent urinary leakage). The second is to size the catheter appropriately; measuring guides are available from most manufacturers and are designed so the penile diameter can be discreetly measured at the base. The third is to ensure a dry skin surface free of hair. The penis should be washed and dried and loose hairs clipped or shaved before application of the catheter. Liquid barrier films are often used before the application of self-adhesive catheters to protect the penile skin from the repetitive application and removal of an adhesive device. Although this practice is widely advocated and theoretically sound, there are no research studies that validate the need for this practice.

An additional factor to be considered in catheter selection for the patient with intact erectile function is the potential for constriction. This is particularly relevant if the patient is using a nonadhesive

sheath secured by a double-sided adhesive strip. There are two categories of double-sided adhesive strips: adhesive-coated foams and adhesive barrier strips. Foam strips lack elasticity and are generally contraindicated for patients who retain erectile function. Barrier strips, conversely, have the capacity to stretch and have variable degrees of memory (the capacity to return to original size and shape).

Wear time for an external catheter varies from 24 to 72 hours, depending on product design, patient tolerance, and manufacturer's specifications. Specific detailed instructions on application technique and early recognition of problems are indicated for the novice user, as well as routine scheduled follow-up examinations. For example, the uncircumcised man should be instructed to leave the foreskin down over the head of the penis when he applies the external catheter.[39] One external device that is now available and that represents an alternative to an external catheter incorporates a fitted cotton brief with an ergonomically designed, latex-free collection device attached to a drainage bag (Afex Incontinence Management System, Arcus Medical, Inc., Charlotte, NC). For nighttime management of UI, a pad can be inserted into the washable brief (Fig. 11-3).

Men with short or retracted penises commonly have difficulty obtaining a secure seal with an external catheter. The man with a short penis can frequently be managed with the use of a sport sheath, which is designed to adhere securely to a short penile shaft. For the man with penile retraction, a system has been designed to adhere to the glans penis as opposed to the penile shaft, the BioDerm (Bioderm Inc., Largo, Fla.) external collection device (see Fig. 10-8). This system includes a drainage tube connected to thin hydrocolloid leaflets configured in the shape of a flower; the leaflets are pressed into place over the glans penis and are secured with a hydrocolloid strip. The drainage tube is then connected to a leg bag or bedside bag and is changed as needed. Wear time is variable but averages 2 or 3 days.

Another option for the patient with a short or retracted penis is an adhesive urinary pouch, either one piece or two piece. One type of retracted penis pouch (Hollister, Inc., Libertyville, IL.) consists of a hydrocolloid skin barrier that adheres to the skin and conforms to body contours. The drainage port

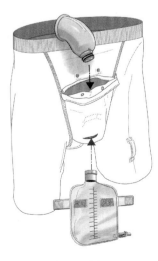

Fig. 11-3 Afex Incontinence Management System. (Courtesy of Arcus Medical, Inc.)

connects to a urinary drainage bag. Preparation for pouch application includes skin cleansing and removal of the pubic hair at the base of the penis. The base of the penis is measured, and a comparably sized opening is created in the adhesive surface; if the patient retains erectile function, radial "darts" may be cut around the opening in the adhesive surface to prevent penile constriction in the event of an erection. The skin at the base of the penis is held taut to provide a smooth surface for pouch application. The pouch is then applied. If a two-piece system is used, the adhesive wafer with flange is first pressed into place, and the pouch is then snapped onto the flange. The pouch is usually connected to straight drainage; alternatively, the spout may be closed, and the patient may be allowed to empty the pouch as needed. Wear time for a urinary pouch varies from 24 to 72 hours for a one-piece system to 5 to 7 days for a two-piece system. Longer wear times are typically obtained when the patient is bedfast or has limited ambulation.

External Devices for Women

External devices for women are very limited. Despite technologic advances and multiple attempts to develop a watertight, nonirritating, comfortable, and cleanable device that fits women of different body types and with different activity levels, no such device is currently available.[40] There is an external pouch that may be used for short-term urine collection in the bedfast patient (for example, for a 24-hour urine collection); however, this device is not feasible for long-term management because of the difficulty in applying an adhesive device to a moist, pliable, irregular, and hairy surface. Therefore, at this time, female devices are limited to those intended to prevent urinary leakage, as opposed to those intended to contain urinary leakage.

Urethral Inserts. Female occlusive devices that fit into the urethra (such as FemSoft, Rochester Medical, Rochester, Minn.) are designed for female incontinence. The FemSoft insert is a disposable, single-use device for the treatment of female stress UI (see Fig. 4-5). It consists of a narrow silicone tube enclosed in a soft, thin, mineral oil-filled sleeve that forms a balloon at the tip. At the opposite end, the sterile tube and sleeve form an external retainer.

FemSoft is inserted into the urethra with a disposable plastic applicator. As the device is inserted, the mineral oil in the balloon drains into the external retainer. Once the tip of the device is advanced to the bladder, the oil flows back into the balloon, creating a seal at the neck of the bladder that prevents urine leakage. FemSoft is removed and discarded during voiding, and then a new device is inserted. Urinary tract infection (UTI), bacteriuria, urgency, and urethral discomfort are potential complications of urethral inserts; however, most women tolerate the device well and use it for episodic protection during activities known to increase the risk of leakage, such as aerobic exercise, golf, or tennis.

CATHETERS
Indwelling Catheters

Prevalence studies indicate that indwelling urinary catheters are utilized in 11% to 25% of hospital patients, 5% of nursing home patients, and 4% of patients in home care.[41,42] Indwelling catheters should rarely be used for management of UI. The Centers for Disease Control and Prevention (CDC) and the AHCPR identify the following as appropriate indications for use of long-term indwelling catheters: (1) urinary retention that cannot otherwise be managed, (2) management of terminally ill or severely ill patients, (3) management of patients with stage 3 or stage 4 pressure ulcers on the trunk or pelvis until the ulcer is healed, and (4) management of UI in the homebound patient who is incapable of self-toileting and whose caregiver is unable to manage the incontinence effectively with toileting, containment devices, or absorptive products. In addition, short-term use of catheters is appropriate for monitoring fluid balance in the acutely ill patient.[24,43,44] Neither the CDC nor the AHCPR advocates use of long-term indwelling catheters as a primary approach to the management of UI. The decision regarding placement of an indwelling catheter requires thoughtful consideration on the part of the clinician about the individual needs of the patient. In many cases, alternative treatment approaches can provide better outcomes. For example, alpha blockers may be used to treat retention caused by outlet obstruction and may eliminate the need for catheterization; this approach may be of particular benefit in the management of men with prostatic enlargement and in patients with postoperative urinary retention. However, the existence of treatment options other than an indwelling catheter for management of urinary dysfunction does not necessarily mean that those options are the best choice for an individual patient. For example, intermittent catheterization is typically considered a "better" option than indwelling catheterization for management of urinary retention; however, in a frail elder who responds to intermittent catheterization with combative behavior, an indwelling catheter could alleviate both urinary retention and the distress associated with intermittent catheterization. In a nursing facility where quality care is measured in part by the number of urinary catheters, the use of catheters must be examined on a case-by-case basis with attention to extenuating circumstances, as opposed to automatic sanctions for use of indwelling catheters in patients who fall outside the established categories for approved use.[45] Less invasive treatment options may not be acceptable or appropriate for every patient.

The urinary catheter has been aptly described as a "one-point restraint" whose use is frequently unjustified or excessively prolonged.[42] The comparison is drawn between catheters and restraints because both restrict activities of daily living and ability to move about freely, are physically uncomfortable, and have harmful consequences. To improve appropriate utilization and reduce the indiscriminate use of catheters, Saint and colleagues recommend the following:[42]

- Educate all medical and nursing staff about adverse clinical consequences, patient discomfort, patient embarrassment, and activity restrictions associated with urinary catheterization.
- Educate staff about the appropriate use of indwelling catheters and the availability and efficacy of other strategies and devices to manage UI (for example, condom catheters and special undergarments).
- Use quality control patient audits to design institution-specific programs to decrease inappropriate use of indwelling urinary catheters.
- Develop and evaluate the effectiveness of automatic "stop orders" for indwelling urinary catheters; these

orders should require that the catheter either be removed or reordered after a specified period of catheterization (for example, after 48 hours).

Long-term indwelling catheterization is associated with morbidity and mortality. Long-term indwelling catheters are usually considered those catheters that remain in place 30 days or longer. Urologic complications of long-term catheterization include chronic renal inflammation, chronic pyelonephritis, nephrolithiasis, cystolithiasis, and symptomatic UTI with pyelonephritis. These complications can lead to bacteremia, urosepsis, and death. In contrast, short-term use of indwelling catheters (less than 30 days) is seldom associated with significant problems apart from UTI.

The primary complication of long-term indwelling urinary catheters is UTI; patients with long-term indwelling catheters develop UTIs at a rate of 5% per day. After 30 days of catheterization, there is a 78% to 95% incidence of bacteriuria, despite the provision of meticulous catheter care.[46,47] Although many catheter-associated febrile episodes are self-limiting and resolve within 24 hours without antibiotic treatment,[48] persistent infection is the root of other complications such as prostatitis, epididymitis, cystitis, pyelonephritis, and bacteremia or urosepsis.

Symptomatic UTI is characterized by fever of 100.8∞F or higher, chills, diaphoresis, suprapubic pain, malaise, nausea/vomiting, mental status changes, hypotension, and autonomic dysreflexia in patients with spinal cord injury.[38,46] Changes in the urine include unusually cloudy urine, increased sedimentation, more frequent catheter blockage, and new or increased bladder spasms.[38] Diagnosis of UTI is more difficult in the elderly, because fever may not always be present; in these patients, altered mental status or increased incidence of bladder spasms may be the primary indicators of infection. White blood cells in the urine are considered the best laboratory indicator of UTI,[49] and a urine culture revealing more than 100,000 colony counts of at least one organism is diagnostic.

The presence of microorganisms in the urine does not imply or predict evidence of UTI; therefore, treatment of asymptomatic bacteriuria is not recommended.[44,46,48,50] The American Medical Directors Association's Urinary Incontinence Clinical Practice Guideline advises that bacteriuria, with or without pyuria, should not be treated in incontinent patients in the absence of symptoms of UTI. Antibiotic treatment of bacteriuria in the patient with a long-term indwelling catheter is not recommended because of cost, potential adverse effects, and the role in encouraging antibiotic drug resistance.[50]

Antibiotic treatment of symptomatic UTI should be based on culture and sensitivity data. Infections are usually polymicrobial with organisms such as *Pseudomonas, Proteus, Providencia, Enterobacteriaceae, Morganella,* and *Enterococcus.*[38] The usual duration of treatment is 5 to 14 days or longer. In patients who are not critically ill, single-drug therapy with trimethoprim-sulfamethoxazole or a second-generation cephalosporin can be prescribed, if the culture does not show multidrug-resistant pathogens.[38] Critically ill or septic patients require two-drug combinations and may require hospitalization. Noncatheter causes of systemic infection should also be considered in the assessment of a patient with apparent urosepsis.

General guidelines for prevention of UTI include utilizing aseptic technique when changing and handling the catheter, securing the catheter to minimize urethral and bladder trauma, ensuring unobstructed urine flow, meatal care, and adequate fluid intake.[44,46] Special catheters (silver alloy, hydrogel-coated latex), urine bag decontamination, catheter irrigations, and ingestion of cranberry juice have not yet been shown to offer benefit in the prevention of UTI in the patient with long-term catheterization.[46,51]

Catheter-related bacteremia or urosepsis is diagnosed when the same microorganisms are isolated from both urine and blood cultures in the absence of other sources of infection.[50,52] Bacteremia is uncommon but potentially life-threatening; it is estimated that the risk of bacteremia is approximately 3.6%, or 1 of every 27 patients with bacteriuria.[52] The attributable risk of death in patients with urinary tract–related bacteremia is estimated at 12.7%, when other potential causes of death are excluded.[52] In a multisite prospective study, patients who were catheterized for 76% or more of their days in the nursing home over 1 year were three times more likely to die within a year, and there was a stepwise increase in mortality associated with duration of catheterization.[53] The clinician should routinely reassess the need for continued use of an indwelling catheter, because removal of any unneeded catheter could lead to a reduction in risk for catheter-related complications and mortality.

Prevention and Management of Catheter-Associated Complications

Routine Care. Catheter-related complications can be reduced by appropriate attention to catheter and drainage unit selection, aseptic and atraumatic techniques for catheter insertion, routine stabilization of the catheter to prevent traction on the bladder neck, gentle nonaggressive meatal care, and meticulous attention to technique when emptying the drainage bag. All these care elements are discussed in detail in Chapter 10.

Complication Management. Common and clinically significant catheter care problems include encrustations, blockage, and bladder spasms;[46,49,51] the nurse must continually monitor the catheterized patient for evidence of these complications and must intervene appropriately to ensure continuous unobstructed bladder drainage and to reduce the risk for UTI.

Catheter encrustation is the result of a series of chemical reactions involving gram-negative organisms such as *Proteus mirabilis* and *Providencia,* which proliferate when the urine is alkaline (pH greater than 6.5) (see Fig. 10-7). When encrustations are present, a gravel-like substance can be palpated when the catheter is rolled between the thumb and forefinger. This gravel is composed of calcium oxalate or struvite (magnesium ammonium phosphate) crystals.

Treatment of encrustations is challenging and only modestly successful. Ideally, the urine should be kept acidic, to inhibit growth of the organisms involved. However, maintenance of a low urine pH is difficult in chronically infected urine, especially in the presence of bladder stones, which perpetuate the cycle of bacterial growth and crystal formation.[54] Conventional recommendations for treatment of encrustations include increased fluid intake to dilute the urine and routine administration of vitamin C or cranberry juice to acidify the urine; however, there is no evidence that ingestion of vitamin C or cranberry juice will change the urinary pH.[41,55] In one study comparing cranberry juice and increased fluid intake for the prevention of encrustation, results showed that consuming an additional liter of water over an 8-hour period was more effective than a liter of cranberry juice in reducing catheter encrustation.[41] Some evidence suggests that cranberry juice contains factors that inhibit the adhesion of urinary tract pathogens to urothelial cells; however, no data support the administration of cranberry juice to prevent catheter encrustations or UTI in the catheterized patient.[41,55] At present, evidence suggests that the most important factor in preventing catheter encrustation is high-volume fluid intake spaced fairly evenly throughout the day.[41,46,56] Catheter irrigations are not generally recommended as a strategy for preventing encrustation; however, research suggests that routine irrigation with acidic solutions may reduce the rate of encrustation and prolong catheter life in patients with chronic encrustation.[46,51,54] (Irrigation may damage the urothelium; therefore, the fluid should be instilled and drained via gravity. This strategy is discussed further in Chapter 10.) Patients who experience frequent episodes of encrustation and blockage should have catheter changes scheduled just before the catheter would typically become blocked. For some patients, catheter changes may be as often as every 10 days to 2 weeks.

Stones (urolithiasis) are another potential complication for the patient who requires long-term catheterization. The pH of urine influences the type of stone development. Calcium carbonate stones typically occur when the urine is alkaline, whereas uric acid stone formation is supported by an acidic urine. Stone formation is also influenced by urinary pathogens; urease-producing pathogens such as *Proteus, Klebsiella,* and *Pseudomonas* promote the formation of struvite stones. Another important factor contributing to stone development is dehydration. Under normal conditions, urine has a high concentration of positively and negatively charged ions; in the presence of dehydration, these ions are more likely to combine with salts to from crystals and stones. Increased fluid intake can help to reduce the risk for encrustations and stone formation; the goal is typically production of at least 2 liters of urine per day, which usually requires 2000 to 4000 mL intake per day.[41,57]

Leakage of urine secondary to bladder spasm is a common problem in the patient with long-term urethral catheterization. The force generated by bladder spasms overwhelms the drainage capacity of the catheter, thus creating leakage around the catheter.[38] Common factors associated with leakage include UTI, catheter obstruction, and fecal impaction. Therefore, assessing and treating the underlying or precipitating cause of spasms comprise the first step. If bladder spasms are identified, and potential causes are addressed, then drug therapy with antispasmodics may be considered to suppress the bladder spasms[38] (Table 11-3). The anticholinergic effects of these drugs on bowel function predispose the patient to constipation and fecal impaction; therefore, a concurrent bowel program is recommended. In clinical practice, the tendency to exchange the catheter for a larger-lumen catheter should be avoided because the larger catheter lumen size imposes tension along the urethra, provokes urethral spasms, and exacerbates the problem.[51]

Suprapubic Catheters

Suprapubic catheters are an alternative to urethral catheters. Urinary drainage through the lower abdominal wall has advantages and disadvantages over the urethral route, as illustrated in Box 11-2.[48] Because suprapubic catheterization avoids urethral injury, it is viewed as a preferred treatment option for neurogenic bladder or bladder dysfunction.[58]

However, for patients with unstable bladder or intrinsic urethral sphincter deficiency, suprapubic catheterization is contraindicated.[58]

Suprapubic catheterization is theoretically associated with decreased risk for UTI and upper tract damage, because there are fewer microbes on the abdominal wall than on the perineum.[38,50] Although suprapubic catheters are associated with a lower risk of UTI, are generally more comfortable, and are frequently more acceptable to the patient, they are currently used much less commonly than urethral catheters.[48,59]

Reengineering of indwelling urinary catheters should address the current complications associated with their use. The current urinary catheter is a rigid structure that drains the bladder but blocks and irritates the urethra. Catheter design ideally should approximate the normal physiologic and mechanical characteristics of the voiding system.[60] The catheter of the future should be constructed of a thin-walled, continuously lubricated, collapsible (conformable) catheter to protect the integrity of the urethra; it should also include a system to hold the catheter in place without a balloon, and measures to imitate the intermittent "bladder washout" of normal voiding.[60] Such devices will, of course, need extensive testing to evaluate the efficacy of each component in reducing complications of long-term urethral catheterization.

Intermittent Catheterization

Intermittent catheterization is a therapeutic option for selected patients with neurogenic bladder or other problems with bladder emptying. The goal of intermittent catheterization is to empty the bladder

TABLE 11-3 Anticholinergics for Treatment of Bladder Spasm

MEDICATION	DOSAGE	COMMENTS
Oxybutynin (Ditropan)	2.5 to 5 mg four times daily	May have central anticholinergic effects
Flavoxate (Urispas)	100 to 200 mg four times daily	May have central anticholinergic effects
Dicyclomine (Bentyl)	10 to 20 mg four times daily	Unapproved for bladder spasticity
Hyoscyamine sulfate (Cystospaz)	0.125 to 0.25 mg four times daily	May have central anticholinergic effects
Tolterodine (Detrol)	1 to 2 mg twice daily	Better tolerated but may be less effective

From Cravens D, Zweig S: Urinary catheter management, *Am Fam Physician* 61(2):369-376, 2000.

BOX II-2   Suprapubic Catheterization: Advantages and Disadvantages

Advantages

Reduction in catheter-related pain
Improved patient acceptability
Reduced risk of urinary tract and genital infections
Reduction in penile/urethral injury
Uninhibited sexual performance
Spontaneous urethral voiding as desired
Ease of genital and catheter hygiene

Disadvantages

Urethral urinary leakage
Bleeding at catheter site
Surgical placement and site closure
Renal calculi
Abdominal wall complications: hematoma, cellulitis, dermatitis, fistula formation
Catheter dislodgement

From Gammack JK: Use and management of chronic urinary catheters in long-term care: much controversy, little consensus, *JAMA* 4(suppl):S53-S59, 2003.

periodically, thus reducing bladder distension and restoring blood flow to the bladder wall.[61] Host resistance to infection is preserved when blood flow to the bladder wall is maintained. Clean intermittent catheterization has been shown to be effective, with a low risk for infection and stone formation; however, complications such as creation of a false urethral passage, urethral strictures, and urethritis do occur, and more data are needed regarding long-term complication rates.[58,61,62] In selected cases, intermittent catheterization is viewed as a preferred option for management of neurogenic bladder or bladder outlet obstruction (as compared with indwelling catheterization).[48] Utilization of clean intermittent catheterization has been limited in long-term care facilities, in part because of the cost (of catheters, other supplies, and nursing labor) and in part because of the characteristics of the patient population. Intermittent catheterization may be emotionally traumatic or distressing to frail elders who have limited understanding of the procedure as a result of cognitive impairments or who experience physical pain or discomfort during the procedure. The benefit of intermittent catheterization over indwelling catheterization in the frail elderly or in the long-term care setting requires further randomized control trials.[48]

ABSORBENT PRODUCTS

Absorbent products absorb and contain urine to facilitate social continence. Absorbent pads and garments remain the mainstays of protection against urinary leakage. Absorptive products are available in both disposable and reusable forms and fit into two categories: bedpads or underpads and body-worn products. Body-worn products come in several designs: shields or guards, pant and pad systems, undergarments, and adult briefs (also known as adult diapers, although this term is discouraged). The wide variety of absorbent products provides the individual with numerous viable options for managing daytime and nighttime incontinence with optimal containment and skin protection.

Disposable products generally have three layers: an absorbent core sandwiched between a waterproof polyethylene backing and a water-permeable cover stock that is next to the skin. The primary component of the absorbent core can be a fluffed wood pulp fiber or cellulose core product (as in conventional disposable "diapers") or a cellulose core product that contains absorbent gelling material. The fluff pulp material is a relatively poor absorbent fiber. When wet, the saturated fiber creates moisture and warmth against the skin, thus increasing the risk for skin maceration, infection, and breakdown. Improvements in product design focus on superabsorbent polymers or absorbent gelling materials that wick and retain moisture in their core while keeping the surface of the material, and the skin, dry.[63] The superabsorbent product was introduced in the early 1980s, following its use in feminine hygiene products. The use of superabsorbent materials resulted in absorbent products that were thinner, lighter, and less likely to leak and cause skin rashes. These materials are concentrated in the perineal area of the pad or brief and retain more urine volume per weight than fluff pulp. Numerous advanced products are emerging: biodegradable disposable products, products enhanced with aloe vera and other skin conditioners, products enhanced with antifungal agents, and products with such "user-friendly" features as wetness indicators or "glow in the dark" frontal tapes.

Reusable absorbent products provide a useful alternative to disposable products in certain situations. These products are engineered from cotton or polyester; the absorbent core is usually made from knitted fabric (rayon and/or polyester fibers), and waterproof polymers may be adhered to the outer surface of the product to prevent leakage.[64] Reusable products may be more comfortable for the patient when they are dry, but they increase the risk for skin problems when they are wet; Hu and colleagues found a statistically significant increase in skin rashes among individuals managed with reusable products as compared with those managed with disposable products.[65] In addition, reusable products are less absorptive than disposables, which means that patients with large volume leakage require a waterproof barrier between the reusable product and their clothing. This barrier further increases heat and friction in the perineal area, which are predisposing factors for skin breakdown. Because of this limitation, some authors suggest that reusable products be used primarily for individuals with low-volume leakage,[66] and meticulous

attention to skin care is essential for any patient whose UI is managed with reusable products.

Bedpads or underpads are absorptive pads that are placed under the patient to protect bed linens. They come in disposable and reusable designs. A commonly used, inexpensive underpad is composed of fiberfill fluff with a polyester waterproof backing. This type of pad is not very useful for management of incontinence because it has poor absorptive capabilities and tends to bunch and wrinkle. In addition, this pad design has the disadvantage of creating heat and moisture at the skin surface, thus increasing the risk for skin maceration, dermatitis, infection, and breakdown. A more effective disposable underpad is engineered with three layers: a soft, nonwoven facing that does not retain moisture and keeps the skin drier; a middle layer of absorptive fibers (such as cellulose) and polymers that encapsulate fluids and lock in moisture; and a waterproof outer layer. Reusable underpads are composed of a quilted cotton or cotton/polyester surface, an absorbent middle layer made of polyester/rayon, and a waterproof backing of vinyl polyester. Underpads are designed with various absorptive capacities (from light to heavy).

Shields or guards are disposable absorptive pads with an adhesive strip that adheres to the patient's own underwear; they have variable capacity but in general are intended for episodic and limited leakage, as occurs with stress incontinence. Feminine hygiene pads represent an alternative to shields and guards for the female patient. Although these products were not designed to absorb urine, many women find that they provide adequate protection at a very low cost. Such products may be effective for low-volume incontinence, but skin rashes may develop if the pads are not changed when wet.

There are specially designed absorptive shields for men; these are pocket- or cup-shaped devices designed to be worn over the penis or around the penis and scrotum. In general, these devices have a capacity of about 90 to 120 mL and are intended primarily for the postprostatectomy patient with stress incontinence. Shields tend to be more acceptable because they are similar to athletic protectors and are more discreet (less bulky, bunchy, and noisy) than briefs or pads.

Pant and pad systems are designed for the ambulatory patient who needs more absorptive capacity than is provided by shields or guards, such as the patient with urge incontinence. The pant component is usually made of a lightweight stretch material such as mesh that can be washed and reused; the disposable pad may be affixed to the pant with an adhesive strip, may slip into a retention pocket, or may be secured with fasteners. This system can be very helpful for the patient with heavy leakage who is cognitively intact and involved in bladder retraining or some other type of bladder management program. The pant design facilitates toileting and supports the concept of continence, whereas the pad component provides backup protection. One-piece absorptive undergarments are an alternative to pant and pad systems. These panties or briefs are manufactured with extra absorptive padding in the crotch area. They are designed as an alternative to standard underwear and are available in disposable and reusable materials. The disposable product is similar to a toddler "pull-up" product. This design may be easier for some elders (or their caregivers) to manage because there is no fastening/unfastening required. When soiled, the disposable product can be torn apart at the side seam for removal; in contrast, the reusable product must be removed as a whole, and this may require removal of clothing.

Adult briefs are larger, one-piece absorptive products constructed with tape or Velcro-type attachments on each side. Adult briefs are generally reserved for the immobile or bedbound population or individuals with continuous or heavy UI. Adult briefs are designed to absorb a full incontinent void, approximately 10 to 12 oz, though absorptive capacity varies from product to product. The outer layer of these products consists of a waterproof backing that is designed to contain urine and prevent leakage onto clothing or furniture, but it contributes to an occlusive environment and increased risk for dermal complications such as fungal infections, dermatitis, and skin breakdown. To reduce this risk in immobile patients, the product can be left unsecured at the side seams to allow for air exchange. Newer products engineered as more "breathable"

may reduce the hazardous consequences of an occlusive environment. In one study, it was found that severe diaper dermatitis was reduced by 38% to 50% among infants wearing breathable diapers as compared with infants wearing standard, nonbreathable disposable diapers.[19] In addition, survival of *Candida* colonies was reduced by almost two-thirds in the sites covered with the "breathable" diaper as compared with the control sites. Some adult briefs now have a breathable plastic film outer layer with microporous openings that allow water vapor to pass to the outside while retaining fluid and odors.[62] Individuals prone to dermatitis and yeast infection should use a product that is breathable to reduce the risk for dermal complications.

Product Selection

Patients and caregivers are frequently overwhelmed by the number of products available, and products are often selected through trial and error;[62] to reduce frustration and improve outcomes, the clinician should assist the patient or caregiver to select products that best meet his or her needs. The clinician should determine the patient's leakage pattern and primary management program and should address the patient's and caregiver's concerns when making recommendations. Typically, patients and caregivers report the following expectations when selecting products to contain urinary leakage: effective containment of urine and odor without leakage, simplicity of use, protection against skin breakdown, protection that is discreet, and reasonable cost.

Disposable or Reusable? Reusable absorbent products were the mainstay of incontinence management until the 1960s, when disposable products became more popular and affordable for use with infants.[66] Since then, the disposable product industry has manufactured adult absorbent products that are more diverse in design with improved urine containment and skin health properties. Factors to consider when recommending products are the type and volume of incontinence; as noted, reusable products are less absorptive than disposable products and are most appropriate for individuals with low-volume leakage. In addition, patients with both fecal and urinary incontinence may be best managed with disposable products, because these products provide better odor control and avoid the challenges associated with effectively laundering products soiled with both urine and stool. A second factor to consider is cost. Disposable products are less costly "per product;" however, the higher initial cost for the reusable product may be offset at least partially by the long life span. When calculating the cost of reusable products, laundering costs (including water and energy costs) must also be considered; these costs may significantly reduce the apparent savings provided by reusable products. A third factor to consider is the impact of various products on the environment. Although reusable products contribute to air and water pollution and add further burden to community water and sewage systems, the use of disposables creates additional landfill waste because these products are not completely biodegradable, and disposable products may also be a source of groundwater contamination. Many community landfill operations are close

to maximum capacity, and some communities have enacted landfill regulations that restrict disposal of absorbent products[66-68] (Table 11-4).

Ability to Contain Urine and Odor. The ability of a product to contain urine without leakage also affects odor control and is obviously a major concern for patients and caregivers. The properties and features known to affect a product's ability to contain urine and to prevent leakage effectively include absorption capacity, absorption speed, retention capacity and wet-back properties, product fit, pad shape, and the presence or absence of elastication and barrier cuffs. Some products are equipped with wetness indicators, which assist the caregiver in determining when to change the product. There are also electronic alarm devices, which can be used to notify caregivers of the need to change an absorbent product.

The retention capacity and wet-back properties affect the product's ability to prevent maceration and to protect the skin. Storer-Brown found polymer

TABLE II-4 **Comparison of Disposable versus Reusable/Washable Pads**

DISPOSABLE PADS	REUSABLE/WASHABLE PADS
Less expensive initially (per unit) but can be more expensive long term	Available in styles similar to normal-looking underwear
Useful for trips or short periods	Less bulky to store than disposables because fewer are needed
May be fitted with an adhesive strip for easier positioning in underwear	Should be stored in an airtight container until they can be washed.
Some brands more absorbent for heavy incontinence- and not too bulky when made with superabsorbent gel or polymer	May be guaranteed to last 200 or more washes if the manufacturer's washing and drying instructions are followed
Available with a wetness strip to indicate need for changing	May be softer on the skin, less friction
Recommended for both fecal and urinary incontinence	**Disadvantages**
Disadvantages	More expensive to buy up front; wrong choices can be costly
More costly in the long run	Not recommended for heavy urine loss; large pads may still leak
Problematic for public waste management and landfills; may contribute to groundwater contamination	Not recommended for fecal incontinence, poor containment and staining
Products can be bulky and noisy, causing embarrassment to the wearer	Requires machine washing and following manufacturer's instructions
	Washing wet or soiled pads is unpleasant; need to rinse soiled pads before laundering
	More skin problems associated with some cloth products

products (products that contain a gelling agent that wicks the urine away from the skin and encapsulates it in a gel matrix) to be significantly more effective in containing urine and protecting the skin than nonpolymer products.[69] Superabsorbent products perform better than fluff products, and patients with fragile skin or large-volume incontinence are best managed with these products.

Simplicity of Use. The patient or caregiver must be able to use the product appropriately, and some products require greater dexterity or a higher level of cognitive function than others; for example, some pant and pad systems require the patient to insert the absorptive pad into a retention pocket or to secure the pad to Velcro fasteners or to straps with buttons. Another consideration is the patient's mobility; some products are easier to use with bedbound patients, whereas others are designed with the ambulatory population in mind. Products designed as "briefs" (the adult version of diapers) typically fasten with tapes and are more difficult and time consuming to remove and reapply than shields or pant and pad systems that are simply pulled up and down. The ambulatory patient who is using the absorptive product as an adjunct to a primary bladder management program will in general find a "guard" or "pant and pad" system more conducive to a toileting program and more supportive of "continence" than an adult brief. Conversely, the caregiver managing a bedbound patient typically finds it much easier to use absorbent underpads and briefs that fasten with tapes (because these products can easily be changed when the patient is rolled from side to side) as opposed to a system that must be pulled up and down.

Protection that is Discreet. For the patient who is ambulatory and active, discretion is an important feature of any bladder management program. This patient will benefit from a product that is low profile and formulated with a "quiet" cover film. This type of design prevents pad noise during physical activity, often a sure "giveaway" that the patient is wearing a pad. Many socially active patients are very conscious of this product feature. Most shields and guards meet these criteria, as do many of the pant and pad systems. In contrast, the caregiver managing a bedbound patient is less likely to be concerned with discretion and more likely to be concerned with ease of use and absorptive capacity. A second pad characteristic is bulkiness. Bulky pads are more noticeable to others and may even alter the fit of the individual's clothing. In some instances, the patient may have to restrict the types of clothing worn because the bulk of the product makes clothing too tight. Women may stop wearing slacks or other "fitted" clothing because of bulky pads. This can further increase the stress and anxiety associated with the incontinence. Thus, selection of products should conform to patient preferences.

Cost. The cost of the product is certainly an important factor in product selection. In some situations, cost may be the primary determining factor. In one trial, Hu and colleagues compared the cost of reusable and disposable absorbent products and concluded that the laundry costs associated with disposable products (bed linens, etc.) were significantly lower because the disposables leaked less than reusable products. Because data suggest that efficacy of reusable products is higher when leakage is low volume, reusable products may be a viable alternative for both cost and containment in patients with "light" UI, but disposable products are likely to be more cost effective for patients with "heavy" UI.[65,66] Higher costs associated with dermal complications such as rashes, infections, and breakdown should also be considered. Products should be evaluated and differentiated for daytime and night time use. The clinician should help the patient or caregiver (or the institution) make decisions based on overall cost of management as opposed to cost per unit of product. A more costly product that provides superior absorption, odor control, and skin protection may be more cost effective than a less expensive and less effective product that requires more frequent changes of absorptive product and linen and that is associated with a higher incidence of skin breakdown. Cost can be modified by using just "enough" product; for example, a high-quality absorbent product that is "downsized" from a brief to a pad insert or pad and pant system can contribute to cost savings without compromising wetness protection. Tailoring product use to the individual's lifestyle, mobility, skin condition, and personal preferences can help to achieve optimal utilization at minimal cost.

Other considerations for product selection include product performance (ability to absorb varying volumes of urine and to contain fecal leakage and fecal odor effectively), the environmental cost of product disposal, patients' and caregivers' preferences for different products under different conditions, and the limitations posed by nonavailability of products in some communities; these issues need to be addressed in clinical studies.[68,70]

When advising patients and caregivers about products, the clinician should obtain a careful history of the patient's mobility and manual dexterity, lifestyle (daily physical and social activities, exercise), toileting pattern, frequency and volume of incontinence, history of skin problems and current skin condition, desire for aesthetic discretion, type of clothing usually worn, and access to product resources. Usually, a trial of various types of products is needed to obtain the best match between products and patient/caregiver preferences and to optimize the patient's and caregiver's quality of life and well-being.

BEDSIDE EQUIPMENT

Bedside equipment such as bedside commodes, raised toilet seats, male and female urinals, and bedpans facilitates toilet access and helps to maintain continence. For individuals with impaired mobility, bedside equipment may promote improved continence by eliminating or compensating for environmental barriers to toilet access. In the frail older adult, bedside equipment and other environmental modifications are of great importance because they serve a compensatory role that enables optimal function and prevents excess disability.[64] Research suggests that UI is an independent risk factor for falls in the elderly, and the use of bedside equipment is one way to reduce the risk for falls while enhancing toilet access and continence.[71]

Bedside commodes are portable toilet substitutes that can be situated close to the bed to facilitate voiding in patients with mobility impairments. For patients with nocturia who are also at high risk for falls, a bedside commode for nocturnal voiding may improve both safety and continence.

Bedside commode designs have changed little over the years, although some commodes have drop arms and adjustable heights to accommodate individual needs. Safety issues associated with bedside commode design include difficulties with sideways transfer, ineffective brakes that cause slippage during transfer, and inadequate trunk support.[62]

Raised toilet seats are placed over the regular toilet seat to facilitate transfer onto and off of the toilet. Raised toilet seats are particularly useful for older patients with weak quadriceps muscles, arthritis in the hips or knees, or a history of hip fracture. Raised toilet seats address a functional limitation to toileting and can help an individual maintain independence in toileting.

Grab bars can be affixed to the side of the toilet and/or to the bathroom wall; grab bars on the wall provide support for the patient in ambulating to the toilet, and grab bars assist both ambulatory and nonambulatory patients to get onto and off of the toilet.

Hand-held urinals are available for both men and women. They are a staple in management of male UI, but female urinals have yet to achieve widespread recognition and use. Urinals can be used independently by patients who have impaired mobility but who retain good manual dexterity; patients who lack manual dexterity may still benefit from the use of urinals with the assistance of caregivers. Some urinals have openings with an internal flange that extends into the urinal and does not allow backflow of urine even when they are tilted upside down; these can be very helpful in preventing spillage.[62,70] For the male patient with a retracted penis, there are urinals with a larger funnel opening that fits over the penis. Female urinals are designed with a cup that fits snugly over the urethra to form a seal so leakage does not occur during voiding. Female urinals work best when used in the standing or squatting position; unfortunately, the design is not optimal for women who need to use the urinal while in the bed or chair, because it is difficult to position the urinal in a manner that facilitates drainage of a full void into the urinal without leakage.[62,72] The Futuro female urinal is manufactured with a "bellows" design that conforms to the curvature of the perineum for comfort and for prevention of

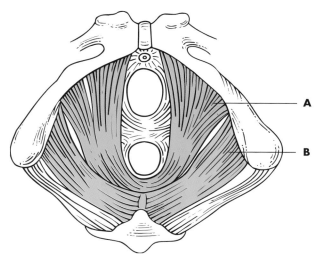

Plate 1 The two segments of levator ani muscle in female. *A,* Thicker U-shaped (pubovisceral) portion arises from pubic bones and attaches to lateral walls of vagina and rectum. *B,* Thinner coccygeal portion originates from pelvic side walls and inserts into bony pelvis behind rectum.

A

B

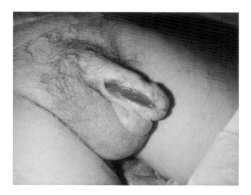

Plate 2 Urethral erosion extending from base of penis to scrotum caused by pressure from indwelling catheter. Urethral catheters should be secured to the lower abdomen or upper thigh in men to reduce pressure at the urethral-scrotal junction. (Courtesy Carolyn Crumley, RN)

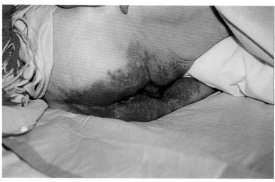

Plate 3 Severe irritant dermatitis, characterized by erythema, edema, epidermal loss, and pain. (Courtesy Debra Thayer, St. Paul, MN)

Plate 4 *Candida albicans* infection, characterized by central confluent erythema and diffuse border with satellite lesions. (Courtesy Coloplast Corp., CEU video program, *Common perineal skin injuries,* Marietta, GA)

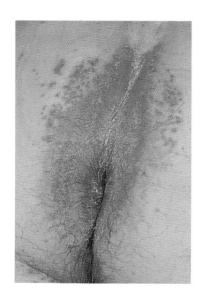
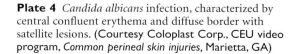

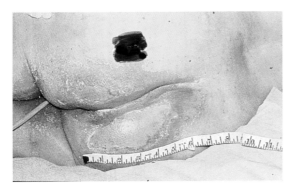

Plate 5 Skin breakdown caused by maceration and friction.

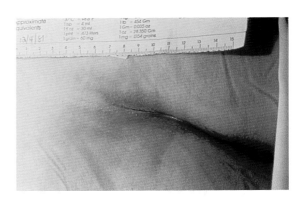

Plate 6 Resolving intertrigo. (Courtesy Debra Thayer, St. Paul, MN)

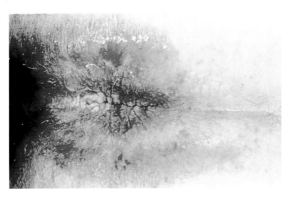

Plate 7 Pruritus ani. (Courtesy Coloplast Corp., CEU video program, *Common perineal skin injuries*, Marietta, GA)

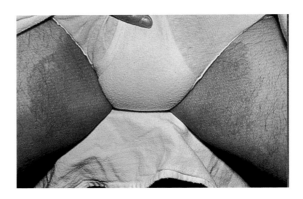

Plate 8 Erythrasma along inner thighs. Notice absence of satellite lesions. (Courtesy Coloplast Corp., CEU video program, *Common perineal skin injuries*, Marietta, GA)

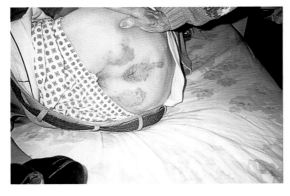

Plate 9 Perineal psoriasis. Notice distinct margins, silvery color, and lack of satellite lesions. (Courtesy Debra Thayer, St. Paul, MN)

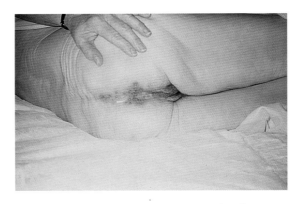

Plate 10 Perianal herpes lesions. Notice distribution along perineal dermatome. (Courtesy Debra Thayer, St. Paul, MN)

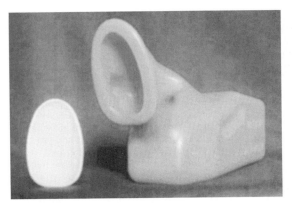

Feminal™

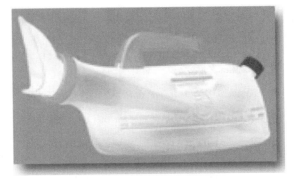

URSEC™

Fig. 11-4 Female urinals. (Feminal™ courtesy Bruce Medical, Waltham, MA; URSEC™, Providence Spillproof Container courtesy Allegro Medical, Providence, RI.)

leakage during use. The Feminal urinal is designed with a handle grip for use in the standing, sitting, or lying position by the patient or caregiver. The URSEC offers a spillproof design with an antireflux system. Fig. 11-4 illustrates female urinal designs.

SUMMARY

Comprehensive management of UI may involve the use of containment devices, absorptive products, catheters, and skin care regimens. For the patient with intractable incontinence, these measures can be essential for the maintenance of skin integrity

and urine containment, preservation of dignity, and promotion of social continence. The utilization of skin care protocols in patients with intractable incontinence reduces the incidence of dermatologic complications such as skin infection, perineal dermatitis, breakdown, and pressure ulcers. Thoughtful utilization of absorbent products, equipment, and devices offers a range of viable alternatives for urine containment. Employment of indwelling urinary catheters, when medically indicated or used as a last resort, requires careful catheter selection and strategies to reduce the risk for symptomatic UTI, obstruction, bladder spasm, and leakage. The clinician must be knowledgeable regarding both the principles of urine containment and skin care and the guidelines for effective use of products, equipment, and devices to provide optimal care for individuals with UI.

SELF-ASSESSMENT EXERCISE

1. Define the term "intractable incontinence," and outline goals for patient management.
2. Explain how each of the following contributes to skin breakdown in the incontinent patient: (a) fecal incontinence, (b) underhydration or overhydration of the epidermis, (c) elevated skin temperature, (d) alkaline pH, (e) cleansing procedures that cause loss of skin lipids.
3. Identify signs, symptoms, and management for each of the following: (a) irritant dermatitis, (b) perineal yeast infection, (c) estrogen deficiency.
4. Explain the value of MSDS sheets in the evaluation of topical products.
5. Explain the role of each of the following in incontinent skin care: (a) cleansers, (b) moisturizers, (c) moisture barriers (creams, ointments, pastes), (d) powders, (e) liquid film barriers.
6. List strategies that improve success in the use of external male catheters.
7. Identify currently accepted criteria for long-term use of indwelling catheters.

8. Identify guidelines for catheter selection.

9. Identify factors the clinician should consider when selecting an absorbent product.

REFERENCES

1. Lekan-Rutledge D, Colling J: Urinary incontinence in the frail elderly, *Am J Nurs* 103(suppl):36-46, 2003.
2. Ouslander J, Johnson T: Continence care for frail older adults: it is time to go beyond assessing quality, *J Am Directors Assoc* May/June:213-216, 2004.
3. Diokno A: Epidemiology of urinary incontinence, *J Gerontol A Biol Sci Med Sci* 56:M3-M4, 2001.
4. Storer-Brown D: Perineal dermatitis risk factors: clinical validation of a conceptual framework, *Ostomy Wound Manage* 41(10):46-48, 50, 52-53, 1995.
5. Ghadially R, Brown BE, Sequeira-Martin SM, et al: The aged epidermal permeability barrier: structural, functional, and lipid biochemical abnormalities in humans and a senescent murine model, *J Clin Invest* 95: 2281-2290, 1995.
6. Schnelle JF, Adamson GM, Cruise PA, et al: Skin disorders and moisture in incontinent nursing home residents: intervention implications, *J Am Geriatr Soc* 45(10):1182-1188, 1997.
7. Schaefer H, Redelmeier TE: *Skin barrier: principles of percutaneous absorption,* Basel, 1996, Karger, pp 43-86.
8. Menczel E: Assessment of delipidization as an enhancing factor in percutaneous penetration, *Curr Probl Dermatol* 22:189-194, 1995.
9. Dikstein S, Slotogorski A: Measurement of skin pH, *Acta Derm Venereol Suppl* (Stockh) 185:18-20, 1994.
10. Berg RW: Etiology and pathophysiology of diaper dermatitis, *Adv Dermatol* 3:75-98, 1988.
11. Lund W: *The pharmaceutical codex: principles and practices of pharmaceutics,* London, 1994, Pharmaceutical Press.
12. Berg RW, Buckingham KW, Stewart RL: Etiologic factors in diaper dermatitis: the role of feces, *Pediatr Dermatol* 3:107-112, 1986.
13. Zimmerer RE: The effects of wearing diapers on skin, *Pediatr Dermatol* 3(2):95-101, 1986.
14. Leyden JJ, Katz S, Stewart R, Kligman AM: Urinary ammonia and ammonia producing organisms in infants with and without diaper dermatitis, *Arch Dermatol* 113:1678-1680, 1977.
15. Andersen PH, Bucher AP, Saeed I, et al: Faecal enzymes: in vivo human skin irritation, *Contact Dermatitis* 30(3):152-158, 1994.
16. Berg RW, Mulligan MC, Sarbaugh FC: Association of skin wetness and pH with diaper dermatitis, *Pediatr Dermatol* 11(1):18-20, 1994.
17. Leyden JJ, Kligman AM: The role of microorganisms in diaper dermatitis, *Arch Dermatol* 114(1):56-59, 1978.
18. Gray M, Ratliffe C, Donovan A: Perineal skin care, *Adv Skin Wound Care* 15(4):170-178, 2002.
19. Akin F, Spraker M, Aly R, et al: Effects of breathable disposable diapers: reduced prevalence of *Candida* and common diaper dermatitis, *Pediatr Dermatol* 18(4): 282-290, 2001.
20. Atherton DJ: The aetiology and management of irritant diaper dermatitis, *J Eur Acad Dermatol Venereol* 15(suppl 1):1-4, 2001.
21. Faria D, Stoia-Davis J, Thayer D: *Common Perineal Skin Injuries.* Coloplast Corporation, Marietta, GA, 1996.
22. Fiers S: Breaking the cycle: the etiology of incontinence dermatitis and evaluating and using skin care products, *Ostomy Wound Manage* 42(3):32-43, 1996.
23. Haugen V: Perineal skin care for patients with frequent diarrhea or fecal incontinence, *Gastroenterol Nurs* 20(3):87-90, 1997.
24. Fantl JA, Newman DK, Colling J, et al: *Urinary incontinence in adults: acute and chronic management,* Clinical practice guideline No. 2, Publication No. 96-0682, Rockville, Md., 1996 update, United States Department of Health and Human Services, Agency for Health Care Policy and Research.
25. Widmer J, Elsner P, Burg G: Skin irritant reactivity following experimental cumulative irritant contact dermatitis, *Contact Dermatitis* 30:38, 1994.
26. Bergstrom N, Allman RM, Carlson CE, et al: *Pressure ulcers in adults: prediction and prevention,* Clinical practice guideline No. 3, Publication No. 92:0050, Rockville, Md., 1992, United States Department of Health and Human Services, Agency for Health Care Policy and Research.
27. Skewes SM: Skin care rituals that do more harm than good, *Am J Nurs* 96(10):33-35, 1996.
28. Larson E: APIC Guideline for hand-washing and hand antisepsis in health care settings, *Am J Infect Control* 23:251-269, 1995.
29. Larson E: Skin hygiene and infection prevention: more of the same or different approaches? *Clin Infect Dis* 29(5): 1287-1294, 1999.
30. Hunter S, Anderson J, Hanson D, et al: Clinical trial of a prevention and treatment protocol for skin breakdown in two nursing homes, *J Wound Ostomy Continence Nurs* 30(5):250-258, 2003.
31. Bale S, Tebele N, Jones V, Price P: The benefits of implementing a new skin care protocol in nursing homes, *J Tissue Viabil* 14(2):44-50, 2004.
32. Byers PH, Ryan PA, Regan MB, et al: Effects of incontinence care cleansing regimens on skin integrity, *J Wound Ostomy Continence Nurs* 22(4):187-192, 1995.
33. Lyder CH, Clemes-Lowrance C, Davis A, et al: Structured skin care regimen to prevent perineal dermatitis in the elderly, *J ET Nurs* 19(1):12-16, 1992.
34. McMullen D: *Candida albicans* and incontinence, *Dermatol Nurs* 3(1):21-24, 1991.
35. Welzel J, Wilhalm KP, Wolff HH: Skin permeability barrier and occlusion: no delay of repair in irritated human skin, *Contact Dermatitis* 35:163-168, 1996.
36. Fisher A: Contact urticaria and anaphylactoid reaction due to cornstarch surgical glove powder, *Contact Dermatitis* 16(4):224-225, 1987.

37. Grove GL, Leyden JJ: *Comparison of the skin protectant properties of various film forming products,* Minneapolis, 1993, 3M Health Care.
38. Cravens D, Zweig S: Urinary catheter management, *Am Fam Physician* 61(2):369-376, 2000.
39. Clinical Practice Committee of WOCN: *Fact sheet on external catheters.* Laguna Beach, Calif., 1996, Wound Ostomy Continence Nurses Society.
40. Pieper B, Cleland V, Johnson D, O'Reilly J: Inventing urine incontinence devices for women, *Image J Nurs Sch* 21(4):205-209, 1989.
41. Morris NS, Stickler DJ: Does drinking cranberry juice produce urine inhibitory to the development of crystalline, catheter blocking *Proteus mirabilis* biofilms? *Br J Urol* 88:192-197, 2001.
42. Saint S, Lipsky BA, Goold DR: Indwelling urinary catheters: a one-point restraint? *Ann Intern Med* 137:125-127, 2002.
43. Agency for Health Care Policy and Research: *Urinary incontinence in adults,* Clinical practice guideline, Rockville, Md., 1992, United States Department of Health and Human Services, Agency for Health Care Policy and Research.
44. Wong ES, Hooton TM: Guidelines for the prevention of catheter-associated urinary tract infections: guidelines for the prevention and control of nosocomial infections, *Am J Infect Control* 11(1):28-36, 1983.
45. Bob H: Chronic indwelling catheters in nursing facilities: are fewer always better? *AMDA Caring Aged* 3(4):3-4, 2002.
46. Wilde MH: Urinary tract infection in people with long-term urinary catheters, *J Wound Ostomy Continence Nurs* 30(6):314-323, 2003.
47. Washington EA: Instillation of 3% hydrogen peroxide or distilled vinegar in urethral catheter drainage bag to decrease catheter-associated bacteriuria, *Biol Res Nurs* 3(2):78-87, 2001.
48. Gammack JK: Use and management of chronic urinary catheters in long-term care: much controversy, little consensus, *JAMA* 4(suppl):S53-S59, 2003.
49. Madigan E, Neff DF: Care of patients with long-term indwelling urinary catheters, *Online J Issues Nurs* 8(3):7, 2003.
50. Saint S, Lipsky BA: Preventing catheter-related bacteriuria: should we? Can we? How? *Arch Intern Med* 159(8):800-808, 1999.
51. Gray M: What nursing interventions reduce the risk of symptomatic urinary tract infection in the patient with an indwelling catheter? *J Wound Ostomy Continence Nurs* 31(1):3-13, 2004.
52. Saint S: Clinical and economic consequences of nosocomial catheter-related bacteriuria, *Am J Infect Control* 28(1):68-75,2000.
53. Kunin CM, Douthitt S, Dancing J, et al: The association between the use of urinary catheters and morbidity and mortality among elderly patients in nursing homes, *Am J Epidemiol* 135:291-301, 1992.
54. Getliffe K. Managing recurrent urinary catheter blockage: problems, promises, and practicalities. *J Wound Ostomy Continence Nurs* 30(3):146-151, 2003.
55. Gray M: Are cranberry juice or cranberry products effective in the prevention or management of urinary tract infection? *J Wound Ostomy Continence Nurs* 29(3):122-126, 2002.
56. Burr RG, Nuselbeh IM: Urinary catheter blockage depends on urine pH, calcium, and rate of flow, *Spinal Cord* 35:521-525, 1997.
57. National Kidney and Urologic Diseases Information Clearing House: National Institute of Diabetes and Digestive and Kidney Diseases (NIDDK). NIH Publication No. 05-2495. Bethesda, Md., 2004, National Institutes of Health.
58. Schnelle JF, Smith RL: Quality indicators for the management of urinary incontinence in vulnerable community-dwelling elders, *Ann Intern Med* 135(8):752-758, 2001.
59. Hebel JR, Warren JW: The use of urethral, condom, and suprapubic catheters in aged nursing home patients, *J Am Geriatr Soc* 38:777-784, 1990.
60. Kunin C: Nosocomial urinary tract infections and the indwelling catheter: what is new and what is true? *Chest* 120(1):10-12, 2001.
61. Lapides J, Diokno AC, Silber SM, Lowe BS: Clean intermittent self-catheterization in the treatment of urinary tract disease, *J Urol* 167(4):1584-1586, 2002.
62. Newman DK: Incontinence products and devices for the elderly, *Urol Nurs* 24(4):316-334, 2004.
63. Lekan-Rutledge D, Doughty D, Moore KN, Wooldridge L: Promoting social continence: products and devices in the management of urinary incontinence, *Urol Nurs* 23(6):416-428, 458, 2004.
64. Lekan-Rutledge D: Urinary incontinence strategies for frail elderly women, *Urol Nurs* 24(4):281-302, 2004.
65. Hu T, Kaltreider DL, Igou J: Incontinence products: which is best? *Geriatr Nurs* 10:184-186, 1989.
66. Macaulay M, Clarke-O'Neill S, Fader M, et al: A pilot study to evaluate reusable absorbent body-worn products for adults with moderate/heavy urinary incontinence, *J Wound Ostomy Continence Nurs* 31:357-366, 2004.
67. Brazilli SE: Absorbent products for containing urinary and/or faecal incontinence in adults, *Cochrane Database Sys Rev* 3:1-26, 2002.
68. Brazilli SE, Shirran E, Vale L: Absorbent products for containing urinary and/or fecal incontinence in adults, *J Wound Ostomy Continence Nurs* 29(1):45-54, 2002.
69. Storer-Brown D: Diapers and underpads. Part I: skin integrity outcomes, *Ostomy Wound Manage* 40(9):20-30, 32, 1994.
70. Newman DK, Fader M, Bliss DZ: Managing incontinence using technology, devices, and products: directions for research, *Nurs Res* 54(6 suppl):S42-S48, 2004.
71. Brown J, Vittinghoff E, Wyman J, et al: Urinary incontinence: does it increase risk for falls and fractures? *J Am Geriatr Soc* 48(7):721-725, 2000.
72. Fader M, Pettersson L, Dean G, et al: The selection of female urinals: results of a multicentre evaluation, *Br J Nurs* 8(14):918-925, 1999.

12 Assessment of Patients with Urinary Incontinence

MIKEL L. GRAY & KATHERINE N. MOORE

OBJECTIVES

1. Construct or use a structured data collection tool to gather and record all critical subjective data from a patient with urinary incontinence.
2. Explain the importance of a bladder chart to the assessment of a patient with urinary incontinence.
3. Identify data to be included in an environmental assessment of the incontinent individual.
4. Describe the specific anatomic and functional factors to be assessed during the physical examination of an individual with urinary incontinence (to include gender-specific factors).
5. Explain why a uroflow study is said to be a screening test for voiding dysfunction but noncontributory to the diagnosis of urinary incontinence.
6. Explain indications, guidelines, and interpretation for provocative maneuvers.
7. Identify indications for complex urodynamic studies in the assessment of an individual with urinary incontinence.
8. Outline information provided by each of the following studies: cystometrogram, voiding cystometrogram (pressure-flow study), videourodynamics, striated sphincter electromyography, abdominal leak point pressure.
9. Identify laboratory tests that should be routinely included in the workup for a patient with urinary incontinence.

The assessment of an individual with urinary incontinence (UI) is influenced by the presence and severity of lower urinary tract symptoms (LUTS), the pathophysiology of the UI, the presence of complicating factors such as urinary tract infection

(UTI), and the goals of management. Nevertheless, some components of the assessment are considered essential when evaluating *any* individual with UI. The International Consultation on Incontinence advocates several essential components for routine assessment of the patient with UI including a focused history, physical examination, urinalysis, and voiding diary.[1] Routine postvoid residual measurement is also advocated in the specialist setting,[1] but in the primary care setting we recommend measurement only in selected cases in which a reasonable suspicion of retention exists. Urodynamic testing is indicated in patients who fail to respond to initial treatment, those with complex UI not adequately evaluated with simpler techniques, and those whose UI is complicated by retention, upper urinary tract distress, significant pelvic organ prolapse, or neurologic disorders. Imaging studies such as ultrasonography, radionuclide scans, or intravenous urography are indicated only in highly selected patients with urinary retention, upper tract distress, hematuria, or inflammatory lesions complicating UI.[2] These patients also may require endoscopic examination or serum studies to further evaluate renal function. This chapter provides a thorough review of the essential elements of assessment for an individual with UI and includes urodynamic testing. In addition, the indications and interpretation of urinary system imaging studies, endoscopy, and serum studies are discussed.

LOWER URINARY TRACT SYMPTOMS

Traditionally, the bladder has been described as an "unreliable witness" and "unable to express its own pathology."[3,4] The basis for these characterizations is the weak correlation between reported symptoms and underlying lower urinary tract disorders.

Although it is true that many of the symptoms expressed by patients do not strongly correlate with the underlying pathophysiology or with the care provider's perceptions of severity and clinical relevance, we must nevertheless remember that these symptoms *are* the barometer that patients use to define severity and bothersomeness. Further, it is the presence of bothersome LUTS, combined with social and media influences, that guide the decision to seek care.[5] Because many lower urinary tract diseases are primarily quality of life disorders, the most direct outcomes of care are based on alleviation of bothersome symptoms rather than indirect measures such as changes in residual urine volumes, bladder capacity, or urodynamic findings.

Therefore, to better understand these symptoms and their relation to lower urinary tract disorders, the term "lower urinary tract symptoms" has been adopted to describe the range of symptoms associated with bladder filling, storage, and emptying. This construct applies to a variety of symptoms associated with multiple disorders affecting urinary continence and voiding efficiency. Table 12-1 outlines common LUTS as defined by the International Continence Society (ICS).[6]

HISTORY

A thorough history is the first component of assessment for any individual with UI. The history is obtained during a face-to-face interview that allows the patient to share his or her concerns related to urinary leakage, although portions may be completed using a standardized form that is reviewed with the patient during the interview.

Chief Complaint

Because the term "incontinence" frequently has negative connotations and has also been used to describe loss of control over sexual behavior, it may be best to ask the patient a more specific question, such as "Do you have bladder control problems?" "Do you have trouble with leaking or dripping urine?" or "Why do you wear pads or absorptive products in your underclothing?" The patient should be allowed time to answer this open-ended question as completely as possible; the clinician may then "follow-up" with specific questions that address

the severity, possible etiologic factors, and treatment options for managing UI.

Onset and Duration of Urinary Incontinence

UI is classified as acute (transient) or chronic (established), and a diagnosis of chronic UI is further subdivided into types such as stress, urge, or mixed. Queries regarding the onset of UI can assist the clinician to determine the type of UI experienced by the individual patient. Acute UI is typically characterized by a sudden onset or exacerbation of urine loss, which often coincides with an acute illness. Acute UI differs from chronic UI, which usually has a gradual or insidious onset and persists for many months or even years before the patient seeks help. Like many chronic conditions, LUTS are likely to undergo periods of exacerbation alternating with periods of remission with milder or fewer symptoms. The exception is chronic UI caused by a paralyzing neurologic disorder such as a stroke or spinal cord injury. In these cases, bladder dysfunction tends to persist over time, even after initial recovery and rehabilitation.

Storage Lower Urinary Tract Symptoms

After determining the onset and duration of the patient's UI, the clinician should query the patient about LUTS. Questions about filling and storage symptoms begin with daytime voiding frequency and nocturia. The questions "How often do you void during the day?" or "How many times do you urinate while awake?" may be difficult to answer with any degree of accuracy. It is often more effective to ask the patient to gauge daytime frequency using an interval example. For example, the patient may be asked whether she or he can sit through a 2-hour movie or meeting before urinating or how long he or she can drive or ride in an automobile before pulling over to urinate. *Increased daytime frequency* is defined as a voiding interval of less than 2 hours during waking hours or more than eight voiding episodes during a 24-hour period. It is associated with multiple lower urinary tract disorders including overactive bladder dysfunction, UI, UTI, and bladder outlet obstruction.[7,8]

TABLE 12-1   **Lower Urinary Tract Symptoms**

SYMPTOM	DESCRIPTION	NORMAL REFERENCE RANGE
Storage Symptoms		
Daytime frequency	Perception of voiding too often during waking hours	Voiding every 2 hours or less often, no more than eight voids over a 24-hour period
Nocturia	Awakening one time or more at night to urinate	Less than 65 years of age: zero to one episode. 65 years of age or older: zero to two episodes
Urgency (sometimes called bothersome urgency)	Sudden and compelling need to urinate that is difficult to defer	Physiologic desire or urgency to urinate that may be deferred or ignored for prolonged periods of time if socially desired
UI	Complaint of any involuntary leakage of urine	Absence of urine loss
Stress UI	Complaint of urinary leakage with physical exertion or with coughing or sneezing	Absence of urine loss with these provocative maneuvers
Urge UI	Complaint of urine loss accompanied or immediately preceded by urgency	Absence of urine loss, even in the presence of urgency
Mixed UI	Complaint of both stress and urge UI symptoms as described above	Absence of urine loss
Continuous UI	Complaint of continuous urine loss	Absence of urine loss
Nocturnal enuresis	Complaint of urine loss while sleeping	Absence of urine loss while asleep
Voiding Symptoms		
Slow stream	Complaint of reduced urine flow as compared with previous patterns or in comparison with others	Continuous urine stream
Splitting or spraying	Complaint of dual urine streams or spraying of urine from urethral meatus	Continuous, single urine stream
Intermittency of urine stream	Complaint that urine stream starts and stops one or more times during single micturition episode	Continuous, single urine stream
Hesitancy	Complaint of difficulty initiating urine stream despite desire to urinate	Prompt onset of urine stream with micturition
Straining	Use of muscular effort (contraction of abdominal muscles) to initiate, maintain, or improve urinary stream	Continuous, single urine stream
Terminal dribble	Description of trickle or dribbling flow near the end of micturition	Continuous, single urine stream
Postmicturition Symptoms		
Postmicturition dribble (postvoid dribbling)	Complaint of urine loss immediately following micturition, when arising from toilet or when replacing clothing	Absence of postmicturition dribble
Feelings of incomplete emptying	Perception of incomplete bladder evacuation despite micturition	Absence of symptom

Continued

TABLE 12-1   Lower Urinary Tract Symptoms—cont'd

SYMPTOM	DESCRIPTION	NORMAL REFERENCE RANGE
Lower Urinary Tract Pain		
Bladder pain	Report of discomfort located in suprapubic or retropubic region, exacerbated by bladder filling; may be relieved or persist after micturition	Absence of pain with bladder filling or micturition
Urethral pain	Discomfort localized to urethra, often exacerbated by micturition	Absence of pain with bladder filling or micturition
Vulvar pain	Discomfort localized to the area in and around the external genitalia	Absence of pain
Vaginal pain	Discomfort localized to vaginal area and above the introitus	Absence of pain
Scrotal pain	Discomfort localized to the testis, epididymis, spermatic cord, or scrotal skin, pain may be difficult to localize	Absence of pain
Perineal pain	Female: discomfort localized to area between the posterior lip of the vaginal introitus and anus Male: discomfort localized between the scrotum and anus	Absence of pain
Pelvic pain	Poorly localized discomfort associated with lower urinary tract and/or fecal elimination cycle	Absence of pain

UI, urinary incontinence.
Data from Abrams P, Cardozo L, Fall M, et al: Standardization Sub-committee of the International Continence Society: the standardization of terminology of lower urinary tract function: report from the Standardization Sub-committee of the International Continence Society. *Neurourol Urodyn* 21(2):167-178, 2002.

Infrequent urination may be defined as a voiding interval of more than 6 hours; this elimination pattern is typical in the individual with a large-capacity bladder. Some individuals consciously adopt this pattern of urination to avoid use of public toilet facilities; others void infrequently because of denervation associated with long-term diabetes mellitus or chronic alcoholism. Infrequent urination is seen in patients with UTI (particularly in children), urinary retention, and occupations that do not allow adequate time for routine urination.[9-12]

Nocturia is defined as the interruption of sleep caused by the urge to urinate. It is important to distinguish true nocturia from incidental nocturnal voiding in the person who was wakened by factors unrelated to the bladder (such as pain or insomnia); one can determine this by asking a question such as, "Is it the urge to urinate that causes you to awaken?" Although many persons are able to sleep through the night (or their equivalent "sleep period") without waking to void, one episode of nocturia is considered normal for individuals less than 65 years of age and up to two episodes of nocturia is considered normal for elderly individuals (that is, those 65 years of age or older). Arising three or more times each night to urinate is considered clinically relevant and is associated with multiple lower urinary tract disorders including overactive bladder, UI, increased nocturnal urine production, obstruction associated with benign prostatic hyperplasia, urinary retention and sleep apnea.[13-15]

Urgency, sometimes referred to as bothersome urgency, should be differentiated from the normal desire to urinate associated with bladder filling.

Although further research is needed to separate these phenomena, it is generally accepted that urgency is a sudden and precipitous desire to urinate that impedes or interrupts the pursuit of all other activities of daily living until it is acted on, whereas the physiologic desire to urinate can be acted on or postponed based on convenience.[16] Bothersome urgency is considered the cornerstone symptom of overactive bladder, and its occurrence defines urge UI.[8]

Pain can be generally defined as an unpleasant sensation and associated emotional response to that sensation associated with tissue damage or distress. Lower urinary tract pain is often characterized as pressure or burning and may be continuous or intermittent in nature. As noted in Table 12-1, pain may be highly localized to the bladder, urethra, or external genitalia, or it may be more diffuse and labeled perineal or pelvic. Descriptions of lower urinary tract pain must include its location, character, intensity, duration, and factors that exacerbate or alleviate the pain. Multiple disorders are associated with pain including UTI, urethritis, trauma, and inflammatory lesions. The etiology and pathophysiology of some pain-related disorders including interstitial cystitis, chronic male pelvic pain syndrome (formerly called prostatodynia or nonbacterial prostatitis), and chronic pelvic pain are largely unknown and are the focus of ongoing research.[17-19] Clear differentiation of lower urinary tract pain and bothersome urgency remains a challenge for both clinicians and researchers.[20]

Urinary Incontinence

The patient is also queried about patterns of urinary leakage and factors that provoke urine loss. This information is important because it allows the clinician to establish an initial diagnosis of UI type, which directs further assessment and management.

Stress Urinary Incontinence. The diagnosis of the symptom of stress UI is based on reports of urine loss provoked by physical activities such as lifting, walking, or running, or by maneuvers that precipitously raise abdominal pressure such as coughing, laughing or sneezing. Pure (sometimes called genuine) stress UI is diagnosed when the patient reports urine loss that occurs with activity and is *not* associated with urgency.

Fortunately, the history has been shown to be a reasonably reliable indicator of stress UI. Diokno, Wells, and Brink[21] compared verbal reports of leakage patterns with urodynamic test results and found that the history permitted accurate prediction of the diagnosis of stress UI in 78% of patients. Jensen, Nielsen, and Ostergard[22] completed a meta-analysis of the clinical evaluation of UI and found a positive predictive value of 0.79 and a negative predictive value of 0.78 when the history was used to diagnose stress UI.

Patients reporting a pattern of stress UI should be further questioned in regard to severity of leakage. Severity may be estimated by determination of the approximate volume of urine lost during a single episode of UI, the approximate volume lost over a period of time, or the activity level required to provoke urine loss. Women with severe stress UI as determined by urodynamic evaluation reported larger volumes of urine loss with each episode and over time as compared with women with mild to moderate stress UI.[23] In addition, women classified by objective testing (urodynamics or pad weight testing) as having severe stress UI are more likely to experience urine loss with mild exertion, such as rolling over while supine or rising from a sitting to a standing position, than women classified as having mild to moderate stress UI.[24]

Urge Urinary Incontinence and Overactive Bladder Dysfunction. The term *overactive bladder* is a comparatively new diagnosis. It is defined as a symptom syndrome characterized by bothersome urgency, and it is usually accompanied by increased daytime voiding frequency and nocturia, with or without urge UI. The NOBLE study revealed that approximately 37% of patients with overactive bladder dysfunction had urge UI and that women were at greater risk for accompanying UI than were men.[25,26] Urge UI occurs when an overactive detrusor contraction leads to partial (or complete) evacuation of urine from the bladder. Traditionally, the diagnosis of urge UI was based exclusively on a report of urinary leakage temporally associated with urgency. However, research has shown that urge UI can be more clearly differentiated from stress UI when reports of urine loss associated with a strong desire to urinate coexist with increased daytime frequency and nocturia. In a study of 200 community-dwelling women, Diokno, Wells, and Brink found that verbal reports of "urge incontinence symptoms" agreed with urodynamic results in only 45% of the cases,[21] and Jensen, Nielsen, and Ostergard found that verbal reports of "urge incontinence" had a positive predictive value of only 0.56 and a negative predictive value of 0.73.[22] Gray and colleagues found that a combination of three LUTS (urgency associated with leakage, increased diurnal frequency, and nocturia) provided a diagnosis of urge UI that more closely correlated with objective measures of testing than the symptom of UI associated with urgency alone.

Mixed Urinary Incontinence. Mixed UI is diagnosed when symptoms of stress and urge UI coexist.

Reflex Incontinence. Reflex UI is caused by neurogenic detrusor overactivity (hyperactive detrusor contractions associated with a disease or lesion affecting the spinal cord). Because these patients typically have reduced or absent sensations of bladder filling, overactive detrusor contractions produce urinary leakage in the absence of urgency. As a result, the patients typically report vague or nonspecific warnings of impending UI, and it is difficult to base the diagnosis on history alone. Nevertheless, reflex UI occurs only in patients with suprasacral spinal cord lesions, and it should be suspected in any patient with a paralyzing spinal disorder and urinary leakage. Patients with reflex UI commonly report the passage of large volumes of urine at regular but unpredictable times. Although most patients describe diminished or absent bladder sensations, some report seemingly unrelated symptoms with UI episodes such as tingling, flushing, palpitations, sweating, and a moderate to intense headache. Sweating, palpitations, and headache are particularly significant because they alert the clinician to the possibility of autonomic hyperreflexia complicating the reflex UI.

Functional Incontinence. Functional UI is characterized by urinary leakage that is partly or entirely attributable to impairment of the patient's mobility, dexterity, or cognition. Patients with functional UI may or may not be able to provide a reliable history; therefore, a care provider or family member may be asked to participate in the interview.

In many instances, the patient with functional UI is managed with an adult containment brief, and no "pattern" of urine loss can be identified. Patients with functional UI and mild or minimal cognitive impairment may describe a leakage pattern similar to that of urge UI; that is, an urge to urinate that occurs with or just before the onset of urinary leakage. Alternatively, the caregiver of an individual with severe cognitive impairment may report periods of dryness interspersed with large volumes of urinary leakage.

Continuous Incontinence. Continuous UI is characterized by ongoing leakage irrespective of physical activity, urgency, or other provocative measures. It is associated with a urinary fistula, ectopia, or surgical reconstruction that bypasses the urethral sphincter mechanism.

Containment Devices. Many individuals with UI wear absorptive devices to contain urinary leakage and to protect clothing. Absorptive devices may be used as a supplement to an overall bladder management program, or they may be used as the primary means to contain uncontrolled urine output. The type of device worn and the frequency with which it is changed may provide clues as to the frequency and severity of the urinary leakage. For example, many patients with mild UI choose to use household products such as tissue or paper towels.[27] Many women, based on their experience with management of menstrual flow, will select a pad intended primarily for that purpose, as opposed to a pad intended for urinary containment. These materials may contain mild urinary leakage, but they have been designed to contain menstrual flow and are not ideal for containing urine loss. Patients who experience frequent or large-volume urinary leakage may choose a pad that is specifically designed to contain urinary leakage. Many such pads are now available and they absorb up to 500 mL of urine while providing protection to clothing and from odor. Containment briefs or pad and pant systems replace standard undergarments; they are useful for patients with very high-volume urine loss or combined fecal incontinence and UI. The frequency with which an absorptive product is changed also provides some indication of the severity of the urinary leakage. However, the person's economic status, personal hygiene patterns, and fear of embarrassment profoundly influence the frequency of change. For example, some individuals are severely distressed by even a relatively small volume of urinary leakage and may change a pad or other protective device as soon as they perceive any urine loss, whereas other patients change their pad only when they perceive it to be "soaked."

A small proportion of patients may use a barrier device such as a urethral insert, penile clamp, or incontinence pessary to prevent urine loss. Because these devices are designed to *prevent* rather than *contain* urinary leakage, the selection of a particular device does not indicate the severity of the underlying UI.

Voiding and Postmicturition Lower Urinary Tract Symptoms

Queries about voiding symptoms focus on the nature of the urinary stream, including its perceived force and duration, and specific symptoms such as hesitancy, splitting, spraying, slowness, or intermittency. We also query patients about postmicturitional symptoms at this point, including postvoid dribbling and feelings of incomplete bladder emptying. Reports of hesitancy, slow stream, intermittency, or feelings of incomplete bladder emptying may indicate poor detrusor contraction strength, obstruction, or simply voiding with a small intravesical volume.[28,29] Patients also may be queried about straining during micturition, but clinical experience and available research suggest that a report of straining during urination does not correlate well with objective evidence of straining or with urinary retention caused by poor detrusor contraction strength or obstruction.[30,31]

Although most patients manage their bladder by spontaneous voiding, a minority will be managed by some form of catheterization. Intermittent catheterization replaces or augments the efficiency of bladder evacuation, while preserving vesicle filling, but indwelling catheterization replaces both phases of lower urinary tract function with ongoing drainage.

Intermittent Catheterization. Growing numbers of patients with voiding dysfunction and related UI manage their bladders with intermittent catheterization. The interviewer should determine both the *prescribed* and the *actual* schedule for catheterization. The patient may be asked whether he or she catheterizes by the clock or in response to suprapubic pressure or urgency; patients who report catheterizing by the clock may be asked the usual frequency (that is, "How often do you catheterize?"). This question typically generates the *prescribed* frequency (such as "every 4 hours"). However, the clinician should be aware that the *actual* frequency is often quite different from the prescribed frequency. Actual frequency is more effectively elicited when the patient is asked to describe a typical day and identify times when she or he would catheterize. It also may be helpful to ask the patient about the usual volume of urine obtained with catheterization (if measured) and about frequency and severity of leakage between catheterizations.

Indwelling Catheter. Some persons manage urinary elimination with an indwelling catheter. Although an indwelling catheter (see Chapter 10) is the best bladder management program in selected cases, it should be viewed as a "last option," and alternatives to its use should be sought whenever possible. Therefore, it is important to ask the patient to identify the reason for initial placement of the catheter and the length of time a catheter has been used to manage urinary elimination. The clinician must then use this information along with the data generated by the overall assessment to determine whether an indwelling catheter truly represents the best option for bladder management and whether the patient desires or is willing to consider another program for bladder management.

Fluid Intake. Many patients modify their fluid intake in an attempt to reduce their problems with leakage; other patients unwittingly contribute to their problems with urinary urgency and frequency by excessive fluid intake. Therefore, the interviewer should ask about the patient's patterns of fluid intake, that is, the approximate volume and types of fluids consumed during a typical day. These questions help the clinician to identify the patient who is consuming an excessive amount of fluids in an attempt to blunt the appetite or in response to a metabolic disorder, such as diabetes mellitus or diabetes insipidus. These questions will also help to identify the patient who strictly limits fluid intake in an attempt to minimize urinary leakage. However, the clinician should remember that the bladder chart (voiding diary) provides a much more accurate and reproducible estimate of fluid consumption than patient recall; data gathered during the interview should not be used as the sole source for assessment of usual fluid intake.

In addition to questions regarding the *volume* of fluid consumed on a daily basis, the patient should be asked about the *type* of fluids consumed. These questions allow the clinician to identify ingestion of bladder irritants, which may contribute to the patient's problems with urinary leakage, sensory urgency, or abnormally frequent urination. Table 12-2 provides a list of substances commonly considered to be bladder "irritants." Table 12-3 focuses specifically on fluids containing caffeine.

Urinary Retention

Urinary retention is defined as the inability to empty the bladder.[32] From a clinical perspective, retention is divided into two types, acute and chronic. Acute urinary retention is characterized by a complete inability to urinate; patients are only able to empty a few mL of urine despite a strong sensation of bladder distension. Patients are intensely aware of the inability to empty their bladder, and they usually report a growing sense of bladder pressure, discomfort, and anxiety as the vesicle becomes increasingly overdistended. In contrast to this clinical situation,

TABLE 12-2   Common Bladder Irritants

SUBSTANCE	PHYSIOLOGIC BASIS FOR ROLE AS BLADDER IRRITANT
Caffeine (refer to Table 12-3)	Stimulates transient smooth muscle contraction (Lee, Wein, Levin, 1993)
	Causes elevated detrusor pressure during filling CMG (Creighton and Stanton, 1990)
Alcohol	Known diuretic and sedative
	Diuretic use associated with UI in community-dwelling elderly men (Umlauf and Sherman, 1996)
	Alcohol intake not a significant risk factor for UI in middle-aged women (Burgio, Matthews and Engel, 1991)
Smoking	Smoking increases lower urinary tract symptoms in adult, community-dwelling men (Koskimaki et al, 1998)

*Possible Bladder Irritants**	
Carbonated beverages	Cheeses
Aspartame, artificial sweeteners	Corned beef
Avocado	Mayonnaise
Soy sauce	Onions
Citrus fruits or juices	Fermented foods
Brewer's yeast	Smoked foods
Sprouts	Foods with molds
Vinegar and vinegar products	Fried foods
Tomatoes and tomato products	Heavily spiced foods
Yogurt	Sour cream
Hydrogenated fats, margarine, shortening	Barbecued foods or sauces

*The evidence for any role as bladder irritant limited to anecdotal reports and clinical experience. Some substances implicated as bladder irritants based on experiences with patients with interstitial cystitis as compared to urinary incontinence.

TABLE 12-3   **Caffeine Content of Common Foods and Beverages**

BEVERAGES AND FOODS	RELEVANT SUBSTANCES AND QUANTITIES
Beverages	
Coffee (brewed; per 5-oz serving)	Caffeinated: 30 to 180 mg
	Decaffeinated: 1 to 5 mg
Tea (brewed)	Hot tea (per 5-oz serving): 25 to 110 mg
	Iced tea (12-oz glass): 67 to 76 mg
Hot cocoa (per 5-oz serving)	2 to 20 mg
Soft drinks (per 12-oz serving)	30 to 59 mg (*highest content:* Sugar Free Mr. Pibb, Mountain Dew; *lowest content:* Canada Dry Jamaica Cola, Canada Dry Diet Cola, caffeine-free colas)
Foods	
Chocolate (per 1-oz serving)	Milk chocolate: 1 to 15 mg
	Dark chocolate: 5 to 35 mg
	Baker's chocolate: 26 mg
	Chocolate syrup: 4 mg

Adapted from Pierson C: Pad testing, nursing interventions and urine loss appliances. In: Ostergard DR, Bent AE, editors: *Urogynecology and urodynamics,* Baltimore, 1991, Williams & Wilkins.

patients with chronic retention (incomplete bladder emptying) frequently have few bothersome LUTS and may be completely unaware that they are unable to empty their bladder despite micturition. LUTS associated with chronic urinary retention include increased daytime frequency, nocturia, and urgency. However, these findings also occur with other types of bladder dysfunction.[33] Voiding LUTS associated with urinary retention include hesitancy, splitting, spraying, slowness, and intermittency, although patients may have adjusted to gradual changes in characteristics of micturition and may not perceive these symptoms as bothersome or even noticeable. The patient suspected of having chronic urinary retention also may be asked about prior episodes of acute urinary retention. However, although these conditions coexist in some patients, the presence of one form is not a reliable predictor of the other. For example, studies in both men and women with acute retention have shown that some patients experience complete resolution after a short-term catheterization program, whereas others experience prolonged difficulty with bladder emptying.[34-36]

Urinary retention may also be associated with urinary leakage. Patients who retain very large volumes of urine may experience *overflow* UI, a condition characterized by a dribbling pattern of urinary leakage. Other patients report leakage immediately after urination; this is commonly known as *postvoid dribble*. Again, these patterns of leakage should not be considered characteristic of urinary retention, and their presence may indicate an unrelated voiding problem. For example, a postvoid dribble in a woman may be caused by a suburethral diverticulum that drains when the woman arises after urination.[37,38] In addition, a postvoid dribble is often seen in young men,[39] and these individuals do not typically exhibit any significant voiding dysfunction.[40,41] Even among elderly men with benign prostatic hyperplasia (BPH), the symptom of postmicturition dribbling does not correlate well with bladder outlet obstruction.[31,42]

Continuous Incontinence. Continuous UI occurs when the anatomic integrity of the urinary system is interrupted, allowing urine to bypass the urethral sphincter mechanism. Patients with continuous UI report ongoing urine loss that is not correlated with the urge to urinate or with physical exertion. The volume of urinary leakage varies from a continuous dribble superimposed on an otherwise normal voiding pattern to constant leakage that replaces any detectable voiding pattern.

Focused Review of Systems

A review of systems is completed to identify conditions that may contribute to UI. Key systems to be included in this review are the genitourinary, gastrointestinal, and neurologic systems. The review of each organ system is typically begun with a general question, followed by specific queries about conditions likely to contribute to voiding dysfunction or UI. In addition, the patient is asked about his or her general medical history, any surgical procedures, and all medications, including both prescription and over-the-counter agents.

Table 12-4 is a structured guide to the review of systems for the individual with UI. Table 12-5 assists the clinician to correlate positive findings with implications for the patient with UI or urinary retention.

Treatment Goals and Motivation

The interview should also include an exploration of the patient's goals for therapy and motivation to achieve these goals. Although it may not be possible to cure the patient's UI completely or to restore bladder function to the "normal" level, it is almost always possible to provide significant improvement in the patient's bladder function. Patients themselves frequently recognize that a "complete" restoration of normal function and continence is not always feasible; when asked, they may report more limited goals, such as elimination of obvious wetness or urinary odor. Skoner and Haylor observed that community-dwelling women resisted defining their UI as a disorder or disease as long as they were able to "normalize" the leakage; normalization was achieved by using self-management techniques to prevent uncontrolled urinary leakage onto clothing or the presence of detectable odors caused by urinary leakage.[43,44]

Similarly, Umlauf and Sherman observed that the majority of a group of community-dwelling elderly men who admitted to UI reported the leakage as "mild;" most of these men chose to manage their UI with household products to contain leakage and prevent odor (as opposed to seeking medical care).[27]

These data support the concept that the clinician should seek a course of treatment that is based on assessment findings *and* on goals that are mutually agreed on by the clinician and the individual seeking care. For some patients, the goal of treatment may be the alleviation of symptoms of urinary urgency and frequency, whereas others may wish to pursue continence at all costs. The importance of the patient's priorities and preferences becomes clear when the options are considered for patients with a combination of urge UI caused by detrusor overactivity and urinary retention caused by impaired detrusor contractility. Some of these patients elect a course of antimuscarinic pharmacotherapy and intermittent catheterization to achieve continence. In contrast, other patients would prefer to cope with some urinary leakage rather than face the prospect of intermittent catheterization. Similarly, some patients with stress or mixed UI may choose to undergo surgery, whereas others pursue behavioral or pharmacologic management. In most situations, there is more than one treatment option. The preferred option can be determined only with the patient or caregiver.

PHYSICAL EXAMINATION

The patient interview is followed by a careful physical examination of the structures and functions affecting voiding and continence. This assessment may be incorporated into a comprehensive physical examination or may be limited to factors specifically affecting urinary continence and bladder function. This discussion addresses only those assessment factors critical to the assessment of UI or voiding dysfunction.

General and Functional Assessment

The examination begins with a general assessment of the patient's cognitive function, mobility, and dexterity. The patient is evaluated for alertness and orientation and for mobility and dexterity; the latter can be evaluated by observation of the ease or difficulty with which the patient moves onto the examination table and carries out the maneuvers necessary to provide a urine specimen. Engberg and colleagues recommended the use of time measurements as a general assessment of functional ability in

TABLE 12-4 Review of Systems

SYSTEM	GENERAL QUESTION	SPECIFIC AREAS OF INQUIRY

Urologic and renal	"Have you experienced problems with your urinary tract or kidneys?"
	
	"Have you ever visited the urology doctor for problems with your urinary tract or kidneys?"
		1. Urinary tract infections
		  a. Frequency
		  b. Febrile versus afebrile
		2. Upper urinary tract problems (vesicoureteral reflux, pyelonephritis)
		3. Urinary tract calculi
		4. Urinary system tumors
		5. Renal insufficiency or renal failure

Neurologic	"Have you experienced problems with numbness, tingling, or weakness caused by back problems or a nerve problem?"	Disorders of the brain 1. Stroke (cerebrovascular accident, brain attack) 2. Tumors 3. Hydrocephalus 4. Dementias (Alzheimer's disease, etc.) 5. Infections (encephalitis)
	"Have you ever visited the nerve conduction doctor for problems with numbness, tingling, weakness, or other nerve problems?"	Disorders of the spinal cord 1. Trauma (level, completeness of injury, neurologic extension) 2. Inflammation or infection (transverse myelitis, Guillain-Barré meningitis, etc.) 3. Spinal column problems (herniated or ruptured disks, stenosis, tethering of spinal cord, etc.) 4. Disorders of peripheral nervous system (metabolic polyneuropathies or autonomic polyneuropathies caused by diabetes mellitus, heavy metal poisoning, chronic alcoholism, cauda equina syndrome, pelvic fracture, pelvic or pudendal nerve trauma) 5. Disorders affecting multiple levels of nervous system (multiple sclerosis, etc.)
Female reproductive	"Are you having any problems with your reproductive organs (womb, ovaries, vagina)?"	1. Obstetric history (gravida/para/AB status, prolonged labor and delivery, breech presentations, forceps-assisted deliveries, tearing, or central episiotomy) 2. Gynecologic history (vaginitis, endometriosis, etc.) 3. Menstrual status (including use of exogenous hormones) 4. Symptoms of pelvic organ prolapse (low back pain exacerbated by standing and relieved by assuming supine position, pressure or perception of "bulge" or "ball" in vagina, stress incontinence or difficulty passing stool with severe rectocele)

Continued

TABLE 12-4 **Review of Systems—cont'd**

SYSTEM	GENERAL QUESTION	SPECIFIC AREAS OF INQUIRY
Male reproductive	"Have you had problems with your prostate, scrotum, or penis?" "Have you had problems with sexual function ("nature")?"	1. Prostate problems (enlarged prostate, prostatitis, prostate cancer) 2. Sexual dysfunction (impotence, ejaculatory dysfunction) 3. Scrotal disorders (epididymitis, orchitis, etc.) 4. Sexually transmitted diseases (urethritis, etc.)
Gastrointestinal	"Have you had problems with your bowel movements?" "Do you have trouble with constipation or controlling your bowels?"	1. Bowel elimination patterns (frequency of bowel movements, consistency and caliber of typical stool) 2. Fecal continence (incontinence of gas, liquid stool, solid stool, frequency and severity of fecal incontinence)
General medical	"Are you being treated for any acute or chronic conditions we have not discussed?"	1. Metabolic disorders (diabetes mellitus, diabetes insipidus) 2. Hypertension 3. Cancer 4. Disorders affecting the sensory organs (hearing loss, visual disorders, etc.)
Surgical history	"What surgeries or operations have you had?"	1. Procedures of the urinary system (including urethral suspension in women) 2. Procedures of the neurologic system (including all procedures on the skull or "back bones") 3. Procedures of the reproductive organs (including hysterectomy, oophorectomy in women, prostate or transurethral procedures in men) 4. Abdominal procedures
Current medications	"Tell me all the medicines you are taking, including everything prescribed by the doctor and everything you use that does not require a prescription."	Dosage, administration, indication for use (if known)

regard to toileting; such measurements document the time required for an elderly patient with UI to move to the bathroom and prepare for urination by manipulating clothing and sitting on the toilet.[45] The examiner should specifically assess the ease with which clothing is removed for toileting, because this is an area for potential intervention.

In most cases, this limited assessment is sufficient to determine the functional ability of the patient in regard to toileting activities. However, patients with paralyzing neurologic disorders or neuromuscular diseases may require a more in-depth assessment of both gross and fine motor abilities before an appropriate bladder management program can be developed. For example, it may be relevant to assess the patient's ability to access the perineum and to hold and control an intermittent catheter (with or without assistive devices). In these cases, it may be beneficial

TABLE 12-5   **Review of Systems: Implications of Positive Findings**

FINDING	IMPLICATION FOR UI
UTIs Upper urinary tract problems Urinary tract calculi Renal insufficiency or failure	Urinary retention (febrile UTI, upper urinary tract problems, renal insufficiency particularly associated with bladder outlet obstruction or low bladder wall compliance)
Urinary system tumor	Urge UI; indication for immediate referral
Disorders of the brain	Urge UI with detrusor hyperreflexia; also altered mobility or cognition, which increases risk of functional UI
Disorders of the spinal cord	Reflex UI with detrusor-sphincter dyssynergia and urinary retention; paralyzing spinal disorders affecting mobility, dexterity, and risk of functional UI
Disorders of the peripheral nerves	Urinary retention with diminished or absent sensations of bladder filling and deficient detrusor contraction strength; may reduce mobility and increase risk of functional UI Denervation is a possible cause of intrinsic sphincter deficiency and stress UI
Disorders affecting multiple levels of the nervous system	Urge or reflex UI; urinary retention
Obstetric history	Multiple deliveries, deliveries requiring forceps assistance, central episiotomy, those complicated by breech presentation, and central tearing increase the risk of pelvic muscle denervation and stress UI
Gynecologic history	Vaginitis and endometriosis may contribute to irritative voiding symptoms and urge UI
Menstrual status	Atrophic vaginitis associated with atrophic urethritis causing irritative voiding symptoms and urge UI
Symptoms of pelvic organ prolapse	Pelvic organ prolapse associated with stress UI; urinary retention possible when prolapse is severe
Prostate problems	Prostate enlargement associated with bladder outlet obstruction and urinary retention Severe bladder outlet obstruction causes detrusor overactivity and urge UI Prostatitis causes irritative voiding symptoms and may produce detrusor overactivity and urge UI
Sexual dysfunction	Erectile dysfunction, ejaculatory dysfunction may be associated with disorders of spinal cord, peripheral nervous system causing urge UI, reflex UI
Scrotal disorders	Epididymitis is a possible indicator of reflux into male reproductive tract from detrusor-sphincter dyssynergia or reflex UI
Sexually transmitted diseases	Gonococcal or nongonococcal urethritis may cause secondary stricture with bladder outlet obstruction and urinary retention
Bowel elimination patterns and fecal continence	Constipation, fecal incontinence may indicate neuropathic bladder dysfunction with urge or reflex UI, urinary retention
Metabolic disorders	Diabetes mellitus most common cause of peripheral polyneuropathies, associated with urgency, frequency, and urge UI in early stages and urinary retention in late stages

Continued

TABLE 12-5 **Review of Systems: Implications of Positive Findings—cont'd**

FINDING	IMPLICATION FOR UI
Hypertension	Hypertension may directly contribute to urinary urgency; medications used to treat hypertension may contribute to transient UI (refer to current medications)
Disorders of special senses (vision, hearing)	Increased risk of functional UI
Cancer	May contribute to urinary retention or UI because of primary effect on urinary system or to secondary effects on nervous system, gastrointestinal system, etc.
Surgical history	**Urologic Procedures** Bladder suspension associated with risk of detrusor overactivity and urge UI or recurrent stress UI and intrinsic sphincter deficiency as well as urethral hypermobility; suspensions also associated with small risk of obstruction and urinary retention Transurethral procedures (TURP, TUIP, etc.) associated with small risk of sphincter damage and subsequent stress UI **Gynecologic Procedures** Hysterectomy carries uncertain risk of subsequent stress UI Cystocele repair may increase the risk of subsequent stress UI **Neurologic Procedures** Risk of urge or reflex UI, urinary retention from preexisting condition and from surgical intervention Abdominal procedures (risk of urinary retention with extensive resection)
Current medications	Anticholinergics, antispasmodics, antidepressants, antipsychotics, sedatives and hypnotics, narcotic analgesics associated with urinary retention or reduced ability to respond to toileting cues with subsequent transient UI Alpha-adrenergic agonists (decongestants) associated with increased risk of urinary retention, particularly in men with prostatic enlargement Beta-adrenergic agonists associated with increased risk of urinary retention, particularly when combined with agents listed above Calcium-channel blockers associated with increased risk of urinary retention, particularly when combined with agents listed above Alpha-adrenergic blockers (antagonists) associated with increased risk of stress UI Diuretics associated with increased risk of urinary frequency, urgency, and urge UI

UI, urinary incontinence; UTI, urinary tract infection.

to have the patient evaluated by a physical therapist, occupational therapist, rehabilitation nurse specialist, or physiatrist.

Female Genitalia and Related Integument

After a thorough explanation of the purpose and specifics of the pelvic examination, the patient is draped, and the examination begins with inspection of the perineal skin. Although little is known about the pathogenesis of perineal dermatitis among adults, it *is* known that UI and fecal incontinence, when combined with use of a containment device, are closely associated factors.[46,47] In its early stages, perineal dermatitis is found in the folds of the skin (intertrigo) and is characterized by redness and erosion of superficial skin layers. More advanced cases are characterized by extensive erosion and secondary infections such as candidiasis or erythrasma. Less commonly, patients may present with linear lesions caused by the elastic bands of containment devices or the straps of a leg bag.

After examination of the perineal skin, the vaginal mucosa is assessed for signs and symptoms of estrogen deficiency. Atrophic vaginitis is characterized by a pale, dry mucosa with absence or flattening of the rugae. The vagina is typically tender to the touch and may bleed easily. In addition, a urethral caruncle (a small red papillary growth) may be evident at the meatal opening. In patients with severe atrophic changes, the labia minora will be small or fused, and the vaginal introitus and vault may be stenotic and difficult to examine. Patients with atrophic vaginitis often report chronic vaginal discomfort and itching. Estrogen deficiency also causes atrophic changes in the urethral mucosa that may produce bothersome LUTS symptoms such as increased daytime voiding frequency, nocturia, and urgency.

After inspection of the vaginal mucosa, the clinician performs a speculum or digital examination to assess for evidence of pelvic organ prolapse. The clinician first places the posterior blade of a Graves speculum, a Sims speculum, or two gloved and lubricated fingers against the posterior wall of the vagina (the vaginal wall adjacent to the rectum) and exerts gentle pressure to prevent movement. The patient is then instructed to perform a slow Valsalva maneuver, and the clinician observes for bulging of the anterior vaginal wall, which is indicative of urethral hypermobility and cystocele. The examiner should also be alert to any urine loss associated with this maneuver, which is indicative of stress UI. The clinician then rotates the speculum or examining fingers to stabilize the anterior wall of the vagina, and the patient is again asked to perform a slow Valsalva maneuver. Bulging of the posterior wall of the vagina is indicative of rectocele. The speculum or fingers are then moved to the distal aspect of the vagina, and the patient is asked to perform a Valsalva maneuver for the third time while the clinician observes for evidence of uterine prolapse, that is, downward movement of the cervix. Ideally, these maneuvers are performed while the patient is in a sitting position, although they may be performed while the woman is supine.

Assessment of Pelvic Muscle Strength

We believe that an assessment of pelvic floor muscle strength is critical to a complete continence examination. The goals of the examination are to assess the baseline neuromuscular function and contractility of the pelvic floor muscles, as well as the patient's ability to identify, isolate, contract, and relax this muscle group. The examiner places one or two gloved fingers into the patient's vagina, and the patient is asked to contract the circumvaginal muscles as if she were trying to interrupt the urinary stream or avoid passing flatus. A brisk contraction of the pelvic floor muscles should produce firm pressure, most appreciable on the posterior and anterior aspects of the fingers but detectable circumferentially. The duration of the contraction should be 3 to 6 seconds, and the fingers should be drawn a short distance toward the posterior aspect of the vaginal vault. With mildly impaired contractility, anteroposterior pressure against the fingers is appreciated, but circumferential contraction is less definite, the duration of the contraction may be reduced, and the fingers are not drawn toward the posterior aspect of the vault. With more profound impairment of pelvic muscle strength, there is little or no perceptible pressure exerted against the fingers, the contraction is typically maintained for less than 3 seconds, and the fingers are not drawn posteriorly. Brink and colleagues and Sampselle and colleagues recommended a four-point scale for evaluating and documenting pelvic muscle strength that is based on three variables: pressure, duration, and finger displacement[48,49] (Table 12-6).

If the patient has evidence of impaired contractility, the clinician should further assess for high-tone versus low-tone dysfunction. High-tone dysfunction is characterized by an elevated resting tone that predisposes the patient to urgency or pain and is frequently associated with UI. It is characterized by tension of the circumvaginal or anal muscles upon palpation, often accompanied by reports of discomfort when palpated. Paradoxically, patients with high-tone dysfunction will have evidence of poor contraction strength and may be unable to identify, contract, and relax the muscles at all, because of the partial state of contraction characteristic of this neuromuscular dysfunction. Low-tone dysfunction, in contrast, is characterized by evidence of low resting tone. These patients also exhibit evidence of poor contraction strength as a result of underlying weakness. The clinician should also determine symmetry of the pelvic floor muscles by noting the bulk of muscle tissue on the right and left aspects of the vaginal wall and/or the clockwise symmetry of the anal sphincter muscle.[1]

Inspection of the perineum also provides clues to pelvic floor contraction strength.[1] Specifically, the patient can be asked to contract the pelvic floor muscles, which are expected to cause visible elevation of the perineal body. Similarly, a visible contraction (sometimes called a wink) of the anus should be observed during pelvic muscle contraction.

Sampselle also advocated a urine stream interruption test for assessing pelvic floor muscle strength.[50] The patient is asked to interrupt the voided urinary stream, and a stopwatch is used to determine the time from verbal prompt to complete interruption of the stream (that is, a flow rate of 0 mL/second). Sampselle found that a "stop time" of 2 seconds or less was associated with good pelvic muscle strength and a lower risk for UI; in contrast, a stop time of greater than 2 seconds was associated with impaired pelvic muscle contractility and a significantly higher risk for moderate to severe UI.[50]

Computer-Based Evaluation of Pelvic Floor Muscle Contractility. Pelvic floor muscle contractility may be assessed or measured via computer-based biofeedback equipment or during complex urodynamic testing. Two techniques are commonly used to assess pelvic floor muscle function, electromyography (EMG) and pressure. A pressure-sensitive probe may be placed into the vagina or the rectum and the patient is then asked to contract the pelvic floor muscles. The peak contraction pressure and the duration of the contraction are recorded over one or more contractions. Dougherty found that maximum pressure among women with normal pelvic muscle function typically ranges from 35 to 42 cm H_2O.[51] Pressure manometry offers several advantages when compared with digital assessment. It quantitatively measures the amplitude (maximum

TABLE 12-6   Pelvic Muscle Strength Rating Scale

	1	2	3	4
Pressure	None	Slight pressure, not perceived around circumference of finger	Moderate pressure, perceived around circumference of finger	Strong pressure, perceived circumferentially
Duration	None	Less than 1 second	1 to 3 seconds	More than 3 seconds
Displacement of finger	None	Slight incline, base of fingers slightly elevated	Greater incline, entire finger elevated	Fingers moving up and inside, toward posterior vault

Adapted from Sampselle CM, Brink CA, Wells TJ: *Nurs Res* 38:135, 1989.

squeeze) of the contraction and its duration, and it provides a visible record for both the patient and clinician that can be used to determine maximum strength, duration and muscle fatigue with repeated exercise. Disadvantages include the need to place and maintain a fluid-filled manometric probe, which may be technically challenging (particularly in the male patient).

Alternatively, EMG may be used to assess pelvic floor muscle strength. This technique measures electrical activity at the level of the striated muscle membrane as opposed to the force of contraction. Although this measure closely correlates with contraction force, it does *not* allow measurement of contraction strength. Nevertheless, it does provide a visual record for the clinician and patient that can be used to assess maximum strength, duration, and fatigue with repeated exercise. Another advantage of EMG is the ability to assess resting pelvic floor muscle tone. We have observed that patients with normal pelvic floor muscle tone and those with low tone pelvic floor dysfunction tend to have resting tones of 2 microvolts or less, whereas those with high resting tone dysfunction tend to have much higher values, often 5 microvolts or considerably higher.

Rectal Examination in Female Patients. A rectal examination is an optional component of the focused physical examination for a female patient with UI, although it is an essential component of any *comprehensive* pelvic evaluation and of the focused physical examination for a female patient with both UI and fecal incontinence. The rectal examination serves two primary purposes; it allows assessment of anal sphincter (and pelvic floor muscle) strength, and it provides an opportunity to assess for masses or the presence of impacted stool in the rectal vault. (Pelvic masses are evaluated with a bimanual examination, a detailed description of which is beyond the scope of this chapter. Additional information is provided by Seidel and colleagues.[52])

Male Genitalia and Related Integument. As with female patients, the pelvic examination in the male patient begins with a thorough inspection of the perineal skin. The penile skin is initially inspected, and the foreskin (when present) is pulled back to permit inspection of the underlying glans penis.

The examiner should be alert to any evidence of phimosis; that is, difficulty retracting and restoring the foreskin. The scrotum and perineal skin are then inspected for rashes or lesions; the examiner should pay close attention to skin folds such as the interface of the scrotum and adjacent integument.

After skin inspection, the patient is prepared for a testicular examination, and each testis is gently palpated for symmetry, evidence of inflammation, or masses. Special attention is paid to the palpation of each epididymis; the presence of fibrosis and scarring is indicative of previous infections and often accompanies long-standing detrusorsphincter dyssynergia or prostatitis with associated bladder outlet obstruction.

Rectal Examination in Male Patients. A digital rectal examination (DRE) is an essential component of the physical examination of the male patient with UI. Within the context of a continence evaluation, the primary purpose of the rectal examination is to evaluate pelvic floor muscle strength and function, although it also provides an immediate opportunity to identify the presence of stool in the rectum and to assess prostate size and symmetry. The clinician first prepares the patient with a thorough explanation of the procedure and then gently inserts a gloved lubricated finger into the rectum. The patient is asked to contract the pelvic floor muscles, and the clinician evaluates muscle tone and endurance. Normal strength of the anal sphincter is evidenced by a strong circumferential contraction in response to a verbal instruction to the patient to "tighten your muscles around my finger as if you are trying not to pass gas or stool." Reduced contractility of the anal sphincter is most commonly seen in men with neurologic lesions or a history of trauma to the anorectal area.

The prostate can be palpated just proximally to the anal sphincter through the anterior rectal wall. The normal prostate is felt as a heart-shaped gland with two distinct lobes separated by a central depression; it is approximately the size of a large chestnut.[53] Each lobe should be symmetric and nontender; normal prostatic tissue is frequently described as having a "rubbery" consistency.[54] Prostatitis causes symmetric enlargement of the prostate gland and sensitivity to palpation. The degree of sensitivity varies from mild to exquisite; severe pain is typically associated with an acute infection. BPH also causes symmetric enlargement of the gland, but patients with BPH do not experience discomfort during the DRE. Prostatic cancer produces asymmetric enlargement of the gland and also produces changes in the consistency of the tissue; the prostate may be indurated, with a hardened or stony consistency, and discrete firm nodules may further distort the normal anatomic structures.

The DRE is also used to assess the presence of stool in the rectal vault and the strength of the anal sphincter. Although a small amount of soft stool in the rectal vault is considered normal, the presence of large-caliber, hardened stools is significant for impaction or constipation, both of which adversely affect lower urinary tract function.

Focused Neurologic Examination

Normal neurologic function is critical to continence; therefore, the focused neurologic examination is a critical component of the physical assessment for any individual with UI. The neurologic examination begins with the assessment of mobility, dexterity, and cognition. These factors are evaluated during the patient interview and the preparatory phase of the physical examination (that is, removal of clothing and positioning on the examining table). Additional components of the neurologic assessment are integrated throughout the physical examination. After the patient's clothing has been removed and before the pelvic examination, the back, buttocks, and lower extremities are examined for signs of denervation. The patient's back is inspected for signs of spinal dysraphism such as a lipomatous area, a hairy tuft, or a skin tag near the lumbosacral spinal segments.[55] The buttocks are evaluated for asymmetry or signs of muscle atrophy. The cheeks of the buttocks are then gently spread, and the anus is inspected for prolapse, gaping, or asymmetric closure. Finally, the lower extremities and feet are examined for muscular asymmetry, atrophy, or other obvious signs of neurologic abnormality.

Neurologic assessment is also incorporated into the examination of the perineum and genitalia. Perineal sensation is assessed in terms of sensitivity to light touch and discrimination between sharp and dull stimuli; testing for two-point discrimination is typically added to the examination whenever there is a suspicion of altered sensory function. Reflex motor activity is assessed by evaluation of the bulbocavernosus reflex (BCR). An intact BCR is indicative of a grossly intact nerve pathway between the motor neurons in the sacral spinal cord and the pelvic muscles. The BCR can be tested during the rectal examination or as a separate maneuver. A gloved lubricated finger is gently inserted into the anal canal, and the clinician stimulates the reflex by gently squeezing the glans penis or tapping the clitoris; a positive reflex response is evidenced by contraction of the anal sphincter around the gloved finger. (For patients with an indwelling catheter, the reflex can also be elicited by gentle traction applied to the catheter, which pulls the balloon against the bladder neck.) Some clinicians use visual inspection of the anus as an alternative to digital examination when assessing the BCR; in this case, the anus is *observed* to contract ("wink") when the clitoris is tapped or the glans penis is gently squeezed. An absent BCR, in addition to other neurologic deficits, may be indicative of an underlying neurologic disorder; however, an absent BCR does not in and of itself indicate a serious neurologic abnormality.

As noted with the BCR, neurologic deficits in the perineal area may or may not be significant clinically; many patients who have no problems with urinary leakage display equivalent findings. Thus, any neurologic "deficit" must be considered in light of the entire assessment, and the patient should be evaluated carefully for additional indicators of neurologic dysfunction. Patients whose leakage is attributable to neurologic abnormalities typically present with additional symptoms of perineal denervation. For example, women with neurologic voiding dysfunction are also likely to complain of chronic constipation or fecal incontinence and of vaginal dryness or dyspareunia that is not explained by estrogen deficiency. In men, the neurologic triad usually includes voiding dysfunction, chronic constipation or fecal incontinence, and erectile or ejaculatory dysfunction. Although the presence of such a triad or of multiple other "neurologic" signs does not necessarily indicate a significant neurologic deficit, such findings do mandate a neurologic consultation and further evaluation of bladder and sphincter function by multichannel urodynamic testing.

ENVIRONMENTAL ASSESSMENT

The assessment of an individual with UI usually includes an evaluation of the home environment, which is particularly critical when the patient is elderly or disabled. The examiner begins by inspecting or asking about the bathroom: its proximity to living areas and the bedroom, its lighting, and the presence of environmental obstacles such as rugs on the floor or a door frame that is too narrow to permit wheelchair entry. Evaluation of the toilet itself should include the presence of supportive bars or handles and the height of the toilet seat in comparison with the patient's status and needs; specifically, the clinician should determine the need for a raised toilet seat, additional supportive bars, or additional assistive devices to facilitate safe toileting.[56,57]

The assessment then moves to the bed area; in addition to evaluating the distance from the bed to the toilet, the examiner looks for or asks about barriers such as stairs. The bed is evaluated for the presence of protective coverings or a padded draw sheet. The examiner also determines whether the bed is single or double, whether the patient sleeps alone or with a partner, and whether a bedside commode or hand-held urinal should be used to facilitate toileting and continence at night.

It may also be helpful to evaluate environmental support for management of absorptive products. The examiner should consider the availability of laundry facilities when determining the feasibility of reusable padding and should address options for containing and discarding disposable products when recommending disposable products for elderly or disabled patients. If an on-site evaluation is done, the examiner should be alert to the overall cleanliness and ventilation of the home environment and the presence of any urine-related odor.[57]

The environmental assessment should also include an assessment of the availability and responsiveness of caregivers. Because UI in the homebound or dependent individual affects caregivers as well as the patient, it is important to evaluate available resources for assistance with care and the perceived burden of the care provided by significant others.[58,59] In assessing available resources, the clinician should consider both community resources and family resources. Community resources include delivery services for incontinence management supplies, laundry services, home health care agencies, and voluntary organizations. A combination of these resources may be required to provide relief to a care provider, who may also have disabilities and health care needs.[34]

ASSESSMENT OF SYMPTOM SEVERITY, EFFECT, AND QUALITY OF LIFE

The number and quality of instruments used to measure voiding-related symptom severity and the effect of UI on activities of daily living and quality of life have grown significantly (Table 12-7). A detailed discussion of these instruments or an exhaustive list of the available tools is beyond the scope of this chapter; however, several instruments that have gained widespread use in the assessment of patients with UI or voiding dysfunction are briefly presented.

International Prostate Symptom Score

The International Prostate Symptom Score (IPSS), also called the AUA-7, was developed to measure the symptoms associated with BPH.[60] This instrument comprises seven items designed to measure the irritative and obstructive symptoms associated with BPH; an eighth item is usually attached to the instrument and is intended to quantify the bothersomeness of these symptoms and their effect on the individual's quality of life (Fig. 12-1). This instrument has been submitted to intensive testing with reference to its psychometric properties;[61] it has been found to be reliable and to possess both content and predictive validity. However, it was not found to possess adequate concurrent validity. Specifically, it has been observed that age is more predictive of the variability in IPSS scores than is the degree of prostatic enlargement,[62,63] that the IPSS score does not correlate with objective evidence of obstruction,[64] that men with detrusor hyperreflexia and *no* obstruction scored higher on the IPSS than men with obstruction caused by BPH,[65] and that the IPS scores were essentially equivalent for men and women within the same age group.[66]

TABLE 12-7 **Other Instruments Designed to Measure Lower Urinary Tract Symptoms, Psychosocial Impact, and Quality of Life***

NAME	PRIMARY PURPOSE AND LIMITATIONS OF CLINICAL UTILITY	REFERENCE
Urge UDI	LUTS, specifically designed for urge UI in women	Lubeck DP, Prebil LA, Peebles B, Brown JS: *Qual Life Res* 8(4):337-344, 1999.
King's Health Questionnaire	HRQOL specific to UI, validated in women and men	Kelleher CJ, Cardozo LD, Khullar V, Salvatore S: *Br J Obstet Gynecol* 104(12):1374-1379, 1997.
Incontinence Severity Index	UI severity in women, two items used mainly in epidemiologic research	Sandvik H, Hunskaar S, Seim A, et al: *J Epidemiol Commun Health Med* 47(6):497-499, 1993.
ICS Male Questionnaire	LUTS in men, available in original and short forms (ICS male SF)	Donovan JL, Abrams P, Peters TJ, et al: *Br J Urol* 77(4):554-562, 1996.
Bristol Female LUTS	LUTS in women, partly based on development process used for ICS male	Jackson S, Donovan J, Brookes S, et al: *Br J Urol* 77(6):805-812, 1996.
ICSQoL	Six-item questionnaire addresses general and continence-related HRQOL	Donovan JL, Kay HE, Peters TJ, et al: *Br J Urol* 80(5):712-721, 1997.

HRQOL, health-related quality of life; ICS, International Continence Society, ICSQoL, International Continence Society quality of life; SF, short form; UDI, Urogenital Distress Inventory; UI, urinary incontinence.
*The reader is referred to Donovan JL, Corcos J, Gotoh M, et al: Symptom and quality of life assessment. In: Abrams P, Cardozo L, Khoury S, Wein A, editors: *Incontinence,* Second International Consultation on Incontinence, Plymouth, United Kingdom, 2002, Plymbridge, pp 267-316, for an excellent and detailed review of these instruments.

Incontinence Impact Questionnaire

The Incontinence Impact Questionnaire (IIQ) originated as a 26-item questionnaire by Wyman and colleagues from the Continence Program for Women Research Group,[67] and it was later revised and validated as a 30-item instrument[68] to measure health-related quality of life in female patients with UI. A shortened version of the IIQ was developed and tested by Ubersax and the Continence Program for Women Research Group,[69] to reduce respondent burden when completing the instrument and to minimize time and economic burden associated with instrument administration, scoring, and interpretation of results (Fig. 12-2). It consists of seven items from the 30-item instrument: two query UI impact on physical activity, two focus on travel, and two on emotional health, and a single item queries its impact on social relationships. Extensive clinical use has shown that the IIQ-7 is reliable, valid and responsive to improvement following treatment in both men and women.

Urogenital Distress Inventory

The Urogenital Distress Inventory (UDI) is a 19-item questionnaire that can be divided into three subscales: (1) LUTS associated with overactive bladder dysfunction, (2) LUTS associated with stress UI, and (3) discomfort or voiding LUTS related to pelvic organ prolapse.[68] A short version of the instrument, the UDI-6, was subsequently developed and validated and is useful for measuring LUTS and discomfort in women (Fig. 12-3). Like the IIQ-7, it has been found to be reliable, valid, and responsive to treatment outcome in women.[69,70]

International Prostate Symptom Score (I-PSS)

Patient's Name

Date of Birth   Date Completed

	Not at all	Less than 1 time in 5	Less than half the time	About half the time	More than half the time	Almost always	Your score
1. Incomplete emptying Over the past month, how often have you had a sensation of not emptying your bladder completely after you finished urinating?	0	1	2	3	4	5	
2. Frequency Over the past month, how often have you had to urinate again less than two hours after you finished urinating?	0	1	2	3	4	5	
3. Intermittency Over the past month how often have you found you stopped and started again several times when you urinated?	0	1	2	3	4	5	
4. Urgency Over the past month, how often have you found it difficult to postpone urination?	0	1	2	3	4	5	
5. Weak stream Over the past month, how often have you had a weak urinary stream?	0	1	2	3	4	5	
6. Straining Over the past month, how often have you had to push or strain to begin urination?	0	1	2	3	4	5	

	None	1 time	2 times	3 times	4 times	5 times or more	
7. Nocturia Over the past month, how many times did you most typically get up to urinate from the time you went to bed at night until the time you got up in the morning?	0	1	2	3	4	5	
Total I-PSS Score							

Quality of Life Due to Urinary Symptoms	Delighted	Pleased	Mostly satisfied	Mixed-about equally satisfied and dissatisfied	Mostly dissatisfied	Unhappy	Terrible
If you were to spend the rest of your life with your urinary condition just the way it is now, how would you feel about that?	0	1	2	3	4	5	6

Fig. 12-1 International Prostate Symptom Score. Scores of 7 or less indicate mild to no symptoms, scores of 8 to 19 indicate moderate symptoms, and scores of 20 to 35 indicate severe symptoms. (Leaflet copyright EMIS and PIP 2005, as distributed on www.patient.co.uk.)

Incontinence Impact Questionnaire—Short Form (IIQ-7)	Not at all (0)	Slightly (1)	Moderately (2)	Greatly (3)
1. Has urine leakage affected your ability to do household chores?				
2. Has urine leakage affected your ability to participate in physical recreation activities?				
3. Has urine leakage affected your ability to participate in entertainment activities (going to a movie or play)?				
4. Has urine leakage affected your ability to travel more than 30 minutes from home?				
5. Has urine leakage affected your ability to participate in social activities?				
6. Has urine leakage affected your emotional health (nervousness, depression, etc.)?				
7. Has urine leakage caused you to feel frustrated?				

Fig. 12-2 Incontinence Impact Questionnaire Short Form (IIQ-7). Items are scored on a scale of 0 to 3, and the mean score is multiplied by 33, providing an overall score ranging from 0 to 100.

Urogenital Distress Inventory—Short Form (UDI-6)	Not at all (0)	Slightly (1)	Moderately (2)	Greatly (3)
Do you experience, and if so, how much are you bothered by:				
Frequent urination				
Urine leakage related to a feeling of urgency				
Urine leakage related to physical activity, coughing or sneezing				
Small amounts of urine leakage (drops)				
Difficulty emptying your bladder				
Pain or discomfort in the lower abdominal or genital area				

Fig. 12-3 Urogenital Distress Inventory Short Form (UDI-6).

VOIDING DIARY (BLADDER CHART)

A voiding diary is used to document patterns of urinary elimination and leakage. We advocate its use as a routine component of initial UI assessment with repeated measurement as indicated during treatment. Various bladder charts are available. The most basic provide information regarding times and patterns of urinary elimination and urinary leakage, whereas more detailed charts can be used to assess average and maximum voided volumes, the volume and type of fluids consumed, and factors precipitating urinary leakage. Selection of a voiding diary is determined by the type of information desired, the motivation and knowledge of the person completing the chart, and the type of voiding dysfunction being assessed. When a clinician is selecting a tool, he or she should remember that simpler diaries provide less information but are easier to complete and maintain over time, whereas more complex instruments generate more detailed information but mandate greater adherence and motivation to complete accurately.

The bladder chart (diary) may be kept by the patient or by lay or professional caregivers. It may be designed to be carried in a pocket or purse, or it may be placed at the bedside or near the toilet. A 7- to 14-day diary has been shown to produce reliable results, with or without intensive instruction.[71,72] However, our clinical experiences support the view that voiding diaries maintained for 1 to 3 days also produce valuable results.

Regardless of the time period for which the bladder diary is maintained, it is essential to discuss the results of the document with the patient and participating caregivers. This discussion provides an opportunity to clarify details of lower urinary tract function, fluid intake, and current bladder management techniques. It also provides reinforcement for compliance with future requests to maintain such records as a means of evaluating response to treatment.

Selection of a Voiding Diary

The simplest voiding diary limits documentation to the patterns of urinary elimination and urinary leakage (Fig. 12-4). It typically contains two columns; the patient is instructed to place a check mark or × in the column labeled "Voided" each time he or she urinates and a similar mark in the column marked "Leaked" each time UI is perceived. This diary can be used to assess diurnal voiding patterns, nocturia, and the frequency of UI. It is easily maintained in the home setting or during work, and little expertise or judgment is required to complete the record accurately. This type of bladder chart is particularly unobtrusive; it can even be designed as an insert for the pocket, which facilitates compliance in public places such as a work setting.

A more sophisticated diary requires the individual to record voided volumes as well as voiding frequency (Fig. 12-5). To complete this type of diary, the patient or recorder must have a graduated urinal, graduated beaker, or "high hat" urine collector. During part or all of the data collection period, the patient is instructed to void into the measuring device and to record each voiding in terms of time and volume. The patient may also be asked to provide a more quantitative estimate of the volume of urine lost during episodes of UI. Typically, urine loss is categorized according to an ordinal scale using such terms as minimal, moderate, or large. "Minimal" is usually defined as several drops of urine, insufficient to stain clothing. "Moderate leakage" usually indicates several teaspoons or tablespoons of urine,

Time	Sunday		Monday		Tuesday		Wednesday		Thursday		Friday		Saturday	
	Voided	Leaked	Voided	Leaked	Voided	Leaked	Voided	Leaked	Voided	Leaked	Voided	Leaked	Voided	Leaked

Fig. 12-4 A simple voiding diary.

Time	Amount voided	Leakage	Amount of fluid consumed

Fig. 12-5 Voiding diary for calculating functional bladder capacity and fluid intake.

easily contained by a small pad, and "large-volume urine loss" generally means sufficient volumes to soak the clothing or to saturate a large pad or containment brief (that is, several ounces or more of urine).[73]

The voiding diary may also be used to assess the effect of fluid consumption on urine elimination patterns and UI. The patient is usually asked to record the type and the approximate volume of fluid consumed. Because it is not feasible for most patients to actually measure the fluids they consume, the voiding diary should include a table of estimated fluid volumes (such as coffee cup = 6 ounces; soft drink can = 12 ounces). It is important to provide sufficient space on the chart for the patient to record the type of fluid consumed, because this information provides important insights concerning the intake of bladder irritants such as caffeine or alcohol.

There are also diaries tailored for use in the various care settings; that is, acute care, rehabilitation, or long-term care settings (Fig. 12-6). These diaries are maintained over a more prolonged period of time to provide ongoing evaluation of bladder function and the patient's response to management programs. They may be used to compare the voided volume with the residual volume obtained by intermittent catheterization or the percentage of continent voids with the percentage of incontinent episodes.

Voiding diaries may also be used to evaluate behavioral and environmental factors influencing continence. These instruments usually provide a space for comments, and the patient or caregiver is asked to describe the circumstances surrounding each episode of urinary leakage. For example, the incontinent patient may be asked to describe whether leakage occurred with physical exertion, shortly after perceiving the urge to urinate, or during sleep. The caregiver for a cognitively impaired patient may be instructed to check the patient hourly and to record the patient's status as "wet" or "dry" at each of these checks; the caregiver may also be asked to record the patient's response to being informed of incontinent episodes during these routine checks. Alternatively, the caregiver may be instructed to take the patient to the toilet on a set schedule and to record the patient's response to each request to use the toilet (Fig. 12-7). This type of diary can be very helpful in evaluating a patient's response to a prompted or scheduled voiding program. (See Chapter 6 for a discussion of these voiding programs.)

Interpretation of Data

The value of the data obtained from a voiding diary is influenced by the type of instrument used, the period of time over which data were collected, and the completeness and accuracy of the recorded data. Its value is enhanced by a detailed and unhurried discussion of the results with the patient or caregivers. This discussion not only provides an opportunity to obtain additional insights from the patient concerning the data recorded, but also enables the patient to gain added insight into the function of the bladder and the influence of environmental and dietary factors on urinary leakage.

Patterns of Urine Elimination. The voiding diary provides a reasonably reliable record of patterns of urinary elimination.[71,72] This information can be used to determine diurnal voiding frequency and the presence and severity of nocturia. To assess these factors accurately, the clinician needs to establish the patient's usual patterns of sleep and wakefulness. The clinician

Name _____   Date _____

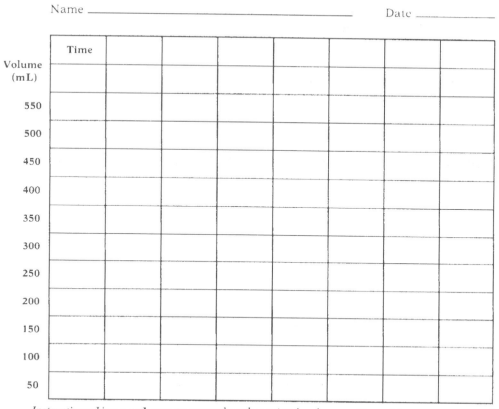

Instructions: Use a **red** pen to record catheterized volumes. Use a **blue** pen to record voided volumes.

Fig. 12-6 Voiding diary for determining voided volume and residual urine volume.

should never assume that a specific patient awakens during the early morning and sleeps during nighttime hours, because work requirements or other factors may profoundly alter patterns of sleep and wakefulness. After determining sleep-wake patterns, the clinician determines the diurnal voiding frequency by noting the longest and shortest intervals between trips to the bathroom and by calculating the average interval between micturition on 1 or more days. The physiologically normal individual usually voids no more often than every 2 hours and no less frequently than every 4 to 6 hours. An average voiding interval of less than 2 hours (more than eight episodes per 24 hours) indicates increased daytime voiding frequency.

The clinician identifies patterns of nocturia by counting the number of times the patient voided during sleeping hours and dividing this number by the number of nights over which data were recorded. Because nocturia can be confused with incidental voiding or with enuresis, the patient should be asked whether it was the urge to urinate or factors such as pain or insomnia that caused him or her to awaken. Nocturia is defined as awakening caused by the urge to void. Any episodes of urine loss occurring during sleep should be considered as enuresis, not nocturia. The patient who is awakened by the urge to urinate and who then experiences leakage before reaching the toilet is considered to have nocturia associated with urge UI. Three or

Name _____   Date _____

Time toilet is offered	Leakage (yes or no)	Was patient aware of urge? (yes or no)	Did patient void? (yes or no)	Comments
0800				
1000				
1200				
1400				
1600				
1800				
2000				

(2200 and so forth)

Fig. 12-7 Prompted voiding diary.

more episodes of nocturia per night are considered excessive.

Patterns of Urinary Leakage. The clinician assesses patterns of urinary leakage by noting the frequency of incontinent episodes, their relation to patterns of voluntary controlled urination, and their relation to documented "precipitating factors." The more detailed voiding diaries contribute to the clinician's ability to determine leakage patterns because they provide estimates of the volume of leakage as well as data regarding the patient's fluid intake and factors associated with incontinent episodes. For example, episodes of stress UI are typically associated with relatively low-volume leakage that occurs during waking hours with physical exertion. In contrast, episodes of urge UI usually cause larger volumes of urine loss, occur during waking hours or at night, and are associated with a precipitous desire to urinate. Extraurethral UI is continuous and is not associated with either physical exertion or the urge to urinate. Unfortunately, no predictable pattern of UI has been described for urinary retention and overflow UI.

Fluid Consumption. Fluid intake is evaluated in terms of overall volume, patterns of intake, and intake of bladder irritants. The United States Food and Nutrition Board has established the recommended dietary allowance (RDA) for fluid intake as 30 mL/kg of body weight. If these figures are converted to ounces and pounds, the RDA for fluid intake is approximately 1/2 ounce per pound of body weight. A significantly lower fluid intake can negatively affect bladder function; dehydration is associated with constipation, an increased risk for bacteriuria, and an increased osmolality (concentration) of urine, each of which can act as a bladder "irritant." A daily volume of fluid intake that is significantly higher than the RDA may also contribute to bladder dysfunction because it produces polyuria and may increase the frequency and volume of any UI.

In addition to evaluating the total volume of fluid consumed during a 24-hour period, the clinician should assess the timing of fluid intake. Consumption of a particularly large volume of fluid over a brief time may precipitate a diuretic effect that results in UI. In addition, there is some evidence that consumption of fluids close to the hour of sleep increases the risk of nocturia or nocturnal UI in the elderly.[74,75]

The clinician should also evaluate the documented intake of substances that are considered bladder irritants. The term *bladder irritant* is typically used to describe a group of dietary substances believed to increase urinary urgency, bladder pain, or the risk of UI in susceptible individuals. Caffeine has been demonstrated to increase voiding frequency and the number of UI episodes, and its restriction has been found to alleviate these effects.[76] Additional research supports recommendations that smoking may affect continence, although the strength of the evidence base is significantly less than that for caffeine.[77,78] Large numbers of additional substances, such as citrus fruits and juices, have also been identified as bladder irritants;[79] however, these substances were studied in a group of women with interstitial cystitis, and it remains unclear whether these substances act as primary bladder irritants or whether their effect is limited to exacerbation of interstitial cystitis pain.

Caution is required when one is interpreting the potential contributions of bladder irritants to UI in a particular patient. Although it is easy to associate perceptions of heightened urinary urgency with the intake of a variety of foods or beverages, multiple factors contribute to these perceptions, and excessive food and fluid restrictions may detract from rather than enhance compliance with an effective bladder management program. Nonetheless, a physiologic basis for the bladder-irritating properties of certain dietary substances has been identified, and patients may be appropriately advised to eliminate or reduce their intake of these substances to reduce symptoms of urgency, frequency, and UI (see Table 12-1). We recommend eliminating potential irritants one at a time to determine the effect of each substance on the individual patient.

Bladder Capacity. Bladder capacity may be defined within three contexts. *Anatomic capacity* is the volume of fluid that the bladder is capable of holding at the limit of its viscoelastic or accommodative properties. It is assessed while the patient is anesthetized or sedated during a cystoscopic examination. The bladder is filled until the inflow of fluid stops, indicating a loss of compliance as the viscoelastic properties of the bladder wall have been reached. *Cystometric capacity* is the volume of urine held by the bladder during urodynamic testing. It is affected by the fill rate, type of fluid used for testing, the patient's anxiety level, and the clinician's judgment. *Functional capacity* is the amount of urine stored in the bladder before a sense of bladder fullness, urgency, or urinary leakage prompts the individual to urinate. One can assess functional capacity by evaluating the patient's bladder chart. The clinician may identify the functional capacity by determining the highest and lowest voided volumes or by determining the "average" voided volume. (The ICS now recommends use of the term "average voided volume" as opposed to "functional bladder capacity.") In physiologically normal adults, the average voided volume ranges from 300 to 600 mL; in children, the "normal" average voided volume is calculated by the following equation:

$$\text{Capacity (mL)} = (\text{Age in years} + 2) \times 30.$$

Prompted Voiding Diary. Unlike most diaries, which rely on self-report, the prompted voiding diary is designed to document the functional and environmental aspects of UI for the patient with functional UI. The data from the chart can be used to assess patterns of urinary elimination, response to prompted toileting, and timing of incontinent episodes. This information can be used to predict the probability of success with prompted voiding and to suggest modifications in the prompted voiding schedule.[45]

Urinary Retention Diary. A bladder chart can also be used to monitor patients in urinary retention who are being managed with intermittent catheterization. For these patients, the bladder chart is used to compare voided volumes with catheterized volumes; these data enable the clinician to assess the patient's ability to void effectively and to modify the catheterization schedule to maximize bladder function while minimizing catheterization frequency. Such a chart also provides the information needed to determine when intermittent catheterization is no longer needed.

LABORATORY STUDIES

In most cases, UI occurs as a result of a structural or functional defect and poses minimal risk to the patient's physical health, although it is associated with significant psychosocial consequences. However, in some cases UI is associated with a neurologic, metabolic, or obstructive disorder that poses a significant threat to the person's overall physical health. Therefore, the number and type of laboratory studies required for the evaluation of a patient with UI vary and are determined by the nature of the UI, the presence of complications such as UTI or altered skin integrity, and the coexistence of urologic, reproductive, neurologic, or metabolic disorders.

Urine Studies

A urinalysis is an essential component of the evaluation of any patient with UI. A dipstick or laboratory analysis should be conducted to determine the specific gravity of the urine and to detect the presence of abnormal substances such as glucose, protein, hemoglobin or red blood cells, white blood cells, and nitrites or bacteria. In addition to dipstick analysis, a microscopic examination is completed whenever feasible. Table 12-8 summarizes urinalysis findings that are common in individuals with UI

TABLE 12-8   Urinalysis: Normal and Significant Findings and their Implications

NORMAL VALUE	SIGNIFICANCE OF ABNORMAL FINDING	FOLLOW-UP STUDY
Specific gravity: 1.003 to 1.029	Low *specific gravity:* excessive water intake, diabetes insipidus	Low *specific gravity:* obtain serum electrolytes; arrange for follow-up evaluation by primary care physician or nephrologist
	High *specific gravity:* dehydration, diabetes mellitus with glucosuria	High *specific gravity:* bladder chart including fluid intake; evaluation for diabetes mellitus if glucosuria present
Glucose: absent	*Glucose present:* uncontrolled or undiagnosed diabetes mellitus	Refer to primary care physician for diagnostic evaluation or alteration in current management
Nitrites and leukocytes: absent	*Nitrites present, no leukocytes:* bacteriuria	Microscopic evaluation for presence of bacteria and white blood cells, urine culture and sensitivity for pyuria and bacteriuria, and culture and sensitivity based on clinical judgment when bacteriuria present but pyuria (leukocytes) absent
	Nitrites and leukocytes present: bacteriuria and pyuria (urinary tract infection)	
Hemoglobin: negative	*Positive hemoglobin:* hematuria	Microscopic examination, urine culture and sensitivity if other signs of infection present (pyuria, bacteriuria), urine cytologic test and referral to urologist if hematuria present without coexisting infection
Protein: negative	*Positive result:* "normal" finding when leukocytes present; otherwise may indicate renal disease	Refer to physician or nephrologist unless urinary tract infection coexists

and the additional diagnostic studies indicated for each finding. Culture and sensitivity testing are indicated only when the urinalysis or other assessment findings raise a suspicion of UTI. UTI should always be treated because treatment may significantly reduce or even eliminate the individual's urinary leakage.

Serum Studies

Serum studies are indicated when UI is complicated by a neurologic, reproductive, metabolic, or obstructive condition. For example, the continence nurse should obtain serum creatinine and blood urea nitrogen (BUN) values when evaluating the patient with BPH, because this condition poses a risk of bladder outlet obstruction and upper tract damage. We believe that serum creatinine and BUN values should also be determined when the clinician is evaluating patients who present with other obstructive processes (such as vesicosphincter dyssynergia) or any evidence of upper tract distress (such as recurring pyelonephritis, hydronephrosis, vesicoureteral reflux, or known renal insufficiency). Prompt consultation

with a urologist is indicated whenever the serum creatinine or BUN levels are elevated.

Other blood studies, such as specific electrolytes, complete blood count, hemoglobin A1c, blood cultures, or prostate specific antigen, may be indicated for selected patients with specific medical problems. Consultation with a physician is essential in these cases, and most patients are referred for complete medical evaluation and management.

Measurement of Postvoid Urinary Residual Volume

The Agency for Health Care Policy and Research Guidelines Panel defined the measurement of a postvoid residual urine volume as an optional component of the assessment for an individual with UI. This recommendation is based on the finding that urinary retention is not common among most patients with UI, and particularly among women with stress, urge, or mixed UI. No absolute guidelines for the diagnosis of urinary retention have been developed; however, Box 12-1 includes a list of risk factors that should prompt the clinician to

---

BOX 12-1   Risk Factors for Urinary Retention

Associated Conditions

Recurrent urinary tract infections
Febrile urinary tract infection
History of acute urinary retention
Enlarged prostate on digital rectal examination
Urethral stricture
Pelvic organ prolapse with grade 3 cystocele
Known history of elevated urinary residual
Paralyzing disorder of the spine (trauma, multiple sclerosis, spinovascular disorders, transverse myelitis, etc.)
Diabetes mellitus
Chronic alcoholism
Stool impaction

Medications

Antidepressants (reduce contractility)
Antipsychotics (reduce contractility)
Sedatives and hypnotics (reduce contractility)
Alpha-adrenergic agonists (increase urethral resistance)
Anticholinergics (reduce contractility)
Calcium-channel blockers (reduce contractility)

evaluate carefully for retention. Postvoid residual volume should be measured on any patient in whom urinary retention is suspected.

There are two approaches to the measurement of postvoid residual volume: catheterization and ultrasonographic imaging. Catheterization offers several potential advantages when compared with ultrasonography. It is relatively inexpensive and accurate, and it can be completed quickly, provided the clinician has experience and competence in the procedure. Nonetheless, catheterization is associated with a low risk for UTI (about 2%)[80] and with discomfort that ranges from mild to significant, depending on the status of the lower urinary tract. In contrast, ultrasonographic imaging is more expensive than catheterization, but it is often preferred because it is noninvasive, carries no risk for infection or discomfort, and is reasonably accurate when compared with catheterization.[81] Regardless of the method used for measurement of postvoid residual, it is important to conduct the study as soon as possible after micturition.

The evaluation of urinary residual volume is deceptively complex. No absolute number can be defined as being indicative of significant urinary retention. The residual volume is usually considered significant if it exceeds 250 mL. When interpreting residual urine volumes, the clinician must be cognizant that opinions vary according to the clinical relevance of urinary residual volumes and that certain patients may carry large residual volumes without experiencing adverse results, whereas others experience recurring UTI or upper tract distress despite the presence of comparatively small residual volumes.

URODYNAMIC EVALUATION

The term *urodynamics* refers to a group of tests designed to evaluate the transport, storage, and elimination functions of the middle and lower urinary tract. Urodynamic evaluation of the lower urinary tract typically comprises a combination of tests that assess bladder filling and storage, urethral sphincter activity during bladder filling, and the function and relationship of the bladder and its outlet during micturition. As with all diagnostic tests, standardization of testing techniques and quality

assurance are critical for the generation of accurate and reproducible results. A survey of urodynamic services in North America revealed both a lack of standardization and resulting variability in the quality of data produced during evaluation.[82,83] Fortunately, attention has been focused on this issue on a global level, resulting in the promulgation of best practice standards for urodynamic testing[84] and raising long-overdue discussions about the need for certification of urodynamic clinicians.

Hydrodynamic Principles

Regardless of the techniques used, urodynamic information is gained by measurement of specific physical properties of fluid within the urinary tract while the fluid is at rest and in motion. A fluid is defined as any substance that deforms or reshapes itself continuously in response to the application of any tangential force (shear), regardless of its magnitude.[85] Thus, it is apparent that both liquids (such as saline and water) and gases (such as carbon dioxide) qualify as fluids. In the physiologic state, the only fluid in the middle and lower urinary tract is urine that has been created by the nephrons. However, for the purposes of urodynamic testing, alternative liquids (such as water, saline solution, or a radiographic contrast solution) or gases (carbon dioxide) have been used to approximate the effects of urine within the urinary system. Two physical properties, *pressure* and *flow,* are measured within this fluid to determine the dynamic function of the lower urinary tract.

Pressure. Pressure is defined as the force per unit area.[85,86] Pressure measurements represent the kinetic or potential energy within the lower urinary tract, and they reflect a combination of detrusor forces and abdominal forces acting on the bladder vesicle and urethral lumen. Kinetic energy is evidenced by the movement of fluid from the bladder to the urethra and then to the outside of the body during micturition. In contrast, potential energy is created when abdominal forces act on urine within the bladder in the presence of a closed outlet. As long as the urethral sphincter mechanism remains closed, urine remains confined within the bladder. However, if the urethral sphincter is incompetent, urine is expelled from the bladder, thus creating the condition known as stress UI.

Three pressures are routinely measured during urodynamic testing: intravesical, abdominal, and detrusor. Intravesical pressure (Pves) is measured by inserting a fluid-filled tube into the bladder or inserting a transducer directly mounted on the catheter. Pves represents the sum of the abdominal and detrusor forces acting on the contents of the bladder. To separate the effects of abdominal forces from the effects of detrusor forces, it is necessary to measure abdominal pressure (Pabd). Pabd is measured by inserting a tube into the rectal vault or posterior vagina. The computer subtracts Pabd from Pves to yield the detrusor pressure (Pdet).

When urodynamic data are being generated or interpreted, it is essential to understand the relation of these pressures to the forces they are intended to measure. *Abdominal forces* are generated when gravity, external forces, or physical exertion affect the abdominal and pelvic viscera. These forces normally act on both the intravesical contents (urine within the bladder) and the sphincter simultaneously. As a result, they do not produce leakage in the continent individual (Fig. 12-8). Abdominal forces are provoked when the patient is asked to rise to a sitting or standing position, to perform Valsalva's maneuver, or to cough during urodynamic testing.

Detrusor forces represent both active and passive tension elements within the bladder wall (Fig. 12-9). Like abdominal forces, detrusor forces act on the contents of the bladder. However, these forces are *not* equally distributed to the urethral sphincter mechanism. Instead, detrusor forces act selectively on the bladder outlet and its two inlets (the paired ureterovesical junctions). Active forces within the bladder wall are attributable to the tone of the detrusor smooth muscle bundles. The passive forces within the bladder wall are attributable to collagen, elastin, and other proteins that ensure the structural integrity of the bladder; collectively, these forces are termed the viscoelastic properties of the bladder wall. The clinician evaluates active detrusor forces by measuring the pressure created by detrusor muscle contraction during micturition and assesses the viscoelastic forces of the bladder by measuring the pressures within the bladder wall during bladder filling.

During urodynamic testing, the measurement of Pves alone does not provide the data needed regarding bladder wall pressures because it reflects the *combined* actions of abdominal and detrusor forces. However, if Pabd is measured simultaneously, it is possible to subtract the contribution of abdominal forces and thereby to calculate Pdet. This permits distinction between the effect of abdominal forces

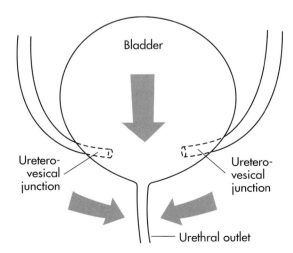

Fig. 12-8 Abdominal forces equally affect the bladder and urethral outlet.

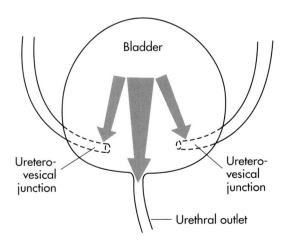

Fig. 12-9 Detrusor forces act selectively on the urethral outlet and the ureterovesical junctions.

and the effect of detrusor forces, which is necessary because each acts on the lower urinary tract in a unique way. For example, stress UI occurs when abdominal forces created by physical exertion cause a rise in Pves that overwhelms the incompetent sphincter and produces urinary leakage in the absence of a detrusor contraction. In contrast, detrusor forces produce urge UI when an overactive detrusor contraction forces the sphincter open, resulting in urgency and leakage of urine. Overflow UI occurs when passive (viscoelastic) elements of the bladder wall are stretched to a point that Pdet rises enough to force urine past the sphincter mechanism, leading to dribbling urinary leakage in the absence of a detrusor contraction.

Physiologic pressure measurements are usually reported as one of three units: millimeters of mercury (mm Hg), centimeters of water (cm H_2O), or kilopascals; 1 mm Hg represents the force required to raise a column of mercury 1 mm; it is the unit used to measure intravascular pressures, including blood pressure; 1 cm H_2O is the force required to raise a column of water 1 cm; 1 mm Hg is equal to approximately 13 cm H_2O. The ICS recommends use of the kilopascal to measure pressure, but this recommendation is seldom followed in the clinical setting. Instead, pressure is measured in "cm H_2O," primarily because the parameter "mm Hg" is sometimes too large to detect subtle but clinically relevant pressure changes during micturition, which may be 10 to 15 cm H_2O or less.

Measuring Pressures. Urodynamic pressures may be measured by a manometer or an electronic transducer. Continence nurses performing simple cystometry use an open syringe attached to a catheter that is placed into the bladder. If the syringe is graduated in centimeters, it acts as a simple manometer and allows for measurement of pressure within the bladder. The nurse completes the bedside cystometrogram (CMG) by slowly filling the bladder in a retrograde manner while observing the level of water within the syringe. If the patient experiences a rise in Pves, the nurse will observe that the inflow of fluid stops and the fluid level in the syringe rises as the detrusor contraction builds toward its maximum amplitude. Provided the nurse discontinues the inflow of water whenever this fluid level is

observed to rise, each centimeter rise within the syringe represents a 1 cm H_2O rise in Pves.

Unfortunately, this technically simple approach to cystometry has disadvantages when it comes to accurate interpretation of results. Simple cystometry does not generate a graphic record of pressure changes observed during bladder filling and micturition. In addition, it does not provide for simultaneous measurements of Pves and Pabd. This lack of simultaneity means that the differential action of abdominal forces and detrusor forces cannot be easily identified using this simple approach. Therefore, most urodynamic testing is now accomplished by the use of electronic transducers attached to a computer-based recording system.

The electronic transducer converts pressure into an electronic signal that is transformed into a graphic representation or tracing. A stereo speaker is an example of a commonly used electronic transducer. The stereo receiver or amplifier transmits signals to the transducer, and the transducer in the speaker converts these signals into sound waves that we appreciate as music or the spoken word. A pressure transducer uses similar electronic principles; it receives pressure signals from the bladder or abdomen and converts them into an electrical signal that generates a plot comparing pressure and volume.

Several types of pressure transducers are used for urodynamic testing. External dome transducers are filled with a fluid and are positioned parallel to the symphysis pubis (Fig. 12-10). These transducers contain a membrane that responds to pressure changes by deforming slightly. This deformity alters the electrical output of the transducer, which is recorded as a change in pressure by the computer. Microtip transducers are located within the catheter itself; they also contain small membranes that respond to changes in pressure by deforming their surfaces (Fig. 12-11, *A*). A third catheter-mounted transducer contains a titanium diaphragm and an optical fiber. Changes in pressure cause changes in the light reflected from the titanium diaphragm onto the optical fiber[87] (Fig. 12-11, *B*). A fourth type of transducer uses tiny air filled balloons to measure urethral pressure and Pves, thus avoiding many of the disadvantages associated with fiber-optic or microtip transducers.

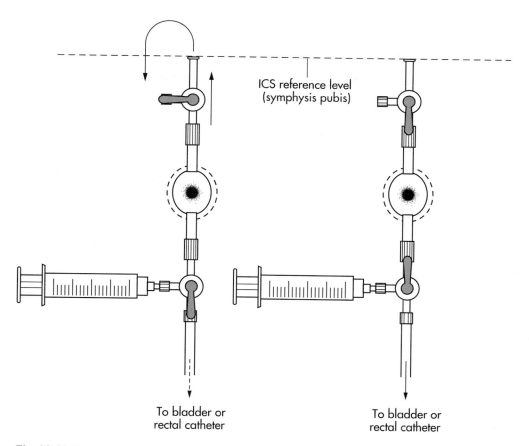

Fig. 12-10 Dome pressure transducers commonly used for urodynamic testing.

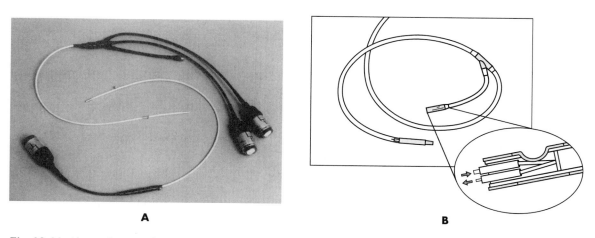

A   **B**

Fig. 12-11 Alternative transducers used for urodynamic testing. **A,** Transducers are mounted directly onto these microtip catheters. **B,** Fiberoptic transducer system relies on changes in deflection of laser-emitted light to measure pressure. Both catheter technologies require a change in reference level from superior border of symphysis to level of catheter. (A, From Walters MD, Karram MM: *Clinical urogynecology,* St. Louis, 1993, Mosby.)

Pressure measurements during urodynamic testing must conform to certain standards to ensure valid (accurate) and reliable (reproducible) results. Further, because pressure is a physical rather than a urodynamic concept, it is essential to comply with those standards of measurement used by the scientific and clinical communities in a variety of settings. Three standards are particularly important when the clinician is completing or evaluating urodynamic testing: (1) pressure must be measured within a reservoir that contains fluid, (2) pressure measurements must be zeroed with reference to atmospheric pressure, and (3) pressures must be measured with reference to some common point (in this case the upper margin of the symphysis pubis).[84]

Application of the first principle to the measurement of Pves is relatively simple, because the bladder is a fluid-filled reservoir that deforms itself according to the volume of fluid it contains. Therefore, insertion of a fluid-filled tube with an open end directly into the bladder vesicle permits measurement of Pves. In contrast, the abdomen is *not* a fluid-filled chamber. Therefore, Pabd is measured by creation of a small fluid-filled reservoir around the pressure monitor. One can create this fluid reservoir by inserting an open-ended tube into the rectum or posterior aspect of the vagina and then perfusing a small "bleb" of liquid, or by covering the open end of the tube with a fluid-filled balloon.

The second and third requirements are to adjust to zero all pressures with reference to atmospheric pressure and to measure all pressures with reference to some common point.[84] To ensure that all pressures are zeroed with reference to atmospheric pressure, all transducers are exposed to atmospheric pressure (that is, opened to air) before the pressure lines are inserted into the patient. To meet the requirement that all pressures be measured with reference to some common point, the external pressure transducers are placed parallel to the superior margin of the symphysis pubis before the procedure is begun because the symphysis pubis has been established as the standard reference level by the ICS.[88] Unfortunately, microtip, fiberoptic, and air-charged catheters record pressure from the tip of the catheter itself, and so the symphysis pubis cannot be used as a reference point for these measurements.

The ICS has determined that the catheter serves as the reference level when this technologic method is used.[89] Whether the variability created by this practice is clinically significant remains controversial.

Urethral Pressure. Although most North American urodynamic services routinely measure Pves, Pabd, and/or Pdet, few routinely measure urethral pressure.[83] There are many reasons for this, including some of the unique physical challenges inherent in the measurement of urethral pressure in the clinical setting. One difficulty is the challenge of creating a fluid bleb around a urethral pressure line or transducer. During bladder filling, the urethra is closed, and any fluid infused into the urethral lumen through an open-ended tube either enters the bladder or drips from the distal end of the urethra. During micturition, the urethra is transformed into a fluid-filled conduit, and pressure measurements are profoundly affected by detrusor forces *and* by the transducer's location within this complex, collapsible tube. Several alternative techniques for urethral pressure measurement have been advocated.[89] One approach is to use microtip transducers or fiberoptic sensors to measure urethral pressure; these methods supposedly bypass the need to perfuse fluid during evaluation. Unfortunately, they are also more likely to measure the force created between the somewhat stiff catheters and the urethral wall than to measure urethral pressures accurately. A more recent and attractive alternative is to use an air-charged catheter that combines catheter-mounted technology with a tiny air-filled chamber to measure urethral pressures.[90]

Flow. Flow is defined as the volume of a fluid that passes a given location within a given unit of time.[89] For the purposes of urodynamic testing, flow is measured as milliliters per second (mL/second). The urinary flow rate is typically measured by use of one of three electronic techniques: rotating disk, electronic dipstick, or gravimetry.[91] Rotating disk technology requires the patient to void directly onto a disk that spins at a given rate; the passage of urine across the disk creates inertia, which is recorded as a flow rate. An electronic dipstick is created when an electrical capacitance disk is mounted into the collecting chamber of a uroflowmeter. The changes in capacitance that occur during urine flow are expressed as the urinary flow rate. Gravimetric uroflowmeters determine flow by measuring the weight of the voided urine as it collects in a container positioned on top of the gravimetric device.

Techniques and Interpretation

Although a detailed discussion of urodynamic testing is beyond the scope of this text, a brief review of fundamental techniques is included because adherence to these principles determines the accuracy of the data and the limitations of data interpretation. The primary emphasis of this discussion is on the interpretation of urodynamic data, because it is this interpretation that assists the continence nurse to identify the pathophysiologic characteristics of UI in a specific patient and to design an individualized plan for management. Whenever possible, the nomenclature in this section conforms to the standards established by the ICS.[88]

Simple, or Bedside, Cystometry. Bedside, or simple, cystometry involves the use of a manometer to assess bladder pressures at a given volume. The patient is typically placed in a supine or semi-recumbent position. A catheter is inserted into the bladder, or an existing, indwelling catheter is used to introduce fluid into the bladder.[92] The catheter is then attached to a Toomey syringe or a manometer and is positioned just above the superior margin of the symphysis pubis. The bladder is slowly filled with saline or sterile water suitable for irrigation. During the process of bladder filling, the clinician observes the fluid level within the syringe. It should remain fairly consistent, indicating the bladder's accommodation of fluid without a simultaneous rise in pressure. If a steady rise in bladder pressure is observed during bladder filling, low bladder wall compliance is suspected, and a multichannel urodynamic study is indicated. The patient is instructed to report sensations of bladder filling, bladder fullness, and urgency. A precipitous but sustained rise in *P*ves accompanied by a reported urge to void is interpreted as a detrusor contraction. A rise in *P*ves associated with an urge to void and with leakage of fluid around the catheter is interpreted as an unstable detrusor contraction accompanied by urge UI.

Simple cystometry has been used to assess bladder sensation and the occurrence of involuntary or unstable detrusor contractions among frail elderly patients.[93] When compared with multichannel urodynamic techniques, it was found to have a sensitivity of 88% and a specificity of 75% for detrusor overactivity. The advantages of simple cystometry include its portability, ease of testing, and application to the home setting. Disadvantages include its exclusive reliance on *P*ves to evaluate detrusor and abdominal forces acting on the lower urinary tract and the limited range of diagnoses that can be made using this technique.

Complex Urodynamic Testing. Complex urodynamic testing typically refers to techniques that rely on electronic recording devices to produce a graphic representation (plot) of some aspects of lower urinary tract function. The most commonly used techniques include uroflowmetry, filling CMG, sphincter EMG, voiding pressure study, urethral pressure studies, and videourodynamic studies.

Uroflowmetry. Invasive urodynamic testing is typically preceded by measurement of a "free" urinary flow rate. The clinician conducts the study by asking the patient to come to the laboratory with a comfortably full bladder and to void into a uroflow device. It is critical to provide the patient with privacy during this screening test. After uroflowmetry, postvoid residual urine may be obtained by catheterization or bladder ultrasonography to determine the effectiveness of bladder emptying. Data from uroflow studies are typically displayed as a combination of numeric values and a chart that displays the flow rate (expressed as milliliters per second) and the time required to complete urination (expressed as seconds). The most significant numeric values provided by uroflowmetry are the maximum flow rate *(Qmax),* the average flow rate *(Qave),* and the voided volume. Other values of interest include the voiding time (time elapsed from the beginning to the end of micturition), the flow time (total time during which urinary flow is recorded), and the postvoid residual volume (the volume of fluid remaining in the bladder after micturition is completed). The normal values for Qmax and Qave vary according to the patient's gender and age and the voided volume. Because of this variability, many clinicians use a flow-rate nomogram to compare the values from a specific uroflow study to age-and gender-matched persons. The volumes on these nomograms usually vary from 100 to 500 mL (Fig. 12-12).

In addition to evaluating the numeric values provided by a uroflow study, the clinician also assesses the flow pattern. A *normal flow pattern* in a male patient resembles a bell curve that may be skewed to the left (Fig. 12-13, *A*). Qmax is typically 12 mL/second or more, particularly among men 50 years of age and younger, and the Qave should be greater than 50% of the maximum flow value. Ideally, the voided volume should be at least 250 mL but not more than 600 mL. The voiding time

should closely mirror the flow time (indicating a lack of intermittency within the urinary stream). The residual urinary volume is expected to be less than 100 mL or 25% of the total bladder volume (voided volume + residual urinary volume). When compared with the normal values for younger men, Qmax and Qave are typically lower for males more than 50 years of age. In addition, some intermittency may be observed, although the residual volume should remain low.

Because of anatomic differences in the length and configuration of the urethra, the normal flow pattern among women is somewhat different from that observed in men (Fig. 12-13, *B*). In women, the Qmax and Qave values tend to be higher and the

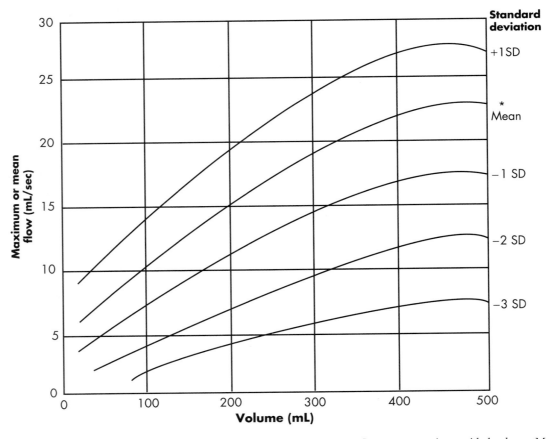

Fig. 12-12 Flow-rate nomogram allows comparison of peak and mean flow rates at a given voided volume. Many computerized systems automatically plot a gender- and age-matched nomogram when a uroflowmetry study is completed.

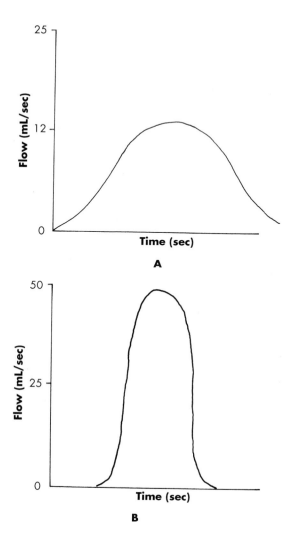

Fig. 12-13 Normal flow rates. **A,** Male. **B,** Female.

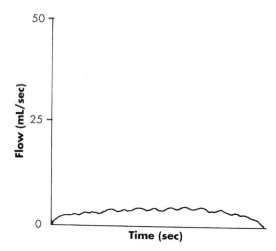

Fig. 12-14 Prolonged (poor) flow pattern indicating either poor detrusor contraction strength or bladder outlet obstruction.

flow and voiding times tend to be shorter than those in men; however, the residual volumes should remain less than 100 mL or 25% of the total bladder volume. Because the Qmax and Qave are particularly high among certain women, especially those with stress UI, a normal flow pattern may be referred to as *explosive.* Although the explosive flow pattern is common among women with stress UI, it is not pathognomonic of this condition.

Two abnormal flow patterns may be observed on uroflowmetry. The *prolonged flow pattern* is characterized by a low Qmax and Qave and a prolonged voiding time and flow time (Fig. 12-14). This flow pattern is also referred to as a "poor" flow pattern. The voided volume may be low, and the postvoid residual volume may be significant. The prolonged flow pattern is frequently associated with bladder outlet obstruction, particularly among men with BPH; however, it also occurs in patients who have poor detrusor contraction strength. Therefore, a prolonged flow pattern should be interpreted as representing either bladder outlet obstruction or poor detrusor contraction strength; a pressure flow study is required to differentiate between these two conditions.

The *interrupted* (sometimes called intermittent) *flow pattern* is characterized by a sawtooth configuration; the Qmax is usually within normal limits, but the Qave is typically low (Fig. 12-15). The voiding time is prolonged, but the flow time may be much shorter, indicating periods during which the individual is straining to void but producing no flow, or periods when detrusor-sphincter dyssynergia prevents urinary flow. The voided volume may be low, and the residual volume may be elevated. Although this flow pattern is usually associated with abdominal straining, it also occurs with bladder

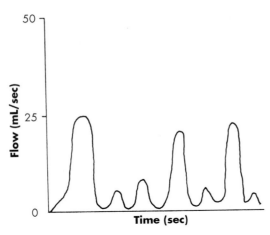

Fig. 12-15 Interrupted (intermittent) flow pattern indicating either poor detrusor contraction strength or bladder outlet obstruction.

outlet obstruction. Therefore, the intermittent flow pattern, like the poor flow pattern, should be interpreted as representing either poor detrusor contraction strength or bladder outlet obstruction, with a pressure flow study required to differentiate between the two.

Filling Cystometrogram. The CMG provides a graphic representation of bladder pressures as a function of volume. During the filling CMG, the bladder is filled with fluid at a specific infusion rate, and corresponding changes in bladder pressure are recorded. During the second phase of the study, the patient is asked to urinate, and bladder pressures are compared with flow rates. This portion of the CMG is typically referred to as a "voiding pressure (or pressure flow) study" and is discussed separately.

The CMG requires catheterization and emptying of the bladder. One of several catheters may be used for cystometry. Multiple-lumen urodynamic catheters are manufactured by several companies, and they are preferred for complex urodynamic testing.[84] These catheters are manufactured with two and three lumina and in sizes 5 to 12 French. Dual-lumen catheters are available in sizes 5 to 8 French; the two lumina permit simultaneous filling of the bladder and measurement of Pves. Triple-lumen catheters vary in size from 7 to 12 French; the three lumina permit measurement of both urethral pressure and Pves, in addition to providing a line for bladder filling. Smaller catheters reduce artifact during the voiding pressure study[94] and during measurement of sphincter competence.[95] We therefore recommend a 7-French dual-lumen catheter for urodynamic testing on adults and a 5-French dual-lumen catheter for urodynamic testing on children or infants.

After insertion of the urodynamic catheters, a tube is inserted to measure Pabd. This catheter may be inserted into the posterior portion of the vagina in women or into the rectum. The catheter may contain a small balloon that is filled with a liquid medium, or fluid may be perfused as needed to ensure that pressure measurements are obtained in a liquid medium. Currently, several manufacturers offer rectal tubes, including some that are latex free, that are designed to measure rectal pressure. Because many of the women we test have significant vaginal vault prolapse, we prefer to use a 6- to 12-French rectal tube for the measurement of Pabd in both women and men.

Once all filling and pressure monitoring lines have been placed, the clinician must select the medium for infusion. Carbon dioxide has been employed for urodynamic testing in some settings but it is no longer recommended or widely used.[96,97] Several types of liquid media are commonly used for urodynamic testing: (1) sterile water for irrigation, (2) sterile saline, and (3) radiographic contrast. Water provides an adequate medium for an intact bladder, but it should be avoided in patients who have undergone augmentation with a segment of bowel or stomach because water is hypotonic and provokes depolarization of smooth muscle cells leading to an artifactually low cystometric capacity. In contrast, normal saline is isotonic and it is appropriate for any urodynamic testing that does not include radiographic imaging. Radiographic contrast material is reserved for videourodynamic studies. However, this hypertonic medium tends to hyperpolarize smooth muscle cells within the augmented bladder and leads to a high cystometric capacity.

Pressure transducers should be zeroed with reference to atmospheric pressure (by manipulating a stopcock) (Fig. 12-16), and positioned parallel to the superior border of the symphysis pubis.[84] The stopcock is then turned so the transducer is closed

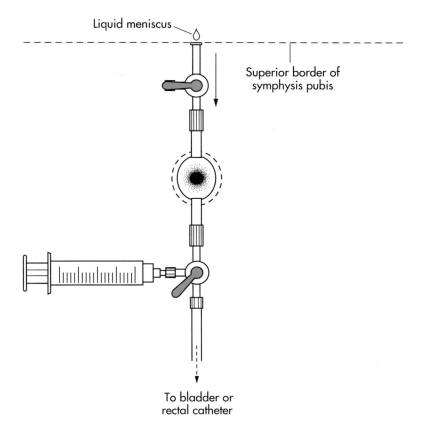

Liquid meniscus

Superior border of symphysis pubis

To bladder or rectal catheter

Fig. 12-16 The external, "dome" pressure transducer is set to zero when stopcock is manipulated so that a drop of water is exposed to air, and system is set to zero electronically. Pressures should be zeroed with reference to atmospheric pressure.

with respect to the surrounding atmosphere but open to the bladder vesicle and rectum, respectively. Initial observation will reveal that Pves is *not* 0 cm H_2O. This observation may create confusion, and some clinicians choose to zero the transducers for a second time to ensure that Pves = 0 cm H_2O. However, this procedure is not recommended. Instead, the clinician should remember that Pves represents the combination of abdominal and detrusor forces acting on the bladder. Because the bladder is empty, the contribution of detrusor forces is negligible. However, abdominal forces continue to act on the empty bladder. These forces are produced by the surrounding viscera, adipose tissue, and muscle within the abdomen. Because Pves is a combined measure of Pabd and Pdet, it follows that Pves = Pabd in the empty bladder. Further consideration reveals that Pdet, which is derived by subtraction of Pabd from Pves, is expected to equal 0 cm H_2O.

Typically, the bladder is filled at a supraphysiologic rate. The ICS has divided fill rates into three categories: slow (0 to 30 mL/min), medium (31 to 100 mL/min), and rapid (greater than 100 mL/min). The faster fill rates tend to cause sensory urgency, compromise bladder wall compliance, and reduce cystometric capacity; therefore, we strongly recommend slow fill rates for children and persons with irritative voiding symptoms and a medium fill rate (typically 40 to 60 mL/min) for adults.

Interpretation. The interpretation of the CMG requires accurate differentiation between detrusor and abdominal forces as they are reflected in simultaneous recordings of Pves, Pabd, and Pdet. Based on the principles discussed in the hydrodynamic principles section in this chapter, it is evident that abdominal events are reflected in the Pabd and Pves pressure recordings but not in the detrusor recording. Similarly, it follows that detrusor events are reflected in the intravesical and detrusor recordings but not in the abdominal recording. Fig. 12-17 depicts these events and their appearance on an actual urodynamic tracing.

In addition to recognizing and differentiating abdominal and detrusor events reflected by the urodynamic recording, the clinician must recognize artifacts. Artifacts may occur as a result of physiologic events or because of inaccurate technique. Physiologic artifacts usually occur because of the difficulties inherent in measuring Pabd in the

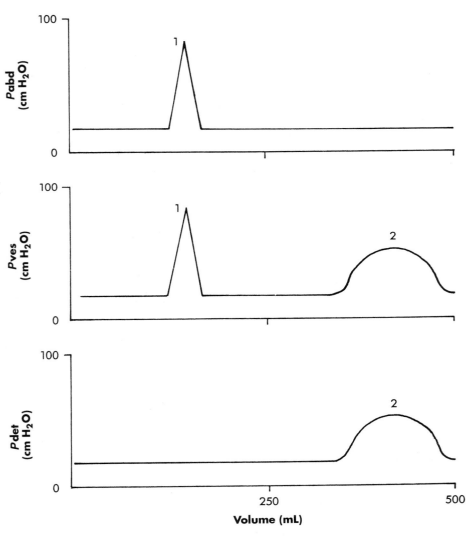

Fig. 12-17 Abdominal and detrusor events as reflected on a multichannel urodynamic tracing.

clinical setting. Although the bladder is a fluid-filled organ that changes its size to accommodate the volume of urine within its vesicle, the abdomen is filled with solid organs, liquids, air, and stool. Therefore, the measurement of *Pabd* represents a best approximation of abdominal forces that act on the bladder. Fig. 12-18, *A*, illustrates what happens when the smooth muscle of the rectal vault contracts during urodynamic testing, which is a relatively common event. In this case, the spontaneous rise in *Pabd* causes a reduction in *Pdet*, whereas *Pves* remains unaffected. Fig. 12-18, *B*, illustrates a transient reduction in resting *Pabd* after a cough. In this case, the spontaneous drop in *Pabd* causes a *rise* in *Pdet*, which is explained by the computer's subtraction of *Pabd* from *Pves* to generate *Pdet*.

Other artifacts occur because of improper technique. For example, air bubbles or "kinks" in the pressure monitoring tubing may cause poor pressure transmission. Fig. 12-19 illustrates two typical artifacts, one caused by a kink in the pressure line and one caused by an air bubble in the pressure line.

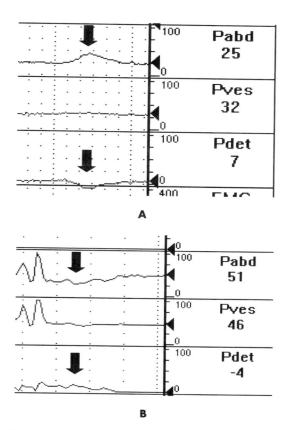

Fig. 12-18 Urodynamic artifacts. **A,** A rectal contraction causes a decline in detrusor pressure (*Pdet*) tracing, **B,** A spontaneous reduction in abdominal pressure (*Pabd*) causes an increase in *Pdet* because the computer is subtracting negative numbers. This phenomenon has sometimes been mistaken for cough-induced detrusor overactivity.

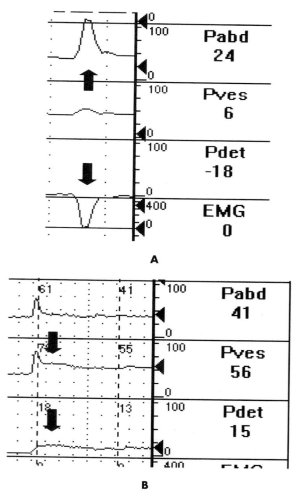

Fig. 12-19 Urodynamic artifacts. **A,** Kink in intravesicular pressure (*Pves*) prevents transmission of pressure from cough. Notice the negative spike produced in the detrusor pressure (*Pdet*) tracing. **B,** Air bubble causes a characteristic stair-step configuration in the base line.

The interpretation of the filling CMG should address five aspects of bladder and sphincter function: capacity, compliance of the bladder wall, competence of the sphincter, sensory function, and detrusor response to bladder filling. Table 12-9 provides a correlation between each of these factors, the relevant urodynamic variable, the range of normal values, and the clinical significance of abnormal findings.

Capacity. Cystometric bladder capacity is based on the patient's subjective report and the clinician's judgment. Generally, the cystometric capacity is recorded as either the volume at which the patient perceives a sense of bladder fullness (that is, a

TABLE 12-9   Interpretation of the Filling Cystometrogram

FILLING CYSTOMETROGRAM (CCSD MNEMONIC)	NORMAL RANGE	CLINICAL SIGNIFICANCE
Capacity	Adults: 300 to 600 mL Children: (Age + 2) $\times$ 30 mL	Large capacity (greater than 600 mL): chronic overdistension, sensory or motor denervation Small capacity (less than 300 mL): low compliance, detrusor overactivity, irritation or inflammation of bladder wall
Compliance	Greater than 30 mL/cm H_2O, sustained Pdet remaining below 20 cm H_2O	Values less than 10 mL/cm H_2O, or sustained Pdet 40 cm H_2O or greater: imminent risk of upper urinary tract distress (febrile urinary tract infection, hydronephrosis, reflux, renal insufficiency) Values sustained Pdet 30 to 39 cm H_2O: moderate risk for upper urinary tract distress
Competence (of the sphincter)	Infinity (abdominal LPP above measurable range)	Any measurable abdominal LPP is an indicator of stress incontinence Abdominal LPP lower than 90 cm H_2O an indicator of intrinsic sphincter deficiency
Sensations	First sensation: 90 to 200 mL Strong urge: 250 to 450 mL Fullness: 300 to 600 mL	Sensory urgency implying small cystometric capacity Delayed or diminished sensations indicators of large cystometric capacity
Detrusor response (detrusor stability)	Absence of overactive detrusor contractions; low pressure rises possible but contractions that cause leakage or bothersome urgency (defined as overactive and clinically relevant) are absent	Overactive detrusor contractions associated with urge or reflex urinary incontinence

LPP, leak point pressure.

strong urge to urinate) or the volume at which an overactive detrusor contraction causes premature voiding. In the patient with low compliance, cystometric capacity is recorded as the point at which overflow UI occurs (as measured by detrusor leak point pressure [det LPP]). Normal cystometric capacity in the infant varies from 15 to 60 mL, and normal capacity in children is determined by the formula: Capacity = (Age in years + 2) × 30.[98,99] Normal cystometric capacity in the adult varies from 300 to 700 mL.[100,101]

An abnormally low cystometric capacity is associated with bothersome urgency, detrusor overactivity, or low bladder wall compliance. Bothersome urgency may be caused by inflammation resulting from bacterial, fungal, or parasitic infections. Urinary calculi and bladder tumors (particularly carcinoma in situ and transitional cell carcinoma) are also associated with bothersome urgency. External-beam radiotherapy for the treatment of cancer causes chronic bladder inflammation in approximately 30% to 40% of patients, and many chemotherapeutic agents are also known to cause acute or chronic bladder inflammation resulting in sensory urgency and possibly urge UI. Acute inflammation occurs with intravesical chemotherapy, particularly bacille Calmette-Guérin (BCG). The systemic administration of cyclophosphamide or ifosfamide may also produce bladder inflammation and hematuria, which may persist for 12 to 18 months after treatment.[102]

Bladder capacity may also be compromised by detrusor overactivity and overactive bladder syndrome. In this situation, the overactive bladder contractions produce a precipitous desire to urinate at relatively low bladder volumes and urge UI, unless the patient is able to reach the toilet quickly.

An abnormally large bladder capacity typically indicates reduced bladder sensations. Complete sensory loss may occur with a spinal cord lesion that interrupts the afferent pathways from the sacral cord or with trauma to the peripheral sensory nerves of the lower urinary tract. Diabetes mellitus can cause reduced sensory awareness of bladder filling, probably because of the combined effects of polyuria and denervation caused by peripheral and autonomic polyneuropathies.[103] These findings are common among patients with long-standing diabetes mellitus. Long-term alcoholism is associated with vitamin B_{12} deficiencies and peripheral polyneuropathies, and it may produce a similar clinical picture.[104]

Behavior patterns may also contribute to diminished sensations of bladder filling, an abnormally large bladder capacity, and urinary retention. Infrequent voiding may ultimately lead to partially or totally irreversible distension of the bladder; this pattern of voiding is commonly observed among professionals who are unable to void when the desire occurs (such as nurses, teachers, and surgeons). Individuals who chronically struggle to control their weight may develop a pattern of excessive fluid intake, which may lead to polyuria and chronic overdistension.

Sensory Awareness of Bladder Filling. Evaluation of the patient's sensory awareness of bladder filling is based on the patient's subjective report of urgency, pressure, or pain. These sensations may be difficult to assess during urodynamic testing because they are profoundly affected by the individual's level of anxiety, discomfort from catheterization, and desire to cooperate with testing and to please the examiner. There are many points at which sensory awareness of bladder filling may be reported. We have found that the first sensation of bladder filling, the first urge to urinate, the strong desire (urge) to urinate, and the sensation of bladder fullness are the most reproducible and useful indicators of sensory function. When documenting sensory awareness, the clinician should record both the volume and the location of the sensation. The first urge to urinate, the strong desire to urinate, and bladder fullness are normally perceived at the level of the urethra. We recommend asking the patient to point to the area at which the sensation of filling is perceived; individuals with normal or exaggerated sensory awareness tend to indicate the urethra near the meatus or some other point on the perineum where the urethra travels in proximity to the skin. In contrast, those with diminished sensation typically point to the lower abdomen, indicating sensory awareness of bladder filling only when the bladder is full enough to impinge on adjacent structures and to produce a sensation of pressure.

The specific causes of increased or decreased sensory awareness of bladder filling are similar to the factors causing abnormally high or low cystometric capacity and have already been discussed. However, a person with a large bladder capacity may also have sensory urgency; this condition is sometimes seen among individuals with bladder outlet obstruction, large residual urine volumes, and detrusor overactivity. Similarly, an individual with a low-capacity bladder may have total loss of the sensation of bladder filling; this is seen among patients with reflex UI caused by a complete spinal cord injury.

Compliance. Bladder wall compliance is defined as its ability to accommodate a large range of bladder volumes (often varying from 1 to 700 mL) while maintaining the low Pdet essential to normal upper urinary tract function. Compliance is a function of the passive (viscoelastic) and active properties of the bladder wall, as discussed earlier in this chapter. In the normal bladder, the relationship between Pdet and bladder volume can be described by application of Laplace's law.[89] This is illustrated by the equation $P\text{det} = F\pi R^2$, where Pdet represents the Pdet measured during urodynamic testing,

F represents the detrusor force acting on the bladder wall, and R represents the radius of the bladder and is a constant. During bladder filling, both F (detrusor force) and R (the radius of the bladder) increase proportionally with volume and tend to cancel out one another. As a result, Pdet remains low, provided the bladder filling is within physiologically tolerable limits. This relationship accounts for the nearly flat slope of the Pdet measurement during filling CMG in the physiologically normal individual (Fig. 12-20). However, when the viscoelastic properties of the bladder are compromised because of fibrosis of the bladder wall or the deposition of collagen, the slope of Pdet rises in direct proportion to the volume infused into the bladder (Fig. 12-21). This loss of compliance is sometimes seen in individuals with reflex UI (neurogenic bladder overactivity) and is discussed in Chapter 7.

Bladder wall compliance may be expressed in milliliters per centimeter of water (mL/cm H_2O) and is calculated by the equation: Compliance (mL/cm H_2O) = ΔVolume/ΔPdet. Bladder wall compliance may also be reported as the end filling pressure, or the value of Pdet obtained at cystometric capacity. However, this approach is based on the

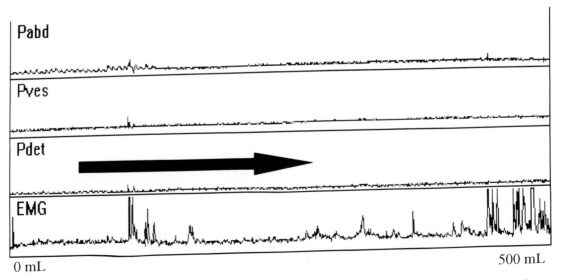

Fig. 12-20 Normal bladder wall compliance. Notice the nearly flat line in the detrusor pressure (Pdet) tracing caused by active and passive accommodation of bladder wall despite filling to 500 mL.

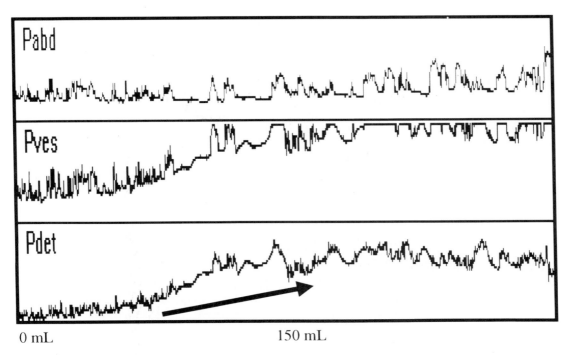

Fig. 12-21 Low bladder wall compliance. Notice the proportional relationship between detrusor pressure (*Pdet*) and volume causing the characteristic steep slope of a low-compliant bladder. In addition, notice the persistence of an elevated pressure after the infusion is stopped at 150 mL.

assumption that normal cystometric capacity is at least 450 mL. Because it is known that a cystometric capacity of 300 mL or less is common among children and the elderly, the clinical application of this approach is limited.

In the normal adult, bladder wall compliance is at least 50 mL/cm H_2O. Even higher values are frequently encountered in persons with a large bladder capacity and among individuals with normal bladder function. Therefore, no clinical significance is attached to a high bladder wall compliance value.[61] In contrast, low bladder wall compliance (including values of 10 mL/cm H_2O or less) *is* clinically significant because the rapid rise in *Pves* associated with bladder filling compromises upper tract function and is associated with stasis, infection, ureterohydronephrosis, and vesicoureteral reflux. Wahl and colleagues[105] have suggested an alternative to the assessment of bladder wall compliance. They noted that sustained *Pdet* values of 20 cm H_2O or less

produce a negligible risk of upper urinary tract changes, whereas sustained pressures of 21 to 30 cm H_2O are associated with a moderate risk, and those 40 cm H_2O and higher produce an imminent risk for upper urinary tract distress. Low compliance may occur in patients with sacral spinal denervation, severe bladder outlet obstruction, bladder wall trabeculation, schistosomiasis, urinary tuberculosis, or fibrosis caused by pelvic radiotherapy.[106-108]

Because bladder wall compliance represents detrusor forces acting on the intravesical contents, it is necessary to consider compliance in conjunction with the resistance provided by the bladder outlet. When bladder wall compliance is low and urethral resistance is high, a substantial detrusor force is required to force urine through the outlet, and the risk of upper tract distress is significant. However, when *both* bladder wall compliance and urethral resistance are low, the risk of upper tract distress is also low. The reason is that the incompetent sphincter permits the urine to escape before the detrusor forces acting on the bladder wall rise to a level that leads to ureteral stasis and upper tract distress.

To quantify the relationship between compliance and urethral resistance, McGuire and colleagues defined a variable known as the *detrusor leak point pressure* (det LPP).[109] The det LPP is the magnitude of Pdet required to drive urine across the urethral sphincter. In the physiologically normal individual, Pdet remains low, and urine crosses the sphincter only during micturition. However, among persons with low compliance, detrusor forces ultimately force the bladder outlet open, causing overflow UI. When the det LPP exceeds 40 cm H_2O and compliance is less than 10 mL/cm H_2O, the risk of upper urinary tract distress approaches 100%.

The relationship between compliance and the det LPP can be observed among children with myelodysplasia and neuropathic bladder function. Some children exhibit low bladder wall compliance and a low det LPP. The low det LPP signifies low urethral resistance, which means that these children have severe UI between catheterizations but are spared from upper tract distress. In contrast, other children present with low bladder wall compliance and a high det LPP, which signifies high urethral resistance. These children remain relatively dry between catheterizations, but their high levels of urethral resistance expose them to high Pdet levels during filling, which increases their risk of upper tract distress. The relationship between compliance and urethral resistance also accounts for the observation that surgical procedures to increase urethral resistance, such as a suburethral sling procedure or implantation of an artificial urinary sphincter, may lead to upper tract distress, unless the low compliance is corrected by a simultaneous augmentation enterocystoplasty.

Energy-Dissipation Phenomenon. Close scrutiny of Fig. 12-22 demonstrates that detrusor forces act on more than the bladder outlet.

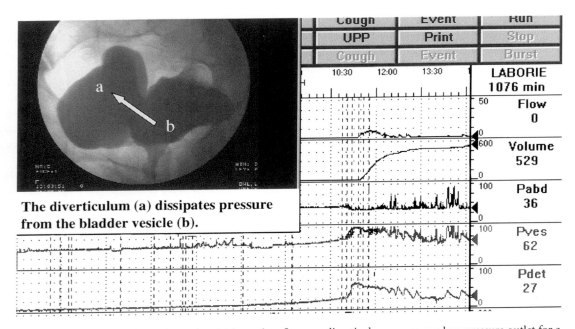

The diverticulum (a) dissipates pressure from the bladder vesicle (b).

Fig. 12-22 Energy dissipation occurs when high-grade reflux or a diverticulum serves as a low-pressure outlet for a bladder with low compliance. In this case, a large diverticulum causes urinary retention but preserves upper urinary tract health by dissipating energy from this obstructed and low-compliant bladder. (Laborie, Courtesy of Laborie Medical Technologies, Toronto.)

Specifically, these forces are also directed against the bladder's two inlets, the ureterovesical junctions. Low compliance combined with an elevated det LPP frequently leads to vesicoureteral reflux because of the deleterious effects on one or both of these inlets. In the presence of vesicoureteral reflux, detrusor forces are dissipated into the upper urinary tracts, which dilate and exhibit ureterohydronephrosis. This dilatation, in turn, tends to raise the bladder wall compliance value as measured during the filling CMG and expressed in milliliters per centimeter of water. Similarly, a bladder diverticulum (herniation of the bladder mucosa through the muscular tunic of the bladder wall) leads to a dissipation of force that raises the compliance values measured during urodynamic testing. Consideration of the effect of this energy dissipation is essential when surgical correction of vesicoureteral reflux or repair of a diverticulum is contemplated in a patient with low bladder wall compliance.

Competence of the Sphincter. Traditionally, the clinician measured competence of the sphincter mechanism by means of a Brown-Wickham urethral pressure profile (UPP) or by measuring urethral pressure and Pves during coughing and using these values to calculate a pressure transmission ratio.[110] The abdominal leak point pressure (abd LPP) was developed as an alternative to this method. The abd LPP is defined as the magnitude of *abdominal* force required to drive urine across the sphincter during bladder filling.[111] In the physiologically normal person, the abd LPP cannot be measured, and leakage does not occur during usual activities. Therefore, any measurable LPP indicates some degree of stress UI. Low abd LPP values indicate sphincter incompetence (formerly called intrinsic sphincter deficiency) and are correlated with more severe UI, whereas higher values are correlated with less severe UI.[112]

Techniques for measuring abd LPP have not been completely standardized, but investigators agree on the general techniques.[110,113] A dual- or triple-lumen catheter of size 8 French or less should be used for testing.[114] A smaller, multiple-lumen catheter is preferred because it allows for measurements of the abd LPP without requiring repeated catheterizations, and the degree of urethral obstruction caused by its presence is minimal. (Significant urethral obstruction could artificially block leakage from stress UI.) The bladder should be filled with a moderate volume of urine, usually between 150 and 200 mL in adults. When the detrusor is overactive or the patient is a child, the bladder should be filled to one half of the functional capacity or one half of the volume observed to elicit an overactive contraction. Excessive filling is avoided because it increases the detrusor forces on the outlet, which could yield an artifactually low abd LPP. Pves is used to measure the abd LPP whenever possible. Alternative pressure measurements (such as rectal or intravaginal pressures) have been described,[111] but we have found them to be less than optimal alternatives because they provide a more indirect evaluation of the abdominal forces acting on the bladder and because of the intrinsic artifacts affecting pressure measurements within these organs. The clinician measures abd LPP by asking the patient to complete a slow Valsalva maneuver and then recording the Pves at which leakage is observed. In addition, the patient may be asked to cough and the LPP measurement may be repeated. Research has demonstrated that the LPP produced by performing Valsalva's maneuver is not identical to that provoked by coughing, and performance of both maneuvers may provide a more comprehensive assessment of sphincter competence.[115] The abd LPP should *never* be measured during a detrusor contraction because the purpose of this test is to quantify the effect of *abdominal* (rather than detrusor) forces acting on the bladder outlet.

Detrusor Response. Detrusor overactivity is characterized by uninhibited or hyperactive detrusor contractions that compromise functional capacity or cause urge UI.[61] An overactive detrusor contraction is observed during the filling CMG as a spontaneous rise in both Pves and Pdet, indicating a contraction of the detrusor muscle, followed by a return to baseline pressure, indicating muscle relaxation (Fig. 12-23). When one is documenting overactive detrusor contractions during the filling CMG, it is essential to record whether the contraction provoked urgency or leakage, or both, and to differentiate overactive from subclinical or filling detrusor contractions.

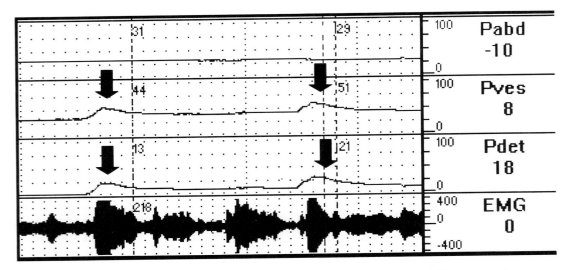

Fig. 12-23 Detrusor overactivity. Two contractions are indicated by *arrows*. Notice rapid elevation of pressure indicating detrusor muscle contraction followed by a return to baseline pressures indicating muscle relaxation. Compare this with persistently elevated pressures characteristic of low bladder wall compliance.

Subclinical or filling detrusor contractions occur in many physiologically normal persons.[61,116] They are typically low pressure (often 10 cm H_2O or less) and produce minimal or no desire to urinate. Although the mechanism that causes these contractions is unclear, recent research evidence suggests that subclinical contractions may be attributable to localized areas of smooth muscle bundle contractions, whereas clinically relevant overactive contractions occur when a contraction involves the entire detrusor.[117] Overactive detrusor contractions cause urgency and/or UI. The urodynamic diagnosis for urine loss associated with this phenomenon advocated by the ICS is detrusor overactivity UI,[6] but most clinicians prefer the label urge UI when the contraction is associated with bothersome urgency, or reflex UI when the contraction occurs with no detectable urgency. The ICS subdivides clinically relevant overactive contractions into two categories: neurogenic detrusor overactivity is associated with a known neurologic disease affecting the central nervous system and detrusor overactivity refers to contractions that occur in the absence of a neurologic explanation.[6]

Sphincter Electromyography. Sphincter EMG is a graphic representation of the electrical activity recorded from the pelvic floor muscles.[118,119] EMG is used to assess neuromuscular function of the pelvic floor muscles; it is usually measured by a transcutaneous patch or a vaginal or anal probe, thus allowing assessment of kinesiology (gross motor movements) only. However, needle electrodes also may be placed for the evaluation of individual action potentials from local striated muscle motor units.

A skeletal muscle, such as the levator ani or periurethral striated muscle, contains a large number of motor units. The motor unit consists of an anterior horn cell, its axon, and the several muscle fibers innervated by the horn cell (Fig. 12-24). The motor unit is activated by depolarization of the anterior horn cell, which initiates transmission of an action potential along the myelinated motor axon. When this action potential reaches the myoneural junction (the small gap between the nerve and the muscle fiber), it causes the release of a neurotransmitter; this neurotransmitter then causes depolarization of the membrane of the muscle fiber. It is this depolarizing electrical current (also known as the motor unit potential) that propagates along the muscle membrane and is measured and recorded by the EMG electrode.

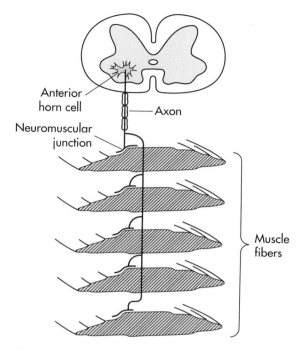

Fig. 12-24 Motor unit comprises the anterior horn cell, myelinated axon, and skeletal muscle fibers it innervates.

Various electrodes are used for EMG studies. During urodynamic testing, a needle electrode may be placed within the pelvic or periurethral muscles[118] or within the circumvaginal muscles.[120] If the electrical signals are transmitted to an oscilloscope type of recording device, individual action potentials can be observed, and the integrity of pelvic muscle innervation can be evaluated. Wire electrodes provide an alternative to needle electrodes; these narrow-gauge electrodes are made of stainless steel, platinum, or copper wires and are insulated. A short length of the wire is stripped of its insulation and is hooked into a small-gauge needle that is inserted into the muscle and subsequently withdrawn. Because of the hook, the wire is left behind. Although wire electrodes, like needle electrodes, require percutaneous placement, they are sometimes preferred to needle EMG because the wires permit much greater patient mobility during urodynamic testing.

Surface electrodes are frequently used as an alternative to the invasive electrodes. Surface electrodes offer several advantages when compared with needle or hooked wire electrodes. In addition to being less invasive, they record the activity of a larger number of motor units (as compared with percutaneous electrodes) and are available in a variety of styles including anal, vaginal, and urethral electrodes and transcutaneous patches. One disadvantage to surface electrodes is the increased risk for artifact (as compared with percutaneous needles and wires). The risk of artifact and the large number of motor units assessed by a single surface electrode make these devices unsuitable for measuring individual action potentials. Instead, surface electrodes are used to assess gross muscle activity (kinesiology).

The placement of an EMG electrode is influenced by the type of electrode selected and the gender of the patient.[118] Needle or hooked wire electrodes are typically inserted into the perineum beneath the scrotum in male patients; in female patients, they are generally inserted approximately 5 mm into the periurethral tissue at the 11 o'clock and 2 o'clock positions (with respect to the meatus). Because of the discomfort and technical difficulty associated with percutaneous electrode placement in women, Lowe and associates described an alternative technique using a transvaginal approach.[120] Their approach is to place the patient in a left side-lying position and to use a Sims speculum to expose the vaginal wall; the urethral sphincter is then palpated, and an EMG needle or wire electrode is inserted. They reported that this technique produces less discomfort and provides satisfactory EMG tracings.

Surface electrodes are usually placed adjacent to the anus. We prefer using a Duoderm or karaya gum-based patch because we find that they provide better adherence to the perianal area than do foam patches. It is important to place the perianal patches immediately adjacent to the anal opening because more distal placement produces EMG tracings of motor unit potentials from the hip muscles as opposed to pelvic floor muscle fiber activity. Anal or vaginal plugs may be used as an alternative to perianal patches. Several manufacturers have designed small foam patches that are easily combined with the anal or vaginal probes used to measure *Pabd*. When using surface patches or plug electrodes, the clinician must place a reference electrode over an area that is free of underlying muscle. This electrode serves as a ground and also provides a reference for the electrical signals received from the active electrode or electrodes.

Urethral electrodes have also been used for sphincter EMG studies.[118] A concentric ring electrode is typically mounted on a reusable catheter, which is placed into the urethra. Unfortunately, the catheter's tendency to "float" in the urethra as it fills with urine during micturition produces significant artifact; therefore, this device is no longer widely used.

Interpretation. The interpretation of sphincter EMG results is based on the type of electrode used and the expertise of the clinician in the analysis of an individual action potential. For example, surface electrodes can be used to assess gross muscle activity, but they cannot provide data regarding pelvic muscle strength or the integrity of pelvic muscle innervation. The clinician assesses the gross activity of the muscle by observing the voltage of the motor unit potentials; this voltage is typically measured in microvolts. An increase in voltage correlates positively with contraction of motor units and recruitment of adjacent units. In contrast, a reduction in voltage is indicative of relaxation of the surrounding motor units.

As noted, changes in voltage correlate with gross muscle activity (that is, muscle contraction); however, voltage does *not* provide any measurement of muscle tone or strength. To measure muscle *strength*, the clinician must evaluate the magnitude of force achieved by a muscle during contraction. For example, the clinician assesses the strength of the skeletal muscles in the arms, legs, or chest by asking the individual to displace a barbell or related device with a known weight. It is obviously not possible to measure the strength of the periurethral striated muscles by having the patient use the muscles to displace a weight. However, it *is* possible to measure the force of contraction by inserting a fluid-filled balloon into the vagina, anal canal, or urethra. The patient can then be asked to contract the pelvic and periurethral muscles, and the pressure (that is,

force per unit area) produced within the balloon can be recorded. The clinician must remember to differentiate between muscle contraction and muscle strength when conducting urodynamics *and* when implementing and evaluating a pelvic muscle reeducation program.

If the sphincter EMG is conducted by use of a needle or hooked wire electrode, it may be possible to evaluate the integrity of the innervation to the pelvic muscles as well as the gross muscle activity (muscle contraction). The integrity of the nerve pathways is assessed by evaluation of the individual action potential. Damage to the anterior horn cell, the axon, or the muscle fiber can be inferred based on this evaluation, and this information can be used (with caution) to predict the general innervation of the pelvic floor. Although use of needle or hooked wire electrodes provides more detailed information than can be obtained from surface electrodes, several features limit clinical application within the urodynamic laboratory. First of all, placement of a needle or wire electrode produces discomfort that may affect the patient's mobility and ability to urinate. In addition, the interpretation of individual action potentials requires considerable expertise that is not inherent within the educational background of most continence nurses, urologists, or urogynecologists. Finally, a needle or wire electrode measures only a small number of motor units as compared with surface electrodes. The information obtained from placement of the needle within a single location cannot be reliably used as a basis for diagnosing the neurologic integrity of the entire pelvic floor muscle group.

Because only a few urodynamic laboratories use needle or wire electrodes and therefore have some capability for assessing the integrity of pelvic muscle innervation, this discussion is limited to the evaluation of EMG tracings obtained from surface electrodes. During the filling CMG, two primary phenomena may be observed. The first is the BCR, which reflects the gross integrity of pelvic muscle innervation. The clinician elicits this reflex by gently tapping on the clitoris in the female patient, gently squeezing the glans penis in the male patient, or placing gentle traction against the bladder neck if an indwelling catheter with a retention balloon is in place. In the individual with a normal BCR, a brief surge of EMG activity is observed in response to these maneuvers (Fig. 12-25). The presence of the BCR indicates grossly intact innervation between the anterior horn cells of the sacral cord and the fibers of the pelvic floor muscles. Absence of the BCR is suggestive of some compromise in this innervation, but it does not provide a measure of the magnitude or clinical relevance of the denervation. The second phenomenon that can be observed on sphincter EMG is recruitment, that is, the steady increase in contracting motor units in response to bladder filling. Recruitment is more likely to be observed during provocative (rapid) bladder filling; its absence has relatively little clinical significance (see Fig. 12-25).

In addition to these maneuvers, we strongly recommend evaluation of the patient's ability to identify, contract, and relax the pelvic floor muscles. This maneuver, long ignored during urodynamic testing in many services, is critically important when pelvic floor muscle rehabilitation is integrated into UI management.

The response of the sphincter muscles to micturition, which is reflected by the sphincter EMG, is critical to a comprehensive EMG evaluation. In the physiologically normal individual, neurons within the pons coordinate detrusor and sphincter activity so the striated muscles of the sphincter mechanism relax in reflex fashion during micturition. Therefore, the sphincter EMG in a "normal" individual will reflect a reduction in voltage during a voluntary detrusor contraction (Fig. 12-26, *A*). However, this relaxation may be overridden by the brain, and sphincter EMG activity during micturition must be interpreted with caution. The most common physiologic reason for sphincter EMG activity during micturition is probably the guarding reflex.[121] "Guarding" refers to voluntary contraction of the striated sphincter in an attempt to prevent urinary leakage during an involuntary detrusor contraction. Sphincter EMG activity may also be observed during micturition as a result of abdominal straining or environmental artifacts.

Detrusor-sphincter dyssynergia refers to the involuntary contraction of the striated sphincter during detrusor contraction. Because the pontine micturition center is responsible for coordination of the detrusor and the sphincter, dyssynergia is indicative of a neurologic process affecting the spinal

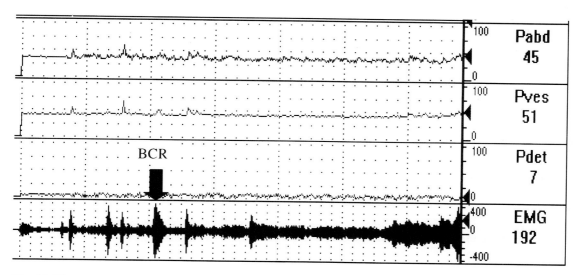

Fig. 12-25 Normal sphincter electromyographic tracing during bladder filling. The bulbocavernosus reflex (BCR), *arrow*, is elicited by gentle squeezing of the glans penis or tapping of the clitoris.

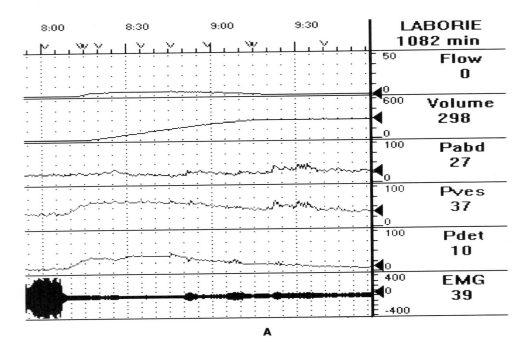

A

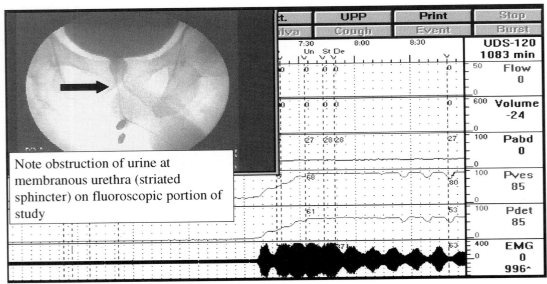

B

Fig. 12-26 A, Normal relaxation of pelvic floor muscles in response to detrusor contraction. **B,** Dyssynergia (uncoordinated contraction of pelvic muscles) during a detrusor contraction.

segments below the pons and above the sacral micturition center (Fig. 12-26, *B*). In addition, pseudodyssynergia may occur when an individual fails to relax the sphincter because of an unconscious or learned behavior pattern. Chapter 7 contains a more detailed discussion of the etiology and management of detrusor-sphincter dyssynergia.

Artifacts. Because the sphincter EMG records extremely weak electrical signals from the muscle fiber membrane, it is particularly prone to both physiologic and environmental artifacts. Physiologic artifacts typically arise from the electrical impulses generated by distant muscle groups. For example, it is not unusual to record the patient's ECG through patch or plug electrodes. Environmental artifacts are those produced by improper electrode placement or by extraneous factors that interfere with the recording of EMG data. Radio broadcast towers, fluorescent lights, rheostat (dimmer) devices, microwaves, or low-volume noise from a drill may produce high-hertz interference. In addition, artifactual EMG activity is often generated when the patient is inadvertently allowed to urinate over the wires or when there is loss of electrode contact during micturition.

Because the sphincter EMG is prone to artifacts, the experienced urodynamicist interprets these tracings with caution. The intermittent occurrence of artifacts is recognized as inevitable, and the focus is on rapid recognition and prompt removal of environmental sources of artifact whenever feasible. When the artifact cannot be eliminated, the urodynamic clinician must rely on interpretation of pressure and flow data to infer the presence or absence of detrusor-sphincter dyssynergia.

Voiding Pressure Study. The filling CMG should be followed by a voiding pressure (micturition) study. The voiding pressure study is a graphic representation of urodynamic pressures (including Pabd, Pves, and Pdet), the urinary flow, and typically the sphincter EMG. The voiding pressure study is usually considered "routine" for a patient undergoing filling CMG, because it provides significant additional information about lower urinary tract function, requires little additional time, and requires no additional invasive instrumentation for the patient. If a two-catheter system is used for

urodynamic testing, the larger filling catheter is removed, and the patient is assisted onto a uroflow device and is asked to urinate. If a multiple-lumen catheter is used, the patient is asked to urinate around the catheter and is reassured that this is both feasible and comfortable. Maximum privacy must be provided for the patient during the voiding pressure study.

Interpretation. Interpretation of the voiding pressure study requires qualitative analysis of the urinary flow pattern, detrusor contraction strength, and sphincter EMG, ideally supplemented by quantitative comparisons of pressure versus flow and voided volume to determine the magnitude of urethral resistance and efficiency of detrusor contractility. Pressure flow nomograms, currently available on all high-quality computer-based urodynamic systems, are critical to the detailed evaluation of the voiding pressure study.

Qualitative Analysis. The urinary flow pattern is identified and (ideally) compared with a free uroflowmetry (one that has been completed before the study and free from the presence of any urethral catheter). If the flow *pattern* for the voiding pressure study matches that observed on the free uroflow tracing, the voiding pressure study is judged to be valid. However, if the study pattern does not match the free urinary flow pattern, the voiding pressure study should be repeated until this pattern is reproduced. Fig. 12-27 illustrates a normal voiding pressure study in a man and a woman. As explained earlier in this chapter, the maximum and mean flow rates tend to be higher in women, and the voiding pressure tends to be lower, reflecting the low resistance provided by the comparatively short and straight female urethra. In these "normal" studies, the sphincter EMG remains quiet throughout voiding for both the male and the female. Fig. 12-28 illustrates the high pressure and poor or intermittent flow pattern characteristic of bladder outlet obstruction. This voiding pressure study should be compared with the study illustrated in Fig. 12-29; in the latter study, the poor or intermittent flow pattern is associated with low voiding pressures and abdominal straining, indicating poor detrusor contraction strength as opposed to bladder outlet obstruction.

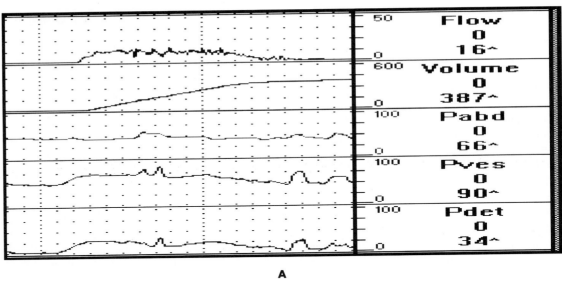

A

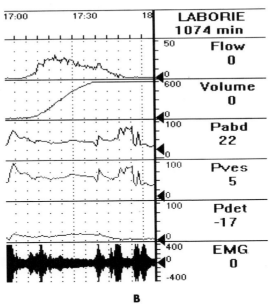

B

Fig. 12-27 Normal pressure-flow relationships. **A,** Male. **B,** Female.

Pressure-Flow Nomograms. Four nomograms have been developed to assist the urodynamic clinician in synthesizing pressure and flow data. Abrams and Griffiths[122] designed a nomogram that plots Pdet on the y (vertical) axis and Q (flow) on the x (horizontal) axis. It has been modified and is now referred to as the ICS nomogram[116] (Fig. 12-30). The chart is divided into three areas: an obstructed zone, an unobstructed zone, and an intermediate (equivocal) zone. (The equivocal zone indicates

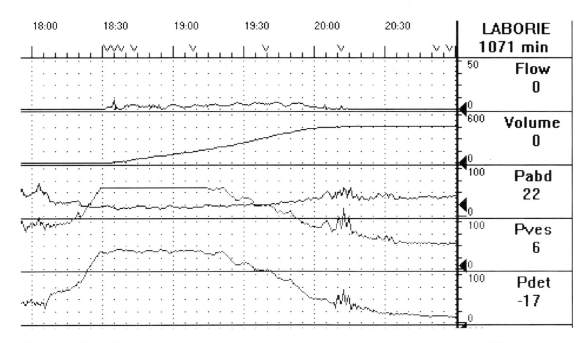

Fig. 12-28 This voiding pressure study shows high detrusor contraction pressure and a prolonged flow pattern, indicating bladder outlet obstruction.

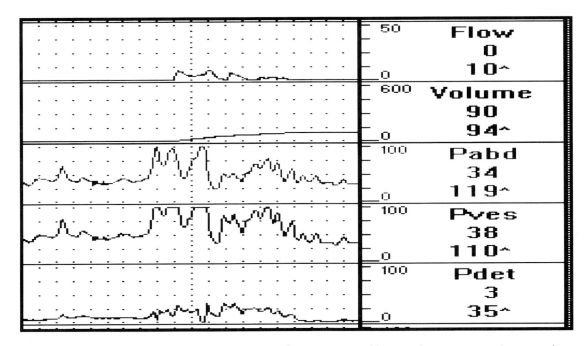

Fig. 12-29 In this case, an interrupted or intermittent flow rate is caused by poor detrusor contraction strength.

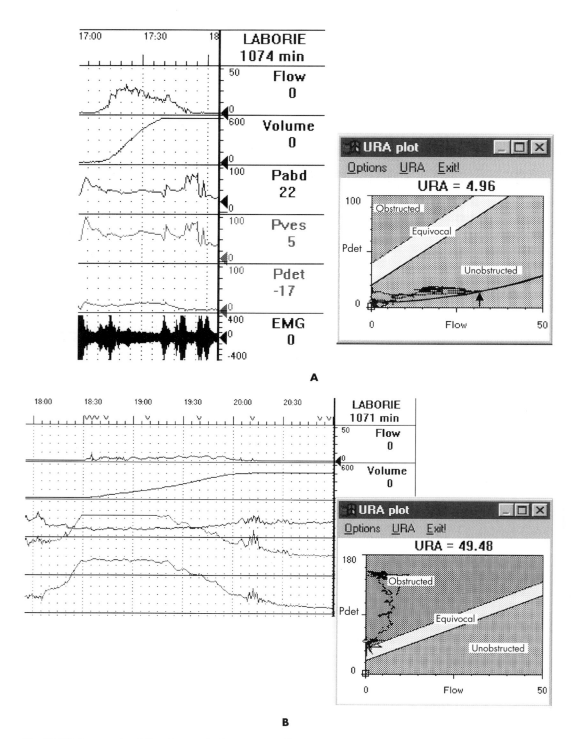

Fig.12-30 International Continence Society pressure flow nomogram. **A,** Normal pressure-flow relationship. The urethral resistance algorithm (URA) score is 4.96. **B,** Obstruction, with a URA score of 49.48.

obstruction of minimal to moderate magnitude.) A urethral resistance algorithm (URA) is calculated based on a comparison of flow rates at maximum detrusor contraction pressure to determine bladder outlet obstruction. Among men, URA values of 20 cm H_2O or less imply normal urethral resistance, values between 21 and 39 cm H_2O are considered equivocal (indicating low magnitude obstruction), and values greater than 40 cm H_2O are consistent with moderate to severe bladder outlet obstruction. Fig. 12-30 depicts an obstructed and an unobstructed voiding pressure study plotted on an ICS nomogram. Chassagne and colleagues[123] examined urodynamic findings in women with bladder outlet obstruction and proposed distinctive cut points for women. They define URA values of 15 cm H_2O as

indicating normal urethral resistance, values between 16 cm H_2O and 29 cm H_2O indicating low magnitude obstruction, whereas values of 30 cm H_2O or higher are consistent with moderate to severe bladder outlet obstruction.

Schafer also developed a nomogram comparing *Pdet* and *Q* (flow) that he described as a graphic representation of the "linearized passive urethral relationship" (linPURR).[124] The elements of this nomogram are similar to those of the nomogram designed by Abrams and Griffiths, but *Pdet* is plotted on the *x* axis and *Q* (flow) on the *y* axis (Fig. 12-31). In addition, this nomogram is divided into six grades of urethral resistance. The range of grades 0 to II includes patients with normal urethral resistance and minimal (that is, not clinically significant)

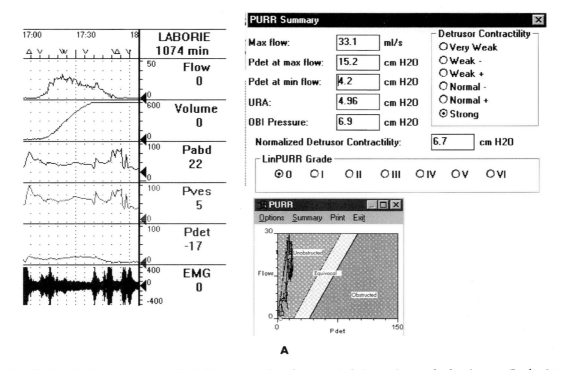

A

Fig. 12-31 Schafer nomogram is divided into six grades of progressively increasing urethral resistance. Grades 0 to I indicate no significant obstruction, grades II to III indicate low-grade obstruction, and grades IV to VI indicate obstruction that is clearly clinically significant and severe. This nomogram also subdivides the detrusor contraction strength into four broad categories, including very weak, weak, normal, and strong. **A,** Normal voiding pressure study in a female patient. Notice the strong detrusor contractility rating despite the low detrusor contraction pressure, indicating low urethral resistance.

Continued

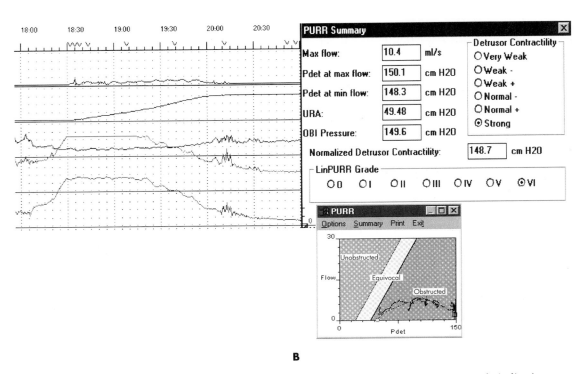

B

Fig. 12-31, cont'd B, Bladder outlet obstruction. Notice the strong detrusor contraction strength, indicating compensation despite the presence of an obstruction at the level of the prostatic urethra.

obstruction; grades III to VI imply varying degrees of clinically significant obstruction. The linPURR nomogram can also be used to assess detrusor contractility and is divided into three broad categories: weak, normal, and strong. Although the linPURR nomogram provides more grades of obstruction than the ICS or Abrams-Griffiths nomogram, a comparison demonstrates that they provide essentially analogous analyses when applied to a specific voiding pressure study.[116]

The CHESS nomogram was developed and designed to quantify obstruction in men with BPH.[125] This two-dimensional nomogram can be displayed as a chess board containing 16 squares. Analysis of a voiding pressure flow study is based on identification of the footprint and curvature of an X-Y plot of pressure versus flow and incorporates the entire micturitional event (from the beginning of measurable flow to the point that flow ceases) as compared with the single-point evaluations used to generate the URA or obstruction grade in the ICS and Schafer plots, respectively. Experience with this nomogram in the United States is limited, and its role in routine *clinical* voiding pressure flow analysis has not yet been established.

Detrusor contractility may be quantified using the CLIM plot.[91,126] The CLIM software generates a contractility factor (WF) that is modeled on Hill's equation and accounts for the continuous volume present in the urinary bladder during micturition.[127,128] Although this software has been reported as useful in selecting treatment options for men undergoing evaluation of voiding dysfunction associated with BPH,[91,128] it was normalized in young adult women and is the only nomogram specifically designed to evaluate detrusor contraction strength in female patients.

Urethral Pressure Studies. Several urethral pressure studies have been described and widely used during urodynamic testing. The Brown-Wickham UPP provides an assessment of urethral resistance.[129] With this approach, the clinician measures urethral resistance by slowly withdrawing a catheter through the urethra while measuring urethral pressure and Pves. By subtracting urethral pressure from Pves, it is possible to calculate the maximum urethral closure pressure, which is used to assess urethral resistance. Unfortunately, the clinical utility of this study is limited, primarily because it fails to evaluate the sphincter's response to abdominal forces such as a cough or a Valsalva maneuver. As a result, the UPP has not proved to reliably differentiate women who have stress UI from those who do not.[130] However, the presence of a very low maximum urethral closure pressure *was* found to correlate with the presence of intrinsic sphincter deficiency.[131]

Because of the limitations inherent in the Brown-Wickham UPP study, other urodynamicists have expanded this test to compare the ratio of pressure to transmission in the urethra and the bladder during a provocative maneuver.[132] To perform this test, the clinician obtains simultaneous measurements of intravesical and urethral pressures, both at rest and during a cough. In the physiologically normal individual, the pressures transmitted to the abdominal urethra (that is, the portion of the urethra extending from the bladder neck to the point of maximum urethral closure pressure) should exceed Pves. In contrast, Pves will exceed the urethral closure pressure in the woman with stress UI. This relationship is expressed as a pressure-transmission ratio; it is calculated by dividing the change in urethral pressure during a cough by the change in Pves during a cough and multiplying the result by 100. A pressure-transmission ratio of 100% or greater indicates that the urethral pressure exceeds Pves during a cough, which maintains sphincter competence and continence. A pressure-transmission ratio of less than 100% implies some degree of sphincter incompetence.

Urethral pressures may also be measured during micturition. The clinician completes the micturitional UPP by withdrawing the catheter during voiding and simultaneously measuring urethral pressure and Pdet.[133] When combined with fluoroscopic monitoring, this technique can be used to localize the level of bladder outlet obstruction.

Videourodynamics. Videourodynamic studies combine pressure, flow, and EMG data with simultaneous lower urinary tract imaging. Fluoroscopy is used in most settings because it provides a dynamic and reliable image of the lower urinary tract.[134,135] Ultrasonic imaging techniques have been explored as an alternative to fluoroscopy,[136,137] but they have failed to gain widespread acceptance because of the limitations to the area imaged when compared with fluoroscopy.

Although no formal document concerning the indications for videourodynamic testing has been promulgated by the ICS or the Society for Female Urology and Urodynamics, there is a growing consensus that this is the preferred technique in several situations. For example, videourodynamics are preferred for the evaluation of specific patients with stress UI, that is, when surgical management is contemplated, when UI is complicated by significant pelvic organ prolapse or urinary retention, and when UI recurs after surgical repair. Videourodynamics are also indicated for patients with urinary retention, particularly when it is believed to be caused by obstruction or when it is complicated by upper tract distress. Patients with potentially hostile neuropathic bladder dysfunction (such as patients with spinal cord injuries or multiple sclerosis) are also best served by videourodynamic testing, as are patients with voiding dysfunction that cannot be diagnosed or adequately managed using simpler techniques.

Stress urinary incontinence. Videourodynamic testing allows the clinician to gain insights into the underlying causes of stress UI. Comprehensive evaluation using videourodynamic techniques combines measurement of the abd LPP with assessment of bladder base descent. The bladder base is assessed at 150 to 200 mL with the patient in an upright (sitting or standing) position. The position of the bladder base is first noted at rest and during Valsalva's maneuver or a cough. In the physiologically normal woman, the bladder base is found above the inferior margin of the symphysis pubis at rest. In severe cases, bladder descent may create a "pressure sink" effect, alleviating stress UI despite the presence of

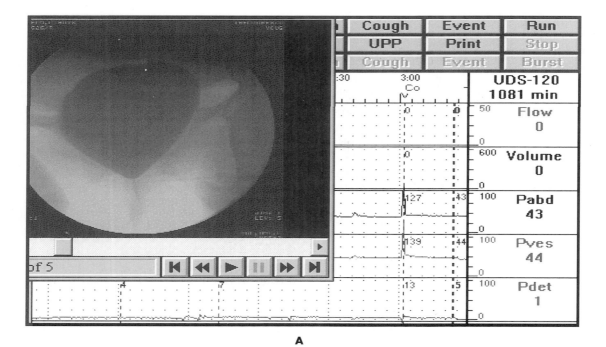

A

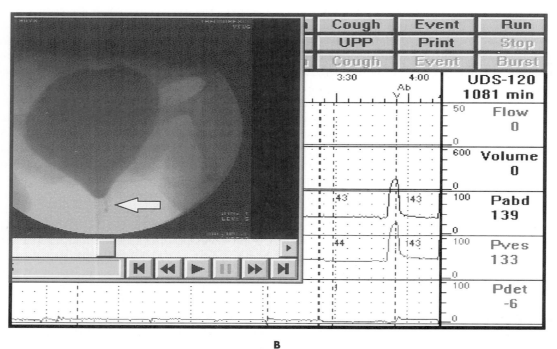

B

Fig. 12-32 Urodynamic stress urinary incontinence with descent of the bladder base. **A,** The bladder at rest is slightly below the inferior margin of the symphysis pubis, indicating a small cystocele. **B,** With abdominal straining, the bladder descends more than 2 cm, and stress urinary incontinence occurs.

significant intrinsic sphincter deficiency (Figs. 12-32 and 12-33). Knowledge of this is clinically relevant because correction of the cystocele, without simultaneous correction of the sphincter deficiency, is likely to exacerbate rather than alleviate stress UI, whereas correction of stress UI without repair of the cystocele may produce postoperative obstruction. Videourodynamic testing in the patient with severe prolapse of the vaginal walls also may reveal bladder outlet obstruction and upper urinary tract distress (Fig. 12-34).[138]

Videourodynamic testing is also useful for the patient with persistent or recurrent voiding dysfunction despite surgical repair. In one series of 52 women with UI despite previous urethral suspension, it was found that UI was attributable to detrusor overactivity in 25%, recurrent urethral hypermobility in 19%, and intrinsic sphincter deficiency in 12%.[139] However, the remaining 44% had a combination of these factors and would have been very unlikely to receive an accurate diagnosis had they been evaluated with techniques that did not combine urodynamic data with dynamic anatomic imaging.

Urinary Retention. Urinary retention can be caused by either bladder outlet obstruction or deficient detrusor contraction strength, or by a combination of these factors. When urodynamics are performed primarily to differentiate between these factors, a voiding pressure study is usually sufficient. However, videourodynamic testing is indicated when the characteristics of the obstructing lesion are unclear or when obstruction is associated with upper urinary tract distress. Imaging of the bladder base and urethra is performed during

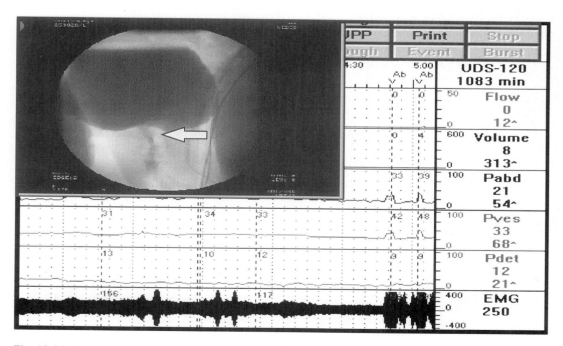

Fig. 12-33 Urodynamic stress urinary incontinence with severe incompetence of the sphincter mechanism (formerly called intrinsic sphincter deficiency). In this case, the bladder neck is found above the inferior margin of the symphysis pubis, but the proximal urethra remains open at rest, and the patient leaks with minimal abdominal pressure (abdominal leak point pressure, 9 cm H_2O).

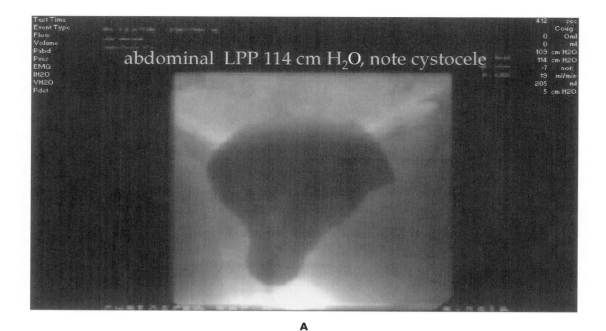

Fig. 12-34 Urodynamic stress urinary incontinence in a patient with severe vaginal wall prolapse and descent of the bladder base. **A,** Large cystocele serves as a pressure sink and minimizes the severity of urinary incontinence. **B,** With support of the prolapsed vaginal wall, however, the bladder neck is observed to be open, and the abdominal leak point pressure falls from 114 to 68 cm H_2O.

the voiding pressure study to determine the location of the obstruction. Figs. 12-35 to 12-37 demonstrate obstruction at the bladder neck, prostatic urethra, and membranous urethra, respectively. Differentiation among these lesions is essential because each is managed differently, from both a pharmacologic and a surgical perspective.

Videourodynamic testing is also necessary to determine the characteristics of bladder outlet obstruction in women. Fig. 12-38 demonstrates the study of a woman who underwent urethral suspension without simultaneous repair of a significant cystocele, and Fig. 12-39 illustrates the study of a woman who is obstructed because of excessive tension on the urethra. Each of these women had undergone cystoscopy, which had failed to reveal the cause of the obstruction.

Hostile bladder dysfunction. Videourodynamic testing is useful when the bladder behaves in a manner that is deleterious to upper urinary tract function. In these situations, fluoroscopic imaging is used to assess the severity of bladder trabeculation, to identify the anatomic characteristics of

any obstruction, and to diagnose and grade vesicoureteral reflux. Simultaneous urodynamic testing is necessary to identify the type of UI and to identify conditions known to contribute to upper tract distress, such as low bladder wall compliance, bladder outlet obstruction, and an elevated det LPP. Fig. 12-40 illustrates the study of a patient with myelodysplasia and right-sided vesicoureteral reflux caused by low bladder wall compliance and a det LPP greater than 40 cm H_2O.

ENDOSCOPY AND IMAGING STUDIES

Although imaging studies are not routinely indicated as a component of the workup for a patient with UI, they provide essential information for some patients. Endoscopic examination is necessary when there is suspicion of a urothelial tumor or when UI is complicated by an inflammatory process or anatomic defect such as a suburethral diverticulum.

A renal bladder ultrasonogram or an intravenous pyelogram is essential for any patient with voiding dysfunction associated with upper tract distress.

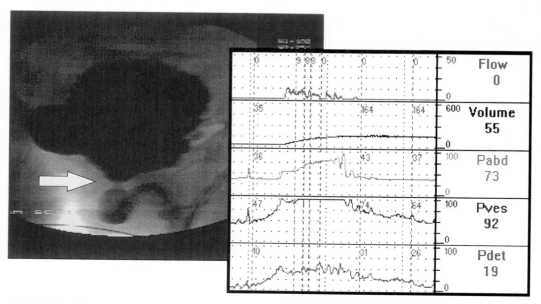

Fig. 12-35 Videourodynamic testing shows an obstruction at the level of the bladder neck in a male patient.

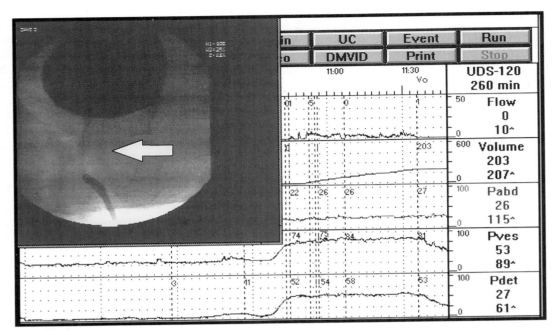

Fig. 12-36 Videourodynamic testing shows an obstruction at the level of the prostatic urethra in a male patient.

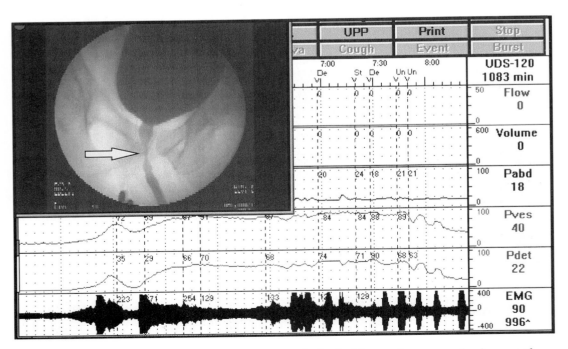

Fig. 12-37 Videourodynamic testing shows an obstruction at the level of the membranous urethra because of detrusor-sphincter dyssynergia in a male patient.

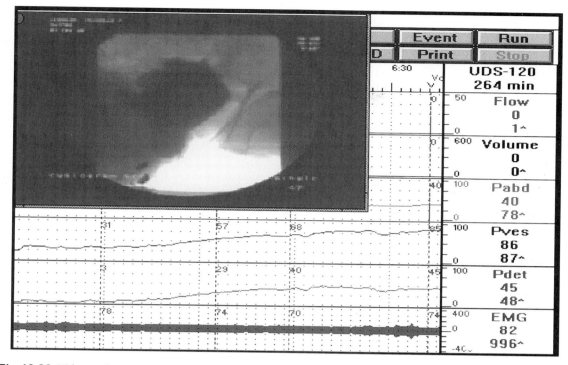

Fig. 12-38 Videourodynamic testing shows an obstruction in a woman after urethral suspension. In this case, the cystocele remains at the level of the resuspended bladder, causing mechanical outlet obstruction.

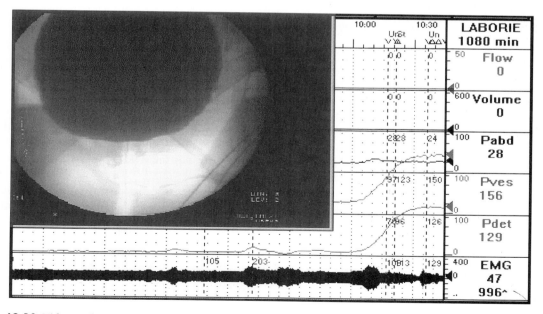

Fig. 12-39 Videourodynamic testing shows an obstruction in a woman after urethral suspension. In this case, increased urethral resistance occurs because of increased compression from suspension acting directly on the urethra.

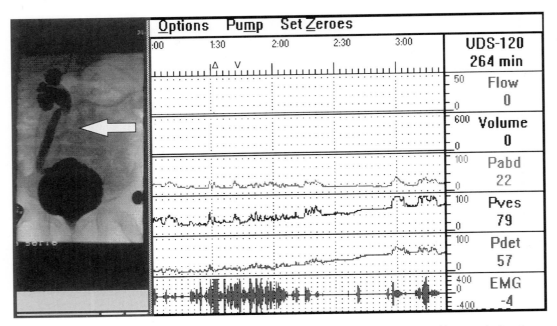

Fig. 12-40 Hostile neurogenic bladder function reflected by increased urethral resistance (detrusor leak point pressure, 43 cm H_2O) and low bladder wall compliance (8 mL/cm H_2O), which contribute to upper urinary tract distress. Notice the grade 4 right reflux, indicated by the *arrow* and the open bladder neck. The bladder neck is forced open not by abdominal forces from straining but by detrusor forces that act selectively on the urethral outlet and ureterovesical junctions.

This includes patients with a history of one or more febrile UTIs, an abnormal serum creatinine or BUN, or evidence of detrusor-sphincter dyssynergia, low bladder wall compliance, or severe bladder outlet obstruction. Selected patients with UI may also benefit from a nuclear medicine study (such as the MAG_3 [technetium 99m-mercaptoacetyl-triglycine] radionuclide scan) to assess renal function and to identify the presence of obstruction within the upper urinary tracts. These studies should be completed under the supervision of a urologist, and we strongly recommend immediate referral of any patient with UI who is determined to be at risk for upper tract distress.

SUMMARY

The assessment of the patient with UI varies from a routine evaluation, which comprises a history, focused physical examination, and bladder chart, to a complex process involving videourodynamics, upper urinary tract imaging studies, and multiple laboratory studies. This chapter provides a review of the most common diagnostic studies used by continence nurses and other clinicians when evaluating UI, and Table 12-10 provides a guide to the specific evaluation strategies indicated for a given patient, based on presenting clinical manifestations. However, the continence nurse must remember that the optimal assessment for a specific patient is based on knowledge of the patient's goals and motives for seeking care, the resources available to that patient (including family support and economic resources), the possible outcomes if a certain management plan is implemented, and the expected outcomes if *no* treatment is pursued.

TABLE 12-10   Evaluation of Urinary Incontinence Based on Clinical Manifestations

SUSPECTED UI TYPE	HISTORY AND PHYSICAL EXAM AND BLADDER CHART	URODYNAMICS AND VIDEOURODYNAMICS	OTHER STUDIES
Stress UI	All cases	Multichannel or videourodynamics when contemplating surgical management or when stress UI is complicated by urinary retention or associated neurologic disease	Renal and bladder ultrasonogram or IVP and serum creatinine and BUN test when associated with severe pelvic organ prolapse, urinary retention, and an elevated risk for upper urinary tract distress
Urge UI	All cases	Multichannel urodynamics when UI is refractory to conservative management or when complicated by urinary retention, neurologic disease; videourodynamics when upper urinary tract distress, suspected obstruction or urinary retention of unknown origin	Renal and bladder ultrasonogram or IVP and serum creatinine and BUN test when complicated by febrile UTI or vesicoureteral reflux
Reflex UI	All cases; bladder chart comparing voided with catheterized volumes may be Indicated	Multichannel or videourodynamics in all cases	Renal and bladder ultrasonogram or IVP and serum creatinine and BUN test in all cases
Functional UI	All cases; prompted voiding bladder chart typically preferred	Urodynamics rarely indicated	Upper urinary tract imaging studies when associated with significant urinary retention
Overflow UI	All cases; bladder chart comparing voided with catheterized volumes may be indicated	Multichannel urodynamics with voiding pressure study to differentiate deficient detrusor contraction strength from bladder outlet obstruction; videourodynamics to identify level of obstruction and to evaluate hostile bladder dysfunction	Renal and bladder ultrasonogram or IVP and serum creatinine and BUN test when upper urinary tract distress is suspected and when obstruction is severe
Continuous UI	All cases; bladder chart may not be feasible or helpful, particularly if UI is severe	Urodynamics not indicated	IVP when ureteral ectopia suspected, cystoscopy or methylene blue/tampon test when vesicovaginal fistula suspected

BUN, blood urea nitrogen; IVP, intravenous pyelography; UI, urinary incontinence; UTI, urinary tract infection.

SELF-ASSESSMENT EXERCISE

1. Identify critical elements to be included in the assessment of an individual with UI.

2. Outline essential information to be obtained in the history of a patient with UI.

3. Rate the following statement as true or false and explain your answer: Stress, urge, and mixed UI can generally be diagnosed based on a careful patient history.

4. Describe key factors to be included in the physical assessment of a patient with UI, to include gender-specific factors.

5. Identify at least two options for assessing pelvic muscle strength in the female patient.

6. Outline the information generated by a voiding diary and guidelines to be included in patient instruction.

7. List two techniques for obtaining postvoid residual urine volume and two "values" for abnormally high residual volumes.

8. Define the term "simple bedside cystometry" and identify at least one situation in which it is appropriate.

9. Briefly describe each of the following tests and identify its clinical relevance:

   a. Uroflowmetry
   b. Filling CMG
   c. Sphincter EMG
   d. Abd LPP
   e. Voiding pressure study
   f. Videourodynamics

10. Identify patients who should be referred for complex urodynamic studies.

REFERENCES

1. Shull BL, Hurt G, Laycock J, et al: Physical examination. In: Abrams P, Cardozo L, Khoury S, Wein A, editors: *Incontinence,* Second International Consultation on Incontinence, Plymouth, United Kingdom, 2002, Plymbridge, pp 373-388.

2. Artibani W, Andersen JT, Gajewski JB, et al: Imaging and other investigations. In: Abrams P, Cardozo L, Khoury S, Wein A, editors: *Incontinence,* Second International Consultation on Incontinence, Plymouth, United Kingdom, 2002, Plymbridge, pp 425-478.

3. Abrams PH: Editorial comment, Neurourol Urodyn 15(5):457, 1996.

4. Blaivas JG: Editorial: the bladder is an unreliable witness, Neurourol Urodyn 15(5):443-445, 1996.

5. Wolters R, Wensing M, van Weel C, et al: Lower urinary tract symptoms: social influence is more important than symptoms in seeking medical care, BJU Int 90(7): 655-661, 2002.

6. Abrams P, Cardozo L, Fall M, et al:Standardization Sub-committee of the International Continence Society. The standardization of terminology of lower urinary tract function: report from the Standardization Sub-committee of the International Continence Society, Neurourol Urodyn 21(2):167-178, 2002.

7. Andersson KE: Storage and voiding symptoms: pathophysiologic aspects, Urology 62(5 suppl 2):3-10, 2003.

8. Wein AJ: Diagnosis and treatment of the overactive bladder, Urology 62(5 suppl 2):20-27, 2003.

9. Hellerstein S, Linebarger JS: Voiding dysfunction in pediatric patients, *Clin Pediatr* 42(1):43-49, 2003.

10. Koff SA, Wagner TT, Jayanthi VR: The relationship among dysfunctional elimination syndromes, primary vesicoureteral reflux and urinary tract infections in children, *J Urol* 160(3):1019-1022, 1998.

11. Mazzola BL, von Vigier RO, Marchand S, et al: Behavioral and functional abnormalities linked with recurrent urinary tract infections in girls, *J Nephrol* 16(1):133-138, 2003.

12. Swinn MJ, Fowler CJ: Isolated urinary retention in young women, or Fowler's syndrome, *Clin Auton Res* 11(5): 309-311, 2001.

13. Asplund R: Nocturia, nocturnal polyuria, and sleep quality in the elderly, *J Psychosom Res* 56(5):517-525, 2004.

14. Guilleminault C, Lin CM, Goncalves MA, Ramos E: A prospective study of nocturia and the quality of life of elderly patients with obstructive sleep apnea or sleep onset insomnia, *J Psychosom Res* 56(5):511-515, 2004.

15. Masuda M, Nakayama K, Hiromoto Y, et al: Etiology of nocturia and clinical efficacy of naftopidil on nocturia in patients with benign prostatic hyperplasia: analysis of frequency volume charts, *Hinyokika Kiyo* 50(5):309-314, 2004.

16. Hunt J: Psychological approaches to the management of sensory urgency and idiopathic detrusor instability, *Br J Urol* 77(3):339-341, 1996.

17. Butrick CW: Interstitial cystitis and chronic pelvic pain: new insights in neuropathology, diagnosis, and treatment, *Clin Obstet Gynecol* 46(4):811-823, 2003.

18. Pontari MA, Ruggieri MR: Mechanisms in prostatitis/chronic pelvic pain syndrome, *J Urol* 172(3):839-845, 2004.

19. Williams RE, Hartmann KE, Steege JF: Documenting the current definitions of chronic pelvic pain: implications for research, *Obstet Gynecol* 103(4):686-691, 2004.

20. Ueda T, Sant GR, Hanno PM, Yoshimura N: Interstitial cystitis and frequency-urgency syndrome (OAB syndrome), *Int J Urol* 10(suppl):S39-S48, 2003.

21. Diokno AC, Wells TJ, Brink CA: Urinary incontinence in elderly women: urodynamic evaluation, *J Am Geriatr Soc* 35:940-946, 1987.
22. Jensen JK, Nielsen R, Ostergard DR: The role of the patient history in the diagnosis of urinary incontinence, *Obstet Gynecol* 85(5):904-909, 1994.
23. Nitti VW, Combs AJ: Correlation of Valsalva leak point pressure with subjective degree of stress urinary incontinence in women, *J Urol* 155:281-285, 1996.
24. Black N, Griffiths J, Pope C: Development of a symptom severity index for stress incontinence in women, *Neurourol Urodyn* 15:630-640, 1996.
25. Stewart WF, Van Rooyen JB, Cundiff GW, et al: Prevalence and burden of overactive bladder in the United States, *World J Urol* 20(6):327-336, 2003.
26. Wagner TH, Hu TW, Bentkover J, et al: Health-related consequences of overactive bladder, *Am J Managed Care* 8(19 suppl):S598-S607, 2002.
27. Umlauf MG, Sherman SM: Symptoms of urinary incontinence among older community dwelling men, *J Wound Ostomy Continence Nurs* 23:314-321, 1996.
28. Tan T, Lieu PK, Ding YY : Urinary retention in hospitalised older women, *Ann Acad Med Singapore* 30(6): 588-592, 2002.
29. Vesely S, Knutson T, Damber JE, et al: Relationship between age, prostate volume, prostate-specific antigen, symptom score and uroflowmetry in men with lower urinary tract symptoms, *Scand J Urol Nephrol* 37(4):322-328, 2003.
30. Jensen KM, Bruskewitz RC, Iversen P, Madsen PO: Abdominal straining in benign prostatic hyperplasia, *J Urol* 129(1):44-47, 1983.
31. Reynard JM, Peters TJ, Lamond E, Abrams P: The significance of abdominal straining in men with lower urinary tract symptoms, *Br J Urol* 75:148-153, 1995.
32. Gray M: Urinary retention: management in the acute care setting, Part 1, *Am J Nurs* 100(7):40-48, 2000.
33. Gray M: Psychometric analysis of the International Prostate Symptom Score, *Urol Nurs* 18:175-183, 1998.
34. Blaivas JG, Labib KB: Acute urinary retention in women: complete urodynamic evaluation, *Urology* 10:383-389, 1977.
35. Kalarskov P, Andersen JT, Asmussen CF, et al: Acute urinary retention in women: a prospective study of 18 consecutive cases, *Scand J Urol Nephrol* 21:29-31, 1987.
36. Taube M, Gajraj H: Trial without catheter following acute retention of urine, *Br J Urol* 63:180-182, 1989.
37. Gillon G, Kessler O, Servadio C: [Surgery for women with urethral diverticulum], *Harefuah* 131(7-8): 242-243, 295, 1996 (in Hebrew).
38. Jensen LM, Aabech J, Lundvall F, Iversen HG: Female urethral diverticulum: clinical aspects and presentation of 15 cases, *Acta Obstet Gynecol Scand* 75:748-752, 1996.
39. Furuya S, Ogura H, Tanaka M, et al: Incidence of post-micturition dribble in adult males in their twenties through fifties, *Acta Urol Japon* 43:407-410, 1997.
40. Corcoran M, Smith G, Chisholm GD: Indications for investigation of post-micturition dribble in young adults, *Br J Urol* 59:222-223, 1987.
41. Furuya S, Yokoyama E: Urodynamic studies in post-micturition dribble, *Acta Urol Japon* 29:395-400, 1983.
42. Beier-Holgersen R, Braun J: Voiding pattern of men 60 to 70 years old: population study in an urban population, *J Urol* 143:531-532, 1990.
43. Skoner MM: Self-management of urinary incontinence among women 31 to 50 years of age, *Rehabil Nurs* 19:339-343, 1994.
44. Skoner MM, Haylor MJ: Managing incontinence: women's normalizing strategies, *Health Care Women Int* 14:549-560, 1993.
45. Engberg S, McDowell BJ, Weber E, et al: Assessment and management of urinary incontinence among homebound elderly adults: a clinical trial protocol, *Adv Pract Nurse Q* 3:48-56, 1997.
46. Gray M: Preventing and managing perineal dermatitis, *J Wound Ostomy Continence Nurs* 31(suppl 1):S2-S12, 2004.
47. Gray M, Ratliff C, Donovan A: Perineal skin care for the incontinent patient, *Adv Skin Wound Care* 15(4): 170-178, 2002.
48. Brink CA, Sampselle CM, Wells TJ, et al: A digital test for pelvic muscle strength in older women with urinary incontinence, *Nurs Res* 38:196-199, 1989.
49. Sampselle CM, Brink CA, Wells TJ: Digital measurement of pelvic muscle strength in childbearing women, *Nurs Res* 38:134-138, 1989.
50. Sampselle CM: Using a stopwatch to assess pelvic muscle strength in the urine stream interruption test, *Nurse Pract* 18:14-20, 1993.
51. Dougherty MC: Current status of research on pelvic muscle strengthening techniques, *J Wound Ostomy Continence Nurs* 25:75-83, 1998.
52. Seidel HM, Ball JW, Dains JE, Benedict GW: *Mosby's guide to physical examination,* ed 4, St. Louis, 1998, Mosby.
53. Grayhack JT, Kozlowski JM: Benign prostatic hyperplasia. In: Gillenwater JY, Grayhack JT, Howards SS, Duckett JW, editors: *Adult and pediatric urology,* ed 3, St. Louis, 1996, Mosby, pp 1501-1574.
54. Bushman W, Wyker AW: Standard diagnostic considerations. In: Gillenwater JY, Grayhack JT, Howards SS, Duckett JW, editors: *Adult and pediatric urology,* ed 3, St. Louis, 1996, Mosby.
55. Bauer SB: Neuropathic dysfunction of the lower urinary tract. In: Walsh PC, Retik AB, Vaughan ED, Wein AJ, editors: *Campbell's urology,* ed 8, Philadelphia, 2002, WB Saunders, pp 2231-2261.
56. Brink CA, Wells TJ: Environmental support for geriatric incontinence: toilets, toilet supplements, and external equipment, *Clin Geriatr Med* 2:829-840, 1986.
57. Dolman M: Continence in the community. In: Norton C, editor: *Nursing for continence,* ed 2, Buckinghamshire, United Kingdom, 1996, Beaconsfield.
58. Flaherty JH, Miller DK, Coe RM: Impact on caregivers of supporting urinary function in noninstitutionalized, chronically ill seniors, *Gerontologist* 32:541-545, 1992.
59. Ouslander JG, Zarit SH, Orr NK, Muria SA: Incontinence among elderly, community dwelling

dementia patients: characteristics, management, and impact on caregivers, *J Am Geriatr Soc* 38:440-445, 1990.

60. Barry MJ, Fowler FJ, O'Leary MP, et al: The American Urologic Association symptom index for benign prostatic hyperplasia, *J Urol* 148:1549-1557, 1992.

61. Gray M: *Urodynamic evaluation of the unstable detrusor,* doctoral dissertation, University of Florida, College of Nursing, Gainesville, Fla., 1990.

62. Kojima M, Naya Y, Inoue W, et al: The American Urological Association symptom index for benign prostatic hyperplasia as a function of age, voided volume, and ultrasonic appearance of the prostate, *J Urol* 157:2160-2165, 1997.

63. Lepor H, Machi G: Comparison of AUA symptom index in unselected males and females between 55 and 79 years of age, *Urology* 42(1):36-41, 1993.

64. Ko DS, Fenster NH, Chambers K, et al: The correlation of multichannel urodynamic pressure flow studies and American Urological Association symptom index in the evaluation of benign prostatic hyperplasia, *J Urol* 154:396-398, 1995.

65. Chancellor MB, Rivas DA: AUA symptom index for women with voiding symptoms: lack of index specificity for BPH, *J Urol* 150(5):1706-1709, 1993.

66. Chancellor MB, Rivas DA, Keeley FX, et al: Similarity of the American Urological Association symptom index with benign prostatic hyperplasia (BPH), urethral obstruction not due to BPH, and detrusor hyperreflexia without outlet obstruction, *Br J Urol* 74:200-203, 1994.

67. Wyman JF, Harkins SW, Choi SC, et al: Psychosocial impact of urinary incontinence in women, *Obstet Gynecol* 70(3):378-381, 1987.

68. Shumaker SA, Wyman JF, Ubersax JS, et al: Health related quality of life measures for women with urinary incontinence: the incontinence impact questionnaire and the urogenital distress inventory, *Qual Life Res* 3: 291-306, 1994.

69. Ubersax JS, Wyman JF, Shumaker SA, et al: Short forms to assess quality of life and symptom distress for urinary incontinence in women: the incontinence impact questionnaire and the urogenital distress inventory, *Neurourol Urodyn* 14:131-139, 1995.

70. Hagen S, Hanley J, Capewell A: Test-retest reliability, validity, and sensitivity to change of the urogenital distress inventory and the incontinence impact questionnaire, *Neurourol Urodyn* 21(6):534-539, 2002.

71. Robinson D, McClish DK, Wyman JF, et al: Comparison between urinary diaries with and without intensive patient instructions, *Neurourol Urodyn* 15:143-148, 1996.

72. Wyman JF, Choi SC, Harkins SW, et al: The urinary diary in evaluation of incontinent women: a test-retest analysis, *Obstet Gynecol* 71:812-817, 1988.

73. Sampselle CM: Teaching women to use a voiding diary, *Am J Nurs* 103(11):62-64, 2003.

74. Griffiths DJ, McCracken PN, Harrison GM, Gromley EA: Characteristics of urinary incontinence in elderly patients studied by 24-hour monitoring and urodynamic testing, *Age Ageing* 21:195-201, 1992.

75. Griffiths DJ, McCracken PN, Harrison GM, Gromley EA: Relationship of fluid intake to voluntary micturition and urinary incontinence in geriatric patients, *Neurourol Urodyn* 12:1-7, 1993.

76. Gray M, Marx RM, Peruggio M, et al: A model for predicting motor urge urinary incontinence, *Nurs Res* 50:116-122, 2001.

77. Hannestad YS, Rortveit G, Daltveit AK, Hunskaar S: Are smoking and other lifestyle factors associated with female urinary incontinence? The Norwegian EPINCONT Study, *Br J Obstet Gynaecol* 110(3): 247-254, 2003.

78. Tampakoudis P, Tantanassis T, Grimbizis G, et al: Cigarette smoking and urinary incontinence in women—a new calculative method of estimating the exposure to smoke, *Eur J Obstet Gynecol Reprod Biol* 63:27-30, 1995.

79. Whitmore KE: Self-care regimens for patients with interstitial cystitis, *Urol Clin North Am* 21:121-130, 1994.

80. Walter S, Vejlsgaard R: Diagnostic catheterization and bacteriuria in women with urinary incontinence, *Br J Urol* 50:106-108, 1978.

81. Bent AE, Nahhas DE, McLennan MT: Portable ultrasound of urinary residual volume, *Int Urogynecol J Pelvic Floor Dysfunct* 8:200-202, 1997.

82. Gray M, Krissovich M: Characteristics of North American urodynamic centers: measuring lower urinary tract filling and storage function, *Urol Nurs* 24(1):30-38, 2004.

83. Krissovich M, Gray M: Characteristics of North American urodynamic laboratories and clinicians, *Urol Nurs* 22:179-182, 2002.

84. Schafer W, Abrams P, Liao L, et al: International Continence Society: good urodynamic practices: uroflowmetry, filling cystometry, and pressure-flow studies, *Neurourol Urodyn* 21(3):261-274, 2002.

85. Fox RW, McDonald AT: *Introduction to fluid mechanics,* ed 3, New York, 1985, John Wiley & Sons.

86. Hinman F: *Hydrodynamics of micturition,* Springfield, Ill., 1968, Charles C Thomas.

87. Belville WD, Swierzewski SJ, Wedemeyer G, McGuire EJ: Fiberoptic microtransducer pressure technology: urodynamic implications, *Neurourol Urodyn* 12:171-178, 1993.

88. International Continence Society: *The standardization of terminology of lower urinary tract function,* Glasgow, United Kingdom, 1984, Glasgow Department of Clinical Physics and Bioengineering.

89. Griffiths DJ: Hydrodynamics and mechanics of the bladder and urethra. In: Mundy AR, Stephenson TP, Wein AJ, editors: *Urodynamics: principles, practice, and application,* London, 1994, Churchill Livingstone.

90. Pollak JT, Neimark M, Connor JT, Davila GW: Air-charged and microtransducer urodynamic catheters in the evaluation of urethral function, *Int Urogynecol J* 15(2):124-128, 2004.

91. Rollema HJ, van Mastrigt R: Improved indication and follow-up in transurethral resection of the prostate using the computer program CLIM: a prospective study, *J Urol* 148:115-116, 1992.

92. Rayome RG: Simple urodynamic techniques, J Wound Ostomy Continence Nurs 22(1):17-26, 1995.

93. Fonda D, Brimage PJ, D'Astoli M: Simple screening for urinary incontinence in the elderly: comparison of simple and multichannel cystometry, Urology 42(5): 536-540, 1993.

94. Neal DE, Rao CNS, Ng R, Ramsden PD: Effects of catheter size on urodynamic measurement in men undergoing elective prostatectomy, Br J Urol 60:61-68, 1987.

95. Klingler HC, Madersbacher S, Schmidbauer CP: Impact of different sized catheters on pressure flow studies in patients with benign prostatic hyperplasia, Neurourol Urodyn 15:473-481, 1996.

96. Proceedings of the first joint meeting of the International Continence Society and the Urodynamics Society, Prog Clin Biol Res 78:1-413, 1981.

97. Wein AJ, Barrett DM: Controversies in neurourology, New York, 1984, Churchill Livingstone.

98. Kaefer M, Zurakowski D, Bauer SB, et al: Estimating normal bladder capacity in children, J Urol 158(6): 2261-2264, 1997.

99. Koff SA: Estimating bladder capacity in children, Urology 21(3):248, 1983.

100. Pauwels E, De Wachter S, Wyndaele JJ: Normality of bladder filling studied in symptom-free middle-aged women, J Urol 171(4):1567-1570, 2004.

101. Schmidt F, Shin P, Jorgensen TM, et al: Urodynamic patterns of normal male micturition: influence of water consumption on urine production and detrusor function, J Urol 168(4):1458-1463, 2002.

102. Gray M: Functional alterations: bladder. In: Johnson BL, Gross J, editors: Handbook of oncology nursing, St. Louis, 1998, Mosby.

103. Sasaki K, Yoshimura N, Chancellor MB: Implications of diabetes mellitus in urology, Urol Clin North Am 30(1):1-12, 2003.

104. Tjandra BS, Janknegt RA: Neurogenic impotence and lower urinary tract symptoms due to vitamin B1 deficiency in chronic alcoholism, J Urol 157(3):954-955, 1997.

105. Wahl EF, Lahdes-Vasama TT, Lerman SE, Churchill BM: Prototype system for enhancing cystometric analysis with special emphasis on the pediatric population, J Endourol 15(8):873-880, 2001.

106. Bagli DJ, van Savage JG, Khoury AE, et al: Basic fibroblast growth factor in the urine of children with voiding pathology, J Urol 158:1123-1127, 1997.

107. Susset JG, Ghoneim GM: Effect of bilateral sacral decentralization in detrusor contractility and passive properties in dogs, Neurourol Urodyn 3:23-33, 1984.

108. Susset JG: Cystometry. In: Krane RJ, Siroky MD, editors: Clinical neurourology, Boston, 1991, Little, Brown.

109. McGuire EJ, Woodside JR, Borden TA, Weiss RM: Prognostic value of urodynamic testing in myelodysplastic patients, J Urol 126:205-209, 1981.

110. Gray M, King CJ: Urodynamic evaluation of the intrinsically incompetent sphincter, Urol Nurs 13(2):67-69, 1993.

111. McGuire EJ, Cespedes RD, O'Connell HE: Leak-point pressures, Urol Clin North Am 23:253-262, 1996.

112. Fleischmann N, Flisser AJ, Blaivas JG, Panagopoulos G: Sphincteric urinary incontinence: relationship of vesical leak point pressure, urethral mobility and severity of incontinence, J Urol 169(3):999-1002, 2003.

113. McGuire EJ: Urodynamic evaluation of stress incontinence, Urol Clin North Am 22(3):551-555, 1995.

114. Flood HD, Alevizatos C, Liu JL: Sex differences in the determination of abdominal leak point pressure in patients with intrinsic sphincter deficiency, J Urol 156(5):1737-1740, 1996.

115. Kuo HC: Videourodynamic analysis of the relationship of Valsalva and cough leak point pressures in women with stress urinary incontinence, Urology 61(3):544-549, 2003.

116. Griffiths DJ: Pressure-flow studies of micturition, Urol Clin North Am 23:279-297, 1996.

117. Fry CH, Sui GP, Severs NJ, Wu C: Spontaneous activity and electrical coupling in human detrusor smooth muscle: implications for detrusor overactivity? Urology 63(3 suppl 1):3-10, 2004.

118. Siroky MB: Electromyography of the perineal striated muscles. In: Krane RJ, Siroky MD, editors: Clinical neurourology, ed 2, Boston, 1991, Little, Brown, pp 245-264.

119. Snooks SJ, Swash M: Neurophysiological techniques for assessment of pelvic floor and striated sphincter muscles and their innervation. In: Urodynamics: principles, practice, and techniques, London, 1994, Churchill Livingstone.

120. Lowe EM, Fowler CJ, Osborne JL, Delancey JO: Improved method for needle electromyography of the urethral sphincter in women, Neurourol Urodyn 13:29-33, 1994.

121. Park JM, Bloom DA, McGuire EJ: The guarding reflex revisited, Br J Urol 80:940-945, 1997.

122. Abrams PH, Griffiths DJ: The assessment of prostatic obstruction from urodynamic measurements and residual urine, Br J Urol 51:129-134, 1979.

123. Chassagne S, Bernier PA, Haab F, et al: Proposed cutoff values to define bladder outlet obstruction in women, Urology 51(3):408-411, 1998.

124. Schafer W: Analysis of bladder-outlet function with the linearized passive urethral resistance relation, lin PURR, and a disease specific approach for grading obstruction: from complex to simple, World J Urol 13: 47-58, 1995.

125. Hofner K, Kramer AEJL, Tan HK, et al: CHESS classification of bladder outflow obstruction, Urology 13: 59-64, 1995.

126. Rollema HJ, van Mastrigt R, Janknegt RA: Urodynamic assessment and quantification of prostatic obstruction before and after transurethral resection of the prostate: standardization with the aid of the computer program CLIM, Urol Int 47(suppl 1):52-54, 1991.

127. Griffiths DJ, Constantinou CE, van Mastrigt R: Urinary bladder function and its control in healthy females, Am J Physiol 251(2):R255-R330, 1986.

128. Svihra J, Bos R, Rollema HJ, Janknegt RA: [Determination of infravesical obstruction in men with benign prostatic hyperplasia using pressure-flow measurement and analysis with the Dx/CLIM software program], *Bratislavske Lekarske Listy* 98: 28-31, 1997.

129. Brown M, Wickham JE: The urethral pressure profile, *Br J Urol* 41:211-217, 1969.

130. Versi E: Discriminant analysis of urethral pressure profilometry for the diagnosis of genuine stress incontinence, *Br J Obstet Gynecol* 97:251-259, 1990.

131. Bergman A, Ballard CA, Koonings CA: Comparison of three different surgical procedures for genuine stress incontinence: prospective randomized study, *J Obstet Gynecol* 160:1102-1106, 1989.

132. Richardson DA: Value of the cough pressure profile in the evaluation of patients with stress incontinence, *Am J Obstet Gynecol* 155:808-811, 1986.

133. Asklin B, Erlandson BE, Johansson G, Petersson S: The micturitional urethral pressure profile, *Scand J Urol Nephrol* 18:269-276, 1984.

134. Einhorn CJ: Videourodynamic techniques, *J Wound Ostomy Continence Nurs* 22:34-43, 1995.

135. McGuire EG, Cespedes RD, Cross CA, O'Connell HE: Videourodynamic studies, *Urol Clin North Am* 23: 309-321, 1996.

136. Bidair M, Teichman JM, Brodak PP, Juma S: Transrectal ultrasound urodynamics, *Urology* 42(6):640-645, 1993.

137. Shapeero LG, Friedland GW, Perkash I: Transrectal sonographic voiding cystourethrography: studies in neuromuscular bladder dysfunction, *AJR Am J Roentgenol* 141:83-90, 1983.

138. Cross CA, Cespedes RD, McGuire EJ: Treatment results using pubovaginal slings in patients with large cystoceles and stress incontinence, *J Urol* 158:431-434, 1997.

139. Gray M: *Persistent urinary incontinence following urethral suspension*, Wound, Ostomy and Continence Nurses Society annual conference, Seattle, June 1996 , Laguna Beach, Calif., 1996, Wound, Ostomy and Continence Nurses Society.

13 *Physiology of Bowel Function*

MARGARET McLEAN HEITKEMPER

OBJECTIVES

1. Identify the major anatomic sections and functions of the colon.
2. Explain the role of intrinsic and extrinsic neural innervation in regulation of colonic motility.
3. Compare and contrast the internal anal sphincter and external anal sphincter in regard to type of muscle, innervation, response to rectal distension, degree of voluntary control, and role in continence and defecation.
4. Describe the role of the pelvic musculature in continence and defecation.
5. Define the following and explain their role in defecation and continence: rectoanal inhibitory reflex, sampling reflex, and peristaltic contractions.
6. Explain the significance of intact sensory pathways to the maintenance of continence.
7. Describe the role of rectal capacitance and compliance in the maintenance of continence.
8. Describe the flap valve and flutter valve theories of continence.

Continence is defined as the ability to retain feces until a socially appropriate time and place for elimination; defecation refers to the forceful expulsion of fecal material from the colon. Both continence and defecation are complex physiologic functions, neither of which are completely understood at this time. Both these functions involve voluntary regulation by the central nervous system as well as involuntary intrinsic reflex mechanisms. For example, defecation requires the individual to use the Valsalva maneuver to voluntarily increase intra-abdominal pressure while relaxing the external anal sphincter and pelvic floor muscles; defecation also involves reflex stimulation of colonic motility to deliver stool to the rectum and anal canal and reflex relaxation of the internal anal sphincter to permit fecal elimination. In contrast, continence is partly dependent on the individual's ability to voluntarily contract the pelvic floor muscles and external anal sphincter in response to sudden rectal distension and partly dependent on reflex relaxation of the rectal walls to provide temporary fecal storage. Thus, problems related to fecal continence and defecation can arise either from an extrinsic disorder involving the central or peripheral nervous system, from an intrinsic disorder involving the colon, rectum, or anal sphincters or from some combination of problems. In most cases, incontinence results from several interacting factors, as opposed to one single etiologic factor.[1] This chapter provides a review of the physiology of continence and defecation, including anatomy and physiology of the colon and the pelvic floor musculature.

ANATOMY AND PHYSIOLOGY OF THE COLON

It is extremely important for the clinician caring for patients with bowel dysfunction or fecal incontinence to have a clear understanding of colonic physiology and the physiology of normal fecal elimination. Unfortunately, few studies have focused on the normal function of the human colon; thus, clinical practice is at this time necessarily based on an incomplete understanding of the processes governing continence and defecation.

Anatomy of the Colon

The colon of the human adult measures approximately 1.2 to 1.5 m in length (3.9–4.9 feet) and can be subdivided into the following sections: cecum (and its appendage, the appendix); ascending colon; transverse colon; descending colon; sigmoid colon; rectum; and anal canal (Fig. 13-1). Such "section" designations are based more on anatomy than on physiologic differences.

Anatomically, the ileum of the small intestine joins the large intestine at the junction of the cecum and ascending colon. The *cecum* is the proximal 5 to 8 cm (2 to 3 inches) of the large intestine; the *appendix* arises off the cecum. The *ileocecal valve* permits contents to move distally, that is, from the small intestine into the colon, but it prevents retrograde movement of intestinal contents from the colon back to the small intestine; this is an important factor in limiting bacterial contamination of the small bowel. The *ascending colon* lies between the cecum and the hepatic flexure and is the portion of the colon that lies in a vertical position on the right side of the abdomen. The *transverse colon* lies in a horizontal position across the abdomen between the hepatic flexure and the splenic flexure; the upper surface of the transverse colon extends upward to the lower border of the liver, stomach, and spleen. The transverse colon

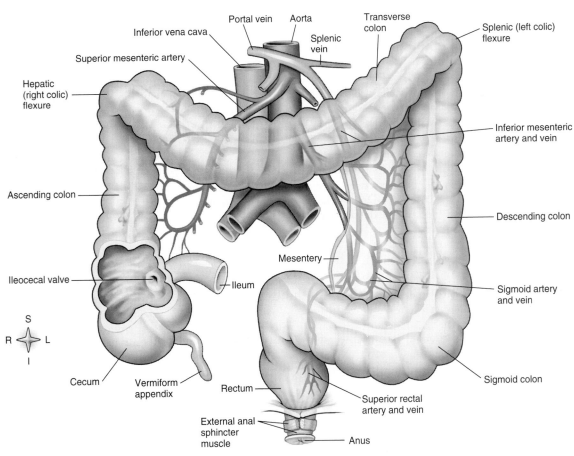

Fig. 13-1 Sections of large intestine. (From Erlandsen SL, Magney J: *Color atlas of histology,* St. Louis, 1999, Mosby.)

plays a major role in the storage and mixing of colonic contents. At the end of the transverse colon, the large intestine takes a 90-degree turn into the *descending colon.* Like the ascending colon, the descending colon lies in a vertical position but on the left half of the abdomen, extending from a point below the stomach and spleen to the level of the iliac crest. The *sigmoid colon* extends from the iliac crest to the rectum. This section of the colon is called "sigmoid" because of its S-shaped curvature. The distal portion of the S curves to the left, which provides the rationale for placing a patient on the left side during an enema or endoscopic exam. The descending colon and rectosigmoid colon act primarily as fecal conduits, delivering stool from the transverse colon to the rectum before defecation.

The remaining portions of the large intestine include the *rectum* and the *anal canal.* The rectum is similar anatomically to the preceding colonic sections, although it is wider in diameter. The rectum is approximately 15 cm (6 inches) in length. The anal canal is the last segment of the large intestine. It is a short canal, usually about 3 cm in length, but plays a very important role in maintenance of fecal continence. The anal canal is surrounded by two sphincter mechanisms that work together to maintain continence and to permit voluntary defecation, the internal and external anal sphincters. These sphincters are illustrated in Fig. 13-2 and are discussed in greater detail later in this chapter.

Structure of the Bowel Wall. The wall of the colon is similar to that of the proximal portion of the gastrointestinal (GI) tract in basic composition and in innervation. First of all, the wall is composed of the same four layers: the inner mucosal lining, the submucosa, the muscularis (muscle), and the outer serosa (Fig. 13-3). The mucosa is the innermost layer and the layer exposed to colonic contents. It contains epithelial cells, which are absorptive, and mucus-secreting cells (goblet cells), which produce mucus that serves to neutralize the acids produced by colonic bacteria and also to facilitate the movement of fecal material through the colonic lumen. The submucosal layer contains connective tissue, blood vessels, lymphatics, reticuloendothelial cells,

and nerve fibers (Meissner's, or submucous, plexus). The muscle layer is actually a double layer of smooth muscle, an inner circular layer and an outer longitudinal layer; these layers coordinate the mixing and propulsion of colonic contents from the cecum to the anal canal. Between the two muscle layers is a second major nerve plexus, Auerbach's plexus (also known as the myenteric plexus). The outermost layer is the serosa, which is continuous with the visceral peritoneum and mesentery.

The colon, like the small intestine, is controlled by both extrinsic and intrinsic neural influences. Intrinsic innervation is provided via the enteric nervous system, which is composed of Meissner's and Auerbach's plexuses, and nerve fibers originating in receptors in the colon wall. The enteric nervous system plays the major role in regulation of colonic motility and is most responsive to local factors, such as distension (stretch) or intraluminal irritants. Extrinsic innervation serves to modulate colonic motility and is provided by the two branches of the autonomic nervous system, the sympathetic and the parasympathetic nervous systems. Innervation of the colon is discussed in greater detail in the next section.

Although the colonic wall is similar to the wall of the small intestine in basic composition and innervation, there are some distinct differences that are significant. One difference is in the longitudinal muscle layer; it does not uniformly encircle the colon but instead forms three muscle bands known as the *taeniae coli,* which run the length of the colon. Because these muscle bands are actually shorter than the colon to which they attach, they gather the colon wall into sacculations known as *haustrations.*

Neural Innervation. As noted earlier, the neural innervation of the large intestine includes both intrinsic and extrinsic components and both sensory and motor elements.

Intrinsic Innervation. The entire GI tract contains intramural nerve plexuses that are known as the enteric nervous system. The plexuses are composed of ganglia (that is, clusters of nerves) as well as nerve processes that interconnect the ganglia and provide communication between the receptors in the bowel

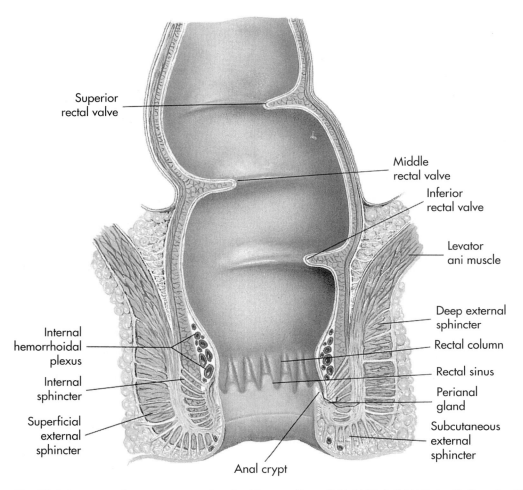

Fig. 13-2 Anatomy of rectum, anus, and anal sphincters. (From Seidel HM, Ball JW, Dains JE, Benedict GW: *Mosby's guide to physical examination,* ed 5, St. Louis, 2003, Mosby.)

wall and the ganglia. These neuronal connections allow for communication and coordination along the length of the colon. It is the myenteric plexus that appears to play the major role in regulation of colonic motility.

In the proximal portion of the colon (the ascending colon and right half of the transverse colon), the anatomic arrangement of the intrinsic nerve pathways is similar to that seen in the small intestine. However, the distribution of fibers changes in the distal portion of the colon. This section of

the colon contains neuronal fibers called *ascending fibers,* which most likely are involved in the coordination of reflex activity (such as colocolonic and colorectal reflexes).

Extrinsic Innervation. As noted earlier, the primary mediator for peristaltic activity is the intrinsic, or enteric nervous system; however, extrinsic innervation plays an important modulating role. Extrinsic innervation is provided by fibers of the autonomic nervous system and includes both parasympathetic and sympathetic input. These extrinsic

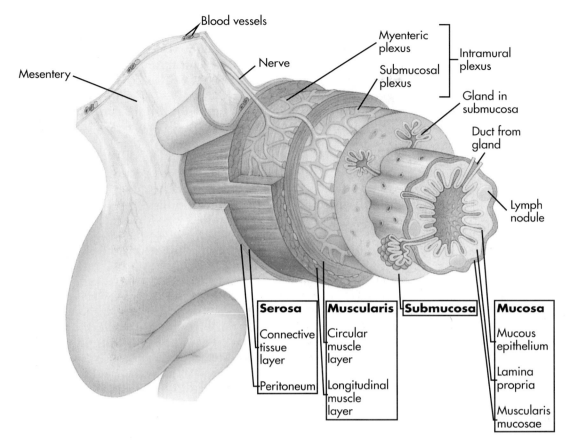

Fig. 13-3 Layers of the colon wall. (From Seeley RR, Stephens T, Tate P: *Anatomy and physiology,* ed 3, St. Louis, 1995, Mosby, figure copyright, McGraw-Hill.)

fibers terminate on neurons of the intrinsic plexuses, and stimulation of these fibers serves either to increase or to decrease peristaltic activity. Sympathetic pathways arise from the thoracolumbar region of the spinal cord, and sympathetic stimulation has an inhibiting effect on GI tract activity, reducing both secretion and motility. Parasympathetic stimulation, conversely, acts to promote peristalsis; parasympathetic input to the proximal portion of the colon is provided via branches of the vagus nerve, whereas parasympathetic input to the descending colon and sigmoid is provided by fibers exiting the cord at the sacral level. Mechanical stimulation of the colon results in coordinated reflex contraction of the rectum and

may elicit defecation. This reflex activity is coordinated by the sacral parasympathetic center and its outflow tract; afferent fibers from the colon enter the cord at the sacral level and activate the parasympathetic efferent fibers, which trigger reflex contractions in the colon. The effect of parasympathetic stimulation can be further illustrated by the inhibiting effect of *anticholinergic* agents such as propantheline (Pro-Banthine) on colonic activity.

Although the enteric nervous system is able to maintain a base level of peristaltic activity without extrinsic (autonomic) innervation, the importance of autonomic innervation should not be underestimated. Patients who lack autonomic innervation (such as patients with spinal cord injuries at the sacral level) frequently experience colonic inertia and severe constipation.

Sensory function is critical to continence and involves two distinct components: awareness of rectal distension and accurate identification of rectal contents. Awareness of rectal distension is facilitated by the fact that the rectum is more sensitive to distension than the remainder of the colon. Distension causes stimulation of afferent receptors in the rectum and pelvic floor musculature that carry the message to the spinal cord; the message is then relayed to the cerebral cortex, triggering conscious recognition of rectal distension and the need to defecate. Accurate identification of rectal contents is provided primarily by the portion of the anal canal just distal to the anorectal junction. This region of the anal canal contains multiple sensory receptors that are able to distinguish solid from fluid from gaseous contents. The distal portion of the anal canal includes a transition zone where the anal epithelium meets the perianal skin. There is a pronounced increase in sensory receptors in this area, and the portion of the canal lined by skin is sensitive to light touch, to temperature differences, and to pinprick.

Physiology of the Colon

Absorption. The human colon plays an important role in the absorption of water and electrolytes (including endogenous secretions) and a minor role in the absorption of some nutrients. The colon has significant reserve in terms of absorptive capacity; under normal conditions, the colon absorbs 1 to 2 liters of water and salts per day, but under conditions of dehydration or fluid loss, the colon can absorb up to 5 or 6 liters of water and salts per day. Numerous hormones and neuropeptides produced by cells in the GI tract (such as vasoactive intestinal polypeptide, neuropeptide Y, and somatostatin) and by other endocrine tissues (such as aldosterone) modulate the ability of the colon to absorb fluids. The absorption of fluid plays an important role in the conversion of stool from a liquid to a solid.

Motility of the Colon. The smooth muscle of the colon, like the smooth muscle in the small intestine, has a basic rhythmic pattern. There are two basic types of muscle contractions in the intestine, haustral contractions and peristaltic waves (sometimes referred to as "mass movements"). Haustral contractions involve simultaneous contraction of the longitudinal muscle bands and a section of circular muscle. These contractions are called *haustral contractions* because they cause the haustra to bulge outward. These contractions serve to increase exposure of the intestinal contents to the mucosal surface and to *gradually* move the intestinal contents distally; it can take as long as 8 to 15 hours to move colonic contents from the ileocecal valve to the transverse colon, during which time the stool is converted from a semifluid to a semisolid consistency. Colonic movement in the left colon is typified by series of propulsive peristaltic waves that rapidly propel stool from the point where the peristaltic waves originated (usually a point of distension or irritation) toward the rectum. These peristaltic waves typically persist for about 10 to 15 minutes two to three times per day, most commonly after a meal. When the stool reaches the rectum, the distension of the rectal walls triggers the urge to defecate. However, continence is supported by muscle contractions in the anal canal that increase in response to rectal distension; this increased contractility produces higher intraanal pressures and helps to prevent the movement of rectal contents into the anal canal.

Colonic motility is decreased during sleep and markedly increased during waking hours.[2] Colonic motility is further increased by eating; this increase in colonic motor activity may be perceived by the individual as an urge to defecate. At one time, this was referred to as the "gastrocolonic reflex;" however, this term is a misnomer because the stimulus is not confined to the stomach and the resulting increase in motility is not confined to the colon. Colonic dysmotility can result in prolonged colonic transit time and constipation, although this delay in transit can also occur without a measurable change in colonic motility.

Internal Anal Sphincter. The internal and external anal sphincters are actually continuations and condensations of the muscles of the colon wall; this merging of the smooth muscle with the internal and external sphincters is important in the coordination of defecation (see Fig. 13-2). The internal anal sphincter is a continuation of the circular muscle layer; it is approximately 3 cm long and encircles the anorectal junction and the proximal 2 cm of the anal canal. The internal anal sphincter is composed predominantly of slow-twitch smooth muscle fibers, which are fatigue resistant; this type of muscle is well equipped to maintain tonic contraction, which contributes significantly to the resting pressure (and closure) of the anal canal. The internal anal sphincter is innervated by both branches of the autonomic nervous system: the sympathetic nervous system via the hypogastric plexus, which exits the cord at T10 – L2 and the parasympathetic nervous system via the pelvic plexus, which originates from the sacral cord (S1 to S3).[3] Alpha-adrenergic (sympathetic) stimulation by the neurotransmitter norepinephrine results in contraction of the internal anal sphincter. The effects of acetylcholine (the parasympathetic neurotransmitter) on the internal anal sphincter are less certain. In addition, the internal anal sphincter receives input from noncholinergic, nonadrenergic pelvic nerves.[2] Greater understanding of the neurochemistry of the internal anal sphincter has resulted in pharmacologic research focused on enhancing sphincter tone. For example, nitric oxide is known to be inhibitory to the internal anal sphincter, resulting in relaxation. Based on this, nitric oxide synthesis inhibitors have been tested in animal models and in humans. Topical phenylephrine, an alpha-adrenoreceptor agonist, has also shown some promise in increasing internal anal sphincter pressure.[3-5]

Relaxation of the internal anal sphincter occurs in response to rectal distension; this is a reflex neurogenic response elicited by the stimulation of mechanoreceptors in the rectum and possibly the sigmoid colon. (This reflex relaxation of the internal sphincter in response to rectal distension is known as the *rectoanal inhibitory reflex* and is explained further later in this chapter.) It is important to understand that the internal anal sphincter is composed of smooth muscle and is therefore not under voluntary control.

External Anal Sphincter. The external anal sphincter is unique in that it is composed of both smooth and striated muscle. Anatomically, it can be divided into superficial and deep components, although such distinctions are not universally accepted. The smooth muscle component is a continuation of the longitudinal muscle layer, which merges with the external anal sphincter in the anal canal. The striated muscle component merges with the puborectalis muscle to form a functional unit that permits voluntary contraction or relaxation of the external anal sphincter. The smooth muscle of the external sphincter is innervated only by the enteric nervous system; it does not receive extrinsic autonomic innervation. Innervation of the striated component of the external anal sphincter is primarily through branches of the pudendal nerve, a somatic nerve that exits the cord at the level of S2, S3, and S4. (The pudendal nerve also contains sensory fibers.) Fortunately, there is bilateral motor innervation of the external anal sphincter, and this provides for maintenance of function even if neurologic damage or destruction of one of the nerves occurs.

Under rest conditions, including sleep, the external anal sphincter remains tonically contracted; this contraction is mediated by a reflex arc. The degree of reflex contraction is increased in response to any activity that increases rectal pressures, such as change to an upright position or rectal filling. The striated component of the external anal sphincter can be voluntarily contracted, and such contraction significantly increases anal canal pressures and helps to maintain continence during internal anal sphincter relaxation. Finally, the external anal sphincter can be voluntarily relaxed, a state critical to normal defecation. Failure to relax the external anal sphincter produces obstructed defecation and chronic constipation, which is common in patients with nonrelaxing puborectalis syndrome.

The external anal sphincter can be stimulated to contract by mechanisms other than rectal distension; for example, electrical stimulation of the perianal skin can induce reflex activation of the external sphincter. The contractile strength of the external anal sphincter and the puborectalis muscle are measured clinically by "squeeze-pressure" readings obtained during anorectal manometry studies.[4]

PELVIC FLOOR MUSCULATURE

The muscles of the pelvic floor play an important role in continence and defecation. These muscles are striated and are therefore under voluntary control. Innervation to these muscles is provided by branches of the sacral plexus and by the perineal branches of the pudendal nerve. These fibers exit the cord at the sacral level (S2 to S4). The *levator ani* muscle and the *puborectalis* muscle combine to form the muscular sheath known as the *pelvic floor.*

The levator ani is composed of two symmetric muscle sheets. These broad, thin sheets arise from the pelvic sidewalls and the sacrospinous ligaments laterally and then run downward and posteriorly to form a funnel. This funnel is crossed in the midline by the pelvic viscera as they exit the pelvis (the anal canal, the urethra, and, in the female, the vagina); thus, these muscle fibers are in close contact with the sidewalls of the pelvic organs (Fig. 13-4). The levator ani muscles receive innervation from the fourth sacral nerve.

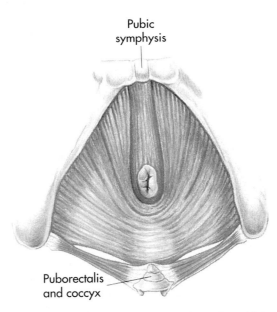

Pubic
symphysis

Puborectalis
and coccyx

Fig. 13-4 Puborectalis and levator ani muscles, which forms pelvic floor. (From Doughty DB, Jackson DB: *Gastrointestinal disorders,* Mosby's clinical nursing series, St. Louis, 1993, Mosby.)

The puborectalis muscle provides a ring of support around the anal canal at the outlet of the funnel created by the levator ani muscle. The U-shaped puborectalis muscle originates along the posterior aspect of the symphysis pubis, passes posteriorly to form a sling around the anorectal junction, and returns to the posterior side of the symphysis pubis (see Fig. 13-4). The orientation of the puborectalis muscle toward the symphysis pubis and the "slinglike" configuration around the anorectal junction create an angle between the anal canal and the rectum. Under resting conditions this angle is 90 degrees, but during straining and defecation this angle straightens to 135 degrees. As stated earlier, the puborectalis and the external anal sphincter muscles form a functional unit with fibers that attach to the perineal body and the coccyx.

CONTINENCE

Continence refers to the ability to control the elimination of feces until a socially acceptable time and place can be secured. Continence is a complicated physiologic phenomenon that is not yet completely understood. Continence requires a combination of competent internal and external anal sphincters, intact pelvic floor musculature, adequate rectal capacitance and compliance, intact intrinsic and extrinsic neural pathways (autonomic, sensory, and motor), and intact cognition and social awareness to provide conscious control. Other factors that affect bowel function and therefore continence include colonic motility and transit time and stool consistency and volume.

Sphincter competence refers to the normal characteristics and responses of the internal and external anal sphincters. Continence is maintained so long as the anal canal pressure is greater than the rectal pressure. The ability of the sphincters to generate adequate anal canal pressure is therefore critical to the maintenance of continence. Approximately 70% to 85% of the anal canal pressure *at rest* is provided by the internal anal sphincter;[1] the remainder of the pressure is provided by tonic (reflex) contraction of the external anal sphincter and by the anal cushions (hemorrhoids). (This ability of the external anal sphincter to provide tonic contraction by means of sacral reflex activity is unique among striated muscles.) Normal anal canal pressures range from 30 to 80 mm Hg,[2] providing a passive barrier to movement of rectal contents into the anal canal. During periods of increased intra-abdominal and increased intrarectal pressure (such as standing, coughing, sneezing, or performance of a Valsalva maneuver), the tonic activity of the external anal sphincter increases because of a compensatory increase in reflex stimulation. *Voluntary* contraction of the external anal sphincter dramatically increases the anal canal pressure to double the pressure at resting levels. However, the maximum amount of time that the external sphincter can be actively contracted is no more than 1 to 3 minutes.

The fact that voluntary contraction of the external anal sphincter can double the resting pressure of the anal canal points to the significance of its role in maintenance of fecal continence during periods of rectal distension and increased rectal pressure. However, voluntary contraction can be sustained for a very limited time, and this points to the significance of the rectum's ability to serve as a temporary reservoir for stool; this ability to stretch and to store stool at relatively low pressures is known as *compliance,* and it is rectal compliance that preserves continence past the point at which the external sphincter relaxes. It is well documented that the continent rectum is able to store stool, but whether this storage capacity is attributable to receptive relaxation of the bowel wall or to some other mechanism remains to be demonstrated. As the rectum fills with stool, its compliance or capacitance decreases. The initial sensation of rectal distension occurs between 11 and 68 mL, and the highest tolerated rectal volume ranges from 250 to 510 mL. In the individual with normal compliance (the ability to stretch and store with minimal increase in pressure), the intraluminal rectal pressure begins to increase at a filling point of about 300 mL. Individuals with rectal disorders often have reduced compliance and are therefore unable to store normal volumes of stool; these individuals experience increased stool frequency, fecal urgency, and sometimes even incontinence. Some individuals experience low compliance even though no pathologic condition can be demonstrated.

In some aspects, the anorectum performs as a functional unit. For example, rectal distension causes stimulation of afferent fibers in the pelvic floor; these fibers, in turn, cause receptive relaxation of the internal anal sphincter. This inhibitory reflex is named the *rectoanal inhibitory reflex.* The reduction in resting anal tone likely facilitates normal defecation by reducing the pressure gradient.[2] Intermittent relaxation of the internal anal sphincter permits stool to move into the proximal area of the anal canal, which allows the rectal contents to contact the numerous sensory receptors located in the upper anal canal. These receptors provide for differentiation among gas, solid, and liquid. This is referred to as the *sampling reflex.*[1] Normally, the external anal sphincter is both reflexively and voluntarily contracted in response to rectal distension. This contraction occurs at the same time as internal anal sphincter relaxation and serves to maintain fecal continence while permitting identification of rectal contents. Once the peristaltic wave has passed, the rectal wall relaxes, the rectal pressures drop, and the internal anal sphincter then resumes normal tone, which maintains closure of the anal canal. Of clinical relevance is the realization that fecal impaction results in persistent rectal distension and persistently elevated rectal pressures, which, in turn, stimulate persistent relaxation of the internal anal sphincter; this explains the frequent seepage of stool commonly seen in patients with stool impaction.

The *flutter valve theory* and the *flap valve theory* are two different theories related to the maintenance of fecal continence during periods of rectal distension. The flutter valve theory was proposed in 1965.[6] According to this theory, intraabdominal pressure applied to a high-pressure area within the lower rectum causes the lower rectum to close and prevents passage of stool into the anal canal (Fig. 13-5). The flap valve theory postulates that increased intraabdominal pressure causes the anterior rectal wall to press down into the anal canal, thus occluding the anal canal and blocking the movement of stool. In this situation, the rectal wall acts as a plug (Fig. 13-6).

Neural control of continence is clearly complex and involves the reflex activity coordinated by the intramural plexuses, sensory input from the pelvic musculature and the anal canal, spinal reflex pathways, and the higher brain centers, which coordinate voluntary muscle activity. This complexity is

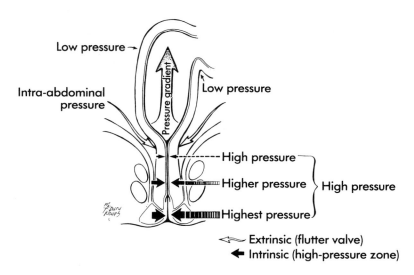

Fig. 13-5 Flutter valve theory of anal continence.

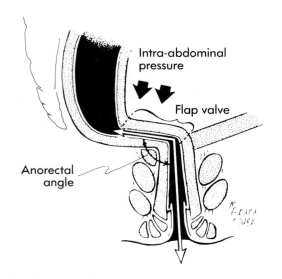

Fig. 13-6 Flap valve theory of anal continence.

reflected in the clinical presentation of patients with neurologic lesions affecting bowel function, such as spinal cord injury. Even if all autonomic innervation is lost, these individuals retain peristaltic activity because the enteric nervous system is the primary modulator of peristaltic activity, and this system is unaffected by spinal cord injury. However, patients with lesions at the level of the sacral cord may suffer from significant constipation because they lose the additional stimulus to colonic motility normally provided by parasympathetic stimulation. (The parasympathetic nerves innervating the left colon exit the cord at S2–S4.) In addition, individuals with spinal cord injuries typically lack both sensory awareness of rectal distension and the ability to delay defecation via contraction of the external sphincter; they usually require an aggressive bowel management program to prevent incontinent episodes. (See Chapters 14 and 15 for further discussion of bowel management in the patient with spinal cord injury.)

DEFECATION

Defecation is initiated when there is sufficient stool in the left side of the colon to initiate peristaltic contractions. These peristaltic waves propel colonic contents into the rectum, which under normal conditions is empty. Stimulation of peripheral afferent nerve fibers in the rectal wall results in the rectoanal inhibitory reflex and relaxation of the internal anal sphincter. At the same time, activation of stretch receptors in the rectum, pelvic floor musculature, and proximal area of the anal canal results in conscious awareness of rectal filling and the need to defecate, and receptors in the anal canal provide information on the characteristics of the rectal contents, that is, whether solid, liquid, gaseous, or mixed. Coinciding with the relaxation of the internal anal sphincter and the movement of fecal contents into the anal canal is a reflex increase in external anal sphincter tone and, in the continent individual, voluntary contraction of the external anal sphincter; these events maintain continence during internal sphincter relaxation. The individual responds to sensory signals regarding the need to defecate and determines whether the timing and place are appropriate for defecation. If the timing and place are acceptable, the individual assumes a squat position. This straightens the anorectal angle and allows movement of rectal contents into the anal canal. Straining causes reflex relaxation of the puborectalis muscle and the external anal sphincter; this permits descent of the pelvic floor and further straightens the anorectal angle. (The anal canal becomes shorter and more funnel-shaped than before.) Voluntary contraction of the abdominal muscles and diaphragm by means of the Valsalva maneuver increases intraabdominal pressure and supports rectal evacuation. Once evacuation has occurred, the anal canal pressure and the angle of the anorectal junction return to normal, and the puborectalis muscle regains normal tone.

Defecation is also affected by stool size and consistency. The ideal stool diameter (in terms of facilitating defecation) is about 2 cm. Small, dry, hard stools require greater effort to eliminate. Therefore, the time and effort required for elimination of stool is inversely related to the size of the stool.

CHANGES WITH AGING

Aging is a gradual process that begins after puberty. With aging, there is some atrophy of the intestinal wall, some reduction in blood supply, and some intrinsic neuronal changes, all of which may contribute to delayed intestinal transit and decreased stool water content.[7,8] For the most part, however,

the GI tract does not show significant functional changes with aging. For example, both secretion and absorption remain relatively constant, and the subtle declines that do occur do not usually result in clinical problems. This constancy is attributable in large part to the redundancy in each segment of the intestinal tract. However, environmental factors and extraintestinal disease states or conditions may greatly affect GI tract function and fecal continence; for example, diet, life style, hereditary predisposition, disease states such as diabetes mellitus, cognitive impairment, and obstetric injuries in women may produce problems that become clinically evident in the individual's later years. Medications taken by older adults for a variety of chronic illnesses can also affect sphincter pressures and may therefore affect continence.

It is well established that anal function declines with age. Women experience a greater decrease in squeeze pressures with aging as compared with men. At menopause, a marked decrease occurs. Studies have demonstrated that injury during obstetric delivery does increase the risk for declining anal function;[9,10] however, a significant portion of the decline results from aging alone. In a series of descriptive studies involving women across the life span, Ryhammer and colleagues found that the sensitivity of the anal mucosa and the rectum were affected by age. However, they also found that repeated vaginal deliveries were associated with long-term adverse effects, such as increased threshold for anal mucosal electrosensitivity and increased pudendal nerve terminal motor latency.[11-,13] These adverse effects increase the potential for fecal incontinence caused by delayed recognition of rectal filling or a delay in external anal sphincter contraction.

SUMMARY

Normal bowel function and fecal continence are dependent on many interrelated structures and functions. Disease or injury affecting any aspect may negatively affect normal function and continence. Effective management of the individual with bowel dysfunction or fecal incontinence requires careful assessment based on an understanding of normal function and interventions to compensate for the dysfunctional component.

SELF-ASSESSMENT EXERCISE

1. Explain the intrinsic and extrinsic innervation of the colon and the implications for management of the patient with fecal incontinence or bowel dysfunction.

2. Describe the two components of normal sensory function and the relevance of each to continence.

3. Compare and contrast the internal and external sphincters in terms of voluntary control, response to rectal distension, and role in continence.

4. Explain the role of the pelvic floor muscles in creating an anorectal angle and the change in angle that occurs during defecation.

5. Explain the maximum length of time the external sphincter can be contracted and the role of rectal capacity and compliance in maintenance of continence.

6. Briefly explain the events that occur during normal defecation.

REFERENCES

1. Rao SS: Pathophysiology of adult fecal incontinence, *Gastroenterology* 126(1 suppl 1):S14-22, 2004.
2. Crowell MD, Lacy BE, Schettler VA, Dineen TN, et al: Subtypes of anal incontinence associated with bowel dysfunction: clinical, physiologic, and psychosocial characterization. *Dis Colon Rectum* 47(10):1627-1635, 2004.
3. Cook TA, Brading AF, Mortensen NJ: The pharmacology of the internal anal sphincter and new treatments of ano-rectal disorders, *Aliment Pharmacol Ther* 15:887-898, 2001.
4. Tuteja AK, Rao SS: Review article: recent trends in diagnosis and treatment of faecal incontinence, *Aliment Pharmacol Ther* 19:829-840, 2004.
5. Cheetham MJ, Kamm MA, Phillips RK: Topical phenylephrine increases anal canal resting pressure in patients with faecal incontinence, *Gut* 48:356-359, 2001.
6. Phillips SF, Edwards DAW: Some aspects of anal continence and defecation, *Gut* 6:395-405, 1965.
7. Orr WC, Chen CL: Aging and neural control of the GI tract: IV. Clinical and physiological aspects of gastrointestinal motility and aging, *Am J Physiol* 283:GI226-GI231, 2002.
8. Hanani M, Fellig Y, Udassin R, Freund HR: Age-related changes in the mor-phology of the myenteric plexus of the human colon, *Auton Neurosci* 30:113(1-2):71-78, 2004.
9. Fenner DE, Genberg B, Brahma P, et al: Fecal and urinary incontinence after vaginal delivery with anal sphincter disruption in an obstetrics unit in the United States, *Am J Obstet Gynecol* 189:1543-1549, 2003.
10. Nygaard IE, Rao SS, Dawson JD: Anal incontinence after anal sphincter disruption: a 30-year retrospective cohort study, *Obstet Gynecol* 89(6):896-901, 1997.
11. Ryhammer AM, Laurberg S, Bek KM: Age and anorectal sensibility in normal women, *Scand J Gastroenterol* 32:278-284, 1997.
12. Ryhammer AM, Laurberg S, Hermann AP: Long term effect of vaginal deliveries on anorectal function in normal perimenopausal women, *Dis Colon Rectum* 39:852-859, 1996.
13. Ryhammer AM, Laurberg S, Sørensen FH: Effects of age on anal function in normal women, *Int J Colorectal Dis* 12(4):225-229, 1997.

DONNA ZIMMARO BLISS, DOROTHY B. DOUGHTY, & MARGARET McLEAN HEITKEMPER

OBJECTIVES

1. Define the following terms: diarrhea; constipation, total incontinence, partial incontinence, and seepage and soiling.
2. Outline data to be gathered when you are interviewing a patient who presents with "diarrhea."
3. Explain the difference between acute and chronic diarrhea in terms of definition and management approach.
4. List three categories of disorders that may produce diarrhea.
5. Differentiate between secretory and osmotic diarrhea in terms of usual causes, volume of stool, stool pH, response to fasting, and stool osmolality "gap."
6. Explain why individuals who are continent for formed stool may leak liquid stool.
7. List at least two factors contributing to diarrhea in the patient with acquired immunodeficiency syndrome.
8. Explain the relationship between constipation and each of the following: female gender, age greater than 70 years, low-calorie and low-fiber diets, and activity level.
9. Identify prescription and over-the-counter medications that may contribute to constipation.
10. Identify comorbid conditions that significantly increase the risk of constipation.
11. Describe each of the following in terms of pathology and clinical presentation: normal-transit constipation, slow-transit constipation, obstructed defecation.
12. Identify key elements of assessment for the patient who presents with constipation.
13. Identify strategies used by patients with obstructed defecation to facilitate stool elimination.

14. Explain why fiber therapy is an essential element of management for the patient with normal-transit constipation but may be contraindicated for the patient with slow-transit constipation and may have no effect on the patient with obstructed defecation.
15. Outline guidelines for initiation of fiber therapy.
16. Explain the differences among bulk laxatives, osmotic laxatives, and stimulant laxatives, and identify indications and guidelines for each type of laxative.
17. Describe the use of biofeedback in the management of patients with obstructed defecation resulting from pelvic floor dyssynergia.
18. Define the term irritable bowel syndrome (IBS), and explain the current theories regarding etiology and pathology.
19. Identify options for management of the patient with IBS.
20. Explain the role of each of the following in maintenance of fecal continence: stool volume and consistency, sensory awareness of rectal distension, sphincter function, and rectal capacity and compliance.
21. Explain the potential impact of spinal cord injury on sensory awareness and sphincter function and the implications for management.
22. Describe the role of vaginal delivery and chronic defecatory straining in the development of pudendal neuropathy and the effect on bowel function and fecal continence.
23. Compare the patterns of fecal leakage associated with internal versus external anal sphincter incompetence.
24. Describe the effect of reduced rectal capacity and compliance on fecal continence.

DIARRHEA: DEFINITION AND ASSESSMENT

Diarrhea is a prominent problem worldwide. The World Health Organization estimates that the prevalence of chronic diarrhea in children ranges from 3% to 20%. In the United States, chronic diarrhea affects 5% of the population.[1] Diarrhea is responsible for more than 200,000 hospitalizations per year.[2] Severe or persistent diarrhea can cause fluid and electrolyte imbalance and significant alterations in nutritional status, activities of daily living, and quality of life.

Diarrhea is generally used to refer to any increase in stool frequency, liquidity, or amount. In talking with a patient who complains of diarrhea, it is first necessary to clarify the meaning of the word "diarrhea." Because any individual's perception of *abnormal* frequency, liquidity, or amount is based on his or her "usual" bowel function, "diarrhea" as commonly used is an imprecise and subjective term. Even in clinical research studies, there is a lack of consensus about a standard definition of diarrhea. In a recent review of diarrhea definitions used in studies of tube feeding tolerance, 31 different definitions were identified, more than twice the number from a similar review of the literature 10 years earlier.[3] The duration of diarrhea (24 hours or longer) is sometimes included in a definition, as seen in several definitions of diarrhea associated with tube feeding or *Clostridium difficile* infection.[3,4] Some definitions of diarrhea include an increase in stool weight to more than 200 or 300 g/day.[5,6] However, many patients with chronic diarrhea have less than 200 g of stool/day, and many persons have large stools equaling more than 200 g/day but do not complain of diarrhea, so this criterion may not apply in all cases.[7,8] In addition, it is not feasible on a routine basis to obtain a 24-hour stool weight; therefore, a careful history is required to determine the specifics behind a patient's complaint of "diarrhea." Using an acronym such as "OLDCART" can assist in questioning the patient about the characteristics of diarrhea in a systematic manner (Box 14-1). The clinician should also inquire about the patient's ability to control elimination. Some patients with primary fecal incontinence report their problem as "diarrhea," perhaps because diarrhea is more socially acceptable than fecal incontinence. Again, the patient interview is critical to accurate diagnosis.

Classification of Diarrheal Conditions

Diarrhea is a symptom of a variety of illnesses, is caused by numerous pathologic processes, and manifests a range of severity. Classification systems typically categorize diarrheal conditions according

---

BOX 14-1 Guide to Systematic Interview about Characteristics of Diarrhea

Onset of diarrheal symptoms: When did symptoms start? Was onset abrupt or gradual? Recent travel? Proximity to ingestion of suspicious or contaminated food or beverage? Change in medications? Contact with ill persons?

Location of symptoms: Abdominal quadrant of any pain, discomfort, distension, or tenesmus

Duration of symptoms: More than 4 weeks (chronic diarrhea)? Improvement, persistence, or worsening of severity of symptoms?

Character: Fever, bloody stools, abdominal pain or distension, prostration?

Consistency and volume of stools? "Explosive defecation"? Pus, greasy stools, foul-smelling stools, color of stools (gray, black, red)? Symptoms of volume depletion (thirst, tachycardia, orthostasis, low urine output, dry mucous membranes, diminished sensorium)?

Aggravating factors: Diet, such as dairy products, alcohol, caffeinated beverages, sugar substitutes, spicy foods, gas producing foods (such as cabbage), medications, stool softeners? Underlying medical conditions (human immunodeficiency virus infection, intestinal resection)?

Relieving factors: Does diarrhea cease when oral intake is discontinued? What over-the-counter medications have been taken, and what was the response?

Timing: Frequency of stooling? Temporal association with meals, medications, smoking, anal intercourse, binge drinking of alcohol?

to duration, pathologic mechanism, or etiologic factor.[9]

Duration. On a clinical basis, diarrheal disorders may be classified as either acute or chronic. Acute diarrheal conditions are defined as those lasting 4 or fewer weeks, whereas chronic diarrhea persists past that point.[1] The value of classification according to duration is that it helps to direct the clinician in terms of workup and management. Acute diarrheal conditions in the nonhospitalized patient are typically self-limiting and are appropriately managed on a symptomatic basis unless there are indicators of significant volume depletion, toxicity, or bleeding. A more extensive clinical evaluation is recommended after 7 days of acute diarrhea in the following patients: (a) those who are immunosuppressed following transplant or as a result of the human immunodeficiency virus (HIV) or acquired immunodeficiency syndrome (AIDS); (b) elderly persons more than 70 years of age; and (c) individuals with worsening health status as indicated by dehydration, fever higher than 38.5°C, abdominal pain, bloody stools, acid-base or electrolyte imbalance, or prostration.[10,11]

Most cases of acute diarrhea result from infections caused by viruses, protozoa, or bacteria (Table 14-1).[2] Inflammatory diarrhea results whenever organisms invade the intestinal mucosa or produce a toxin that damages epithelial cells; this type of diarrhea is characterized by stools that contain guaiac, blood, leukocytes, pus, or mucus.[12] Other symptoms associated with infectious/inflammatory diarrhea are fever higher than 38.5°C and prostration. Risk factors for infectious diarrhea include recent travel, ingestion of unusual foods or fluids or foods/fluids that may have been contaminated, exposure to sick people, and anal sexual intercourse; thus, the history must include queries regarding each of these.[13] *C. difficile* is the organism responsible for the majority of cases of acute diarrhea in patients in a hospital or nursing home; therefore, clinical evaluation of acute diarrhea in these patients should include testing for *C. difficile* toxin.[4,14,15] Other causes of acute diarrhea in the hospitalized patient include antibiotics, other medications (Box 14-2), and initiation of tube feeding.[16-18]

Chronic diarrhea mandates a thorough workup to determine causative factors and pathologic mechanism. Stools should be analyzed for blood,

TABLE 14-1   **Infectious Diarrhea Organisms**

NO INFLAMMATORY RESPONSE	INFLAMMATORY RESPONSE
Viruses	
Rotovirus	Cytomegalovirus
Norwalk virus	Adenovirus
	Herpes simplex virus
Bacteria	
Staphylococcus aureus	*Shigella*
Clostridum perfringens	*Plesiomonas shigelloides*
Vibrio cholerae	*Salmonella*
Enterotoxigenic	*Chlamydia*
Escherichia coli	*Neisseria gonorrhoeae*
(ETEC)	*Listeria monocytogenes*
	Campylobacter jejuni
	Clostridium difficile
	Escherichia coli
	O157:H5
Protozoa	
Giardia lamblia	*Entamoeba histolytica*
Cryptosporidium	
Isospora belli	
Microsporidia	

Adapted from McQuaid KR: Alimentary canal. In: Tierney, LM, McPhee, Papadakis MA eds: *CMDT 2003 Current medical diagnosis and treatment*, New York, 2003, McGraw-Hill.

white blood cells, pus, fat, osmolality, microbes and toxins, pH, electrolytes, and laxatives. Serum chemistry values should also be measured, and the patient may need to undergo visual or radiographic examination of the intestinal tract.[1] In selected cases, testing for malabsorption and pancreatic function may be indicated. Some patients continue to have altered bowel patterns for weeks after an acute diarrheal illness. These individuals may appear to have a chronic condition, but in fact they are merely experiencing gradual recovery from the acute episode.[8] This underscores the importance of a careful history of the onset of the illness and any gradual changes or improvements.

Pathologic Mechanisms. The classification of diarrhea according to pathologic mechanism is

BOX 14-2 Medications Causing Diarrhea

Alzheimer's Disease Medications
Acetylcholinesterase inhibitors (such as donepezil, velnacrine)

Antibiotics
Ampicillin, cefazolin, cephalexin, ceftriaxone, ciprofloxocin, clindamycin, ceftazidime, erythromycin

Cardiac Medications
Angiotensin-converting enzyme (ACE) inhibitors
Digoxin
Beta blockers
Methyldopa
Quinidine
Procainamide

Chemotherapies and Combinations
5-fluorouracil and leucovorin, capecitabine, irinotecan, oxaliplatin, methotrexate

Histamine H$_2$-Receptor Antagonist
Ranitidine

Magnesium- and Phosphate-Containing Antacids

Nonsteroidal Antiinflammatory Drugs

Neuropsychiatric Drugs
Fluoxetine
Lithium
L-Dopa

Oral Hypoglycemic Agents
Alpha-glucosidase inhibitors (such as acarbose)

Osteoarthritis Medications
Colchicine
Diacerein

Polyethylene Glycol–Containing Elixirs
Lorazepam

Prokinetics
Metoclopramide

Sorbitol-Containing Elixirs or Suspensions
Acetaminophen, cimetidine, potassium chloride, theophylline

Stool Softeners

based on the physiologic processes that normally prevent diarrhea, that is, secretory, absorptive, and motility (both peristaltic and transit) functions (Fig. 14-1). Diarrheal states represent some alteration in the normal balance among secretion, absorption, and motility, and in some cases the pathologic features involve more than one of these processes.[9] Patients with diarrhea for which there is no identifiable cause are said to have an idiopathic diarrhea.

Under normal conditions, approximately 7 liters of fluid are secreted into the upper intestinal tract to support the digestion and absorption of nutrients. About 1 liter of fluid typically passes through the ileocecal valve into the colon, which is well within the healthy colon's absorptive capacity. The healthy colon can actually absorb up to 5 or 6 liters of fluid/day. Normal bowel function produces a formed but not overly hard stool.

Secretory disorders. Secretory diarrhea results when the volume of water and electrolytes secreted *into* the lumen of the bowel is increased enough to overwhelm the bowel's absorptive capacity. It may occur along with compromised absorptive function or in the patient with normal absorptive function. Secretory diarrhea is most commonly caused by infectious agents (such as *Vibrio cholerae* or enterotoxigenic *Escherichia coli*); however, it can also be caused by any substance that acts as a secretagogue (a stimulant to secretion). The effect of secretagogues on intraluminal secretion can be illustrated by the effect of cholera. The toxin secreted by cholera binds to the membrane of the enterocyte and irreversibly increases the production of cyclic adenosine monophosphate (cAMP); the increased production of cAMP increases the net secretion of water and electrolytes (especially sodium) into the lumen of the bowel.[17,19]

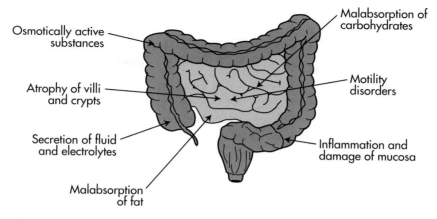

Fig. 14-1 Pathologic processes contributing to diarrhea.

Noninfectious secretagogues include certain malabsorbed substances (such as bile acids and fatty acids), substances produced by selected malignant tumors (such as villous adenoma, medullary carcinoma of the thyroid, non–beta cell pancreatic islet cell tumors, and Zollinger-Ellison syndrome), and prostaglandins produced by the colonic mucosa in patients with colitis.[17,20] Excess levels of bile acids and fatty acids stimulate secretion of chloride ions by the mucosal cells in the colon to produce a secretory diarrhea. Excessive levels of bile acids in the colonic lumen are common after extensive ileal resection; this is attributable to loss of bile salt reabsorption, which normally occurs in the terminal portion of the ileum. Interestingly, the effect of extensive ileal resection and the severity of "bile acid diarrhea" are partly determined by the length of colon retained. If most or all of the colon remains, the patient may experience less bile acid diarrhea.[21,22] This is because short-chain fatty acids are produced throughout the colon by bacterial metabolism of dietary fiber and malabsorbed carbohydrates; the short-chain fatty acids promote absorption of sodium and water,[23] and they also maintain an acid pH in the colon. The acid pH keeps the bile acids from becoming soluble in water, which also keeps them from exerting their secretory effects.[24]

Secretory diarrhea is characterized by elimination of a large volume of fluid (usually more than 1 liter/day), neutral stool pH, failure to respond to fasting with reduced stool volume, sodium losses in excess of potassium losses resulting in hyponatremia, and a stool osmotic gap less than 50 mOsm/kg.[11,25] The osmotic gap is one way to differentiate secretory from osmotic diarrhea. The osmotic gap refers to the difference between the osmolality of the stool, which is a measure of all osmotic substances in the stool, and the concentration of ions in the stool (one type of osmotic substance). Sodium and potassium represent the main cations, which are positively charged; these values are multiplied by two to account for the anions or negatively charged ions. An osmotic gap greater than 50 mOsm/kg indicates osmotic diarrhea, meaning that osmotic substances *other than* electrolytes are causing retention of water in the intestine. An osmotic gap less than 50 mOsm/kg indicates secretory diarrhea, and a gap equal to 50 mOsm/kg is an inconclusive finding.[11,25] The formula used to calculate the osmotic gap is as follows: stool osmolality − 2([sodium cation] + [potassium cation]). In practice, a value commonly used for stool osmolality is 290 mOsm/kg, which is the osmolality of plasma.[1,25] The osmolality of the distal colon is assumed to be in equilibrium with the osmolality of plasma. (Measuring stool osmolality accurately and quickly before colonic bacteria ferment residual carbohydrates into osmotically active substances is difficult and not routine.)

Absorptive disorders. Diarrhea can also be caused by any condition that compromises absorption within the intestine. Reduced absorption directly increases the volume of stool; in addition, the unabsorbed substances create an osmotic force that pulls water out of the bloodstream and into the intestinal lumen, which further increases stool volume and liquidity.[17,20] This explains the term osmotic diarrhea, which is sometimes used to differentiate diarrheal states caused by inadequate absorption from those caused by increased secretion (the secretory diarrheas). Table 14-2 contrasts secretory and osmotic diarrhea. Osmotic diarrhea will cease when the causative factor is eliminated.

Two types of pathologic states can cause compromised absorption: (1) those causing alterations within the intestinal mucosa that compromise its absorptive status and (2) those producing intraluminal substances that interfere with the transport of ions across the intestinal epithelium. Some pathologic conditions have a dual influence on absorptive capacity; that is, they alter the intestinal mucosa and also produce intraluminal substances that block absorption into the intestinal epithelial cell.

Conditions that alter the absorptive capacity of the intestine include those that compromise the bowel's absorptive *function,* that is, the ability to transport nutrients into the intestinal epithelial cell, and those that compromise the bowel's absorptive *surface.* Common examples include protein-calorie malnutrition, prolonged NPO (nothing by mouth) status, hypoproteinemia, extensive bowel resection, and inflammatory conditions such as inflammatory bowel disease or intestinal infections. Protein-calorie malnutrition and prolonged NPO status (that is, for more than 5 to 7 days) can cause reversible atrophy of the villi and brush border. This atrophy causes both a reduction in the absorptive surface and a reduced ability to transport intraluminal substances into the intestinal epithelial cell (because the brush border contains enzymes and carrier substances critical to the absorptive process).[18,26] Hypoproteinemia results in a reduced concentration of the intravascular proteins that normally serve to "attract and hold" fluid within the intravascular compartment. The result is interstitial edema that extends to the bowel wall and may interfere with absorption. There are contradictory data regarding the effect of

TABLE 14-2   Comparison of Secretory and Osmotic Diarrhea

CLINICAL CHARACTERISTIC	SECRETORY DIARRHEA	OSMOTIC DIARRHEA
Underlying disorder	*Increased secretion* of water and electrolytes into lumen of bowel	*Reduced absorption* of water and electrolytes into intestinal epithelial cell
Average stool volume	More than 1 liter/day	Less than 1 liter/day
Average stool pH	Neutral (7.0)	Acidic (less than 7.0)
Stool osmolality gap	Less than 40 mOsm/kg	More than 50 mOsm/kg
Other characteristics	Sodium lost in excess of potassium No reduction in stool volume with fasting	Potassium lost in excess of sodium Stool volume reduced with fasting
Examples (clinical)	Bacterial infections Substances secreted by selected tumors Malabsorbed substances such as bile acids	Bowel resection Bowel wall edema Atrophy of villi Lactose intolerance Inflammatory processes Sorbitol Fat malabsorption

hypoalbuminemia on diarrhea. Some studies indicate that diarrhea is common in individuals with serum albumin levels of less than 2.5 mg/dL, whereas other studies show no consistent relationship between albumin levels and development of diarrhea.[18]

Extensive bowel resection significantly reduces the absorptive surface of the bowel. Extensive ileal resection may also contribute to *malabsorption,* either because of the effects of unabsorbed bile acids on colonic absorption or because of the effects of fat malabsorption, which is caused by the loss of bile acids. (Bile acids are needed for fat breakdown and absorption; when large amounts of bile acids are lost as a result of ileal resection, the liver is unable to produce enough bile to provide for digestion and absorption of fats.[24,27]) Inflammatory and infectious conditions of the bowel can alter absorptive capacity by causing mucosal edema and damage to the intestinal epithelial cells. Colonic involvement is characterized by cramping abdominal pain, tenesmus, and mucus or blood in the stools, whereas small bowel disease typically produces high-volume watery diarrhea, nausea, and vomiting.[28]

Several conditions cause chronic "osmotic" diarrhea through the production or ingestion of nonabsorbable substances; these hyperosmolar substances within the lumen of the bowel block transport of water and electrolytes out of the bowel and into the intestinal epithelial cell and actually serve as an osmotic force that pulls water and electrolytes *into* the lumen of the bowel. Osmotic diarrhea is characterized by fairly low-volume stool (usually less than 1 liter/day), with an acid pH (less than 7), and with potassium loss in excess of sodium, leading to the potential for hypokalemia. Stool volume is reduced with fasting because the malabsorbed substance causing diarrhea is eliminated. The stool osmolality gap is greater than 50 mOsm/kg because much of the osmotic component of the stool is provided by the unabsorbed substances in the stool.[9,25,29] Table 14-2 highlights the major differences between secretory and osmotic diarrhea.

The most common etiologic factors for osmotic diarrhea include intolerance to sugars such as sorbitol, fructose, and lactose, and fat malabsorption syndromes. Sorbitol is commonly used as a nonnutritive sweetener for foods and medications;

it produces a strong osmotic effect within the lumen of the bowel and can even be used as a laxative. Some common medications that contain sorbitol and can cause osmotic diarrhea are listed in Box 14-2. The clinician should always question any patient with complaints of diarrhea about *all* medications (including over-the-counter (OTC) agents that have laxative effects, such as magnesium-based antacids) and should also ask about the intake of "dietetic" foods that might contain sorbitol.[29] Similarly, high-fructose syrup is a primary sweetening agent for many foods. Toddlers consume the highest body-weight adjusted amount of fructose, primarily from apple juice. High fructose intake contributes to chronic nonspecific diarrhea in this age group of children and may be an unrecognized contributor to diarrhea in adults, because the symptoms and mechanisms of diarrhea are similar to the diarrhea caused by lactose intolerance and by sorbitol.[30,31] Lactose intolerance is a very common and frequently unrecognized etiologic factor for diarrhea. Many individuals who tolerated milk products well as children develop a lactase deficiency later in life. These individuals have reduced ability to metabolize lactose to absorbable monosaccharides. The persistence of lactose within the lumen of the bowel causes osmotic diarrhea. In addition to the diarrhea, these individuals frequently experience cramping pain and explosive gas caused by the fermenting action of colonic bacteria on the undigested and unabsorbed lactose.[32]

Fat malabsorption is another etiologic factor for osmotic diarrhea. Fat malabsorption is most commonly caused by bile acid deficiency, which can occur as a result of extensive ileal resection. The terminal portion of the ileum normally provides for reabsorption of bile salts; loss of this segment may result in bile salt wastage sufficient to cause bile acid deficiency.[9,27] Fat malabsorption may also occur as a result of bacterial overgrowth within the small intestine or as a result of an enzyme deficiency. Any condition that interferes with the normal solubilization and metabolism of fat causes high intraluminal levels of fat, reduced absorption of water and electrolytes in the colon, and diarrhea characterized by malodorous, "greasy" stools (steatorrhea).[9,27]

Patients receiving tube feedings also commonly experience diarrhea, usually primarily because of inability to absorb the feeding. Diarrhea associated with tube feeding can also be caused by factors such as the composition of the enteral formula (nutrient complexity or lack of fiber), concomitant exposure to antibiotics, administration of liquid medications containing sorbitol through the feeding tube, and contamination of the formula or delivery system.[17,18,26] Other contributing factors to diarrhea in the tube-fed patient are protein-calorie malnutrition, atrophic villi, and the rate of feeding.

Continuous administration of an enteral formula is indicated when patients are fed into the small bowel. If the patient is tube fed intermittently into the stomach, migration of the tip of the feeding tube into the small intestine can result in diarrhea.

Motility disorders. Diarrhea can also result from alterations in bowel motility. The most common alteration is *increased* motility, which significantly reduces the contact time between intraluminal contents and intestinal mucosa and increases the rate at which stool is delivered to the rectum for evacuation. Increased motility is believed to play a role in the diarrhea associated with inflammatory bowel disease, irritable bowel syndrome (IBS), and infectious diarrheas.[20,29] Conditions resulting in rapid gastric emptying may also contribute to diarrhea.[33]

Diminished motility may also contribute to liquid stool and fecal incontinence. Probably the most common example is seepage of liquid stool around an obstructing mass of feces in the rectum referred to as an impaction. Diminished bowel motility produces severe constipation and fecal impaction. Bacterial action on the fecal mass produces liquid stool. The persistent rectal distension causes internal sphincter relaxation and allows seepage of liquid stool that may be interpreted as "diarrhea."

Diminished motility may cause diarrhea even in the absence of constipation or impaction. This type of diarrhea is believed to be secondary to bacterial overgrowth in the distal small intestine caused by reduced motility and fecal stasis, and it is particularly common in the elderly population (more than 75 years of age).[9,34] The precise mechanisms by which bacterial overgrowth produce diarrhea are not clear. It is believed that the high bacterial counts may compromise normal digestive processes and produce osmotic diarrhea; for example, the bacteria may deconjugate bile, resulting in fat malabsorption. Another theory is that the bacterial toxins act as secretagogues.[9]

Diarrhea associated with disordered motility is usually characterized by low-volume stools (unless there is a coexisting problem with secretion or absorption) and is frequently accompanied by cramping pain.[29] However, in many situations, disordered motility is only one component of a complex clinical picture that also includes alterations in secretion or absorption. This is true of patients with inflammatory bowel disease, massive bowel resection, and infectious diarrhea.

Mixed disorders. As noted earlier, some diarrheal syndromes are caused by pathologic conditions that involve alterations in secretion or absorption in addition to disordered motility. Examples of mixed disorders include laxative abuse, *C. difficile* infections, cancer treatment–induced diarrhea, and AIDS-related diarrhea.

Laxative abuse typically causes increased intestinal motility in addition to reduced absorption. In addition, patients typically conceal their laxative intake so the causative factor is not at all evident. Laxative abuse should be suspected in anorexic or bulimic patients, in patients who obtain primary or secondary benefits from illness, in the elderly, and in dependent children with hovering parents. When laxative abuse is suspected, the stool should be analyzed for evidence of laxatives.[35]

Infectious diarrhea caused by *C. difficile* is another example of mixed-pathology diarrhea. Multiple factors contribute to *C. difficile*–associated diarrhea (Box 14-3).[15,36,37] It is thought that antibiotic therapy alters the profile or metabolism of the normal intestinal flora and allows the *C. difficile* organism to proliferate. *C. difficile* produces toxins that cause a secretory diarrhea and also produces pseudomembranes that significantly alter intestinal absorptive function.[36,37]

The types of chemotherapeutic agents associated with diarrhea are listed in Box 14-2. The diarrhea

BOX 14-3 **Risk Factors for** *Clostridium difficile*–**Associated Diarrhea**

Age more than 65 years
Extended stay in hospital or nursing home
Recent antibiotic exposure, multiple antibiotics
Recent chemotherapy
Recent gastrointestinal surgery
Gastrointestinal intubation including postpyloric tube feeding

resulting from cancer treatment is caused in part by direct biochemical toxicity to the rapidly dividing crypt cells of the gastrointestinal tract, which frequently results in cell death.[38] Immature crypt cells are then produced to replace the lost cells, but the newly produced cells are secretory. In addition, the damaged cells are less able to absorb nutrients and fluids, and the inflammation caused by cell damage leads to secretion of substances that stimulate further fluid secretion, such as prostaglandins and leukotrienes.[38]

AIDS-related diarrhea is a common and complex condition. Studies indicate that 60% of HIV-infected patients in the United States develop diarrhea at some point during their illness and that diarrhea significantly affects their quality of life.[39] In addition to the multiple enteric pathogens that are common in AIDS, there seem to be noninfectious mechanisms that cause diarrhea. Diarrhea occurring in the absence of identifiable infection is known as AIDS enteropathy.[29] One mechanism contributing to AIDS-related diarrhea is malabsorption,[39,40] which seems to be particularly common and severe in patients infected with microsporidial organisms, and there is currently no effective treatment for this pathogen.[41] Bacterial overgrowth in the small intestine (caused by impaired gastric acid secretion) and inflammation of the intestinal mucosa also contribute to diarrhea in HIV-infected patients. Patients with AIDS are also at risk for secretory diarrhea, which may be caused by enteric pathogens or by AIDS enteropathy; in severe cases, patients can experience stool volumes of 4 to 6 liters/day, resulting in extreme wasting and weight loss.[29,39]

Diarrhea and Fecal Incontinence

Diarrhea does not necessarily cause incontinence, especially in the individual with intact continence mechanisms; however, diarrheal conditions definitely *stress* the continence mechanism. Loose or liquid stool is more difficult to retain than solid stool,[42,43] and large-volume diarrheal stools can overwhelm the strongest sphincter and cause episodic incontinence. Individuals with diminished sensory awareness or compromised sphincter function may routinely experience incontinence whenever the consistency of their stool becomes liquid or mushy. In addition, studies suggest that pelvic muscle exercises with biofeedback are less successful at reducing fecal incontinence when stool consistency is liquid.[44]

MANAGEMENT OF DIARRHEAL CONDITIONS

Symptom Management

Because most acute diarrheal conditions are self-limiting viral diseases, initial management of any diarrheal state is typically symptomatic and directed toward maintenance of fluid-electrolyte balance and screening for signs of systemic toxicity or bacterial diarrhea. OTC medications commonly used for symptomatic relief of mild traveler's diarrhea are bismuth subsalicylate and loperamide; the maximum 24-hour adult dose for bismuth subsalicylate is approximately 2 g (8 tablets or 16 tablespoons), and the maximum 24-hour OTC adult dose for loperamide is 8 mg. Severe traveler's diarrhea may be treated with ciprofloxacin or trimethoprim-sulfamethoxazole.[37,45] Patients who present with bloody diarrhea, acute abdominal pain, and fever require close monitoring and additional diagnostic studies. Depending on the specific pathogen, antibiotic therapy may be indicated. For example, patients with *C. difficile* infections should be treated with oral metronidazole or vancomycin.[37,46]

Correction of Underlying Cause

Management of chronic diarrheal conditions includes treatment of the underlying etiologic factors, measures to modify the consistency and volume of stool, strategies to decrease the frequency of stools, and/or measures to adjust the profile of intestinal bacteria. Measures to treat the underlying etiologic factors are obviously quite variable. For dietary intolerances, intake of the diarrhea-producing substances (such as sorbitol, fructose, or lactose) should be restricted; individuals with lactose intolerance may be able to tolerate some lactose with the addition of Lactaid and may also be able to tolerate yogurt containing live bacterial cultures.[47,48] A low-fat diet is indicated for patients with fat malabsorption, and bile acid–binding agents, such as cholestyramine, can be effective for bile acid diarrhea.[9] Antibiotic therapy is appropriate for patients with evidence of bacterial overgrowth syndromes.

Other Dietary Measures

Measures to modify the consistency and volume of stool primarily include dietary modifications, fiber supplements, and antidiarrheal medications. Dietary modifications include specific restrictions based on etiologic factors and general measures such as increased intake of fluids and restriction of caffeine, spices that make food taste "hot," and foods such as nuts that are high in insoluble fiber (roughage).[48] Foods and supplements containing soluble dietary fiber, such as oats, pectin, guar gum, germinated barley, and psyllium, may be beneficial because they are thought to absorb water, thicken the stool, and promote the health and absorptive function of the colon; a firmer stool is easier to retain. The addition of guar gum fiber to rehydration solutions has improved rehydration and reduced diarrhea in children with cholera,[49] and banana flakes containing pectin fiber have reduced diarrhea among tube-fed patients.[50] Tube-fed patients with protein-calorie malnutrition and hypoalbuminemia may also benefit from slower rates of formula administration or from use of "elemental" formulas (formulas with nutrients that require less digestion); however, it is critical to continue feedings in these patients despite the associated diarrhea, because feeding is required to reverse the malnutrition and to reestablish the villi.

Complementary Therapies

In patients receiving antibiotics, the addition of probiotics is an effective strategy for reducing diarrhea. Probiotics are live microbial supplements that exert beneficial health effects and improve microbial balance in the intestine.[51] Probiotics containing yeast (*Saccharomyces boulardii*) or bacteria (lactobacilli or enterococci) have been shown to reduce antibiotic-associated diarrhea.[52] There is also growing interest in complementary therapies, and several of these modalities have been used for managing diarrhea. For example, acupuncture and moxibustion (warming acupuncture points with smoldering herbs) have been pilot tested in HIV-infected patients with chronic diarrhea and have been shown to reduce diarrhea in these patients.[39] The effects of these and other complementary therapies require more research.

Medications

Antidiarrheal medications include opioid derivatives, octreotide, and bismuth subsalicylate. The opioid derivatives work by binding with opiate receptors in the intestine to reduce motility, and some agents may also affect secretion and absorption. The most commonly used opioids include codeine, diphenoxylate, and loperamide. Codeine is a very effective agent, but it is the least frequently used because of its side effects (including nausea) and addicting potential. Diphenoxylate hydrochloride with atropine sulfate (Lomotil) is a commonly used opioid that works primarily by reducing intestinal motility; the opioid derivative (diphenoxylate) is coupled with an anticholinergic (atropine), which further contributes to reduction of intestinal motility. (The combination of these two antimotility agents provides effective control of diarrhea at relatively low doses, which is important because high doses of diphenoxylate produce opiumlike central nervous system effects and are therefore contraindicated.) The one opioid derivative that is available in an OTC formulation is loperamide (Imodium). This agent works by reducing motility and increasing anal sphincter pressure. It is effective in a variety of diarrheal conditions and has been shown to be safe in patients with cancer chemotherapy–induced diarrhea even at high doses (16 capsules/day).[48] Somatostatin is a gastrointestinal hormone that reduces intestinal secretion; its synthetic analogue, octreotide, has been used to treat a variety of diarrheal disorders, including chemotherapy–induced diarrhea. Initially this drug had a relatively short duration of action and required frequent subcutaneous injections. However, a longer-acting formulation has been developed that is given intramuscularly at weekly or monthly intervals.[53] Octreotide is expensive and typically reserved for patients who have not responded to other agents.[54] Bismuth subsalicylate is widely available OTC and is most effective in treating traveler's diarrhea; it is believed to act by binding bacterial toxins.

DISORDERED DEFECATION: CONSTIPATION

Constipation is a very common disorder in Western countries; estimates of prevalence range from a low of 2% to a high of 28%, depending on survey method and definition.[55,56] One challenge in accurately determining prevalence is the lack of a single widely accepted definition for constipation. Patients commonly define constipation as any difficulty with fecal elimination; symptoms reported as constipation include hard stools, infrequent bowel movements, difficulty with stool elimination, straining, and a sense of incomplete evacuation.[56-59] Health care personnel have typically defined constipation primarily as infrequent bowel movements, a definition that fails to capture many of the complaints perceived by patients as constipation and may lead to inaccuracies in diagnosis and management. To improve recognition and treatment of this very common condition, an international panel developed a set of criteria (the Rome II criteria) for the diagnosis of constipation that incorporates symptoms of difficult defecation (straining, use of manual maneuvers, sensation of incomplete evacuation, or sensation of blockage with bowel movements), as well as infrequent bowel movements or hard stools.[56,58-60] (Box 14-4). Interestingly, patient self-reports of constipation consistently yield much higher prevalence rates (27% to 28%) than use of the objective Rome II critiera, which typically produce prevalence rates of about 14%.[56]

Constipation is generally thought to be a minor problem in terms of overall health status and quality of life, but there is increasing recognition that constipation can cause significant impairment in quality of life, especially among individuals with severe constipation that is refractory to medical management.[56,60]

BOX 14-4   Rome II Criteria for Constipation

Any two (or more) of the following symptoms for at least 12 weeks during the past 12 months in patients who do not meet the criteria for irritable bowel syndrome (see Box 14-7 for criteria):

Straining with more than 25% of bowel movements

Lumpy or hard stool with more than 25% of bowel movements

Sensation of incomplete evacuation with more than 25% of bowel movements

Sensation of obstruction or blockage with more than 25% of bowel movements

Manual maneuvers to facilitate stool evacuation required with more than 25% of bowel movements

Less than three bowel movements per week

Risk Factors

Epidemiologic studies have identified the following as risk factors for constipation among residents of North America: female gender; nonwhite racial origin; lower socioeconomic status; and advanced age, with marked increase in constipation among individuals more than 70 years of age. Life-style factors associated with increased risk of constipation include low-calorie diets, low-fiber diets, and sedentary life style/less exercise, although studies indicate that increased fiber and exercise fail to correct constipation in a large percentage of patients. Some of the strongest risk factors for constipation are comorbid medical conditions; neuromuscular disorders such as multiple sclerosis, vertebral fracture, sprains and strains of the sacroiliac region, and spinal cord injury are all highly associated with constipation, as is herpes zoster affecting the sacral dermatomes. Affective psychotic disorders are also highly correlated, as is use of opioid analgesics, even among patients also taking medications to prevent constipation. (Nonsteroidal antiinflammatory drugs may also contribute to constipation.) Interestingly, diabetes mellitus was not found to be associated with constipation in North American studies, in contrast to studies done in other countries. Finally, some studies demonstrate a strong correlation between reported sexual abuse and constipation, although this finding has been challenged by other investigators. In summary, comorbid neuromuscular disorders, affective psychoses, and opioid analgesics seem to be the most important risk factors for constipation; female gender and advancing age are also significant indicators.[55,56,61]

Etiology and Pathology

Effective management of any condition depends on an accurate understanding of the underlying pathophysiologic mechanisms. This is particularly challenging in the management of constipation, because there seem to be at least three distinct subtypes: normal-transit constipation, also sometimes known as "functional" constipation; slow-transit constipation; and obstructed defecation syndromes. (Some authors identify a fourth subtype, constipation-predominant IBS; this type of constipation is covered in the section on IBS.) An additional challenge for the clinician is that many patients present with an overlap of one or more of the constipation subtypes; for example, as many as 50% of patients with slow-transit constipation also suffer from obstructed defecation.[55,57-59,62] This section includes a brief description of the pathologic features of each of the subtypes of constipation.

Normal-Transit Constipation. This type of constipation, also known as functional or simple constipation, is the most common type of constipation and also the one most responsive to treatment. As implied by its label, this type of constipation is seen in patients who have essentially normal colon function and no obstruction to stool elimination; the symptoms most commonly reported by patients include hard stools and difficult evacuation, along with associated symptoms such as bloating or abdominal discomfort. Because colonic motility is normal in these patients, the constipation is thought to be caused by factors *extrinsic* to the bowel, such as inadequate fiber or fluid, inactivity, chronic failure to respond to the call to stool, or constipating medications.[55,57,63]

Fiber and fluid intake. Insufficient fiber and fluid intake have long been associated with the development of constipation; although there are

limited data to support this association, fiber and fluid therapy remains the foundation for initial treatment of constipation. Inadequate fiber intake reduces stool volume and results in hard, small-caliber stools, which fail to stimulate the enteric nervous system sufficiently to elicit effective propagating contractions. This diminished peristaltic activity results in prolonged contact between the stool and the intestinal mucosa, which causes further absorption of water from the stools. The hard, narrow stools are much more difficult to propel through the bowel and to eliminate from the rectum, thus producing the classic complaints of hard stools and difficult defecation. Fiber therapy is thought to enhance bowel function in the patient with normal colonic motility by increasing stool weight, volume, and water content; the bulkier stools stimulate peristalsis, thus reducing colonic transit time, and they are also easier to eliminate from the rectum. These theorized benefits are supported by studies demonstrating decreased reports of constipation and reduced use of laxatives and enemas in response to increased fiber and fluid intake.[57,64-66] In addition to benefits related to bowel function, increased fiber intake helps to lower cholesterol levels, improve blood glucose control, and slow or prevent the progression of diverticular disease. Additional arguments for fiber therapy as first-line treatment for constipation include the fact that fiber is both safe and inexpensive.

Activity level. Immobility can contribute to constipation by reducing motility within the gut. In addition, the loss of muscle tone associated with inactivity decreases the facilitative function of the abdominal and pelvic floor musculature in evacuating stool from the rectum. (Straining helps to increase intraabdominal pressure and also causes pelvic floor relaxation and descent; this helps to straighten the anorectal angle and supports evacuation of stool from the rectum.) Immobility may be caused by musculoskeletal disorders, general weakness and debilitation, or sedentary life style; inactivity is thought to contribute to the severe constipation commonly seen in patients who are bedbound or chairbound. Although there are limited data to support inactivity as a significant etiologic factor for constipation, regular activity or exercise

(20 to 30 minutes/day) can increase gut motility and may be helpful in the prevention or treatment of constipation.

Toileting behaviors. Poor toileting behaviors, such as chronically delaying defecation, can eventually lead to problems with bowel elimination. Failure to respond to the "call to stool" actually occurs quite frequently. Many people chronically suppress the urge and delay defecation because they believe that bowel elimination is an intensely private function, and they are uncomfortable having a bowel movement in a public facility or even in any setting other than their own home. When a suitably private setting is later obtained, the peristaltic "push" (call to stool) has subsided, and the individual must compensate by initiating an abdominal muscle contraction of sufficient magnitude to propel stool through the anal canal. Delayed defecation is made even more difficult because the stool has been further dehydrated during the delay, so additional force is typically required for effective evacuation. Hospitalized patients who must use a bedside commode or bedpan may have tremendous difficulty with effective stool elimination, caused by a combination of reduced privacy, embarrassment, and the inability to assume a position that facilitates evacuation.

Position is an important component of effective toileting. Defecation is facilitated by a sitting position, which decreases the acuity of the anorectal angle and promotes the movement of stool into the anal canal. In actuality, the optimal position for defecation is squatting; this position augments abdominal pressure through the compressive action of the thighs against the abdomen. Patients should be taught to sit with their feet flat on the floor or on a step stool; if additional compressive force is needed, they should be instructed to lean forward with the back held straight or to bring their thighs up against the abdomen. In addition, patients should be taught to intersperse moderate-level straining with deep breathing; deep breathing causes descent of the diaphragm and increased abdominal pressure, and it also helps to maintain relaxation of the pelvic floor muscles. In contrast, prolonged straining tends to cause contraction of the pelvic floor muscles, which creates obstruction at the anal outlet.

Constipating medications. Numerous pharmaceutical agents adversely affect colonic motility, either by affecting the autonomic nervous system or by binding directly to receptors within the gut wall. Drugs most commonly associated with constipation include narcotic analgesics, particularly the opioid analgesics; these drugs bind directly to opioid receptors in the bowel wall, thus profoundly inhibiting peristalsis.[67] Opioids are a major contributor to severe constipation among patients with cancer. There are also OTC medications used by many individuals that can contribute to constipation; these include aluminum and calcium-based antacids and nonsteroidal antiinflammatory drugs.[57] Stimulant laxatives have frequently been blamed for chronic constipation, theoretically through damage to the nerve cells within the bowel wall; however, this theory has been challenged. Investigators point out that any enteric nerve damage observed in chronically constipated patients may have been the *initial event,* that is, the cause of the constipation, as opposed to an adverse effect of the laxatives used for treatment. As a result of this reevaluation, there is less reluctance to prescribe stimulant laxatives for patients with chronic constipation.[57] Drugs that contribute to constipation are listed in Box 14-5.

Slow-Transit Constipation. Approximately 15% to 30% of patients with constipation have the subtype known as slow-transit constipation; this type of constipation is characterized by a marked reduction in frequency of bowel movements, to once a week or even less, and by associated bloating and abdominal discomfort.[59] This type of constipation occurs most commonly in young women, who frequently report onset at puberty. Slow-transit constipation is characterized by a marked reduction in the propagating contractions that normally propel stool through the colon and into the rectum; there are fewer propagating contractions in response to the normal stimuli of waking and eating, and the contractions that do occur are of significantly reduced amplitude, velocity, and duration. As a result, stool moves extremely slowly through the colon, resulting in infrequent bowel movements; the slow transit also promotes abnormal dehydration of the stool, which results in difficulty eliminating the stool when it does reach the rectum.[55,57,58] In addition

BOX 14-5   **Medications Contributing to Constipation**

Anticholinergic Medications
Antihistamines
Antispasmodics
Tricyclic antidepressants
Antipsychotics

Cardiovascular Medications
Calcium-channel blockers
Beta-adrenergic antagonists
Diuretics
Antiarrhythmics

Central Nervous System Depressants
Anticonvulsants
Antiparkinsonian drugs

Narcotic Analgesics
Opiates
Barbiturates

Antineoplastics
Vinca alkaloids

Cation-Containing Medications
Antacids
Sucralfate
Calcium, iron, barium

Others
Bile acid binding agents (cholestyramine)
Nonsteroidal antiinflammatory drugs (ibuprofen,
   naproxen)
Oral hypoglycemics
Parasympathetic blockers (oxybutynin)
Acetylsalicylic acid

to the reduction in propagating contractions, patients with slow-transit constipation exhibit *increased* motor activity in the rectosigmoid, which serves to create a high-pressure zone that further impairs transit of stool through the colon.[57,58]

In some patients, the marked reduction in stool frequency can be attributed to a neurologic lesion or condition that interrupts or damages the nerve pathways mediating peristalsis in the distal colon. For example, sacral level cord lesions interrupt the parasympathetic pathways that innervate the left colon; as a result, patients with low-level spinal cord lesions typically experience profound constipation. Severe constipation is also common in patients with Parkinson's disease; this is partly the result of degeneration of the autonomic nervous system, which is a major mediator of intestinal peristalsis, and partly because of the effects of anti-Parkinson's drugs, which further reduce motility. Another neurologic disorder associated with severe constipation is multiple sclerosis; constipation in these patients is caused partly by motor dysfunction involving the bowel itself, partly by sacral level lesions that interrupt the parasympathetic pathways controlling motility in the left colon, and partly by the muscle

weakness and immobility associated with the progressive neurologic impairment.[68]

The etiologic factors for idiopathic slow-transit constipation are not well understood. The finding that this condition is most common among young women and the fact that onset typically coincides with puberty suggest a hormonal link. Other potential causes include genetic, inflammatory, or degenerative disorders causing dysfunction of either the autonomic nerves controlling colonic motility or the nerve cells within the bowel wall. Some studies have shown a marked reduction in the interstitial cells of Cajal, which are thought to control motility in the gut, and others have shown loss of ganglion cells in the myenteric plexus.[55,58,69,70] Another possible cause is some alteration in the release of 5-hydroxy-tryptamine (5-HT) or the interaction of 5-HT with specific receptors in the gut wall; disturbances in 5-HT physiology are thought to contribute to both slow-transit constipation and IBS.[71] This is the basis for the development of 5-HT$_4$ receptor agonists such as tegaserod, a newly developed category of drugs that act to promote peristalsis.[72] Finally, cholecystokinin (CCK) is now known to inhibit colonic motility; CCK(1) receptor antagonists are currently being developed, and it is hoped that these drugs will be useful in the treatment of reduced motility and constipation.[73]

Slow-transit constipation is also sometimes known as colonic inertia; however, Bassotti and colleagues mounted a convincing argument that colonic inertia is a distinct and relatively rare subtype of constipation characterized by significantly prolonged transit time, minimal or no colonic motor activity following eating, and no response to pharmacologic stimulation.[59]

Obstructed Defecation Syndromes. Several disorders result in the inability to effectively eliminate stool from the rectum, even if the stool is of normal consistency; these disorders are collectively termed *obstructed defecation syndromes.* Specific disorders leading to obstructed defecation include *functional pelvic floor disorders,* such as excessive perineal descent and dyssynergic defecation (the inability to relax the pelvic floor muscles and external sphincter or the inability to coordinate sphincter relaxation and abdominal muscle contraction), and *anorectal structural anomalies,* such as rectal prolapse and rectocele.[57,58] Patients with obstructed defecation syndromes have difficulty initiating defecation and do not achieve complete rectal evacuation despite excessive and prolonged straining; they commonly report a "lumplike" sensation or a feeling of "blockage" in the anal area.[58] Patients with obstructed defecation utilize a variety of measures to facilitate stool elimination: manual "splinting" of the perineum; digital evacuation of the stool; and digital pressure against the posterior vaginal wall (which is particularly effective when the obstruction is caused by a rectocele). As noted, obstructed defecation syndromes result in difficult evacuation even if the stool is soft; however, the incomplete emptying characteristic of these syndromes results in prolonged contact between the stool and the rectal mucosa, which produces drying of the retained stool. As a result, many patients present with a combination of hard stools and incomplete evacuation.

Pelvic floor dyssnergia. The most common cause of obstructed defecation is thought to be impaired ability to coordinate pelvic floor and external sphincter relaxation with abdominal muscle contraction, a condition also known as *pelvic floor dyssynergia.*[74] The diagnostic criteria for this condition include the Rome II criteria for functional constipation (described earlier in this section), in addition to at least two of the following:[58]

- Evidence of dyssynergia on anorectal manometry, that is, paradoxical increase in anal sphincter pressure or less than 20% reduction in resting anal sphincter pressure during attempted defecation, with or without an increase in intrarectal pressure
- Inability to expel a balloon or stool-like device (such as a fecom), within 3 minutes
- Prolonged colonic transit time as evidenced by retention of more than five radiopaque markers 120 hours following ingestion of a Sitz Mark capsule containing 24 radiopaque markers
- Inability to expel barium or greater than 50% retention during barium defecography

In addition, as many as two-thirds of patients with pelvic floor dyssynergia also demonstrate impaired rectal sensation.

The underlying cause of pelvic floor dyssynergia is not well understood; in the past, spasticity of the anal sphincter was thought to be the problem, but anal myectomy and treatment with botulinum toxin (to paralyze the anal sphincter) have not been effective. Currently, this condition is thought to be the result of unconscious but dysfunctional muscle contraction and relaxation; the patient inadvertently contracts the anal sphincter when she or he should relax and may also fail to contract the abdominal muscles effectively[58,74] (Fig. 14-2). To date, the most effective treatment seems to be pelvic muscle reeducation using biofeedback techniques.[60,74-76]

Rectocele. Rectoceles are herniations of the anterior rectal wall into the posterior vagina; risk factors for this condition include vaginal delivery, hysterectomy, postmenopausal status, connective tissue disorders, and chronic straining with defecation. Small rectoceles are typically asymptomatic; however, a large rectocele can cause obstructed defecation because straining to defecate pushes the stool into the vaginal pouch rather than into the anal canal (Fig. 14-3). Rectoceles are usually corrected surgically in conjunction with other pelvic floor surgery; because these procedures are typically performed by gynecologists, we lack definitive data regarding functional and clinical outcomes of the

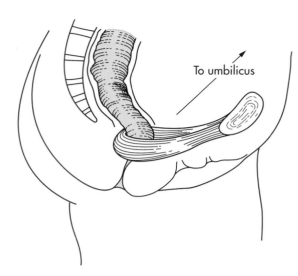

Fig. 14-2 Pelvic floor dyssynergia. Failure to relax pelvic floor muscles during attempted defecation causes obstructed defecation.

various surgical approaches in terms of bowel function.[76,77] Rectoceles may also be managed conservatively with use of pessaries in women who are not surgical candidates.

Assessment Guidelines

Assessment of the patient presenting with constipation is designed to determine the specific etiologic factors and subtypes of constipation; these data are then used to determine an appropriate treatment plan. As is true of most conditions, accurate assessment begins with a thorough history and focused physical examination.

History. The patient interview must include a comprehensive discussion of the patient's symptoms related to constipation and identification of the symptoms the patient finds most problematic; the clinician must ask about the frequency of defecation, the volume and consistency of the stool, any aids to elimination (such as suppositories, laxatives, enemas, or digital support maneuvers), usual fiber and fluid intake, feelings of incomplete evacuation, amount of straining required to eliminate stool, and any associated symptoms (such as abdominal

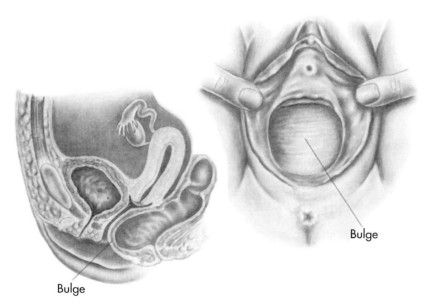

Fig. 14-3 Rectocele causing obstructed defecation. (From Seidel H, Ball JW, Dains JE, Benedict GW: *Mosby's guide to physical examination*, ed 4, St Louis, 1999, Mosby.)

pain, cramping, or bloating). Patients must be specifically asked about the need to use digital support or digital evacuation, because many are too embarrassed to volunteer this information. The nurse should also ask the patient about the frequency with which he or she perceives the urge to defecate (call to stool) and the frequency with which he or she is able to respond promptly. Finally, the patient should be queried regarding all prescription and OTC medications, because many patients are unknowingly contributing to the problem with anti-motility medications.

Physical Examination. The focused physical examination should include screening for evidence of neurologic disease or thyroid disease, an abdominal examination to detect evidence of retained stool, and a careful anorectal exam to detect evidence of rectocele or sphincter dysfunction (such as paradoxical contraction of the anal sphincter in response to the command to "push my finger out").

The history and physical exam provide major clues to the subtype of constipation; for example, patients with normal-transit constipation usually report hard stools that are difficult to eliminate as their major concern, and the anorectal exam indicates normal sphincter function. In contrast, patients with slow-transit constipation typically report infrequent urge to defecate, very infrequent bowel movements, extremely hard stools, and bloating; physical exam findings usually include abdominal distension and evidence of retained stool. This differs from patients with pelvic floor dyssynergia, who typically report normal frequency but major difficulty with stool elimination and feelings of incomplete evacuation; these patients also commonly report the need to use manual measures to eliminate the stool, and the physical exam may reveal either rectocele or the inability to coordinate anal sphincter relaxation and abdominal muscle contraction (in response to the command to push the examiner's finger out). Patients with constipation-predominant IBS are most likely to report cramping pain and bloating as their primary symptoms, and their anorectal exam is usually normal.

Diagnostic Studies. For many patients, a thorough history and physical exam are sufficient to establish a preliminary diagnosis of normal-transit constipation, and no further workup is indicated unless primary therapy with fiber, fluids, and osmotic laxatives is ineffective. However, laboratory studies are indicated whenever the physical exam suggests that the constipation is secondary to a systemic condition, such as thyroid dysfunction, and specific diagnostic studies are frequently needed when the initial workup suggests either reduced motility or pelvic floor dyssynergia. For example, the patient with suspected slow-transit constipation should undergo motility testing, whereas the patient with evidence of pelvic floor dyssynergia may benefit from physiologic testing of the anorectal sphincter mechanism and defecating proctography. The studies most commonly used to evaluate the patient with refractory constipation are briefly described as follows:[55,60]

- Colonic transit study (motility study). Colonic motility can be easily and simply evaluated by the Sitz Marker test. The patient ingests a gelatin capsule filled with radiopaque markers (Sitz Mark, Konsyl Pharmaceuticals, Easton, MD), and a plain abdominal radiograph is obtained 120 to 144 hours (5 to 6 days) following capsule ingestion. Because normal colonic transit time is less than 72 hours, retention of more than 20% of the markers at 120 hours is indicative of prolonged transit time. A cluster of retained markers in the rectosigmoid suggests obstructed defecation.

- Anorectal manometry. Patients with suspected obstructed defecation may benefit from anorectal manometry; this test involves use of pressure-sensitive balloons placed into the rectum and the anal canal to evaluate sensory awareness of rectal distension, anal sphincter tone at rest and with voluntary contraction, the response of the anal sphincters to rectal distension, and the patient's ability to relax the sphincter during straining. The patient with pelvic floor dyssynergia typically exhibits paradoxical contraction (or failed relaxation) of the anal sphincter in response to straining. (See Chapter 15 for a more detailed description of this test.)

- Balloon expulsion test. This simple office-based screening test is used to evaluate a patient's ability to evacuate stool from the rectum (to confirm or rule out obstructed defecation). The test involves insertion of a latex balloon into the rectum;

the balloon is then filled with 50 mL of water, and the patient is asked to expel the balloon into a toilet. The inability to expel the balloon within 2 minutes suggests obstructed defecation and the need for further evaluation.

- Defecating proctography. This test is used to evaluate the patient's ability to evacuate "simulated stool" (barium paste). The barium paste is instilled into the rectum, and the patient is then placed onto a radiolucent commode chair and is instructed to evacuate the barium paste; fluoroscopy is used to evaluate the response of the rectum, anal canal, sphincters, and pelvic floor during the attempted evacuation. This test can be beneficial in identifying structural defects that inhibit defecation, such as rectocele or prolapse of the rectal mucosa. However, it is an embarrassing test for the patient, thus making it difficult to obtain accurate results, and there are no established parameters regarding "normal" findings; in addition, interrater reliability is poor. Based on these limitations, the value of this test has been questioned.[76]

Treatment

Effective management for the patient with constipation is dependent on an accurate determination of the etiologic factors. Patients with normal-transit constipation typically respond well to primary therapy (fiber, fluids, and osmotic laxatives as indicated); in contrast, patients with obstructed defecation require treatment to relieve the obstruction (such as biofeedback for pelvic floor dyssynergia or surgical repair for the patient with a rectocele), and patients with slow-transit constipation require additional medications and possibly surgery (Table 14-3).

TABLE 14-3   Types of Constipation: Presentation, Diagnosis, Management

TYPE OF CONSTIPATION	CLINICAL PRESENTATION	DIAGNOSTIC STUDIES	MANAGEMENT OPTIONS
Normal transit-constipation	Hard stools that are difficult to eliminate Less frequent bowel movements	None required unless additional symptoms present or patient fails conservative management	Fiber and fluids Education about importance of prompt response to urge to defecate/correct position Increased activity as tolerated Osmotic laxatives as needed
Slow transit-constipation	Very infrequent bowel movements Infrequent urge to defecate Minimal or no response to fiber, fluids, osmotic laxatives (fiber may cause increased bloating)	Colonic motility study (Sitz Marker Study)	Fluids and fiber as tolerated Laxatives: osmotic laxatives on routine basis and stimulant laxatives as needed Surgical intervention if inadequate response to laxative therapy
Obstructed defecation	Difficulty with stool elimination even when stool is soft Straining; use of digital maneuvers to evacuate stool	Pelvic exam to rule out rectocele Anorectal exam to assess ability to relax pelvic floor muscles Anorectal manometry Defecography	For patient with rectocele; surgical repair or pessary placement For patient with pelvic floor dyssynergia: biofeedback

Fiber and Fluid Therapy. Fiber and fluid therapy is considered the first step in the treatment of constipation; such measures may effectively "cure" patients with normal-transit constipation, and even patients with obstructed defecation or slow-transit constipation frequently benefit from measures to create soft, bulky stools.[55,57] Before initiation of fiber therapy, patients with retained stool throughout the colon and rectum require removal of any impacted stool and the administration of laxatives and enemas to evacuate the retained stool.[55] (See Chapter 15 for further discussion of strategies for colonic cleansing.)

The recommended goal for fiber intake in adults is 28 to 30 g/day. Fiber should be gradually increased until the desired stool consistency is reached. Patients should be informed of the potential for increased gas production and bloating during the initiation of fiber therapy; the clinician should emphasize to the patient that these symptoms are transient and generally subside as the bowel adjusts to the increase in fiber intake. Patients must also be counseled regarding the importance of adequate fluid intake (30 mL/kg of body weight/day); an increase in fiber intake coupled with inadequate fluid intake places the patient at risk for intestinal obstruction. (Patients who are on fluid restriction should not be prescribed fiber therapy; these individuals are more appropriately managed with softener-stimulant combinations.) Options for increasing fiber intake include *dietary modifications, bulk laxatives, and bran formulas.*

One approach to fiber therapy is to modify the diet to ensure adequate fiber intake; this is an excellent option, but many individuals are unable or unwilling to modify their diet sufficiently to meet daily fiber needs. Patients who prefer to use dietary modifications should be provided with a list of fiber-containing foods and should be assisted to establish specific target goals for fiber and fluid intake. Some patients find that the simplest approach to ensuring adequate dietary fiber is to eat a high-fiber cereal each day; selected cereals (such as Fiber One) contain 27 g of fiber in a 1-cup serving. Chapter 16 includes a table of high-fiber foods.

Bulk laxatives attract and retain water within the fecal mass, thus producing a bulkier and softer stool.

The bulkier stool produces colonic distension, which stimulates the propagating contractions that propel stool through the colon. Bulk laxatives are a very safe way to add fiber on a routine basis, and patients should be taught that long-term use of these agents is safe and beneficial; it may be helpful to refer to these products as fiber supplements as opposed to bulk laxatives, because many individuals have been taught to avoid long-term use of "laxatives." These products are now available in multiple forms, including powders that are designed to be mixed with water or juice, wafers or cookies, and caplets or capsules. In selecting a specific product for an individual patient, the clinician must consider any comorbid conditions that would affect the decision; for example, some products contain significant amounts of sugar or sodium, which would be contraindicated for the diabetic patient or a patient on a sodium-restricted diet. In addition, some types of fiber may be poorly tolerated by the patient with IBS; some studies indicate that soluble fiber (such as psyllium, ispaghula, and calcium polycarbophil) is better tolerated than insoluble fiber (such as bran).[78] Finally, methylcellulose products (such as Citrucel) may be better tolerated by some individuals because these products are associated with less bloating (because methylcellulose does not undergo bacterial fermentation).

Bran formulas made with unprocessed bran and prunes are one way to increase fiber intake for individuals who are unable to consume adequate amounts of high-fiber foods or who prefer an alternate approach to fiber therapy. Box 14-6 provides two examples of bran formulas that can be taken in small amounts on a daily basis to normalize stool consistency.

Biofeedback Therapy. Biofeedback therapy is the recommended treatment approach for patients with obstructed defecation caused by pelvic floor dyssynergia; the patient receives visual feedback regarding pelvic floor and abdominal muscle contraction and is taught to coordinate abdominal muscle contraction with pelvic floor relaxation. Simulated evacuation with a balloon or silicone device filled with artificial stool (a "fecom") can be used to allow the patient to "practice" effective defecation. Specific techniques included in the

BOX 14-6 Fiber Supplement Recipes

Power Pudding	Bran Formula
½ cup prune juice	1 cup unprocessed miller's bran
½ cup applesauce	1 cup applesauce
½ cup wheat bran flakes	¼ cup prune juice
½ cup canned or stewed prunes	
¼ cup per day initially; increase the daily dose by ¼ cup each week until desired results are obtained	1 tablespoon per day initially; increase the daily dose by 1 tbsp each week until desired results are obtained

From Neal LJ: Power Pudding: Natural laxative therapy for elderly who are homebound. *Home Healthcare Nurse* 13(3): 66-71, 1995.

instructional program for patients with dyssynergic defecation include abdominal breathing exercises, abdominal strengthening exercises, pelvic floor relaxation, and coordination of abdominal and pelvic muscle contraction.[55,60,74,75] Biofeedback can also be used to improve sensory awareness of rectal distension.

Laxatives and Other Pharmacologic Agents.

Laxatives remain the primary treatment option for patients with slow-transit constipation and are frequently used to supplement the primary management program for patients with normal-transit constipation and obstructed defecation. Although long-term laxative therapy has traditionally been considered contraindicated and a risk factor for colonic denervation and reduced motility, current data suggest that the colonic dysfunction sometimes attributed to long-term laxative use ("cathartic colon") may actually be the *reason* for long-term laxative therapy as opposed to the *result*.

Laxatives can be classified according to their mechanism of action: bulk-forming laxatives, osmotic laxatives, emollient laxatives, and stimulant laxatives. The American Gastroenterological Association recommends bulk-forming laxatives as first-line therapy for most patients; however, caution must be used in prescribing these agents for patients with severe slow-transit constipation, because bulk agents may actually worsen symptoms

in these individuals. Osmotic laxatives are the second tier in laxative use; they are recommended for use on an as-needed basis but are safe for daily administration in patients with slow-transit constipation. Osmotic laxatives include any agent that "works" by pulling fluid into the bowel to soften the stool and to distend the bowel sufficiently to stimulate peristalsis; saline-based laxatives are inexpensive and effective and are usually considered the first choice (so long as there is no contraindication to a sodium-based agent). Additional osmotic agents include lactulose, sorbitol, and polyethylene glycol solutions; these agents are effective, but lactulose and sorbitol increase gas production, and polyethylene glycol solutions are more expensive. Stimulant laxatives include sennabased products and bisacodyl (Dulcolax); these agents work by stimulating the enteric nervous system to increase peristaltic activity. They are generally considered the most powerful agents and the agents most likely to cause adverse effects; they are typically reserved for constipation that is unresponsive to fiber and osmotic agents.

Additional pharmacologic agents that may be of benefit for selected patients include the following:

- 5-HT$_4$ agonists such as tegaserod have shown benefit in women with constipation-predominant IBS (at 12 mg/day), specifically increased number of bowel movements, fewer days without bowel movements, and reduced abdominal pain and bloating; however, more studies are needed, and currently we have no data regarding the efficacy of these agents in men.[72,79]
- Peripheral opioid-receptor antagonists such as methylnaltrexone are under investigation and show promise in the prevention or treatment of opioid-induced constipation.[80]
- Probiotics such as *Lactobacillus* and bifudobacteria are gaining increasing recognition as vital to bowel health and are being investigated for their effects on a variety of bowel disorders, including constipation; these agents interact with fiber to produce substances that protect the bowel wall and help maintain bowel health.[81,82]
- Prokinetic agents are under investigation for their ability to increase colonic motility; these agents include prostaglandin analogues and neurotrophins.[58]

In summary, laxatives are currently the mainstay of pharmacologic treatment for constipation; the hope is that research currently in process will produce agents that selectively address the underlying pathologic processes.

Surgical Intervention. Surgery is a last-resort treatment option for the patient with severe slow-transit constipation; if the reduced motility is confined to the colon, these patients may benefit from colectomy and ileorectal anastomosis. A thorough workup should be conducted before one considers surgical intervention, because colectomy is of limited benefit for patients with pelvic floor dyssynergia and patients with small bowel dysfunction.[55,58]

DISORDERED DEFECATION: IRRITABLE BOWEL SYNDROME

IBS is a chronic, recurrent functional bowel disorder that is characterized by abdominal pain, bloating and distension, and changes in stool frequency and consistency.[83] IBS can be further classified as constipation-predominant, diarrhea-predominant, or intermittent episodes of each (that is, alternating bowel pattern). The predominant bowel symptom associated with IBS usually influences the treatment approach. The pathology of IBS remains unclear, and there is no biologic marker or diagnostic tool to identify the disorder; however, symptom-based criteria have been developed to aid the clinician in identifying patients with this condition[83] (Box 14-7).

Treatment is focused on management of symptoms and on control of dietary and psychosocial factors that are associated with exacerbation of symptoms.

It is estimated that 40% to 50% of gastroenterology referrals are for symptoms compatible with a diagnosis of IBS. The costs of IBS are high, not only for the individual but also for the health care system; the direct and indirect costs associated with diagnosis and management of IBS were estimated to be 1.66 billion dollars in 2000.[84-89] Excess surgical procedures contribute to the health care costs for patients with an IBS diagnosis.[90]

In addition to increased utilization of health care, the impact of IBS is reflected in the poorer quality of life reported by patients with IBS, as well as missed days at work and school.[91] IBS affects more women than men and typically becomes manifest in late adolescence and early adulthood.[92,93] Patients with IBS commonly report symptoms of diffuse abdominal pain that may be associated with eating, psychologic stress, or any intraluminal stimulation (such as gas, rectal exam, or endoscopy), as well as a change in stool frequency or consistency and feelings of incomplete evacuation. The pain is typically relieved with defecation. Women usually exhibit an increase in symptoms during the late premenses and menses phases of the menstrual

---

BOX 14-7 **Rome II Diagnostic Criteria for Irritable Bowel Syndrome**

At least 3 months of continuous or recurrent symptoms, as follows:

Abdominal Pain or Discomfort
Relieved with defecation, or
Associated with a change in frequency of stool, or
Associated with a change in consistency of stool

Two or More of the Following, on at Least 25% of Occasions or Days
Altered stool frequency (for research purposes, "altered" may be defined as more than three bowel movements each day or less than three bowel movements each week), or
Altered stool form (lumpy/hard or loose/watery stool), or
Altered stool passage (straining, urgency, or feeling of incomplete evacuation), or
Passage of mucus, or
Bloating or feeling of abdominal distension

From American Gastroenterological Association medical position statement; Irritable bowel syndrome, *Gastroenterology* 112(6): 2118-2119, 1997.

cycle; women with IBS also frequently report dysmenorrhea and premenstrual distress syndrome (PMS), as well as extraintestinal conditions such as fibromyalgia and insomnia.[94] Specific foods can also worsen symptoms, particularly those that increase gas production.[95]

Risk Factors

Multiple factors are thought to play a role in the development of IBS; therefore, a biopsychosocial model is often used to characterize the disorder.[96] The pathophysiology of IBS likely involves genetic predisposition factors, visceral hypersensitivity, and altered motility and transit. However, no one discernible motility disorder is common to all patients with IBS,[97,98] and transit time differences are noted when IBS subgroups are compared, such as those with constipation-predominant IBS and those with diarrhea-predominant IBS. Studies utilizing the barostat device to distend the bowel while monitoring patients' perceptions of discomfort and pain have demonstrated that patients with IBS are hyper-responsive to visceral stimuli, a condition known as visceral hyperalgesia. More recent studies utilizing pain imaging techniques such as functional magnetic resonance imaging have demonstrated differences in brain activation patterns in patients with IBS as compared with healthy controls.[99-101] This hypersensitivity of the gut to mechanical distension may be attributable to recruitment of silent receptors, increased responsiveness at the level of the dorsal horns in the spinal cord, or altered central nervous system modulation.

Patients who have experienced an intestinal infection, either viral or bacterial, may exhibit symptoms of IBS following resolution of the primary infection; this phenomenon has been referred to as postinfectious IBS.[102,103] Women are more likely to experience these IBS symptoms following infection as compared with men.

Autonomic nervous system dysfunction may also play a role in IBS. Investigators using both laboratory techniques and 24-hour monitoring of heart rate have demonstrated a link between parasympathetic (vagal) dysfunction and constipation, and alterations in sympathetic innervation are linked to symptoms of diarrhea.[104,105]

Psychologic disturbances have long been linked to IBS, and numerous studies support the effect of psychologic distress on the symptoms associated with IBS.[106,107] However, the question is: "Which comes first?" Does the psychologic disturbance cause or augment the symptom complex of IBS, or is the disease process causing the psychologic problems? As noted previously, these patients miss many more days of work or school and must cope with recurrent or chronic pain, which may cause social isolation; these factors may contribute to a psychologic disturbance. Another potential source of psychologic distress is the fear experienced by many patients that they have a terminal illness. These psychosocial issues may influence the person's behavior or response to IBS; they may complain of symptoms more frequently, seek medical help more often, and subject themselves to additional diagnostic or treatment procedures. Some reports have documented a high incidence of sexual and psychologic abuse in patients with IBS; however, other studies have failed to yield statistically significant results.[108,109] It is known that individuals with posttraumatic stress disorder, such as Gulf War veterans, have higher rates of IBS.[110]

Dietary intolerances, such as lactose intolerance and gluten sensitivity (celiac disease), can give rise to symptoms similar to those of IBS. In addition, dietary factors have long been associated with exaggeration of symptoms in patients with IBS; therefore, dietary intake should be carefully scrutinized for common offenders. Food products that have been reported to aggravate symptoms include cheese, onions, milk, wheat, chocolate, butter, yogurt, coffee, eggs, gas-forming fruits and vegetables, tea, potatoes, and alcohol. Patients should be instructed to complete a "diet, stool, and symptom" diary and should then be counseled to delete any items that tend to aggravate their symptoms, especially fatty foods, caffeine, and gas-producing foods; however, a highly restricted diet is usually not necessary.

Treatment

Current treatment strategies for IBS include behavioral therapies and/or drug therapy. The first step is to provide the patient with education regarding IBS. Patients frequently benefit from maintenance of a symptom diary to help identify factors and situations that act as triggers for their symptoms. Cognitive-behavioral therapies have been shown to be more effective than education alone in reducing symptoms and enhancing quality of life in women with IBS.[111,112] Drugs such as laxatives, antidiarrheals, and smooth muscle relaxants have traditionally been used for symptom management. In the past few years, certain pharmacologic agents designed to modulate the action of serotonin in the gastrointestinal tract have been approved (by the United States Food and Drug Administration) for management of IBS symptoms in women. For example, Alosetron is a $5-HT_3$ antagonist that is indicated for women with refractory diarrhea and pain associated with IBS,[113] and tegaserod is a $5-HT_4$ agonist that has been shown to be effective in the management of women with constipation-prone IBS.[114] Additional drugs are under investigation; these include additional serotonergic agents, the alpha-2-adrenergic receptor agonist clonidine, selective muscarinic receptor blockers, and antidepressants.[115]

Summary

In summary, there appear to be several pathophysiologic mechanisms involved in IBS, including dysmotility, impaired visceral sensation (visceral hyperalgesia), and psychologic disturbances; each of these must be addressed in diagnosing and managing IBS. Because the exact cause is not yet known, treatment is centered around symptom management: pharmacologic support to address pain, diarrhea, constipation, bloating, and distension; behavioral therapy or psychologic analysis to address the psychosocial component of the disorder and to provide emotional support and counseling for living with a chronic illness and coping with stress; and education regarding extraintestinal factors influencing IBS, management options for IBS, and the underlying basis for the symptoms, that is, gastrointestinal dysfunction. Patients need to be reassured that their symptoms are *not* indicative of a terminal illness and that IBS does not place them at higher risk for colorectal cancer.

FECAL INCONTINENCE

Fecal continence is dependent on the individual's ability to recognize rectal distension and to delay defecation until a suitable time and place are found. Fecal *incontinence* has been variably defined. Some authors include a duration factor (such as leakage for a month or longer), and some include a frequency factor (such as fecal leakage occurring twice or more per month), whereas others consider any involuntary passage of stool to be abnormal and to therefore represent incontinence.[116] Incontinence can also be defined and classified according to severity: complete incontinence indicates incontinence of gas, liquid, and solid stool; partial incontinence refers to leakage of gas and liquid stool (but continence for solid stool); and seepage and soiling reflect leakage of small amounts of stool between bowel movements in a patient who is continent of stool and gas and able to delay defecation.[117,118]

Incidence and Prevalence

It is difficult to accurately determine the incidence and prevalence of fecal incontinence, partly because most individuals are reluctant to admit to problems with bowel control, and partly because of differences in definition of the condition (such as the inclusion or exclusion of incontinence for flatus and the inclusion or exclusion of frequency criteria). Published prevalence data for community-dwelling adults range from a low of 2% to a high of more than 10%, but these statistics probably represent underreporting; in the long-term care setting, prevalence approaches 50%.[116,119,120]

Risk Factors

Risk factors for fecal incontinence in young and middle-aged adults include obstetric trauma, IBS, neuromuscular disorders affecting mobility, neurologic lesions or surgical procedures resulting in denervation of the pelvic floor and anorectum, and diarrhea. In the long-term care setting, the primary risk factors are dementia, immobility, and colonic dysfunction (diarrhea or fecal impaction).[119,120]

Etiology and Pathology

There are many different approaches to classification of the etiologic and pathologic factors contributing to fecal incontinence; in this text, a functional classification system is used. Within this context, the factors contributing to fecal incontinence can be grouped as follows: alterations in stool consistency and volume; diminished ability to recognize rectal distension and to identify rectal contents; compromised function of the internal anal sphincter, external anal sphincter, or both; and reduced rectal capacity and compliance. In most patients, the incontinence is multifactorial; for example, the young woman with sphincter damage secondary to obstetric trauma may be fully continent so long as her stool remains formed, but she may be incontinent during episodes of diarrhea.

The pathologic conditions contributing to fecal incontinence are discussed from the perspective of specific etiologic factors, impact on continence, and management goals. Specific treatment options are discussed in the following chapter.

Alterations in Stool Consistency and Volume.
As noted earlier in this chapter, continence is partially dependent on normal stool consistency and volume. Diarrheal conditions are particularly likely to cause temporary or episodic incontinence, because the anal sphincter is much more competent for formed stool.[119] Many individuals with compromised bowel control report the inability to control liquid stool, and high-volume liquid stools can precipitate incontinence in *any* individual who is unable to reach the toilet in a timely manner. On the other end of the spectrum, severe constipation and fecal impaction can result in leakage of liquid stool around the fecal bolus. Both diarrhea and constipation represent primary disorders of defecation as well as potential etiologic factors for incontinence; therefore, they are discussed in detail in the first section of this chapter. They are mentioned again here to stress that normalization of stool volume and consistency is a primary goal in bowel management.

Alterations in Ability to Recognize Rectal Filling and Rectal Contents. Normal anorectal sensation alerts the individual to rectal filling and informs the individual regarding the nature of the rectal contents; the individual can then move to the bathroom to initiate defecation or can contract the external anal sphincter to delay defecation.[121] The individual with normal sensory awareness is able to recognize as little as 10 to 20 mL of air or water in the rectum.[122] This recognition is important

because relatively small volumes of stool or gas can activate the rectoanal inhibitory reflex, which allows rectal contents to pass into the anal canal.[123] Studies have shown that transient relaxation of the internal sphincter is typically stimulated by 20 mL of stool or gas and can occur with as little as 5 mL, whereas persistent relaxation of the internal sphincter is commonly produced by 60 mL of rectal contents.[124,125] Maintenance of continence in the presence of internal anal sphincter relaxation is dependent on external sphincter contraction; this is provided in part by a subconscious reflex contractile response to increases in rectal pressure, but it is primarily dependent on voluntarily contraction (which, in turn, depends on recognition of rectal distension). Any compromise in sensory awareness increases the risk for incontinence because the individual fails to recognize impending defecation and to respond appropriately (either by moving to the bathroom or by contracting the external sphincter). Common pathologic conditions resulting in sensory dysfunction include spinal cord lesions, pudendal nerve damage, chronic rectal distension, and cognitive impairment.[116,123]

Neurologic lesions and conditions may produce severe compromise in sensory awareness of rectal filling. Specific conditions associated with sensory loss include progressive neurologic diseases such as multiple sclerosis and spinal cord lesions such as spinal cord injury or myelomeningocele. Although the severity of the sensory dysfunction is variable, many individuals with spinal cord lesions report total absence of rectal sensation, and these individuals commonly lack voluntary sphincter control as well. This means that any volume of rectal filling sufficient to initiate the rectoanal inhibitory reflex is likely to produce fecal incontinence. Therefore, effective management of these patients is dependent on a program to maintain solid stool consistency (because the passively contracted anal sphincter is most competent for solid stool) and to stimulate defecation on a routine basis before the rectum fills sufficiently to trigger involuntary elimination.

Pudendal nerve damage is believed to be a significant causative factor for fecal incontinence among women and the elderly. Pudendal nerve damage can be caused by prolonged second stage of labor, difficult or instrumental vaginal delivery, and chronic straining resulting from constipation.[123,126] These conditions all cause excessive stretching of the pudendal nerve (stretch neuropathy); stretch injuries result in partial denervation followed by reinnervation, which is associated with delayed transmission of sensory and motor impulses. (This delay is typically evaluated by pudendal nerve terminal motor latency measurements, although the validity and reliability of this test have been challenged.[121]) Stretch neuropathy has been documented in up to 80% of women after initial vaginal delivery; however, most of these women report no problems with fecal incontinence, and pudendal nerve terminal motor latency measurements usually normalize by 6 months following delivery.[126,127] It may be that repetitive damage associated with subsequent vaginal deliveries (or with chronic constipation and straining at stool) causes persistent neuropathy that increases the woman's risk for incontinence later in life.[123] Whatever the mechanism of injury, loss of sensory awareness can contribute to incontinence in one of two ways: by creating a higher threshold for recognition of rectal distension or by creating a time delay in recognition of rectal distension. Individuals with compromised sensory awareness of rectal distension are most likely to experience incontinence when the stool is liquid; therefore, interventions should include measures to maintain formed stool as well as biofeedback therapy to improve sensory awareness of rectal filling.[128]

Cognitive impairment is a common cause of sensory dysfunction in institutionalized elderly individuals.[120] The nerve pathways that signal rectal distension are intact, but the individual is unable to interpret or respond to the message appropriately because of cognitive loss. These individuals are unable to respond to behavioral therapy and are most effectively managed by a program of stimulated defecation, in which stimuli such as suppositories are used to induce defecation on a routine basis.

Chronic rectal distension is another etiologic factor for impaired sensory function. Individuals with chronic constipation may present with a distended rectum but no urge to defecate. Management involves rectal disimpaction and colonic cleansing; however, sensory loss persists in some individuals

despite appropriate management.[124] Patients with persistent sensory loss may require long-term management with stimulated defecation programs.

Some studies suggest that sensory compromise is one cause of the seepage-and-soiling pattern of incontinence. These individuals typically demonstrate adequate voluntary sphincter function and are able to delay defecation, but they leak small volumes of stool with no conscious awareness. Anorectal physiology testing in these patients usually reveals normal squeeze pressures and a normal rectoanal inhibitory reflex but an elevated threshold for recognition of rectal distension; this results in leakage when the volume of stool is high enough to produce internal anal sphincter relaxation but too low to trigger sensory awareness.[117]

Increased rectal sensitivity can also contribute to problems with fecal incontinence; these patients experience intense fecal urgency and may be unable to delay defecation if they cannot reach a toilet facility quickly. This pattern is sometimes seen in patients with inflammatory conditions affecting the rectum, such as inflammatory bowel disease.

Compromised Sphincter Function. Intact sphincter function is clearly essential to maintenance of continence. The internal anal sphincter is primarily responsible for continence at rest, contributing 70% to 85% of resting anal canal pressure. (The blood-filled vascular cushions of the anal mucosa provide additional support for the internal anal sphincter and are thought to contribute up to 20% of resting pressure.[123]) In contrast, the external anal sphincter is primarily responsible for continence during periods of rectal distension; 60% of resistance following sudden distension is provided by contraction of the external sphincter.[123] Any compromise in sphincter function is therefore likely to produce fecal leakage. Dysfunction of the internal sphincter is most commonly associated with leakage of gas and liquid at rest, whereas external sphincter dysfunction is more commonly associated with incontinence associated with fecal urgency or diarrhea.[123] In many patients, both the internal and external sphincters are damaged, resulting in combination patterns of incontinence. Common etiologic factors for sphincter dysfunction include traumatic disruption of the sphincter muscle itself and denervation injuries or processes.

Traumatic disruption of the sphincter muscle is most commonly the result of obstetric trauma (traumatic vaginal delivery), but it may also be caused by anorectal injury or surgery.[123] Sphincteric injury secondary to vaginal delivery is most likely to occur during the first vaginal delivery. Sphincteric "mapping" by anal endosonography and other techniques demonstrated sphincter defects in 30% to 35% of women 6 weeks following delivery, especially among women in whom delivery was complicated by one of more of the following: large-birth-weight infant, forceps delivery, occipitoposterior presentation, prolonged second stage of labor, and perineal tears. Episiotomy also seems to be a risk factor for sphincter dysfunction.[123] Most of the women studied who had evidence of sphincter dysfunction were asymptomatic; however, researchers pointed out that sphincter deficits may increase the individual's risk for incontinence later in life.[123,126] It is important to distinguish between primary sphincter *damage* and compromised sphincter *function* resulting from denervation injuries. Patients with primary sphincter damage usually respond well to surgical correction and/or biofeedback, because the intact components of the muscle are normally innervated, whereas patients with denervation injuries usually respond poorly.[128,129] It is also important to understand that primary repair of obstetric injuries is frequently inadequate. A persistent sphincteric defect can be demonstrated in many of these women, and many of them suffer from fecal incontinence unless a subsequent sphincter repair is performed.[129] Other causes of traumatic sphincter damage include anorectal surgical procedures, such as hemorrhoidectomy, anal dilatation, and sphincterotomy; perineal trauma or pelvic fracture can also damage the sphincter and lead to fecal incontinence.[123] Many clinicians believe that anal intercourse is a potential cause of sphincteric damage; however, Chun and colleagues found no evidence of sphincteric injury from anoreceptive intercourse among homosexual men.[130]

Sphincteric incompetence may also occur as a result of denervation injuries. The most obvious and most complete of these are spinal cord injuries

and lesions; disordered defecation, constipation, and fecal incontinence have been documented in up to 80% of patients with spinal cord lesions.[131] Individuals with complete spinal cord lesions are unable to voluntarily contract the external anal sphincter, and even those with incomplete lesions typically lack adequate sphincter control. In addition, these individuals usually have reduced or absent sensations of rectal filling and are therefore unable to predict, much less control, defecation. However, the rectoanal inhibitory reflex and internal sphincter function are usually retained (because these functions are controlled by the enteric and autonomic nervous systems); thus, rectal distension produces relaxation of the internal sphincter but no compensatory contraction of the external sphincter, and fecal incontinence is typically the result.[123,129,131] A potential complicating factor in the management of patients with sacral-level spinal cord lesions and multiple sclerosis is the profound constipation typically experienced by these patients; this is caused by a significant reduction in peristaltic activity in the left colon (from loss of the parasympathetic pathways that exit the cord at S2 to S4). In some individuals, this reduced peristaltic activity serves to support continence, but significant numbers of these patients develop recurrent fecal impactions, especially if they are not following an effective bowel management program. Effective management for these patients is dependent on maintenance of a bulky formed stool (which is effectively retained by a passively contracted sphincter but can be easily eliminated), and a stimulated defecation program to prevent constipation and incontinence.

A less severe denervation injury is common in women and in the elderly and is attributable to pudendal neuropathy, which may be caused by obstetric trauma, straining at stool, or age-related changes in the pelvic floor.[123] In regard to obstetric trauma, it has been theorized that denervation injury associated with vaginal delivery may be the initial insult in a series of events that eventually results in fecal incontinence. Subsequent deliveries, especially those associated with prolonged labor or forceps delivery, the effects of declining estrogen levels following menopause, and progressive deterioration of pelvic nerve pathways (in part from aging) may all contribute to the eventual development of incontinence.[116,123,126] Whatever the causative factor for pudendal neuropathy, the result is compromised function of the external anal sphincter. (The internal sphincter is unaffected because it is innervated by the autonomic and enteric nervous systems.) Compromised function of the external sphincter is manifest by reduced squeeze pressures and reduced ability to delay defecation, especially when the stool is liquid or mushy; many individuals report intense defecatory urgency and episodes of "urge fecal incontinence."[132,133] Individuals with external sphincter dysfunction must be carefully evaluated to determine whether they have an anatomic sphincter defect in addition to the neuropathic dysfunction. Defects can usually be repaired surgically, whereas neuropathic dysfunction typically requires behavioral management (measures to maintain formed stool and stimulated defecation programs) or surgical procedures to restore anal canal resistance.

The pelvic floor muscles, particularly the puborectalis, have been theorized to contribute to continence by maintaining the anorectal angle (as explained in Chapter 13). Individuals with pelvic floor relaxation and pathologic perineal descent typically lose the normal anorectal angle; this has been thought to contribute to fecal leakage by permitting rectal contents to pass into the anal canal. Some studies suggest that the normal angle may contribute to the retention of solid and semisolid stool; however, other studies failed to demonstrate any relationship between anorectal angle and continence, and these investigators suggest that increased anal canal resistance and fecal continence result primarily from contraction of the external sphincter and the puborectalis muscle and *not* from maintenance of an obtuse anorectal angle.[123]

Compromised Rectal Capacity and Compliance. Normally, the rectum can serve as a temporary storage area for stool, which supports continence during the period between recognition of rectal filling and arrival at an appropriate time and place for defecation. This "reservoir" function requires adequate rectal capacity and normal rectal elasticity, or compliance.[123] Any significant increase or decrease in rectal capacity and compliance can adversely affect bowel function and continence.

Increased rectal capacity sometimes occurs in individuals who habitually delay defecation. These individuals may develop a megarectum characterized by excessive compliance and reduced sensitivity to distension. These individuals no longer sense rectal distension normally and experience no urge to defecate. In addition, the overstretched rectal walls lack normal contractility, and so attempts to defecate may be only partially effective.[129] Management requires disimpaction and colonic cleansing, followed by measures to maintain normal stool consistency and stimulated defecation programs to reestablish normal bowel function. These patients may or may not regain normal sensory awareness and rectal contractility.[134]

Reduced rectal capacity and compliance may occur as a result of inflammatory conditions (such as inflammatory bowel disease or gastroenteritis) or as a result of fibrotic changes within the rectal wall (such as those that occur following pelvic radiation or ischemic injury). Reduced capacity and compliance significantly limit the reservoir function of the rectum and result in severe defecatory urgency with small volumes of stool.[123,134] These patients are at great risk for incontinence despite normal anorectal sensation and normal sphincter function.[123] They can maintain continence only for the period of time that they are able to contract their sphincter maximally, which is usually less than 60 seconds. Because the rectal wall is unable to relax and to accommodate the bolus of stool, the intrarectal pressure remains elevated until defecation occurs; if partial relaxation of the external sphincter reduces the anal canal pressure to a level below rectal pressure, incontinence is inevitable. These individuals commonly report knowing the location of "every bathroom in town," and many live in constant anxiety related to the risk of incontinence. Management depends on effective treatment of the underlying condition or on fecal diversion.

SUMMARY

Disorders of defecation and fecal incontinence are common and extremely distressing conditions that quite negatively affect the individual's quality of life. Effective management is dependent on thorough evaluation and accurate identification of the causative factors, which then direct the management plan.

SELF-ASSESSMENT EXERCISE

1. Compare secretory and osmotic diarrhea in terms of: causative factors, stool volume and pH, response to fasting, and stool osmolality gap.

2. Explain the relationship between diarrhea and fecal incontinence.

3. Explain the role of each of the following in management of diarrhea:
   • Dietary modifications
   • Soluble fiber supplements
   • Probiotics
   • Antidiarrheal medications

4. Explain the difference between "lay" definitions of constipation and health care providers' definitions of constipation.

5. Explain the pathology and presentation of each of the following:
   • Normal-transit constipation
   • Slow-transit constipation
   • Obstructed defecation disorders

6. Explain the role of each of the following in management of patients with constipation:
   • Fiber and fluid therapy
   • Laxatives
   • Biofeedback

7. Describe key factors to be included in assessment of the patient with chronic constipation.

8. Explain current theories regarding the cause of IBS and implications for management.

9. Explain why each of the following patients is at risk for fecal incontinence:
   • 26-year-old man with paraplegia secondary to spinal cord injury at L2
   • 62-year-old woman whose medical history includes four vaginal deliveries, two forceps-assisted, and chronic constipation
   • 18-year-old woman with inflammatory bowel disease and proctitis
   • 83-year-old man with advanced dementia and no history of bowel dysfunction

REFERENCES

1. American Gastroenterological Association: Medical position statement: guidelines for the evaluation and management of chronic diarrhea, *Gastroenterology* 116:1461-1463, 1999.
2. Tamkin GW: An approach to diarrhea, *Emerg Med* 30:16-36, 1998.
3. Lebak K, Bliss D, Savik K, Patton-Marsh K: What's new on defining diarrhea in tube feeding studies? *Clin Nurs Res* 12:174-204, 2003.
4. Simor AE, Bradley S, Strausbaugh C, Crossley K, Nicolle L: SHEA Longterm Care Committee: *Clostridium difficile* in long-term-care facilities for the elderly, *Infect Control Hosp Epidemiol* 23:696-703, 2002.
5. Heimburger D, Geels V, Bilbrey J, Redden D, Keeney C: Effects of small-peptide and whole protein enteral feedings on serum proteins and diarrhea in critically-ill patients: a randomized trial, *JPEN J Parenteral Enteral Nutr* 21:162-167, 1997.
6. Kandil H, Opper F, Switzer B, Heizer W: Marked resistance of normal subjects to tube feeding induced diarrhea: the role of magnesium, *Am J Clin Nutr* 57:73-80, 1993.
7. Wenzl HH, Fine K, Schiller C, Fordtran J: Determinants of decreased fecal consistency in patients with diarrhea, *Gastroenterology* 108:1729-1738, 1995.
8. Fine KD, Schiller LR: AGA technical review on the evaluation and management of chronic diarrhea, *Gastroenterology* 116:1464-1486, 1999.
9. McQuaid KR: Alimentary tract. In: LM Tierney Jr, McPhee SJ, Papadakis MA, editors: *Current medical diagnosis and treatment,* New York, 2003, Lange Medical Books/McGraw-Hill, pp 522-627.
10. Pennachio D: Diarrhea: differentiating the acute from the chronic, *Patient Care* 9:52-56, 2002.
11. McCray W, et al: Diagnosing diarrhea in adults: a practical approach, *Hosp Med* 34:27-30, 32, 35-36, 1998.
12. Bushen O, Guerrant R: Acute infectious diarrhea approach and management in the emergency department, *Top Emerg Med* 25:139-149, 2003.
13. DuPont HL: Guidelines on acute infectious diarrhea in adults: the Practice Parameters Committee of the American College of Gastroenterology, *Am J Gastroenterol* 92:1962-1975, 1997.
14. Alfa MJ, Di T, Beda G: Survey of incidence of *Clostridium difficile* infection in Canadian hospitals and diagnostic approaches, *J Clin Microbiol* 36:2076-2080, 1998.
15. Bliss D, Johnson S, Savik K, Clabots C, Willard K, Gerding N: The acquisition of *Clostridium difficile* and associated diarrhea in hospitalized patients receiving tube feeding, *Ann Intern Med* 129:1012-1019, 1998.
16. Ratnaike RN, Jones TE: Mechanisms of drug-induced diarrhoea in the elderly, *Drugs Aging* 13:245-253, 1998.
17. Sabol VK, Friedenberg F: Diarrhea, *AACN Clin Issues* 8:425-436, 1997.
18. Eisenberg P: An overview of diarrhea in the patient receiving enteral nutrition, *Gastroenterol Nurs* 25:95-104, 2002.

19. Freidman L, Isselbacher K: Diarrhea and constipation. In: AS Fauci, Braunwald E, Isselbacher K, et al, editors: *Harrison's principles of internal medicine,* ed 14, New York, 1998, McGraw-Hill, pp 236-242.

20. Braunwald E, Fauci AS, Kasper DL, Hauser SL, Longo DL, Jameson JL: Diarrhea, constipation, and malabsorption. In: *Harrison's manual of medicine,* ed 15, New York, 2002, McGraw-Hill, pp 77-83.

21. DeMeo M, Kolli S, Keshavarzian A, Borton M, Al-Hosin M, et al: Beneficial effect of a bile acid resin binder on enteral feeding induced diarrhea, *Am J Gastroenterol* 93:967-971, 1998.

22. Cummings J, James W, Wiggins H: Role of the colon in ileal resection diarrhea, *Lancet* 1:344-347, 1973.

23. Topping DL, Clifton PM: Short-chain fatty acids and human colonic function: roles of resistant starch and non-starch polysaccharides, *Physiol Rev* 81:1031-1064, 2001.

24. Potter G: Bile acid diarrhea, *Dig Dis* 16:118-124, 1998.

25. Wilkes J, DiPalma J: Chronic diarrhea: differential diagnosis and management, *Consultant* 41:53-57, 2001.

26. Burns PE, Jairath N: Diarrhea and the patient receiving enteral feedings: a multifactorial problem, *J Wound Ostomy Continence Nurs* 21:257-263, 1994.

27. Jeejeebhoy KN: Short bowel syndrome: a nutritional and medical approach, *Can Med Assoc J* 166:1297-1302, 2002.

28. Kolars JC, Fischer PR: Evaluation of diarrhea in the returned traveler, *Prim Care* 29:931-945, 2002.

29. Fruto LV: Current concepts: management of diarrhea in acute care, *J Wound Ostomy Continence Nurs* 21: 199-205, 1994.

30. Corpe CP, Burant C, Hoekstra J: Intestinal fructose absorption: clinical and molecular aspects, *J Pediatr Gastroenterol Nutr* 28:364-374, 1999.

31. Choi YK, Johlin FC Jr., Summers R, Jackson M, Rao SS: Fructose intolerance: an under-recognized problem, *Am J Gastroenterol* 98:1348-1353, 2003.

32. Tierney L, Saint S, Whooley M: *Essentials of diagnosis and treatment,* ed 2, New York, 2002, McGraw-Hill.

33. Charles F, Phillips S, Camilleri M, Thomforde G: Rapid gastric emptying in patients with functional diarrhea, *Mayo Clin Proc* 72:323-328, 1997.

34. Riordan S, McIver C, Wakefield D, Bolin T, Duncombe V, Thomas M: Small intestinal bacterial overgrowth in the symptomatic elderly, *Am J Gastroenterol* 92:47-51, 1997.

35. Harari D, Gurwitz J, Avorn J, Bohn R, Minaker K: Bowel habit in relation to age and gender, *Arch Intern Med* 156:315-320, 1996.

36. Bignardi GE: Risk factors for *Clostridium difficile* infection, *J Hosp Infect* 40:1-15, 1998.

37. Miller JM, Walton J, Tordecilla L: Recognizing and managing *Clostridium difficile*-associated diarrhea, *Medsurg Nurs* 7:348-349, 352-356, 1998.

38. Viele CS: Overview of chemotherapy-induced diarrhea, *Semin Oncol Nurs* 19:2-5, 2003.

39. Anastasi JK, McMahon DJ: Testing strategies to reduce diarrhea in persons with HIV using traditional Chinese medicine: acupuncture and moxibustion, *J Assoc Nurses AIDS Care* 14:28-40, 2003.

40. Carlson S, Webster C, Craig R: Urinary recovery of lactulose compared to D-xylose absorption kinetics in HIV patients with diarrhea and weight loss, *Dig Dis Sci* 42:2599-2602, 1997.

41. Lambl B, Federman M, Pleskow D, Wanke C: Malabsorption and wasting in AIDS with microsporidia and pathogen-negative diarrhea, *AIDS* 10:739-744, 1996.

42. Bliss DZ, Johnson S, Savik K, Clabots C, Gerding N: Fecal incontinence in hospitalized patients who are acutely ill, *Nurs Res* 49:101-108, 2000.

43. Bliss DZ, Jung H, Savik K, Lowry A, LeMoine M, Jensen L, Werner C, Schaffer K: Supplementation with dietary fiber improves fecal incontinence, *Nurs Res* 50:203-213, 2001.

44. Chiarioni G, Scattolini C, Bonfante F, Vantini I: Liquid stool incontinence with severe urgency: anorectal function and effective biofeedback treatment, *Gut* 34: 1576-1580, 1993.

45. Juckett G: Prevention and treatment of traveler's diarrhea, *Am Fam Physician* 60:119-124, 135-136, 1999.

46. Rao GG, Qzerek A, Jeanes A: Rational protocols for testing faeces in the investigation of sporadic hospital-acquired diarrhoea, *J Hosp Infect* 47:79-83, 2001.

47. Aurisicchio LN, Pitchumoni C: Lactose intolerance: recognizing the link between diet and discomfort, *Postgrad Med* 95:113-120, 1994.

48. Stern J, Ippoliti C: Management of acute cancer treatment-induced diarrhea, *Semin Oncol Nurs* 19:11-16, 2003.

49. Alam NH, Meier R, Schneider H, Sarker S, Bordhan P, Mahalanabis D, et al: Partially hydrolyzed guar gum-supplemented oral rehydration solution in the treatment of acute diarrhea in children, *J Pediatr Gastroenterol Nutr* 31:503-507, 2000.

50. Emery E, Ahmad S, Koethe J, Skipper A, Perlmutter S, Paskin D: Banana flakes control diarrhea in enterally fed patients, *Nutr Clin Pract* 8:119-123, 1997.

51. Cresci GA: The use of probiotics with the treatment of diarrhea, *Nutr Clin Pract* 16:30-34, 2001.

52. D'Souza AL, Rajkumar C, Cooke J, Bulpitt C: Probiotics in prevention of antibiotic associated diarrhoea: meta-analysis, *BMJ* 324:1361, 2002.

53. Anthony L: New strategies for the prevention and reduction of cancer treatment-induced diarrhea, *Semin Oncol Nurs* 19:17-21, 2003.

54. Cope DG: Management of chemotherapy-induced diarrhea and constipation, *Nurs Clin North Am* 36:695-707, 2001.

55. Lembo A, Camilleri M: Current concepts: chronic constipation, *N Engl J Med* 349(14):1360-1368, 2003.

56. Higgins P, Johanson J: Epidemiology of constipation in North America: a systematic review, *Am J Gastroenterol* 99:750-759, 2004.

57. American Gastroenterological Association: American Gastroenterological Association Medical Position Statement: guidelines on constipation, *Gastroenterology* 119(6):1761-1770, 2000.

58. Sao R: Constipation: evaluation and treatment, *Gastroenterol Clin North Am* 32:659-683, 2003.

59. Bassotti G, de Roberto G, Sediari L, Morelli A: Toward a definition of colonic inertia, *World J Gastroenterol* 10(17):2465-2467, 2004.

60. Stessman M: Biofeedback: its role in the treatment of chronic constipation, *Gastroenterol Nurs* 26(6):251-260, 2003.

61. Talley N: Definitions, epidemiology, and impact of chronic constipation, *Rev Gastroenterol Disord* 4(suppl 2): S3-S10, 2004.

62. Prather C: Subtypes of constipation: sorting out the confusion, *Rev Gastroenterol Disord* 4(suppl 2):S11-S16, 2004.

63. Klaschik E, Nauck F, Ostgathe C: Constipation: modern laxative therapy, *Support Care Cancer* 11(11):679-685, 2003.

64. Benton J, O'Hara P, Chen H, et al: Changing bowel hygiene practice successfully: a program to reduce laxative use in a chronic care hospital, *Geriatr Nurs* 18(1): 12-17, 1997.

65. Oullett L, Turner T, Pond S, et al: Dietary fiber and laxation in postop orthopedic patients, *Clin Nurs Res* 5(4):428-440, 1996.

66. Voderholzer W, Schatke W, Muhldorfer B, et al: Clinical response to dietary fiber treatment of chronic constipation, *Am J Gastroenterol* 92(1):95-98, 1997.

67. Holzer P: Opioids and opioid receptors in the enteric nervous system: from a problem in opioid analgesia to a possible new prokinetic in humans, *Neurosci Lett* 361 (1-3):192-195, 2004.

68. Castro D, Cherry D: Extracolonic causes of constipation. In: Wexner S, Bartolo D, editors: *Constipation: etiology, evaluation, and management,* Boston: Butterworth-Heinemann, 1995.

69. Chelimsky G, Chelimsky T: Evaluation and treatment of autonomic disorders of the gastrointestinal tract, *Semin Neurol* 23(4):453-458, 2003.

70. De Giorgio R, Guerrini S, Barbara G, et al: New insights into human enteric neuropathies, *Neurogastoenterol Motil* 16(suppl 1):143-147, 2004.

71. Crowell M, Shetzline M, Moses P, et al: Enterochromaffin cells and 5-HT signaling in the pathophysiology of disorders of gastrointestinal function, *Curr Opin Invest Drugs* 5(1):55-60, 2004.

72. Evans B, Clark W, Moore D, Whorwell P: Tegaserod for the treatment of irritable bowel syndrome, *Cochrane Database Syst Rev* 4, 2004.

73. Varga G, Balint A, Burghardt B, D'Amato M: Involvement of endogenous CCK and CCK1 receptors in colonic motor function, *Br J Pharmacol* 141(8): 1275-1284, 2004.

74. Bassotti G, Chistolini F, Sietchiping-Nzepa F, et al: Biofeedback for pelvic floor dysfunction in constipation, *BMJ* 328(7436):393-396, 2004.

75. Sanmiguel C, Soffer E: Constipation caused by functional outlet obstruction, *Curr Gastroenterol Rep* 5(5):414-418, 2003.

76. Cheung O, Wald A: Review article: the management of pelvic floor disorders, *Aliment Pharmacol Ther* 19: 481-495, 2004.

77. Zbar A, Lienemann A, Fritsch H, et al: Rectocele: pathogenesis and surgical management, *Int J Colorectal Dis* 18(5):369-384, 2003.

78. Bijkerk C, Muris J, Knottnerus J, et al: Systematic review: the role of different types of fibre in the treatment of irritable bowel syndrome, *Aliment Pharmacol Ther* 19:245-251, 2004.

79. Scarlett Y: Medical management of fecal incontinence, *Gastroenterology* 126:S55-S63, 2004.

80. Yuan C: Clinical status of methylnaltrexone, a new agent to prevent and manage opioid-induced side effects, *J Support Oncol* 2(2):111-117, 2004.

81. Goossens D, Jonkers D, Stobberingh E, et al: Probiotics in gastroenterology: indications and future perspectives, *Scand J Gastroenterol* Suppl 239:15-23, 2003.

82. Hamilton-Miller J: Probiotics and prebiotics in the elderly, *Postgrad Med J* 80(946):447-451, 2004.

83. American College of Gastroenterology Functional Disorders Task Force: Evidence-based position statement on the management of irritable bowel syndrome in North America, *Am J Gastroenterol* 97:S1-S5, 2002.

84. Drossman D, Andruzzi E, Temple R, et al: US householder survey of functional gastrointestinal disorders: prevalence, sociodemography, and health impact, *Dig Dis Sci* 38:1569-1580, 1993.

85. Sandler R, Everhart J, Donowitz M, et al: The burden of selected digestive diseases in the United States, *Gastroenterology* 122:1500-1511, 2002.

86. Levy R, Von Korff M, Whitehead W, et al: Costs of care for irritable bowel syndrome patients in a health maintenance organization, *Am J Gastroenterol* 96:3122-3129, 2001.

87. Brandt L, Bjorkman D, Fennerty M, et al: Systematic review on the management of irritable bowel syndrome in North America, *Am J Gastroenterol* 97:S7-S26, 2002.

88. Drossman D, Camilleri M, Mayer E, et al: AGA technical review on irritable bowel syndrome, *Gastroenterology* 123:2108-2131, 2002.

89. Leong S, Barghout V, Birnbaum H, et al: The economic consequences of irritable bowel syndrome: a US employer perspective, *Arch Intern Med* 163:929-935, 2003.

90. Feld A, Von Korff M, Levy R, et al: Excess surgery in irritable bowel syndrome (IBS), *Gastroenterology* 124:388, 2003.

91. Whitehead W, Burnett C, Cook E III, et al: Impact of irritable bowel syndrome on quality of life, *Dig Dis Sci* 41:2248-2253, 1996.

92. Lee O, Mayer E, Schmulson M, et al: Gender-related differences in IBS symptoms, *Am J Gastroenterol* 96:2184-2193, 2001.

93. Chang L, Heitkemper M: Gender differences in irritable bowel syndrome, *Gastroenterology* 123:1686-1690, 2002.

94. Heitkemper M, Cain K, Jarrett M, et al: Symptoms across the menstrual cycle in women with irritable bowel syndrome, *Am J Gastroenterol* 98:420-430, 2003.

95. Floch M, Narayan R: Diet in the irritable bowel syndrome, *J Clin Gastroenterol* 35(1 suppl):S45-52, 2002.

96. Camilleri M, Spiller R: *Irritable bowel syndrome: diagnosis and treatment,* Philadelphia, 2002, WB Saunders.

97. Chey W, Jin H, Lee M, et al: Colonic motility abnormality in patients with irritable bowel syndrome exhibiting abdominal pain and diarrhea, *Am J Gastroenterol* 96(5):1499-1506, 2001.

98. Clemens C, Samsom M, Roelofs J, et al: Association between pain episodes and high amplitude propagated pressure waves in patients with irritable bowel syndrome, *Am J Gastroenterol* 98:1838-1843, 2003.

99. Silverman D, Munakata J, Ennes H, et al: Reginal cerebral activity in normal and pathological perception of visceral pain, *Gastroenterology* 112:64-72, 1997.

100. Mayer E, Naliboff B, Munakata J: The evolving neurobiology of gut feelings, *Prog Brain Res* 122:195-206, 2000.

101. Chang L, Berman S, Mayer E, et al: Brain responses to visceral and somatic stimuli in patients with irritable bowel syndrome with and without fibromyalgia, *Am J Gastroenterol* 98(6):1354-1361, 2003.

102. Spiller R: Postinfectious irritable bowel syndrome, *Gastroenterology* 124(6):1662-1671, 2003.

103. Parry S, Stansfield R, Jelley D, et al: Does bacterial gastroenteritis predispose people to functional gastrointestinal disorders? A prospective, community-based, case-control study, *Am J Gastroenterol* 98(9):1970-1975, 2003.

104. Thompson J, Elsenbruch S, Harnish M, et al: Autonomic functioning during REM sleep differentiates IBS symptom subgroups, *Am J Gastroenterol* 97(12):3147-3153, 2002.

105. Aggarwal A, Cutts T, Abell T, et al: Predominant symptoms in irritable bowel syndrome correlate with specific autonomic nervous system abnormalities, *Gastroenterology* 106(4):945-950, 1994.

106. Lydiard R: Irritable bowel syndrome, anxiety, and depression: what are the links? *J Clin Psychiatry* 62(suppl 8):38-45, 2001.

107. Folks D: The interface of psychiatry and irritable bowel syndrome, *Curr Psychiatr Rep* 6(3):210-215, 2004.

108. Blanchard E, Keefer L, Lackner J, et al: The role of childhood abuse in axis I and axis II psychiatric disorders and medical disorders of unknown origin among irritable bowel syndrome patients, *J Psychosom Res* 56(4):431-436, 2004.

109. Ringel Y, Whitehead W, Toner B, et al: Sexual and physical abuse are not associated with rectal hypersensitivity in patients with irritable bowel syndrome, *Gut* 53(6):838-842, 2004.

110. Dobie D, Kivlahan D, Maynard C, et al: Posttraumatic stress disorder in female veterans: association with self-reported health problems and functional impairment, *Arch Intern Med* 164(4):394-400, 2004.

111. Drossman D, Toner B, Whitehead W, et al: Cognitive-behavioral therapy versus education and desipramine versus placebo for moderate to severe functional bowel disorders, *Gastroenterology* 125(1):19-31, 2003.

112. Heitkemper M, Jarrett M, Levy R, et al: Self-management for women with irritable bowel syndrome, *Clin Gastroenterol Hepatol* 2(7):585-596, 2004.

113. Lembo A, Olden K, Ameen V, et al: Effect of alosetron on bowel urgency and global symptoms in women with severe, diarrhea-predominant irritable bowel syndrome: analysis of two controlled trials, *Clin Gastroenterol Hepatol* 2(8):675-682, 2004.

114. Nyhlin H, Bang C, Elsborg L, et al: A double-blind, placebo-controlled, randomized study to evaluate the efficacy, safety, and tolerability of tegaserod in patients with irritable bowel syndrome, *Scand J Gastroenterol* 39(2):119-126, 2004.

115. Kuiken S, Tytgat G, Boeckxstaens G: The selective serotonin reuptake inhibitor fluoxetine does not change rectal sensitivity and symptoms in patients with irritable bowel syndrome: a double-blind, randomized, placebo-controlled study, *Clin Gastroenterol Hepatol* 1(3):219-228, 2003.

116. Johanson J: Fecal incontinence. In: Johanson J, editor: *Gastrointestinal diseases: risk factors and prevention,* Philadelphia: 1997, Lippincott-Raven.

117. Hoffmann B, Timmcke E, Gaithright J Jr, et al: Fecal seepage and soiling: a problem of rectal sensation, *Dis Colon Rectum* 38(6):746-748, 1995.

118. Sentovich S, Rivela L, Blatchford G, et al: Patterns of male fecal incontinence, *Dis Colon Rectum* 38(3):281-285, 1995.

119. Nelson R: Epidemiology of fecal incontinence, *Gastroenterology* 126:S3-S7, 2004.

120. Schnelle J, Leung F: Urinary and fecal incontinence in nursing homes, *Gastroenterology* 126:S41-S47, 2004.

121. Bharucha A: Outcome measures for fecal incontinence: anorectal structure and function, *Gastroenterology* 126:S90-S98, 2004.

122. Shelton A, Welton M: The pelvic floor in health and disease, *West J Med* 167(2):90-98, 1997.

123. Rao S: Pathophysiology of adult fecal incontinence, *Gastroenterology* 126:S14-S22, 2004.

124. Sagar P, Pemberton J: Anorectal and pelvic floor function: relevance to continence, incontinence, and constipation, *Gastroenterol Clin North Am* 25(1):163-179, 1996.

125. Sangwan Y, Coller J, Schoetz D, et al: Spectrum of abnormal rectoanal reflex patterns in patients with fecal incontinence, *Dis Colon Rectum* 39(1):59-65, 1996.

126. Sultan A: Anal incontinence after childbirth, *Curr Opin Obstet Gynecol* 9:320-324, 1997.

127. Meshkinpour H, Movahedi H, Welgan P: Clinical value of anorectal manometry index in neurogenic fecal incontinence, *Dis Colon Rectum* 40(6):457-461, 1997.

128. Norton C: Behavioral management of fecal incontinence in adults, *Gastroenterology* 126:S64-S70, 2004.

129. Rasmussen O, Christiansen J: Physiology and pathophysiology of anal function, *Scand J Gastroenterol Suppl* 31:169-174, 1996.

130. Chun A, Rose S, Mitrani C, et al: Anal sphincter structure and function in homosexual males engaging in

anoreceptive intercourse, *Am J Gastroenterol* 92: 465-468, 1997.

131. Krogh K, Nielsen J, Djurhuus J, et al: Colorectal function in patients with spinal cord lesions, *Dis Colon Rectum* 40(10):1233-1239, 1997.

132. Gee A, Durdey P: Urge incontinence of faeces is a marker of severe external anal sphincter dysfunction, *Br J Surg* 82:1179-1182, 1995.

133. Roig J, Villosalad C, Lledo S, et al: Prevalence of pudendal neuropathy in fecal incontinence: results of a prospective study, *Dis Colon Rectum* 38(9):952-958, 1995.

134. Rose S, Wald A: Fecal incontinence. In: Snape WJ Jr, editor: *Consultations in gastroenterology,* Philadelphia, 1996, WB Saunders.

CHAPTER

15

Assessment and Management of the Patient with Fecal Incontinence and Related Bowel Dysfunction

DOROTHY B. DOUGHTY & LINDA L. JENSEN

OBJECTIVES

1. Describe the impact of fecal incontinence on quality of life and implications for management.
2. Identify major risk factors for fecal incontinence and explain why fecal incontinence is more common among women and the elderly.
3. Explain the difference between passive incontinence and incontinence associated with fecal urgency.
4. Explain the relationship between fecal incontinence and diarrhea or constipation.
5. Identify critical data to be included in the interview, physical examination, and bowel chart for the patient with fecal incontinence.
6. Identify patients who would benefit from additional testing, such as anorectal physiology testing, defecography, endoanal ultrasonography, or magnetic resonance imaging.
7. Explain the effect of impacted stool on anorectal function and identify options for disimpaction and colonic cleansing.
8. Identify dietary modifications and pharmacologic agents that can be used to reduce stool volume and improve stool consistency in the patient with diarrhea.
9. Identify advantages and disadvantages of perianal pouching systems and internal drainage systems for containment of liquid stool in the incontinent patient.
10. Define the term "elimination diet" and explain its role in management of the patient with chronic diarrhea.
11. Explain why bulking agents may be of benefit to patients with diarrhea and patients with constipation.
12. Describe key elements to be included in behavioral programs designed to improve bowel control and bowel function.
13. Identify indications and key elements of stimulated defecation programs.
14. Explain the role of biofeedback in the management of fecal incontinence.
15. Explain how sacral nerve stimulation improves anorectal function and fecal continence.
16. Identify patients who would benefit from each of the following surgical procedures: sphincter repair, anal encirclement, artificial anal sphincter, antegrade continence enema (ACE) procedure, and colostomy.

Fecal incontinence is the loss of voluntary control of passage of liquid or solid stool.[1] It can be further classified based on sensory awareness and the type and volume of leakage; *passive incontinence* is the term sometimes used to describe unrecognized leakage of stool, *urge incontinence* denotes leakage of stool associated with fecal urgency and occurring despite the individual's efforts to retain the stool, and *seepage and soiling* refer to leakage of small amounts of stool that stain the underwear and that occurs without the individual's awareness.[2-4] Whether or not involuntary passage of flatus should be incorporated into the definition of fecal incontinence is controversial; most authors limit use of the term *fecal incontinence* to loss of stool and use the term *anal incontinence* to include involuntary passage of gas, liquid, or solid stool.[1,2]

PREVALENCE

It is very difficult to accurately determine the prevalence of fecal incontinence, due in large part

457

to patients' reluctance to discuss the problem or to seek medical assistance.[5-7] Population-based prevalence studies yield widely varying prevalence rates, because of differences in survey method, sample population, and the definition of fecal incontinence. The prevalence among the general population is thought to range from 2% to 7%, although prevalence among the community-dwelling elderly may be as high as 17%.[6,8,9] The prevalence is highest among the institutionalized elderly, in whom it approaches 50%;[7,10,11] the high prevalence among this group is partly the result of the effects of dementia and immobility, which are common among these individuals, but it may also be a reflection of the fact that fecal incontinence is a common reason for institutionalization.[5,7,12] Among younger adults, fecal incontinence is much more common in women than in men; however, the prevalence among men rises with advancing age.[7,12]

IMPACT ON QUALITY OF LIFE

Fecal incontinence has a profound impact on quality of life and can result in severe restriction of usual activities such as dining out, engaging in sexual activity, or even going to work or school. Patients report high levels of anxiety related to the threat of recurrent incontinent episodes, embarrassment, and shame over their lack of bowel control, and depression. Some individuals become essentially homebound in their efforts to avoid incontinent episodes and public humiliation.[2,3,5,13] Because incontinence is a "taboo" subject, most individuals do not realize that their condition is both common and treatable; thus, many never seek treatment. The lack of knowledge regarding fecal incontinence among health care providers is a contributing problem; many providers fail to screen for incontinence because they believe they have nothing to offer the patient or because they do not realize that fecal incontinence is fairly common among community-dwelling adults.

RISK FACTORS FOR FECAL INCONTINENCE

Normal bowel function and fecal continence are complex phenomena that involve a number of physiologic mechanisms; fecal *incontinence* occurs when one or more of these mechanisms is disrupted to the extent that the remaining mechanisms are unable to compensate and maintain continence.[14,15] Risk factors for fecal incontinence can be classified as factors interfering with normal bowel motility, factors that interfere with sensory awareness of rectal distension, conditions resulting in damage to the nerves or muscles of the anorectal sphincter mechanism, and conditions that alter rectal capacity or compliance (Table 15-1). Specific risk factors include the following:

- *Diarrhea.* Diarrhea is an independent risk factor for fecal incontinence, especially for the patient with a compromised anorectal sphincter mechanism (because a weak sphincter is more competent for formed stool than for liquid stool); thus, the young woman who has sustained sphincter damage during childbirth is more likely to experience incontinence during episodes of diarrhea. In addition, diarrheal conditions producing large volume liquid stools or intense fecal urgency can overwhelm a completely normal continence mechanism; for example, hospitalized patients with large-volume diarrhea secondary to a *Clostridium difficile* infection and individuals with diarrhea-predominant irritable bowel syndrome may experience fecal incontinence if they are unable to reach the toilet in a timely manner.[7,10,11,15,16]

- *Constipation.* Chronic constipation is also an independent risk factor for incontinence; chronic constipation frequently results in "overflow fecal leakage" caused by a chronically distended rectum and reflex inhibition of the internal anal sphincter. The likelihood of incontinence is further increased by the fact that *chronic* rectal distension fails to activate the nerve pathways that normally create sensory awareness of rectal fullness and the urge to defecate; thus, the individual is unaware of impending leakage.[5,10,11,16]

- *Childbirth injuries to anorectal sphincter mechanism and/or pudendal nerve.* Vaginal delivery is the *major* risk factor for sphincter disruption and traction injury to the pudendal nerve. Obstetric trauma to the anorectal sphincter and pudendal nerve has been documented to occur in up to one-third of primiparous women, although most of these women remain asymptomatic until later in life or experience incontinence only during episodes

TABLE 15-1   **Functional Classification of Risk Factors for Fecal Incontinence**

FUNCTIONAL FACTOR	SPECIFIC RISK FACTORS
Normal bowel motility	Diarrheal conditions (infectious diarrhea; irritable bowel syndrome) Constipation/impaction Diabetes mellitus
Sensory awareness of rectal distension	Obstetric trauma causing pudendal neuropathy Neurologic lesions (spinal cord injury) Chronic rectal distension Dementia Diabetes mellitus
Normal sphincter function	Obstetric trauma causing disruption or denervation of sphincter Anorectal surgery or trauma Neurologic lesions (spinal cord injury) Dementia Aging (possible risk factor)
Normal rectal capacity and compliance	Inflammatory conditions such as radiation proctitis or inflammatory bowel disease Chronic rectal distension
Ability to use the toilet independently	Dementia Immobility

of diarrhea. Specific risk factors for childbirth-related injuries include forceps or suction delivery, infant birth weight greater than 4 kg, delivery of an infant in the occiput posterior position, and episiotomy.[5,7,9,15-17]

- *Anorectal surgery or trauma.* Impalement injuries, pelvic fractures, and anorectal surgical procedures can cause direct damage to the nerves and muscles of the anorectal sphincter mechanism. Surgical procedures that may result in fecal incontinence include sphincterotomy, fistulectomy, anal dilatation, and hemorrhoidectomy.[7,15] The newer sphincter-saving operations, such as low anterior resection and ileal pouch anal anastomosis, also place the individual at increased risk for incontinence (although they eliminate the need for a permanent stoma); the risk of incontinence is related to nerve and sphincter damage incurred during the anorectal dissection and coloanal or ilealanal anastomosis, as well as to loss of the rectal reservoir (in patients undergoing low anterior resection).[5,7,15,16]

- *Neurologic lesions such as spinal cord injury.* Fecal continence is dependent on prompt recognition of rectal distension and on an innervated and normally contractile external anal sphincter; any lesion or condition that interferes with normal transmission of neurologic signals from the anorectum to the cortex (and vice versa) results in loss of the ability to sense and delay impending defecation. Common neurologic lesions resulting in fecal incontinence include spina bifida with myelomeningocele, spinal cord injury, and multiple sclerosis.[5,7]

- *Dementia.* Alterations in mental status compromise the individual's ability to recognize rectal distension and to respond in a socially appropriate manner, by moving to the toilet or by contracting the external sphincter to delay defecation. Dementia and immobility are consistently shown to be the primary risk factors for fecal incontinence among the institutionalized elderly.[11,15]

- *Damage to the pudendal nerve (stretch neuropathy).* As noted, intact nerve pathways and normal innervation are essential to continence; any damage to the nerves signaling rectal distension or providing for external sphincter contraction place the individual at risk for leakage. Stretch injuries to the pudendal nerve are common sequelae of childbirth injury, and they may also occur secondary to excessive perineal descent and chronic straining at stool; these injuries can result in sphincteric weakness and delayed recognition of rectal distension.[5,15]

- *Diabetes mellitus.* Fecal incontinence is much more common among individuals with diabetes mellitus, probably because of a combination of factors including altered sensory function, changes in colonic motility, and changes in anorectal function. The link between diabetes mellitus and fecal incontinence is of particular concern, given the rising incidence of diabetes and the significant impact of fecal incontinence on quality of life and functional status; this is an area in which additional research is desperately needed and of profound importance.[4,7,9]

- *Immobility.* The preservation of fecal continence is dependent in part on the ability to move to the toilet in a timely manner, and studies indicate that general debilitation and immobility are major risk factors for fecal incontinence among the institutionalized elderly. The impact of immobility is further underscored by data indicating that the use of restraints is the most significant risk factor for the new onset of fecal incontinence among nursing home residents.[7,11]

- *Aging.* All epidemiologic studies related to fecal incontinence reflect a marked increase among the elderly, partly because elders are at increased risk for dementia and immobility. However, there is an increased prevalence of fecal incontinence even among mobile and cognitively intact elders living in the community. These data suggest that changes related to aging may compromise sphincter function or other elements essential to continence, and some data do suggest a reduction in maximum "squeeze pressure" among the elderly. Interestingly, squeeze pressures are consistently lower in women than in men, with significant reductions in sphincter contractility following menopause; reduced squeeze pressures in postmenopausal women are consistent with human studies indicating that the external sphincter contains estrogen receptors and animal studies demonstrating atrophy of the striated sphincter following oophorectomy.[9,15]

Successful management of the patient with fecal incontinence requires the clinician to understand normal function and factors contributing to incontinence, to utilize this understanding as a basis for comprehensive assessment of each patient, and to establish an individualized management plan designed to correct or compensate for areas of dysfunction. The continence nurse can play a key role in the assessment and management of these patients.

ASSESSMENT OF BOWEL FUNCTION

The assessment of any individual with fecal incontinence must include a thorough history, a focused physical examination, and completion and analysis of a bowel chart. Patients with complex clinical pictures and patients who are refractory to primary interventions may require additional studies, such as anorectal manometry, endoanal ultrasound, pelvic magnetic resonance imaging (MRI), or defecography (Box 15-1).

Patient History

The assessment begins with a thorough history, which provides much of the data on which the diagnosis and management plan are based. The history should be obtained in a quiet, relaxed environment by someone who understands normal bowel function and is therefore prepared to conduct a meaningful interview. It is important for the interviewer to establish good rapport with the patient and to use simple, clear language and direct, focused questions to elicit a comprehensive picture of the patient's bowel function and continence issues. The clinician must realize that it is very difficult for most individuals to talk openly about problems with bowel control, even to a continence specialist. It is common for patients to report problems with "diarrhea," "itching," or "urgency" rather than incontinence; thus, any report of bowel dysfunction or anorectal symptoms must be followed by direct questions regarding any problems with bowel control. The clinician must also be aware that patients may lack the vocabulary to describe their problem in "medical" terms; it is

BOX 15-1   Key Elements in Patient Assessment

History
- Current problem/impact on quality of life/goals for treatment
- Review of pertinent systems (neurologic, gastrointestinal, endocrine, urologic)

Physical Examination
- Abdominal exam
- Pelvic exam
- Anorectal exam

Bowel Diary

Anorectal Physiology Testing as Indicated
- Anorectal manometry
- Sphincter mapping via endoanal ultrasound and anal magnetic resonance imaging

---

frequently helpful to give the patient "permission" to use nonmedical words such as "fart" and "poop." At times, it may be necessary to involve the patient's family or caregiver in the interview. Again, the intent is to obtain a clear picture of the current problems as well as the relevant history.[3,18]

The history should include both complaint-specific and general health information. It is usually best to begin with an exploration of the current bowel problem, because it is this concern that has led the patient to seek care. The interviewer should inquire about the onset of the problem with incontinence and should obtain detailed information regarding the specifics and severity of the problem, as well as any precipitating factors associated with the onset of the incontinence. Specifically the interviewer should question the patient regarding the usual frequency, consistency, and volume of voluntary bowel movements, the frequency, consistency, and volume of any incontinent stools, and the ability to control flatus. The patient should be asked to compare his or her present bowel function and control to his or her baseline "normal" function, that is, function and control before the onset of the current problem. The patient should also be asked to identify any factors or events associated with the onset of the incontinence, such as surgery, injury, or a change in medications, diet, or activity. The patient should be specifically asked about sensory awareness of the urge to defecate or pass flatus, the ability to delay defecation or to control flatus, and factors that affect the ability to delay defecation (such as the consistency of the stool). It is also important to query the patient regarding any associated symptoms or phenomena, such as intense fecal urgency and frequency or the passage of blood or tissue. All these questions are important because the answers provide insight into the specific mechanisms contributing to *this* individual's incontinence, such as chronic diarrhea, blunted sensation, or the inability to delay defecation. In addition, positive responses to queries regarding associated symptoms may indicate a more serious problem; for example, the patient with severe urgency and frequency may have inflammatory bowel disease, and the patient with altered bowel function and rectal bleeding may have a neoplasm. Any patient with symptoms suggestive of an underlying disorder must be promptly referred for further workup.[3,18]

In addition to gathering data regarding the specifics of the problem, the interviewer must explore with the patient his or her current bowel management plan and the effect of the incontinence on his or her health status and life style. For example, the patient should be asked about any changes in diet or activity resulting from the incontinence and should be asked to describe the measures currently used to deal with the problem; this may include avoidance of food and fluid intake, constipating diets, or enemas to control the time of elimination, laxatives to correct constipation, absorbent products and deodorants for fecal containment, or activity restrictions to prevent incontinence in public. The interviewer should also ask about factors that affect bowel function, such as daily intake of fiber and fluids, prescription and over-the-counter medications, and activity level. Finally, the patient should be encouraged to share his or her feelings about the incontinence, the impact on quality of life, and goals for treatment (Fig. 15-1). It is helpful to use validated severity scales and quality of life scales to quantify the severity of

Control

1. What problems are you having related to bowel control?

   ___Urgency ___Leakage ___Major accidents ___Other (describe)

2. How often do you usually have a bowel movement?

   _____

3. What is the usual consistency of your stool?

   ___Small hard pellets ___Hard lumps ___Formed and firm

   ___Formed and soft ___Mushy ___Liquid ___Variable

4. Can you tell when you need to have a bowel movement?

   ___Always ___Usually ___Sometimes ___Never

5. Can you differentiate between gas, liquid, and solid rectal contents?

   ___Always ___Usually ___Sometimes ___Never

6. Can you "hold" the stool till you get to the toilet?

   ___Always ___Usually ___Sometimes ___Never

   How long can you usually "hold" the stool?

   ___< 1 minute ___1 to 5 minutes ___5 to 10 minutes ___As long as I need to

   Can you "hold" both liquid and solid stool?

   ___Yes ___I can hold solid but not liquid ___I can't hold either solid or liquid

7. How often do you use the following bowel control aids?

	Regularly (> once a week)	Occasionally (< once a week)	Rarely (< once a month)
Enemas	_____	_____	_____
Bulking agents	_____	_____	_____

Fig. 15-1 Screening questionnaire for fecal incontinence.

Antidiarrheal medications			
Pads to manage leakage			

8. How does your bowel problem affect your ability to do the things you like to do?

___Not at all

___A little

___Some

___A lot

9. What are your goals for treatment?

_____

_____

10. Comments:_____

_____

Fig. 15-1, cont'd. Screening questionnaire for fecal incontinence.

the incontinence, and its impact, at baseline; these data provide a basis for determining the effects of treatment. Severity scales assign numeric values to factors such as the frequency and type of incontinence, the need to utilize absorptive products, and the need to make life-style changes; the individual numeric values are then totaled to produce an overall severity score.[5,13,18] Quality of life should be assessed separately, because there is *not* a direct correlation between the severity of the incontinence and its impact on the individual's quality of life. An incontinence-specific quality of life scale is now available that measures the impact of the incontinence on life style, coping and behavior, depression and self-concept, and embarrassment.[5,19]

In addition to the complaint-specific history, the interviewer must obtain a focused medical-surgical history. This should include a brief review of systems and conditions affecting bowel function and includes the following: neurologic conditions, such as back or spinal cord surgery or trauma, or diabetic neuropathy; obstetric history, with a focus on traumatic deliveries and vaginal tears; anorectal surgery or trauma; abdominal or pelvic surgery or radiation; coexisting urinary incontinence; and gastrointestinal disorders affecting intestinal motility or stool consistency. The assessment should include a review of all medications currently being taken by the patient, a thorough dietary history, and an evaluation of the patient's general mobility and dexterity, cognition, and motivation. An environmental assessment is also important, with a focus on toilet access; this is especially important for the patient with limitations in mobility and dexterity.[3,5] Standardized assessment tools assist the interviewer in capturing all the critical information, and there are many of these available.[20,21] One example of a standardized universal health assessment tool is the Short Form (SF)-36. These standardized tools may be used by the professional to guide the history or may be given to the patient to complete.

Bowel diary. A bowel diary provides valuable objective data regarding the patient's bowel elimination patterns (that is, frequency, volume, and consistency of both voluntary and involuntary stools). Fig. 15-2 outlines the data provided. Ideally, the patient maintains the bowel diary for at least 1 to 2 weeks before beginning treatment; the diary is then continued during treatment to permit ongoing assessment of progress in establishing normal bowel patterns and control. Data from the bowel diary can provide much of the information required to generate a severity score.[18]

Physical Examination

As noted earlier, the health history should include data regarding the patient's mobility, dexterity, and cognition. These data should be confirmed during the physical examination. In addition, the examiner should carefully inspect, percuss, and palpate the abdomen to detect any evidence of colonic distension secondary to retained stool; indicators of a "loaded colon" include distension, dullness to percussion in most or all quadrants, and palpable stool in the left lower quadrant. Abdominal palpation is also used to rule out any palpable mass; the patient with a palpable mass is promptly referred for further evaluation. However, the *primary* focus

of the physical examination is a thorough assessment of the perianal area, anal canal, and rectal vault. These components of the physical examination are described in more detail.

Visual Inspection of Perineum and Perianal Skin. The perineum should be assessed for overall anatomic integrity; specifically the clinician should look for a thinned or deformed perineal body (the triangular body of tissue between the vaginal introitus and the anus) and for any scars suggesting previous surgery or trauma. The clinician should then ask the patient to bear down as if attempting to defecate, to rule out pelvic organ prolapse and excessive perineal descent (defined as descent to a level 2 to 3 cm below the ischial tuberosities). The buttocks should then be gently spread to permit inspection of the perianal area and the anus. The perianal area is inspected for fecal soiling, hemorrhoids, and alterations in skin integrity caused by chronic fecal leakage (dermatitis, denudation, erythema, or maceration). The anus is inspected for any evidence of denervation or sphincter damage; normally the anus is closed circumferentially, and a patulous anus is usually indicative of impaired innervation or of sphincter damage. When low resting tone is suspected, as in the patient with postdefecation soiling, the clinician should apply gentle traction adjacent to the anus; gaping is commonly seen in the patient with diminished sphincter tone. The examiner should then gently stroke the perianal skin with a finger or pin at the 9 o'clock and 3 o'clock positions. This maneuver normally elicits the "anal wink," or visible contraction of the anal sphincter, and absence of this response is usually

BOWEL DIARY

Date/time	Voluntary bowel movements (amount and consistency)	Incontinent stools (amount/consistency)	Comments

Fig. 15-2 Bowel diary.

indicative of a neurologic deficit. The patient is then instructed to squeeze or tighten the anus ("as if trying not to pass gas") and to strain or bear down ("as if trying to pass stool") while the examiner watches for any evidence of dysfunction. For example, straining may reveal the presence of rectal prolapse or anterior displacement of the anal canal (which is suggestive of disruption of the sphincter muscle), and an inability to contract the anal sphincter on command may indicate a neurologic deficit or damage to the muscle itself.[3,5,18,22] If rectal prolapse is suspected but not visualized during the Valsalva maneuver with the patient in the supine or sidelying position, the patient should be positioned on the toilet and should be instructed to lean forward and bear down; the clinician can then inspect or palpate for rectal prolapse.[18]

Digital Examination of the Anal Canal and Rectum.

The digital anorectal examination is performed to rule out a possible rectal tumor, to assess for fecal impaction, and to evaluate the function of the pelvic floor musculature. Evaluation of muscle function includes assessment of resting tone, contractile function, and relaxation function. Resting tone is evaluated during finger insertion and before having the patient perform active contraction and relaxation. Normal sphincter tone provides symmetric circumferential resistance to finger insertion and tension around the examining finger. The patient is then asked to "tighten around my finger as if trying to hold my finger in or trying not to pass gas." The normal response is an exaggeration of the resting state, that is, strong symmetric and circumferential contraction; the clinician should assess the patient's ability to maintain the contraction as well as the strength of the contraction. The patient is next instructed to "relax and push down as if trying to push out my finger or have a bowel movement." The normal response is sphincter relaxation and a downward push felt by the examining finger. There are several "abnormal" patterns that indicate the need for further evaluation, such as anorectal physiology testing. These include diminished sphincter resistance and compromised contractility, localized sphincter defects (evidenced by asymmetrical contraction), or abnormalities in pelvic floor function (evidenced by full-thickness rectal prolapse, rectocele, or excessive perineal descent). A careful digital examination may also reveal nonrelaxing puborectalis syndrome, which involves persistent contraction of the sphincter throughout the "bearing-down" (Valsalva) maneuver. This failure of sphincter relaxation is usually responsive to biofeedback therapy, as discussed later in this chapter.[3,5,18,22]

Digital anorectal exam is considered a key element of the physical examination for any patient with fecal incontinence, and it typically yields valuable insight into the mechanisms contributing to the incontinence; for example, reduced strength or duration of voluntary sphincter contraction has been found to correlate with fecal urgency and difficulty in delaying defecation, and absence of voluntary sphincter contraction clearly indicates a damaged or denervated sphincter mechanism. However, the examiner should be aware that clinician estimates of resting tone and squeeze pressures do not correlate well with any *objective* measures of sphincter function, and there are no validated scales for assessing sphincter contractility and endurance. Thus, the clinician should not hesitate to suggest anorectal physiology testing for any patient with inconclusive findings on physical exam and for any patient who fails to respond to conservative management.[18]

Anorectal Physiologic Studies.

Anorectal physiology testing provides a quantitative assessment of the complex mechanisms involved in maintenance of continence.[23] Ideally, these tests should meet the following criteria: (1) provide dynamic information about the function of each mechanism involved in fecal continence; (2) mimic the situations that pose a threat to continence; that is, function as stress tests for the continence mechanisms; (3) provide guidance in selection of treatment options; (4) create little or no discomfort for the patient; and (5) avoid interference with normal anorectal function.

Many different tests can be used to assess anorectal physiology; the tests most commonly used include anorectal manometry, endoanal ultrasonography and MRI to "map" the sphincters, pudendal nerve terminal motor latency (PNTML) and anal electromyography (EMG), and defecography. The most valuable of these tests appear to be anorectal manometry and endoanal ultrasound/MRI imaging of the sphincters; some studies indicate that the addition of these studies to the history and physical either confirm the initial impression or provide a corrected diagnosis in most patients.[3] Accurate identification of the causative factors for the incontinence helps the clinician to determine which patients can be managed with behavioral therapies and/or medications and which patients are likely to benefit from surgical intervention (such as repair of a damaged sphincter, rectal prolapse, or rectocele, or construction of a diverting stoma)[24] (Table 15-2).

Anorectal manometry. Anorectal manometry provides an objective measurement of anorectal sensation, the rectoanal inhibitory reflex, the pressures generated by the sphincter complex, and the length of the anal canal.[5] To obtain these measurements, a small-diameter catheter (usually water perfused or solid state) is inserted through the anal canal into the rectum. This catheter contains pressure transducers that transmit pressure recordings from four points within the anal canal (the anterior wall, the posterior wall, and the left and right sidewalls). The catheter is connected to a computer that records the transmitted pressures. A balloon is attached to the rectal end of the catheter (Fig. 15-3) and is inflated with air after the catheter has been passed into the rectum.

The test of anorectal sensation is conducted as follows: the patient is asked to report the first sensation of rectal filling (or of something in the rectum) and the point at which the rectum feels full and the patient feels the need to defecate. The rectal balloon is then gradually inflated, and the volumes required to trigger "first sensation" and "full sensation" are noted. Normal first sensation occurs at 20 to 40 mL of filling.[13] The rectoanal inhibitory reflex can also be evaluated during the test of rectal sensation; an intact reflex is demonstrated by a drop in resting anal canal pressures in response to rectal distension (inflation of the intrarectal balloon).[5,13]

The pressures generated by the sphincter complex are measured while the patient is "at rest," while the patient is voluntarily "squeezing" the external anal sphincter ("as if to hold in gas or a bowel movement"), and during a Valsalva maneuver.

TABLE 15-2 Anorectal Physiology Testing: Implications for Treatment

FUNCTIONAL FACTOR	ABNORMAL TEST RESULTS	IMPLICATIONS
Anorectal sensation	Anorectal sensory testing: Diminished sensory function/delay in recognition of rectal distension Urgency at low volumes	Sensory reeducation: Biofeedback programs to increase sensory awareness Reeducation to reduce urgency
Sphincter integrity	Endoanal ultrasound and/or anorectal magnetic resonance imaging: Anatomic disruption of one or both sphincters	Surgical repair (sphincteroplasty) OR Sphincter retraining with or without biofeedback OR Sacral nerve stimulation
Sphincter function	Anorectal manometry Diminished resting tone Diminished "squeeze" pressure Inability to "hold" sphincter contraction Total inability to contract sphincter voluntarily	Sphincter retraining with or without biofeedback OR Sacral nerve stimulation OR Phenylephrine gel Stimulated defecation OR Artificial sphincter OR Diversion (colostomy)
Rectal capacity and compliance	Rectal compliance study Marked increase in intrarectal pressure with minimal filling volumes	Treatment of underlying condition Diversion if condition severe/nontreatable

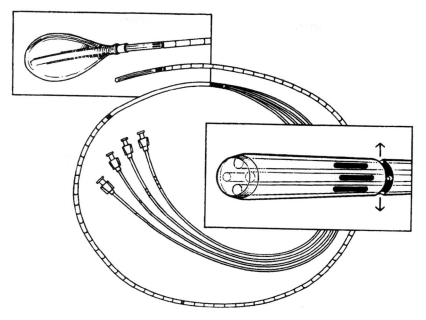

Fig. 15-3 Anorectal manometry catheter with rectal balloon attached.

The clinician obtains pressure measurements either through a "stationary" technique or a "pull-through" technique. With the stationary approach, the catheter is positioned with the balloon tip in the rectum, and resting, squeeze, and Valsalva pressures are recorded without moving the catheter. The manual pull-through technique is generally considered the preferred technique. With this approach, the catheter tip is initially positioned 6 cm proximal to the anal verge, and rectal pressures are recorded; the catheter is then slowly withdrawn until the intraluminal pressures begin to rise, which reflects the beginning of the functional anal canal. The examiner then withdraws the catheter 1 cm at a time and records resting and squeeze pressures at each point. The examiner can also assess reflex contraction of the external anal sphincter in response to sudden increases in abdominal pressure, by having the patient cough forcefully and noting any reflex contraction of the external sphincter (evidenced by increased anal canal pressures).[3,13]

To determine anal canal length, the clinician must first identify the area of highest resting pressure within the anal canal. This "high-pressure zone" is produced by the internal anal sphincter, which is located at the anorectal junction. The distance from the "resting high-pressure zone" (that is, the anorectal junction) to the anus can then be measured. Average anal canal length is about 3 cm, and male patients typically have higher resting pressures and a longer anal canal than female patients.[13]

In a relaxed patient, the resting pressures reflect the tone of the *internal* anal sphincter, whereas the "squeeze" pressures reflect the contractility of the *external* anal sphincter and the pelvic floor muscles. The pressures generated during a Valsalva maneuver reflect the patient's ability to relax the external anal sphincter and pelvic floor muscles while "bearing down" to evacuate stool; a normal response is evidenced by an increase in intrarectal pressure and a simultaneous decrease in the anal canal pressure.

Anorectal manometry testing provides an objective measurement of the pressures within the anal canal during rest, during voluntary contraction, and during voluntary relaxation. (Table 15-3 gives "typical" values in a continent subject.) The values obtained for any individual should be compared

TABLE 15-3 **Typical Anorectal Physiology Test Values in Continent Subject***

PARAMETERS	NORMAL
Anal manometry	
Resting pressure	40 to 80 mm Hg
Maximum voluntary contraction	80 to 160 mm Hg
Squeeze pressure (over resting pressure)	40 to 80 mm Hg
Anal canal length	Female: 2.0 to 3.5 cm Male: 3.0 to 4.0 cm
Rectal anal inhibitory reflex	Present
Rectal sensation	
First sensation	20 to 40 mL
Sensation of fullness	120 to 150 mL
Rectal compliance	16.8 ± 2 mL/cm H_2O
Electromyography	
Pudendal nerve terminal motor latencies	2.0 ± 0.2 milliseconds

*Values should be compared with age- and gender-matched controls because of the lack of normative data.

with age- and-gender matched subjects, because we currently lack normative data and standards for interpreting test results and because women and elders consistently exhibit lower sphincter pressures. Despite the lack of normative data, manometry can help to identify patients with sphincter dysfunction; data to date suggest that maximum squeeze pressure is the test with the greatest ability to differentiate between incontinent patients and continent controls. Unfortunately, manometry cannot reliably differentiate between sphincter dysfunction caused by a specific defect and sphincter dysfunction resulting from a denervation injury; thus, these data should be interpreted in conjunction with endoanal ultrasound or pelvic MRI.[13]

Sphincter mapping with endoanal ultrasonography and magnetic resonance imaging. Sphincter mapping is frequently indicated for the individual with fecal incontinence, because anatomic disruption of the sphincter is the primary indication for surgical intervention. As noted, needle EMG has been used in the past to map the sphincter; however, this has been largely replaced by endoanal ultrasound and MRI. Endoanal ultrasonography involves placement of a sonographic probe in the anal canal; the sonographic probe provides visualization of the thickness and structural integrity of the internal and external anal sphincters and can identify any disruption, scarring, or thinning of the sphincter complex (Fig. 15-4). Endoanal ultrasound is particularly beneficial in mapping the internal sphincter, because this tissue is hyperechoic as compared with the surrounding tissue; it is less effective in mapping the external sphincter, because the echogenicity of the sphincter and that of the surrounding fat are very similar. Mapping of the external sphincter can more effectively be accomplished with MRI, which provides very clear imaging and spatial resolution of the external anal sphincter. Currently, optimal imaging of the internal sphincter is obtained via endoanal ultrasound, and optimal imaging of the external sphincter is obtained via MRI.[3,5] Accurate sphincter mapping is very beneficial in planning treatment; if one or both of the sphincters have been disrupted, surgical repair may provide the best outcome. Conversely, the patient who has an intact but thinning sphincter may benefit from sphincter retraining with or without biofeedback.[25,26]

Pelvic floor and anal electromyography. Pelvic floor and anal EMG studies are sometimes used to assess for pelvic muscle or sphincter injury or denervation; these studies can be performed using needle electrodes, surface electrodes, or an anal plug. Needle electrode studies are particularly beneficial in differentiating between sphincter and pelvic muscle dysfunction resulting from muscle damage and dysfunction caused by denervation. To conduct the study, needles are placed into the external anal sphincter at several points around its circumference, and the patient is asked to contract the sphincter while the muscle response is recorded. (No anesthetic is given.) Although this study can provide valuable information, insertion of the needles is painful; as a result, endoanal ultrasound has largely

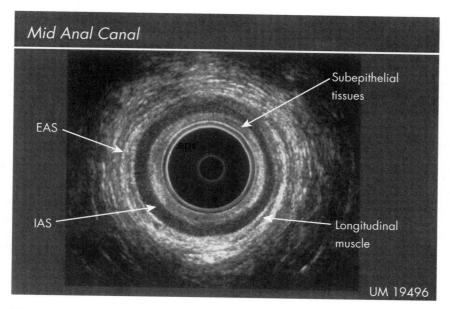

Fig. 15-4 Endoanal ultrasound demonstrating anatomy of sphincter complex.

replaced EMG for sphincter mapping. In contrast, surface or anal plug EMG is painless and can provide the patient with visual biofeedback of sphincter and pelvic muscle function; therefore, these forms of EMG are frequently beneficial in treatment.[3,13]

Pudendal nerve terminal motor latency test. PNTML studies are sometimes used to assess the innervation of the external anal sphincter. PNTML studies are conducted using disposable glove electrodes (Fig. 15-5). The examiner dons the glove and inserts the gloved electrode finger into the patient's anal canal. The pudendal nerves are identified, a low-voltage stimulation is given, and the time from stimulation to contraction of the muscle is recorded. This procedure is repeated for both the right and the left pudendal nerves. This test is not painful; the patient senses the digital exam but feels only a slight contraction of the external anal sphincter with the stimulation. Normal innervation is indicated by a PNTML of 2.0 ± 0.2 milliseconds. Latencies greater than 2.2 milliseconds are indicative of neuropathy and may be associated with diminished recognition of rectal filling.[27] It is important to realize that the normal range of pudendal latency is

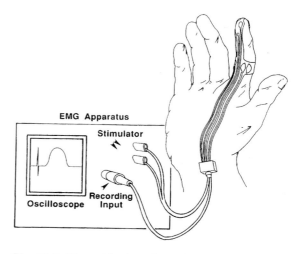

Fig. 15-5 Disposable glove electrode used for pudendal nerve terminal motor latency (PNTML) studies.

very small, which indicates a great need for precision and a significant margin for error. In addition, the significance of "abnormal" findings is questionable; the finding that at least 31% of patients with prolonged PNTML results have *normal* squeeze pressures and almost half of individuals with normal PNTML studies have abnormally *low* squeeze pressures suggests that either this is an insensitive test or pudendal neuropathy is of little clinical significance. Currently, the role of PNTML in assessment of individuals with fecal incontinence is unclear, and some authors now suggest that it provides little relevant data and should be used only in patients in whom the presence of neuropathy could change the management plan (such as a patient scheduled for sphincter repair).[13,14]

Saline continence study. The saline continence study was developed to permit quantification of fecal incontinence. The clinician conducts the study by infusing a body temperature saline solution into the rectum, either with a funnel and graduated cylinder or with a bag of saline solution connected to standard intravenous tubing. The solution is infused at a rate of 60 mL/minute for 25 minutes. The point of first leak (leakage of more than 10 mL) and the total retained volume are recorded. It is generally believed that physiologically normal individuals can retain 1500 mL, whereas incontinent individuals usually leak at less than 500 mL; however, significant numbers of continent individuals are unable to retain 500 mL. Therefore, the validity and reliability of this test are questionable, and it is no longer routinely used.[13,14,21,28]

Rectal compliance study. Rectal compliance refers to the distensibility of the rectum, that is, its ability to stretch and store stool at low pressures. It is tested by insertion of a balloon-tipped catheter with pressure transducers into the rectum (either in conjunction with anorectal manometry or as a "stand-alone" study). The balloon is progressively filled, and the corresponding increases in rectal pressure are recorded. If the rectum tolerates significant filling volumes with minimal increases in pressure, the rectal wall is said to be highly compliant. Low compliance is evidenced by significant increases in pressure with minimal filling volumes. Conditions associated with low compliance include neurologic lesions, rectal fibrosis, and inflammatory conditions such as radiation proctitis or inflammatory bowel disease. In addition, individuals with fecal incontinence often demonstrate lower rectal compliance than normal controls, even when there is no identifiable etiologic factor. Ideally, compliance parameters are compared with age-and-gender-matched controls, because rectal compliance decreases with age, even among healthy subjects.[14]

Defecating proctography. Defecating proctography, also known as defecography, is used to evaluate the *function* of the anorectal unit during defecation. This study is valuable in the assessment of patients who have difficulty evacuating stool from the rectal vault, even when the stool is of normal consistency. For example, defecography is typically recommended when rectal prolapse is suspected as the cause for incomplete evacuation of stool or fecal incontinence.[29] The clinician conducts the test by filling the rectum with a thick barium paste ("pseudostool"); the patient is then positioned on a special radiolucent commode and asked to expel the paste during radiographic examination. The response of the anorectal unit to the Valsalva maneuver is captured both on still films (with the patient at rest, "squeezing" to retain the paste, and "pushing" to expel the paste) and by fluoroscopy. Measurements are taken to determine changes in the pelvic floor occurring during attempted defecation.[3,13]

Defecography allows the clinician to identify pelvic floor dysfunction affecting rectal evacuation. For example, rectal prolapse is evidenced by descent of the rectum into or through the anal canal during a Valsalva maneuver. Patients with rectal prolapse experience incontinence if the prolapse is not reduced, either spontaneously or with manual reduction, because the sphincter mechanism is unable to close when the rectum is occupying the anal canal. In addition, patients with long-standing prolapse may develop neurologic dysfunction resulting from prolonged pressure on the sphincter mechanism and its nerve pathways. Additional examples of obstructive syndromes that can be identified or confirmed by defecography include rectocele and nonrelaxing puborectalis syndrome; however, these conditions do not generally result in incontinence.[13,22]

Although defecography can be helpful in diagnosing occult rectal prolapse and in identifying the etiologic factors for obstructed defecation, in most situations it adds little information to that provided by anorectal manometry and is of limited value in the assessment of fecal incontinence.[5]

Radiographic Studies of the Colon. Radiographic studies of the colon may be indicated for the patient who presents with chronic constipation unresponsive to primary management or for the patient with any evidence of a mass lesion or a chronic inflammatory process. The most commonly performed studies include barium enema and barium enema with both air and contrast medium; these studies permit identification of any structural changes in the colon. Motility studies are indicated for the patient with refractory constipation; these studies are discussed further in Chapter 14.

Laboratory Studies. Laboratory studies are performed selectively, based on the patient's clinical presentation and history. For example, the patient with persistent diarrhea of unknown cause requires a workup including stool analysis for blood, ova, and parasites and stool culture. Patients with evidence of malabsorption require a further workup to identify the specific intolerance.

In summary, a thorough assessment provides the data needed to develop an effective management plan for any individual with fecal incontinence. All patients require a thorough history, completion of a bowel chart with careful assessment of the data, and a focused physical examination. Additional studies are indicated for selected patients: those whose history and physical examination suggest sphincter or pelvic floor dysfunction, those with signs and symptoms of an underlying disease or lesion, and those for whom surgical intervention is contemplated. Additional tests may also be indicated for the individual who fails to respond to initial treatment. The underlying goal of the assessment phase is to identify the factors contributing to this individual's problem, as a basis for development of an appropriate treatment plan.

PRIMARY MANAGEMENT STRATEGIES

As noted, normal bowel function and continence are complex, multifactorial processes; dysfunctional states and incontinence may be equally complex. The critical factors in both normal and abnormal states include stool consistency and volume, anorectal sensory function, the function of the sphincter mechanism, and rectal capacity and compliance. Extraintestinal factors that may be equally contributory are mobility, motivation, cognition, and environmental factors. As discussed earlier in this chapter, comprehensive assessment is utilized to identify the specific dysfunctional components in each patient's condition. Effective management then involves measures to correct or compensate for each of these dysfunctional factors, with the goal of restoring normal or near-normal bowel control and improving the individual's quality of life. Management may involve one or more of the following: strategies to normalize stool consistency; patient education regarding bowel function and bowel control strategies, including environmental modifications for individuals with impaired mobility or cognition; strategies to improve anorectal sensory function; strategies to improve sphincter tone and contractility; strategies to reduce or manage fecal urgency; strategies to compensate for total loss of sensory awareness and sphincter control (caused by a neurologic lesion or dementia); and containment strategies for patients with severe diarrhea and fecal incontinence (Box 15-2). Each of these treatment strategies is discussed in more detail.

Strategies to Normalize Stool Consistency

Stool consistency plays an important role in normal bowel function and fecal continence, with soft formed stool representing the optimal consistency; liquid stool challenges and may overwhelm the competence of the sphincter mechanism, and small-caliber hard stools are very difficult to eliminate.[10] Thus, the first step in establishing both normal bowel function and fecal continence is establishment of normal stool consistency.[9] For the patient with diarrhea, this involves identification and correction of etiologic factors as well as measures to thicken the stool, and for the patient with constipation this involves measures to soften the stool and to reduce intestinal transit time.

Management of Diarrhea. Effective management of the patient with diarrhea involves treatment of the causative agent or process when possible, measures to reduce stool frequency and volume, and possibly measures to contain the stool and protect the skin. Identification and treatment of the causative agent or process have been

BOX 15-2 Measures to Correct Fecal Incontinence

Behavioral Therapies
- Dietary and fluid modifications to correct stool consistency
- Patient education and counseling regarding bowel function and bowel control
- "Urge resistance" training
- Sensory reeducation
- Sphincter retraining with or without biofeedback
- Stimulated defecation programs

Pharmacologic Agents
- Antidiarrheals
- Bulking agents
- Phenylephrine gel to increase anal resistance (experimental)

Neuromodulation/Sacral Nerve Stimulation

Surgical
- Sphincter repair
- Artificial anal sphincter
- Antegrade continence enema procedure
- Colostomy

discussed previously; the focus in this chapter is on measures to improve stool frequency and consistency and to contain the stool and protect the skin.

Identification and elimination of poorly tolerated foods. Chronic diarrhea is frequently the result of some type of dietary intolerance; thus, management of any patient with chronic diarrhea of unknown origin begins with completion of an "intake, fecal output, and intestinal symptom diary" designed to identify and eliminate poorly tolerated foods.[3] The patient is asked to maintain a record of all oral intake and all fecal output for 1 week; the patient is specifically instructed to include the types and volumes of all foods and fluids ingested (including additives such as spices, sugar, and creamer) and the volume and consistency of all stools. In addition, the patient is asked to record any intestinal symptoms, such as cramping or flatulence.[30] The patient is then counseled regarding any

dietary substances found to cause diarrheal episodes (Table 15-4).

An elimination diet is a structured approach to elimination (selected exclusion) of foods and fluids that are poorly tolerated. The initial diet eliminates foods that are *known* offenders, that is, those identified by the food and bowel record, and foods that are *common* offenders, such as chocolate and dairy products. The patient is asked to follow this diet for 2 weeks.[30] If the patient fails to improve during this time, a more restricted diet is tried. Once the patient has demonstrated improvement, the eliminated (excluded) foods are reintroduced one at a time every 3 days. This permits identification and restriction or elimination of poorly tolerated foods and fluids. A registered dietitian can provide very helpful guidance in the implementation of an elimination diet.[31] One of the most common food intolerances is lactose intolerance. Individuals with lactose intolerance are unable to digest lactose (a sugar found in milk and milk products) because of a deficiency of the enzyme lactase. A lactose-free diet is typically recommended for these patients,[32] although some individuals are able to tolerate small amounts of processed or cultured milk products (such as cottage cheese or yogurt). In addition, there are now available some dairy products that contain live *Lactobacillus acidophilus* culture. This milk culture converts the lactose into glucose and galactose, which are more readily tolerated. (Supplements such as Lactaid are also available over the counter.) A much more serious condition is celiac disease. This disease involves an enzyme deficiency in which gluten cannot be detoxified and gluten-containing substances actually damage the intestinal mucosa. Gluten is found in multiple foods and food additives, and a strict gluten-free diet is the only management option for these individuals.[33] Fortunately, gluten-free products are now widely available in health food stores and large grocery stores.

Some food substances alter stool consistency by affecting intestinal motility. Caffeine is known to cause diarrhea in some individuals, and the mechanism is believed to be increased peristaltic activity caused by increased production of gastric acid and pepsin.[34] Because caffeine is an ingredient in many foods, beverages, and drugs, it is important to

TABLE 15-4   Dietary Intake and Bowel Record*

TIME	FOOD OR FLUID	AMOUNT	STOOLS
7:00 AM	Coffee with sugar	2 cups	
	Toast with butter and jam	1 slice	
10:30 AM	Coffee	1 cup	Loose stool
12:15 PM	Ham/cheese sandwich (white bread)	1	
	Potato chips	bag (1 oz)	
	Chocolate chip cookies	2	
	Coffee with sugar	1 cup	
2:30 PM	Diet Coke	8 oz	
6:00 PM	White wine	4 oz	
	Pretzels	10 small	
7:00 PM	Roast turkey	3 oz	
	Gravy	2 tbsp	
	Cranberry sauce	1/2 cup	
	Green beans	1/2 cup	
	Biscuit with butter	1 small	
	Green salad with blue cheese	3 tbsp	
	Chocolate cake	Medium slice	
	Coffee with sugar	1 cup	Loose stool

*Patient is asked to record food and fluid intake, fecal output, and any gastrointestinal symptoms.

identify individuals who are intolerant of caffeine and to counsel them appropriately. Alcohol can also cause diarrhea, especially when it is consumed in large amounts. Again, the individual is assisted to recognize alcohol intake as an etiologic factor and is counseled to reduce or avoid alcohol.

Measures to improve stool frequency and consistency. Reduction of stool frequency and improvement in stool consistency may be accomplished by dietary modifications or pharmacologic agents. Bulk agents and constipating diets are frequently effective in thickening the stool and reducing stool volume, which helps to prevent fecal incontinence.[35,36] For example, the BRAT diet (bananas, rice, applesauce, toast, and tapioca) is commonly prescribed for both children and adults; additional "constipating" foods include yogurt, cheese, marshmallows, some wheat products, and pectin-containing fruits such as apples. All these foods reduce the water content of the stool, and pectin also helps to slow gastric emptying.[37]

Bulk agents such as psyllium or guar gum also help to thicken the stool and to slow intestinal transit time.[35,38] Bulking agents are commonly labeled as "laxatives," and as a result many patients with diarrhea are reluctant to use them. The clinician needs to explain to the patient that these agents work by absorbing fluid. For the patient with constipation, the water-holding effect provides softer stools that are easier to eliminate. However, for the patient with diarrhea, the water-holding effect helps to thicken the stool, and such thickening makes it easier to retain. The usual recommended dosage is 1 to 3 teaspoons three times daily for a total daily dose of 1 to 3 tablespoons. The patient does not need to drink large volumes of fluid with the bulking agent, because the product is intended to absorb the excess fluid within the intestinal tract; rather, the patient is instructed to drink a small glass of water or juice with each dose. Bulking agents are now available in various forms (such as cereal, tablet, and wafer form) and in various flavors. Sugar-free and nongelling agents are also available. The patient who is receiving enteral feedings may benefit from a formula that contains soluble fiber or from the addition of a nongelling bulk agent such as Benefiber.[30]

Pharmacologic agents to improve stool consistency and reduce stool frequency. Some patients require pharmacologic agents to reduce their colonic motility or to improve the consistency of their stool. The most commonly used agents include kaolin-pectin preparations, bismuth-subsalicylate agents, and antimotility drugs.[10,30] Kaolin-pectin preparations "work" by reducing stool fluidity, and bismuth-subsalicylate preparations work by reducing intestinal secretions and microbial proliferation; these agents are most appropriately used for mild episodic diarrhea. The antidiarrheal medications work by reducing intestinal motility and should therefore be used only for noninfectious diarrhea and only if impaction has been excluded. Within the category of antimotility agents, loperamide is the drug of choice because it has an excellent safety profile and has demonstrated efficacy in the treatment of both acute and chronic diarrheal conditions.[10] Loperamide works by reducing peristaltic activity, which reduces fecal urgency, stool frequency, and stool volume. In addition, loperamide increases sphincter tone and may reduce the sensitivity of the rectoanal inhibitory reflex, both of which would support continence during diarrheal episodes.[10,39] However, loperamide can cause abdominal pain and constipation if the dose is not titrated correctly; thus, slow upward titration is critical to optimal outcomes. Several strengths of loperamide (Imodium) are available over the counter.

Disimpaction. Fecal impaction compromises bowel function by creating a mechanical obstruction in the lumen of the distal bowel; in addition, fecal impaction increases the risk for incontinence because the presence of a stool bolus in the rectum creates a persistent stimulus for relaxation of the internal anal sphincter (which permits leakage of liquid stool around the impacted bolus). Thus, assessment of the patient with bowel dysfunction or fecal incontinence always includes a rectal examination, and any patient found to have an impaction is immediately begun on a disimpaction program. There are several approaches to disimpaction and bowel cleansing. If rectal exam reveals a hard mass that is too large for spontaneous elimination, the disimpaction procedure begins with administration of softening and lubricating enemas, followed by manual breakup and removal. Solutions commonly used include mineral oil and a 1:1 solution of milk and molasses. Once the rectal mass has been removed, the patient is given suppositories, enemas, or laxatives to evacuate the colon. Commonly used regimens include bisacodyl given orally and rectally, hypertonic phosphate solutions given orally and rectally, and oral administration of lactulose or mineral oil. The goal is to remove all inspissated stool from the colon, and achievement of this goal is evidenced by the passage of soft mushy stool.

Correction of constipation. Initial management of the patient with constipation involves correction of the common etiologic factors, that is, reduction or elimination of peristaltic inhibitors (such as inactivity and antimotility medications), and measures to produce soft formed stool (such as increased fiber and fluid intake). Ideal fiber intake for the adult is 30 to 40 g of fiber a day; however, for most older adults the goal is simply soft formed stool rather than an absolute amount of fiber. Fiber can be provided by dietary modifications, daily intake of bran, or bulk laxatives. A commonly prescribed bran mixture is 1 cup of unprocessed bran, 1 cup of applesauce, and 1/4 cup of prune juice; there are several variations on this mixture, any of which may be used effectively. The initial dose is typically 1 to 2 tablespoons per day; the daily dose is adjusted weekly as needed (usually by 1 tablespoon) until the desired results are obtained. Bulk laxatives, such as psyllium products, are the third option for providing the needed amount of fiber; the daily dose and titration schedule for these agents are the same as that for bran.

In initiating fiber therapy, it is essential to ensure adequate fluid intake (that is, 30 mL/kg of body weight/day); failure to provide adequate fluid intake with fiber therapy poses a risk for intestinal obstruction. Thus, fluid intake is a *major* concern for patients receiving either bran or bulk laxatives. It is also important to educate patients and caregivers regarding the potential for a temporary increase in bloating, flatulence, and stool frequency. These so-called adverse effects reflect the colon's adaptation response and are transient. The patient should be strongly encouraged to continue the therapy until the colon has adapted, at which time bowel function usually normalizes, as evidenced by regular elimination of soft formed stool. Stool softeners are rarely required for the patient who is receiving adequate volumes of bulk and fluids because the bulking agent attracts fluid and creates a soft formed stool.

As noted, adequate fluid intake is an essential component of safe and effective fiber therapy. This therapy is therefore contraindicated for the patient on fluid restriction (such as the patient in renal failure). One possible approach for these patients is routine administration of prune juice, typically 1 glass twice daily. Another option is the administration of a softener-stimulant combination, such as docusate and casanthranol (Peri-Colace or Doxidan). The softener component retains water within the fecal mass, and the peristaltic stimulant component promotes passage of the stool through the bowel, which prevents prolonged transit times and subsequent drying of the stool. The dose for any given patient is titrated based on response, with the most common starting dose being one tablet two or three times daily.

The patient who fails to respond to the foregoing measures requires further workup, typically motility studies or defecography, or both. Management is then based on the specific etiologic factors. For example, the patient who is found to have a dysfunctional segment of bowel may benefit from a segmental bowel resection; surgical intervention may also benefit the patient with rectal prolapse or rectocele interfering with fecal elimination. In contrast, the patient with a nonrelaxing puborectalis would require pelvic muscle reeducation by biofeedback, which is discussed in Chapter 14. The pathology and management of constipation are discussed in further detail in Chapter 14.

Patient Education Regarding Bowel Function and Bowel Control

Key elements of any program to improve bowel function and fecal continence are patient education and support. Fecal incontinence typically induces feelings of shame, loss of control, intense anxiety, and depression; many individuals live in fear of an accident and respond to any urge to defecate with a sense of panic that they will be unable to reach the toilet in time. Education regarding normal bowel function and control strategies can reduce anxiety and improve the individual's ability to respond appropriately to rectal distension. The clinician explains to the patient that normal bowel function is characterized by intermittent "waves" of muscle activity (peristalsis) that sweep stool toward the rectum, and that a sudden urge to defecate indicates that stool has been delivered to the rectum. The nurse should emphasize that this sudden urge to defecate is actually a "warning" signal, to alert the individual that defecation is imminent unless actions are taken to delay stool elimination. It is helpful to remind the patient that, if at all possible, he or she should move to the toilet, because defecation is accomplished most easily during these peristaltic waves. However, the clinician should also emphasize that the anal canal is surrounded by sphincter muscles that allow him or her to delay defecation when it is socially inconvenient; it is helpful to explain the role of each of the sphincters as well as the rectoanal inhibitory reflex. Specifically, the clinician explains that the internal sphincter is normally closed, but it relaxes briefly in response to rectal distension, which allows the rectal contents to contact the skin in the anal canal. (A good way to explain this to the patient is to ask him or her to recall the fact that the first sensation is simply that of rectal distension, but this is followed almost immediately by an appreciation of rectal contents, that is, solid, liquid, or gas, that is provided by contact between the rectal contents and the anal canal.) The clinician should emphasize the importance of the external sphincter during this period of internal sphincter relaxation; the external sphincter must be contracted to prevent leakage. The clinician should also explain that contraction of the external sphincter delays defecation long enough to allow the rectal walls to relax, which provides for temporary storage of the stool. The clinician should emphasize that the intense urge to defecate is usually relatively transient, and that voluntary sphincter contraction coupled with standing still or sitting and deep breathing are effective "control strategies" (Box 15-3).

Patients with episodic constipation are encouraged to establish a routine schedule for attempted

---

BOX 15-3 **Key Points in Education for Patient with Fecal Urgency**
....
- Normal peristaltic patterns/effects of "mass movements"
- Function of internal anal sphincter and external anal sphincter
- Impact of rectoanal inhibitory reflex
  Permits discrimination rectal contents
  Requires compensatory contraction of external sphincter
- Urge resistance strategies
  Sphincter contraction
  Deep breathing
  Distraction
- Urge resistance program and goals (gradual lengthening of "delay" interval and gradual distancing from
  "safety" of toilet)
- Sphincter-strengthening exercises

---

defecation, based on their previous bowel patterns; for example, the patient whose usual pattern was a bowel movement after breakfast is encouraged to attempt defecation on that schedule and to use any natural stimulants that he or she has found effective in the past, such as hot tea or warm juice. However, the clinician should emphasize to the patient that responding as promptly as possible to the urge to defecate is more important than maintaining a schedule of attempted defecation. The patient is encouraged to work "with" his or her natural bowel activity rather than "against" it.

For patients with impaired mobility, many simple interventions can facilitate toileting and continence. These include measures such as maintaining the bed and chair at heights that facilitate entry and exit, ensuring that bathrooms are well marked and well lit, maintaining unobstructed pathways to the bathrooms, encouraging use of appropriate assistive devices and ensuring that all bathroom facilities are constructed to accommodate such devices, providing side rails on the toilets or the walls, and modifying clothing to facilitate toileting. For the bedbound patient, continence and dignity are supported by leaving a clean bed pan within easy reach and ensuring that the call bell is within reach.

The patient who is cognitively impaired but who retains the ability to follow simple instructions frequently benefits from a routine toileting program coupled with strategies to maintain normal stool consistency, as described earlier. The toileting schedule should be based on the individual's "usual" bowel patterns; for example, the patient who frequently has an incontinent bowel movement after breakfast should be taken to the bathroom routinely following breakfast. Long-term care facilities frequently report positive outcomes from the use of bran formulas to normalize stool consistency and bowel function and from routine toileting to reduce fecal accidents.

Strategies to Improve Sensory Awareness/Sensory Reeducation

Sensory deficits are not uncommon in patients who have sustained nerve damage and repair. In these situations, there is a prolonged period between rectal distension and conscious awareness of rectal filling because of the altered nerve pathways. This delay in recognition of rectal filling causes a delay in sphincter contraction, which may cause leakage of gas or stool. Diminished sensory awareness also occurs in the patient who has habitually ignored the call to stool. In these patients, the rectum is chronically distended with stool, and the sensory response to rectal filling becomes blunted. For the patient with a primary sensory deficit (that is, the patient with nerve damage), sensory reeducation represents primary therapy; for the patient who has diminished sensory response caused by chronic rectal distension, the management program must also include colonic cleansing, measures to normalize stool consistency, and patient education regarding bowel function. Sensory reeducation programs are beneficial only for cognitively intact patients who retain some degree of sensory awareness.

The clinician begins sensory retraining by inserting a catheter with a balloon tip into the rectum and gradually inflating the balloon. The patient is asked to report the first sensation of rectal filling, and the volume required to initiate conscious awareness of rectal distension is noted. The patient is then asked to focus on the sensation of the balloon as the balloon is gradually deflated. The goal is to reeducate the patient to recognize and respond to rectal filling at the normal volume of 15 to 30 mL. Biofeedback can also be utilized to enhance sensory reeducation; this involves placement of an intrarectal balloon with transducers connected to a monitor.[5,40,41] Biofeedback allows the patient to visualize rectal filling while focusing on the sensation of rectal distension. Several studies have documented the efficacy of biofeedback in improving sensory function and fecal continence.[14]

Strategies to Improve Sphincter Function

Compromised sphincter function is a causative or contributing factor for most individuals with fecal incontinence; therefore, strategies to improve sphincter contractility and endurance are key elements of most management programs. Strategies to improve sphincter function include sphincter strengthening programs, medications to enhance sphincter tone, electrical stimulation or sacral nerve stimulation, and surgical procedures to correct or compensate for sphincter deficits.

Sphincter Strengthening. Many patients with fecal incontinence or bowel dysfunction can benefit from sphincter reeducation, either with or without biofeedback.[40-45] This therapy is most commonly used for patients who have diminished sphincter tone but intact nerve pathways. Sphincter retraining may also be indicated for patients with minimal sphincter disruption. In these patients, sphincter exercises are used to strengthen the muscle, and such strengthening helps to compensate for the area of disruption. The patient criteria for sphincter retraining are similar to those for sensory reeducation. The patient must be cognitively intact and motivated, must have sufficient innervation to permit

voluntary contraction of the pelvic floor muscles, and must possess at least minimal rectal sensation.

The simplest approach to sphincter strengthening involves teaching the patient to do pelvic muscle exercises; repetitive contraction of the anal sphincter and pelvic floor muscles improves both contractile strength and the ability to maintain the contraction.[16] Clinically, this improvement in sphincter tone and endurance is manifest as increased anal canal resistance and the ability to delay defecation. Sphincter and pelvic muscle exercises are commonly known as "Kegel exercises" because it was Arnold Kegel who first reported their benefits in 1948.[46]

In teaching the patient to do pelvic muscle exercises, the clinician begins by explaining the benefits of the therapy, the time frame for response, and the importance of diligence in completing the exercises. The patient is then assisted to identify the target muscle group. To ensure isolation of the correct muscle group, the clinician places a gloved finger into the patient's anal canal and instructs the patient to "tighten and lift" or to "squeeze tightly" around the examining finger (as if trying not to pass gas or stool). In assessing the patient's ability to isolate the correct muscle, the clinician must observe for inappropriate contraction of the gluteal or abdominal muscles. Verbal feedback is then given to the patient regarding his or her ability to contract the desired muscle. Once the patient has demonstrated the ability to contract the target muscle group correctly, he or she can be instructed in a specific exercise protocol. There are no evidence-based protocols to guide the clinician in prescribing an effective exercise program; the specific approach and the recommended number of repetitions vary based on clinician and clinical setting.[16] One protocol involves teaching the patient to contract the muscle, to hold the contraction for a count of 10, and then to relax for a count of 10; the patient is instructed to repeat this exercise 15 to 25 times three times daily. However, the clinician should individualize the length of the contraction goal and the number of repetitions based on the patient's baseline muscle function. For example, the patient who has a very weak muscle and who can maintain a contraction for only 2 seconds may initially be instructed to hold the contraction for 3 seconds and to perform 10 repetitions three times daily; once the patient achieves this goal, higher goals are established. Studies suggest that exercises designed to increase endurance (gradual lengthening of the "hold" time) are particularly important to continence; this makes physiologic sense in that contraction of the external sphincter needs to persist longer than the reflex relaxation of the internal sphincter and long enough for the rectum to relax around the bolus of stool.[2]

Kegel exercises may be performed while the patient is standing, sitting, or lying down, and, when the exercises are done correctly, the patient's performance is invisible. This has important implications for patients who need long-term pelvic muscle exercise therapy. Once patients have acquired skill in performing the exercises, they can learn to incorporate them into activities of daily living. This approach supports long-term compliance and the associated reduction in fecal leakage.[46,47]

Biofeedback-Assisted Reeducation Programs.
The term "biofeedback" refers to several techniques used to bring under conscious control bodily processes normally believed to be beyond voluntary command.[16] Within the field of continence care and pelvic muscle reeducation, biofeedback is helpful because many patients have difficulty identifying the target muscle group and performing the exercises properly. Studies indicate that biofeedback can be used to improve success rates and clinical outcomes for patients requiring pelvic muscle reeducation, especially those who have difficulty correctly isolating the sphincter and pelvic floor muscles.[3,41,48]

The two most common approaches to biofeedback are the manometric approach and the EMG approach.[3] Manometric (pressure) biofeedback is typically provided via an air-filled anal probe or three-balloon system with transducers connected to a computer; both these systems provide recordings of the pressures generated at rest, during voluntary contraction, and with voluntary relaxation. The three-balloon system also provides a recording of rectal balloon inflation, which is helpful for the patient who also requires sensory reeducation or who needs to focus on rapidly contracting the sphincter in response to rectal distension. The EMG approach, initially described by MacLeod,[49] is currently the

more popular technique for biofeedback. EMG biofeedback uses an intraanal sensor, intravaginal sensor, or perianal surface electrodes to detect electrical activity in the muscles and to transmit the electrical signals to a computer monitor; the computerized recording provides the patient visual "feedback" regarding sphincter muscle activity at rest, with voluntary contraction, and with voluntary relaxation. Surface electrodes may also be placed on the gluteus maximus muscle or the abdominal muscles to detect and display inappropriate contraction of those muscle groups. The simultaneous feedback regarding pelvic muscle contraction and gluteal or abdominal muscle contraction assists the patient with deficient pelvic muscle strength to isolate and contract the pelvic muscles while keeping the gluteal and abdominal muscles relaxed.[3] (An alternative approach to monitoring for inappropriate contraction of the abdominal muscles is to have the patient place his or her hand on the abdomen and to watch for rising and falling of the hand.)

Biofeedback training programs differ from center to center and can be modified to address various treatment goals.[2,3,16] The simplest programs focus on assisting the patient to identify and strengthen the sphincter and pelvic floor muscles. The patient is instructed to contract his or her muscles as if trying to hold in stool or gas; the patient is then shown the recording of his or her sphincter contraction with explanations of the clinical significance and goals of treatment. For example, the clinician explains to the patient with weak muscles or minimal endurance that the inability to tighten and hold effectively is causing the problem with leakage, and that the goal of treatment is to increase both muscle strength and endurance to delay defecation. (It is frequently helpful to again explain the "basics" of bowel function, specifically the normal transient relaxation of the internal sphincter and the role of the external sphincter and pelvic floor muscles in "compensating" for this transient relaxation and preventing fecal leakage.) The patient is then instructed in an exercise program that includes gradual lengthening of the contraction period. A more advanced biofeedback program focuses on teaching the patient to contract the external sphincter and pelvic floor muscles rapidly *in response to* rectal distension; this requires placement of an intrarectal balloon with transducers connected to the computer so the patient can "visualize" rectal distension (in addition to the intraanal, intravaginal, or perianal sensors that record sphincter function). The balloon is distended with air, and the patient is taught to focus on early recognition of rectal distension and on prompt contraction of the external sphincter and pelvic floor muscles. These programs are based on studies suggesting that a delay in recognition of rectal distension and the subsequent delay in sphincter contraction may be one cause of leakage.[2]

There is controversy regarding the benefits of biofeedback-assisted training as compared with pelvic muscle reeducation without biofeedback. Whitehead's findings indicated that biofeedback-assisted therapy did provide greater improvement in continence than pelvic muscle reeducation without biofeedback,[50] but this remains a controversial issue, and more data are needed. One issue in measuring outcomes is the definition of success. Many authors define success as a reduction in the number of incontinent episodes,[40,42-45] but the criteria for "success" ranges from 50% to 90% reduction in incontinent episodes, and many do not identify the methods used to determine the level of improvement (patient reports versus bowel diaries versus other methods).[2,3] A recent Cochrane review of the efficacy of sphincter exercises and biofeedback in treatment of fecal incontinence concluded that there is insufficient evidence to determine whether these interventions are helpful, which patients are likely to respond, and whether biofeedback-assisted exercise programs are more effective than exercise programs without biofeedback.[2,48] Norton reported on a study in which 171 patients with fecal incontinence were assessed by anal ultrasound and then assigned to one of two groups: those with intact sphincter muscles and those with sphincter disruption. Patients in each of these groups were then randomly assigned to one of four treatment groups; group 1 received intensive education and support, but no instruction in sphincter exercises and no biofeedback; group 2 received education and support combined with verbal and written instructions regarding sphincter exercises; group 3 received education, support, and sphincter exercises supported by

biofeedback at each clinic visit; and group 4 received education, support, instruction in sphincter exercises supported by biofeedback at each clinic visit, and a home biofeedback device. Interestingly, there was no significant difference in outcomes among any of the treatment groups; individuals with sphincter disruption improved as much as those with intact sphincters, and patients receiving only intensive education and support improved as much as those who also received biofeedback-assisted sphincter exercises. Seventy-five percent of the participants reported improvement in their symptoms and the median satisfaction with treatment was 8 on a scale of 0 to 10 (with 10 being the best outcome). Although this study needs to be replicated, these data strongly suggest that conservative treatment programs are successful even when there is anatomic sphincter damage and that education and support are the key elements to success with conservative treatment programs.[2]

Pharmacologic Agents. To date, pharmacotherapy for the management of fecal incontinence has been limited to antidiarrheal agents; however, phenylephrine gel is currently under investigation as a "sphincter-enhancing" agent. Phenylephrine is an alpha-1-adrenergic agonist currently approved for use as a nasal decongestant and a vasopressor; it is now being evaluated for its ability to increase resting tone of the internal anal sphincter via its action on vascular smooth muscle.[10,39] In one small study involving patients with weak internal sphincter muscles, topical application of the gel in concentrations ranging from 10% to 40% increased maximum anal resting pressure to a statistically significant level, and the 30% and 40% concentrations increased the resting tone to normal levels.[51] The only adverse effect was localized stinging, which resolved within 20 minutes. This agent is currently thought to hold promise for individuals with "passive" incontinence resulting from low resting anal canal pressures; however, as noted in a recent Cochrane review, more data are needed, and its use is currently considered experimental.[39]

Electrical Stimulation. Electrical stimulation has been used in a number of centers as a component of a comprehensive program to improve sphincter function; protocols used have differed widely in terms of frequency, duration, and stimulation parameters. As a result, we currently lack any valid data regarding its efficacy in treatment of patients with fecal incontinence, although many clinicians report positive outcomes with its use. The limited data available suggest that it is most effective in strengthening the external sphincter in patients with intact sensation and that stimulation should be provided at 20 to 60 Hz (because this is the natural firing frequency for fast-twitch fibers), with a rest period equal to or greater than the stimulation period. This is an area of treatment in which more study is desperately needed.[16]

Sacral Nerve Stimulation. Sacral nerve stimulation was initially used in the management of patients with urinary incontinence; its use in fecal incontinence is relatively new and is based on observations of improved bowel function and bowel control among patients receiving the therapy for urinary incontinence.[52] Sacral nerve stimulation involves operative implantation of a device that provides chronic stimulation of the sacral nerves innervating the sphincter muscles, at a frequency of 15 Hz, a pulse width of 210 microseconds, and an on-off cycle of 5 seconds to 1 second. Before implantation of the permanent nerve stimulator, patient candidacy for the therapy is determined by acute percutaneous nerve stimulation, followed by a test period of chronic stimulation. Acute stimulation of the various sacral nerves is performed via placement of percutaneous needle electrodes into the foramina of the sacral nerves, followed by application of electrical current to the various electrodes. The goals are to determine the responsiveness of the sacral nerves to electrical stimulation and to identify the specific nerves most important to fecal continence in the individual being evaluated; if the nerve pathways are intact, stimulation via the percutaneous electrodes will generate a visible contraction of the external sphincter . If the nerves are determined to be responsive to acute stimulation, the patient then undergoes a test period of chronic low-frequency stimulation via the percutaneous needle electrodes, to determine whether chronic stimulation provides therapeutic benefit. Once therapeutic efficacy is determined, a pulse generator is implanted (into the abdomen or the gluteal area) and is connected to electrodes placed in the sacral foramen. The patient is taught to use a hand-held programmer to interrupt stimulation when he or she needs to defecate. Data to date indicate that sacral nerve stimulation significantly increases anal squeeze pressure, which translates into a marked improvement in the ability to delay defecation, reduced episodes of fecal incontinence, and improved quality of life.[14,52,53]

Surgical Procedures to Correct Sphincter Defects/Improve Sphincter Function. Several surgical procedures have been introduced with the goal of eliminating fecal incontinence. The most widely used procedures have included sphincter repair, graciloplasty and dynamic graciloplasty, and artificial anal sphincter placement.

Sphincteroplasty. Clinical consensus has held that surgical repair is the most appropriate intervention for individuals with sphincteric disruption, and surgical intervention has also been tried for patients with weak but intact sphincters, in an attempt to increase anal canal resistance. Overlapping sphincteroplasty is generally considered the procedure of choice. This procedure involves dissection of the scarred sphincter back to healthy muscle on each side; the healthy ends of the muscle are then overlapped to form an intact ring of muscle. Sphincter repair following obstetric trauma typically results in resolution of symptoms for up to 80% of patients. However, some studies indicate poor long-term outcomes, especially in patients for whom sphincteroplasty was performed for a weak sphincter, as opposed to sphincteric disruption. Interestingly, no studies have ever been done to compare sphincter repair with conservative management including sphincter exercises with or without biofeedback, and biofeedback is sometimes suggested as the treatment of choice for individuals in whom sphincter repair has failed.[3,5,54] Thus, more data are clearly needed to elucidate the role of sphincter repair in the management of fecal incontinence.

Graciloplasty and dynamic graciloplasty. Other surgical procedures designed to compensate for a weak sphincter mechanism include graciloplasty and dynamic graciloplasty. Graciloplasty involves mobilization of the gracilis muscle (from its attachments in the leg); the muscle is then wrapped snugly around the anus. This "passive graciloplasty" has been reported to improve sphincter resistance and fecal continence in a number of patients. However, this procedure has significant limitations; some patients are unable to voluntarily contract the transposed muscle, and the muscle is typically unable to provide sustained resistance (because it is a skeletal muscle composed primarily of fast-twitch fibers.) Dynamic graciloplasty involves the addition of chronic low-frequency electrical stimulation to the transposed muscle; the electrical stimulation converts fast-twitch fibers to slow-twitch fibers, which improves tonic resistance and also provides for continuous muscle contraction, which obviates the need for volitional contraction. (To defecate, the patient uses a hand-held device to interrupt the electrical stimulus.) Reported success rates range from 54% to 83%; however, these results must be interpreted with caution because the criteria for success and the methods for outcomes measurement varied significantly from study to study. In addition, this procedure is associated with complications in as many as 74% of patients. As a result, it is not widely used, and the hardware for the procedure is not approved for use in the United States.[3,54]

Artificial anal sphincter. The artificial anal sphincter is an alternative to dynamic graciloplasty and is designed to provide continuous occlusion of the anal canal until defecation is desired. The artificial sphincter (Acticon Neosphincter, American Medical Systems, Minnetonka, MN) is a modification of the artificial urinary sphincter and involves comparable components: a cuff placed around the anal canal (the artificial sphincter), a reservoir implanted into the groin or lower abdomen, and a pump implanted into the scrotum or labia (Fig 15-6). The cuff is maintained in an open position for the first 6 to 8 weeks after surgery, and at that time, if proper healing has occurred, the system is activated. After activation, the fluid from the reservoir expands the cuff, which compresses the anal canal to provide continence. When evacuation is desired, the individual squeezes the pump, and this maneuver displaces the fluid from the cuff to the balloon and thereby opens the anal canal. Successful implantation of this device has provided good functional results for a number of patients; in a recent series, 85% of

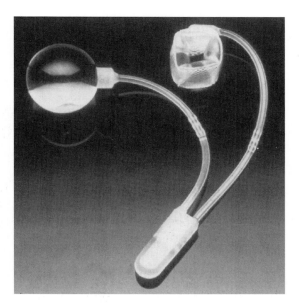

Fig. 15-6 Artificial bowel sphincter with three components: pressure-regulating balloon, cuff, and pump.

the patients who were able to retain the sphincter reported positive outcomes, but 51 of 112 patients required one or more surgical revisions, and 41 required removal of the device.[3,54,55] Thus, this procedure is typically reserved for selected patients with refractory fecal incontinence.

Strategies to Improve Ability to Control Fecal Urgency

In cognitively intact individuals with sensory awareness of rectal distension, incontinence is usually caused by the inability to delay defecation long enough to reach a toilet; many of these individuals complain of "fecal urgency" accompanied by intense anxiety (related to fear of a fecal accident). These individuals typically benefit from behavioral strategies designed to reduce urgency and improve the ability to delay defecation; some may benefit from biofeedback or selected medications.

Instruction in Urge Resistance. Programs to enhance urge resistance include basic education regarding normal bowel function with a focus on strategies to control fecal urgency and to delay defecation. The clinician reviews normal bowel function with the patient and emphasizes the importance of volitional contraction of the external sphincter in response to rectal distension and the urge to defecate (see Box 15-3). The clinician then explains to the patient that he or she needs to regain both voluntary control (and the ability to delay defecation) and *confidence* in his or her ability to delay defecation. The program advocated by Norton involves a series of maneuvers designed to improve voluntary control and "urge resistance." Initially, the patient is instructed to go to the toilet whenever he or she feels the urge to defecate, but is taught to delay defecation for at least 1 minute; strategies used to delay defecation include voluntary sphincter contraction, deep breathing (relaxation), and distraction. Once the patient can delay defecation for 1 minute, he or she is instructed to progressively extend the "delay" interval until he or she is able to delay defecation for 5 minutes. At that point, the patient is instructed to extend the "delay" interval gradually to 10 minutes. Once the patient is able to delay defecation for 10 minutes while sitting on the toilet, he or she is instructed to gradually move *away* from the toilet, that is, to sit on the edge of the bathtub or on a chair outside the bathroom for 5 minutes and to extend the interval gradually to 10 minutes. At this point, the patient is instructed to begin increasing the distance between himself or herself and the toilet. This "stepped" program progressively increases both voluntary control over defecation and *confidence* in one's ability to control defecation. In addition, the individual learns specific strategies that can be used to control intense fecal urgency, such as deep breathing, voluntary contraction of the sphincter muscles, and distraction.[16]

Biofeedback can be used to augment urge resistance programs. Specifically, a balloon-tipped catheter can be inserted into the rectum and inflated to the point of initial urgency; the patient is then encouraged to use "delay" strategies to control the sense of urgency, and the balloon is gradually inflated to simulate increasing levels of rectal distension while the patient uses "delay" strategies to control the associated urgency.[2]

Medications. No medications are currently approved for reduction of fecal urgency, but amitriptyline has shown promise in preliminary studies.

Specifically, this tricyclic antidepressant has demonstrated efficacy in reducing the amplitude and frequency of rectal contractions and fecal urgency and the incidence and severity of incontinence episodes. However, additional studies are required before any recommendations can be made regarding its use in clinical practice.[10]

Strategies to Compensate for Total Loss of Sensory Awareness or Sphincter Control

As described earlier in this chapter, individuals with diminished sensory awareness or sphincter control frequently benefit from behavioral therapies; however, these therapies are not effective for patients who have total loss of sensory awareness and sphincter control resulting from neurologic conditions (such as a spinal cord injury) or advanced dementia. These patients are typically managed with stimulated defecation programs; other options include the antegrade continence enema procedure or colostomy (for individuals with neurologic lesions) or containment and skin care (for patients with advanced dementia).

Stimulated Defecation Programs. Continence for individuals with no sensory awareness or sphincter control requires stimulation of colonic and rectal evacuation at a time convenient for them (or their caregivers) and at sufficient frequency to prevent rectal filling and overflow incontinence, that is, stimulated defecation programs. It is usually *not* sufficient simply to normalize stool consistency and establish a regular schedule for attempted defecation, because propulsive contractions, for most individuals, do not occur at a precise and predictable time, and stool cannot be eliminated until it is delivered to the rectum by these propulsive contractions. Stimulated defecation programs, in contrast, *are* usually effective because they combine the scheduled attempt at elimination with a stimulus that triggers propulsive activity and delivers stool to the rectum "on schedule" (Box 15-4).

The initial steps in a stimulated defecation program involve elimination of impacted stool, colonic cleansing, and establishment of normal stool consistency. For patients with sensory or sphincter compromise, the goal for stool consistency is to maintain formed stool that is firm but not hard;

BOX 15-4   Key Steps in Stimulated Defecation Program

- Educate patient or caregiver regarding program goals (stimulate defecation on a routine basis before the rectum is full enough to empty spontaneously)
- Establish normal stool consistency (formed but not hard)
- Establish regular schedule for elimination (daily or every other day at same time of day)
- Select stimulus
     Digital stimulation
     Suppositories
     Minienema
     Tap water enema given via catheter with retention balloon
- Maintain records and modify program as indicated

---

very soft or mushy stool tends to leak through the compromised sphincter mechanism.

The next step is to establish an appropriate schedule for elimination. The initial *frequency* is usually daily or every other day and is based on the patient's prior bowel patterns. The *timing* for the stimulated elimination is variable also and may be based either on the patient's prior bowel patterns or on convenience factors. For example, a spinal cord–injured patient whose usual pattern was a bowel movement after breakfast may prefer an evening schedule as a result of multiple self-care requirements before work or school. In this situation, an evening schedule may be utilized initially; however, if the patient has frequent morning "accidents," it may be necessary to revise the schedule to coincide with the patient's natural bowel patterns and to shift other morning activities to the evening hours.

The final step in initiation of a stimulated defecation program is to select an appropriate stimulus. The stimulus is designed to trigger propulsive activity in the left colon; options include digital stimulation, suppositories, minienemas, and a low-volume enema with a retention balloon.[20] The stimulus should be selected based on the patient's prior use of stimulants, the patient's or caregiver's preferences, and the patient's response. Digital stimulation is commonly used in rehabilitation settings. The patient is taught to insert a gloved lubricated finger approximately 5 cm into the anal canal and to use circular motions to stimulate relaxation of the internal anal sphincter and peristaltic contractions in the left colon. (A "dilstick" may also be used; this is a wand with a finger-shaped attachment that facilitates digital stimulation for some patients.) The stimulus is continued for up to 20 minutes or until evacuation occurs. Over time, many patients are able to stimulate evacuation in less than 20 minutes. Advantages to digital stimulation include its very low cost, physiologic features, and effectiveness. Disadvantages include difficulty in performing the procedure for some patients with sitting imbalance and occasional problems with patient or caregiver acceptance. A second option is use of a rectal suppository; commonly used suppository formulas include glycerin, bisacodyl, and carbon dioxide. Each of these has a different mechanism of action, as outlined in Table 15-5; this difference means that a patient who responds minimally or unpredictably to bisacodyl may experience consistent effective evacuation with the use of glycerin or carbon dioxide (or vice versa). It is therefore reasonable clinical practice to try various types of suppositories before concluding that suppositories are an ineffective option for a given patient. Because suppositories are inexpensive, readily available, and easy to use, they are a fairly popular option for stimulated defecation. However, many individuals find that their response to suppositories is variable, and such variability contradicts the need for a predictable consistent evacuation in response to the selected stimulus. The third option for stimulated defecation is the use of minienemas, which are gelatin ampules with an enema tip. At this time, the most commonly available minienema is Enemeez (Western Research Laboratories, Phoenix, AZ); this product has an enema

TABLE 15-5   Mechanism of Action for Commonly Used Suppositories

Glycerin suppositories	Exact mechanism of action unknown; exerts lubricating effects and believed to exert laxative effect by dehydration of exposed mucosa and resultant "irritant" effect (probably activates enteric nervous system receptors)
Bisacodyl suppositories (such as Dulcolax)	Stimulates sensory receptors in colonic mucosa to activate parasympathetic reflexes mediating peristalsis; also promotes fluid and ion accumulation in the colon, which further enhances peristalsis (probably acts by combination of enteric nervous system and autonomic nervous system stimulation)
Carbon dioxide–releasing suppositories (such as Ceo-Two by Beutlich)	Sodium bicarbonate ingredient combines with water in bowel to release approximately 175 mL of carbon dioxide, which causes colonic distension and peristalsis; also exerts lubricant effect (activates receptors of enteric nervous system and usually empties the distal 10 to 12 inches of colon)

tip attached to a 4-mL gelatin ampule containing docusate (a stool softener) and soft soap (a mild irritant). The clinician administers the minienema by removing the twist-off tip and then slowly instilling the fluid into the rectum. After administration, the patient is instructed to hold the buttocks together for at least 10 minutes to facilitate retention. The minienema administered in this fashion typically provides very effective evacuation. The advantages of the minienema include patient and caregiver acceptance, ease of use, and therapeutic efficacy; its major disadvantage is the cost (typically $1.00 to $2.00 each). The last option for stimulated defecation is a tap-water enema administered via catheter and retention balloon; this provides for colonic distension, which, in turn, promotes peristalsis and elimination. A commercial device is available that facilitates enema administration (the MIC Bowel Management Kit, by Ballard, Midvale, UT); however, a regular indwelling catheter (with the balloon inflated and pulled taut against the anorectal junction) can be used as well. The volume of water used should be the least amount that effectively stimulates elimination; some individuals may require as little as 250 mL to stimulate evacuation, whereas others require a much greater volume. The enema option is particularly helpful for individuals with sacral spinal lesions because these individuals are dependent on stimulation of the enteric nervous

system (which responds to intraluminal irritants and to bowel wall distension) to achieve emptying.

The patient or caregiver is instructed to maintain a bowel record to monitor response to the program. Generally, the program is continued as initiated for at least 2 weeks, and any modifications are evaluated for at least 2 weeks before decisions are made regarding efficacy. Components of the program that may require modification include measures to produce formed stool, the frequency and timing of stimulated defecation, and the stimulus used. Generally, only one aspect of the program is changed at a time, so the effect of that modification can be accurately evaluated. Compliance with the established program is absolutely essential and must be a key component of patient education and of program evaluation.

Antegrade Continence Enema Procedure. The antegrade colonic enema (ACE) procedure is an option for patients with neurogenic incontinence who cannot be effectively managed with stimulated defecation. This procedure involves creation of a continent catheterizable channel between the abdominal wall and the colon. The catheterizable channel may be created by use of the appendix or a tubularized segment of bowel.[56,57] Continence is maintained by tunneling of the appendix or tubularized segment of bowel through the subcutaneous tissue and into the cecum or by creation of a nipple-shaped valve by intussusception. The one-way stoma is then used to perform regular colonic washouts to maintain continence. The procedure was first used successfully in children and is now being used successfully in adults as well.[3,57,58]

Colostomy. Patients with fecal incontinence that is intractable to all medical, behavioral, and surgical attempts to restore continence should be evaluated for fecal diversion. Although most patients and clinicians consider this a last resort in the management of incontinence, a well-constructed colostomy provides the individual with bowel control and restores their potential for a normal life.[3,59] Many patients are able to regulate fecal output by routine colostomy irrigations; for those who are unable to irrigate or who respond poorly to irrigation, there are many lightweight, odorproof, and easy-to-manage pouching systems for fecal containment. Patients should be counseled and supported by a nurse clinician knowledgeable regarding ostomy management.

Stool Containment and Skin Protection. For patients with intractable or unpredictable incontinence, containment is a critical element of care. Key options for containment include perianal pouches, internal drainage systems, absorptive briefs, and anal plugs. The clinician must consider the volume and consistency of the stool and the goals of care in selecting the best product for the individual patient.

External Collection Devices: Perianal Pouches. For the patient with high-volume liquid diarrhea and fecal incontinence, care is focused on correcting the underlying causes of the diarrhea, effectively containing the stool, and protecting the perianal skin. Two options for containment also provide for skin protection: external collection devices (perianal pouches) and internal drainage systems. External collection devices are drainable pouches attached to a synthetic, adhesive skin barrier; the pouch is constructed to conform to the perianal area and buttocks[60] (Fig. 15-7). The perianal pouch is usually considered first-line therapy because these devices are inexpensive, relatively simple to apply, and pose no safety risks. Application of a perianal pouch is similar to application of an ostomy pouch; the skin is cleaned and dried, any denuded areas are treated by application of a pectin-based powder followed by an alcohol-free skin sealant, the aperture in the pouch is enlarged as needed to "clear" the anal area, and the pouch is pressed into place. The pouch spout may be connected to bedside drainage or closed with a clamp. The pouch is typically changed every 3 to 5 days and as needed.[61,62]

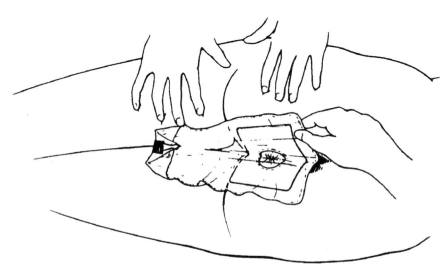

Fig. 15-7 Perianal pouching systems.

TABLE 15-6   Products for Perianal Pouching

Conva Tec Division of ER Squibb and Sons, Inc. Princeton, NJ 08543	Flexiseal Fecal Incontinence Pouch Stomahesive Powder and Paste Allcare Skin Sealant Wipes
Hollister Libertyville, IL 60048	Fecal Incontinence Collector Premium Powder and Paste Skin Gel Sealant Wipes
CR Bard, Inc. Murray Hill, NJ 07974	Fecal Drainage Collector Bard Incontinence Barrier Spray

See Table 15-6 for a listing of companies and products used for perianal pouching.

Internal Drainage Systems. If the patient has severe perianal skin breakdown, it may not be possible to achieve a secure seal with a perianal pouch. In this case, the patient should be evaluated for the use of an internal drainage system. In the past, the only management option for these patients was use of a large-bore balloon-tipped catheter (Foley catheter) connected to bedside drainage; use of these systems is now generally considered contraindicated because of the potential for anorectal necrosis. The two internal drainage systems with demonstrated safety and efficacy are nasopharyneal airways and low-pressure balloon-tipped catheter systems. The nasopharyngeal airway has been used for many years to protect the nasal passages of patients who require nasotracheal suction; this device is now being used to provide drainage of high-volume liquid stool as well. The tubular (shaft) end of a 32-French (8-mm) airway (trumpet) is connected to a bedside drainage bag, and the system is "primed" with mineral oil; the tubing is clamped, mineral oil is instilled through the flange end of the trumpet, and the tubing is opened to allow the mineral oil to drain through the system. The flared end of the airway is then gently inserted into the rectum, and the tubing is stabilized to prevent "pull" on the trumpet. A limited study among intensive care

unit patients demonstrated effective containment of liquid stool and no evidence of anorectal tissue damage with use of this device.[63] Two commercial internal drainage systems are also now available: the Zassi Bowel Management System (Zassi Medical, St. Louis, MO) and the Flexiseal System by Convatec (Princeton, NJ). Both systems involve a large-bore catheter stabilized by a low-pressure balloon, and both have documented safety and efficacy in containment of liquid stool.

Skin protection is another issue for the patient with severe diarrhea because the liquid stool contains enzymes that are extremely damaging to the skin. The goal in management is to create a protective layer between the skin and the stool, and this can be accomplished with plasticizing agents or moisture-barrier products such as zinc oxide preparations. The patient with denuded skin can be managed with an absorptive skin paste or by application of a thin layer of pectin powder followed by a thick layer of moisture-barrier ointment. Skin care is discussed further in Chapter 11.

Absorptive Products. The primary containment option for the individual with chronic fecal incontinence is absorptive products (pads or briefs); individuals with episodic incontinence may also choose to use these products for protection in case of an accident. Individuals who utilize absorptive products for management of fecal incontinence may also benefit from use of oral deodorants, such as bismuth subgallate (Devrom) or chlorophyllin copper complex (Derifil); when taken on a routine basis, these agents tremendously reduce fecal odor. These agents are available over the counter from companies that provide ostomy and incontinent supplies. Absorptive products are discussed further in Chapter 11.

Anal Plugs. For patients with low-volume leakage, such as the patient with passive seepage resulting from internal sphincter damage, anal plugs offer an alternative to absorptive products. These devices consist of a tubular "plug" encased in a water-soluble film and attached to a removal string; when they are inserted into the rectum, the water-soluble film dissolves, and the plug opens into a cup-shaped device that occludes the anal opening. Although these devices have been used effectively by some patients, those with intact sensation frequently find them too uncomfortable to wear. They are currently available in the United Kingdom but not in the United States.[64,65]

SUMMARY

Fecal continence and normal bowel function are complex and multifaceted, and fecal incontinence and bowel dysfunction are underreported but debilitating problems. Effective management of these patients begins with comprehensive assessment that includes a thorough history, focused physical examination, and a bowel chart. Selected patients require additional studies such as anorectal physiology testing, sphincter mapping, or defecography. The assessment data are then used to determine the specific areas of dysfunction and to establish a management plan that corrects or compensates for the dysfunctional component. Specific management strategies include measures to normalize stool consistency, patient education regarding bowel function and bowel management, sensory reeducation programs, strategies to improve sphincter tone and endurance, strategies to reduce fecal urgency, stimulated defecation programs, and surgical procedures to correct specific anatomic defects or to increase anal canal resistance. Patients who are refractory to these strategies may be managed with the ACE procedure and colonic washouts or with fecal diversion. For all patients, available options provide for fecal containment and significantly improve the patient's quality of life.

SELF-ASSESSMENT EXERCISE

1. List critical information to be gathered from the (a) interview, (b) physical examination, and (c) bowel chart of the patient with bowel dysfunction or fecal incontinence.
2. Identify data provided by each of the following studies: (a) anorectal manometry, (b) endoanal ultrasound and MRI of the anal canal, (c) defecography.
3. Explain the effect of fecal impaction on anorectal function and identify options for disimpaction and colonic cleansing.
4. Explain why bulking agents may be used to normalize stool consistency in patients with diarrhea as well as patients with constipation.
5. Explain the following statement: The ideal stool consistency is formed but soft.
6. Identify options for management of high-volume liquid stool and advantages/disadvantages of each.
7. Explain the rationale and basic guidelines for elimination diet therapy.
8. Outline appropriate management for each of the following patients:
   a. A 76-year-old woman with history of chronic constipation who presents with fecal impaction and leakage of liquid stool. On being questioned, she denies any sensation of rectal fullness; her anal wink is intact, and her sphincter tone is normal with good voluntary contractility. She eats mostly starches, dairy products, and meats. She does not eat fruits and vegetables because they bother her stomach. She has used over-the-counter laxatives to induce bowel movements with increasing frequency over the past few years. She reports current use of laxatives as being about once a week and frequency of bowel movements as once or twice a week "with straining." The leakage began just this week, and she is very upset about it. She says she will "do whatever you recommend" to get her bowels working right again.
   b. A 46-year-old woman with complaints of fecal urgency and episodic fecal incontinence, which are more likely to occur when her stool is loose or mushy. History is positive for a third-degree tear during vaginal delivery, which was repaired immediately following delivery. She reports extreme anxiety and depression related to her problems with urgency and leakage and tells you she "doesn't go anywhere unless she can be right next to the bathroom." On examination, her abdomen is soft,

her pelvic is negative for rectocele or prolapse, and her anorectal exam reveals a weak but contractile sphincter. Endoanal ultrasound and anal MRI confirm a small area of scarring involving both the internal and external sphincter, and anorectal manometry reveals sensory awareness of distension at 15 mL but diminished squeeze pressures and very limited ability to "hold" the contraction.

c. A 26-year-old man with low level spina bifida lesion (at S2). He has managed his bowels with a combination of digital stimulation, suppositories, and Fleet enemas but has never had good control. Currently, he is constipating himself during the week so that he maintains continence at work, but on the weekend he uses laxatives to clean himself out. He asks about alternatives to this program but stresses that he would rather continue his present patterns and sacrifice his weekends than risk fecal incontinence. He has no sensory awareness on digital exam and no ability to contract the sphincter voluntarily. His rectum is empty (he scheduled the appointment on Monday so that he would be "cleaned out").

REFERENCES

1. Macmillan A, Merrie A, Marshall R, Parry B: The prevalence of fecal incontinence in community-dwelling adults: a systematic review of the literature, *Dis Colon Rectum* 47(8):1341-1349, 2004.
2. Norton C: The development of bowel control. In: Norton C, Chelvanayagam S, editors: *Bowel continence nursing*, Beaconsfield, United Kingdom, 2004, Beaconsfield Publishers, pp 1-7.
3. Tuteja A, Rao S: Review article: recent trends in diagnosis and treatment of faecal incontinence, *Aliment Pharmacol Ther* 19:829-840, 2004.
4. Miner P: Economic and personal impact of fecal and urinary incontinence, *Gastroenterology* 126:S8-S13, 2004.
5. Madoff R, Parker S, Varma M, Lowry A: Faecal incontinence in adults, *Lancet* 364:621-632, 2004.
6. Johanson J, Lafferty J: Epidemiology of fecal incontinence: the silent affliction, *Am J Gastroenterol* 91:33-36, 1996.
7. Nelson R: Epidemiology of fecal incontinence, *Gastroenterology* 126:S3-S7, 2004.
8. Nelson R, Norton N, Cautley E, Furner S: Community-based prevalence of anal incontinence, *JAMA* 274:559-561, 1995.
9. Bliss D, Norton C, Miller J, Krissovich M: Directions for future nursing research on fecal incontinence, *Nurs Res* 53(6S):S15-S21, 2004.
10. Scarlett Y: Medical management of fecal incontinence, *Gastroenterology* 126:S55-S63, 2004.
11. Schnelle J, Leung F: Urinary and fecal incontinence in nursing homes, *Gastroenterology* 126:S41-S47, 2004.
12. Tariq S: Geriatric fecal incontinence, *Clin Geriatr Med* 20(3):571-587, 2004.
13. Kouraklis G, Andromanakos N: Evaluating patients with anorectal incontinence, *Surg Today* 34:304-312, 2004.
14. Bharucha A: Outcome measures for fecal incontinence: anorectal structure and function, *Gastroenterology* 126:S90-S98, 2004.
15. Rao S: Pathophysiology of adult fecal incontinence, *Gastroenterology* 126:S14-S22, 2004.
16. Norton C, Chelvanayagam S: Causes of faecal incontinence, In: Norton C, Chelvanayagam S, editors: *Bowel continence nursing*, Beaconsfield, United Kingdom, 2004, Beaconsfield Publishers, pp 23-32.
17. Gregory W, Nygaard I: Childbirth and pelvic floor disorders, *Clin Obstet Gynecol* 47(2):394-403, 2004.
18. Chelvanayagam S, Norton C: Nursing assessment of adults with faecal incontinence, In: Norton C, Chelvanayagam S, editors: *Bowel continence nursing*, Beaconsfield, United Kingdom, 2004, Beaconsfield Publishers, pp 45-62.
19. Rockwood T, Church J, Fleshman J, et al: Fecal incontinence quality of life scale: quality of life instrument for patients with fecal incontinence, *Dis Colon Rectum* 43:9-16, 2000.
20. Doughty D: A physiologic approach to bowel training, *J Wound Ostomy Continence Nurs* 23:46, 1996.
21. MacLeod J: Assessment of patients with fecal incontinence. In: Doughty D, editor: *Urinary and fecal incontinence: nursing management*, St. Louis, 1991, Mosby.
22. Cundiff G, Fenner D: Evaluation and treatment of women with rectocele: focus on associated defecatory and sexual dysfunction, *Obstet Gynecol* 104(6):1403-1421, 2004.
23. Coller J, Sangwan Y: Computerized anal sphincter manometry performance and analysis. In: Smith L, editor: *Practical guide to anorectal testing*, ed 2, New York, 1995, Igaku-Shoin.
24. Read N, Sun W: Anorectal manometry. In: MM Henry, M Swash, editors: *Coloproctology and the pelvic floor*, Stoneham, Mass., 1992, Butterworth Heinemann.
25. Sentovich S, Blatchford G, Rivela L, et al: Diagnosing anal sphincter injury with transanal ultrasound and manometry, *Dis Colon Rectum* 40(12):1430, 1997.
26. Wong W: Endorectal ultrasonography for benign disease. In: Staren ED, editor: *Ultrasound for the surgeon*, Philadelphia, 1997, Lippincott-Raven.
27. Orkin B: Fecal incontinence: evaluation. In: Smith LE, editor: *Practical guide to anorectal testing*, ed 2, New York, 1995, Igaku-Shoin.
28. Nicholls T: Anorectal physiology investigation techniques, In: Norton C, Chelvanayagam S, editors: *Bowel continence nursing*, Beaconsfield, United Kingdom, 2004, Beaconsfield Publishers, pp 69-82.

29. Glassman L: Defecography. In: Smith L, ed. *Practical guide to anorectal testing,* ed 2, New York, 1995, Igaku-Shoin.

30. Basch A, Jensen L: Management of fecal incontinence. In: Doughty D, editor: *Urinary and fecal incontinence: nursing management,* St. Louis, 1991, Mosby.

31. Frick O: A sensible approach to food allergy, *Patient Care* 19:48, 1985.

32. Hyams J: Carbohydrate malabsorption. In: Bayless TM, editor: *Current therapy in gastroenterology and liver disease,* Toronto, 1990, BC Decker.

33. Kumar P: Celiac sprue and related problems. In: Bayless TM, editor: *Current therapy in gastroenterology and liver disease,* Toronto, 1990, BC Decker.

34. Leonard T, Watson R, Mohs M: The effects of caffeine on various body systems: a review, *J Am Diet Assoc* 87:8, 1987.

35. Burkitt D, Walker A, Painter N: Effect of dietary fiber on stools and transit times and its role in causation of disease, *Lancet* 12:1408, 1972.

36. Gross J: Elimination: functional alterations of bowel. In: Johnson B, Gross J, editors: *Handbook on oncology nursing,* Bethany, Conn., 1985, Fleshner Publishing Co.

37. Di Lorenzo C, Williams C, Hajnal F, Valenzuela J: Pectin delays gastric emptying and increases satiety in obese subjects, *Gastroenterology* 95:1211, 1988.

38. Bliss D, Jung H, Savik K, et al: Supplementation with dietary fiber improves fecal incontinence, *Nurs Res* 50:203-213, 2001.

39. Cheetham M, Brazzelli M, Norton C, Glazener C: Drug treatment for faecal incontinence in adults, *Cochrane Database Syst Rev* 2005.

40. Cerulli M, Nikoomanesh P, Schuster M: Progress in biofeedback for fecal incontinence, *Gastroenterology* 76:742, 1979.

41. Whitehead W, Burgio K, Engel B: Biofeedback treatment for fecal incontinence in geriatric patients, *J Am Geriatr Soc* 33:320, 1985.

42. Engel B, Nikoomanesh P, Schuster M: Operant conditioning of rectosphincteric responses in the treatment of fecal incontinence, *N Engl J Med* 290:646, 1994.

43. Jensen L, Lowry A: Biofeedback improves the functional outcome after sphincteroplasty, *Dis Colon Rectum* 40:197, 1997.

44. Lowry A, Jensen L: Biofeedback for anal incontinence. In: Schrock TR, editor: *Perspectives in colon and rectal surgery,* St. Louis, 1992, Quality Medical Publishers.

45. Wald A: Biofeedback therapy for fecal incontinence, *Ann Intern Med* 95:146, 1981.

46. Kegel A: Progressive resistive exercises in the functional restoration of the perineal muscles, *Am J Obstet Gynecol* 56:238, 1948.

47. Kegel A: Stress incontinence of women: psychological treatment, *J Int Coll Surg* 25:484, 1956.

48. Norton C, Hosker G, Brazzelli M: Biofeedback and/or sphincter exercises for the treatment of faecal incontinence in adults, *Cochrane Rev* 3:2004.

49. MacLeod J: Management of anal incontinence by biofeedback, *Gastroenterology* 93(2):291-294, 1987.

50. Whitehead W, Schuster M: Anorectal physiology and pathophysiology, *Am J Gastroenterol* 82:487, 1987.

51. Cheetham M, Kamm M, Phillips R: Topical phenylephrine increases anal canal resting pressure in patients with faecal incontinence, *Gut* 48:356-359, 2001.

52. Jarrett M, Mowatt G, Glazener M, et al: Systematic review of sacral nerve stimulation for faecal incontinence and constipation, *Br J Surg* 91:1559-1569, 2004.

53. Matzel K, Stadelmaier U, Hohenberger W: Innovations in fecal incontinence: sacral nerve stimulation, *Dis Colon Rectum* 47(10):1720-1728, 2004.

54. Madoff R: Surgical treatment options for fecal incontinence, *Gastroenterology* 126:S48-S54, 2004.

55. Wong W, Congliosi S, Spencer M, et al: The safety and efficacy of the artificial bowel sphincter for fecal incontinence: results from a multicenter cohort study, *Dis Colon Rectum* 45:1139-1153, 2002.

56. Cromie W, Goldfischer E, Kim J: Laparoscopic creation of a continent cecal tube for antegrade colonic irrigation, *Urology* 47(6):905-907, 1996.

57. Teichman J, Rogenes V, Barber D: The Malone antegrade continence enema combined with urinary diversion in adult neurogenic patients: early results, *Urology* 49(6):963-967, 1997.

58. Herndon C, Rink R, Cain M, et al: In situ Malone antegrade continence enema in 127 patients: a 6-year experience, *J Urol* 172(4 suppl):1689-1691, 2004.

59. McGarity W: Gastrointestinal surgical procedures. In: Hampton B, Bryant R, editors: *Ostomies and continent diversions: nursing management,* St. Louis, 1992, Mosby.

60. Vulhop L, Sommers M, Wolverton C: Containment of fecal incontinence by the use of a perianal pouch, *J Enterostomal Ther* 11:59-62, 1984.

61. Jeter K: The use of incontinence products. In: Jeter K, Faller N, Norton C, editors: *Nursing for continence,* Philadelphia, 1990, WB Saunders.

62. Ross V: The fecal containment device: one answer to a dreaded procedure, *Ostomy Wound Manage* 39:42, 1993.

63. Grogan T, Kramer D: The rectal trumpet: use of a nasopharyngeal airway to contain fecal incontinence in critically ill patients, *J Wound Ostomy Continence Nurs* 29(4):193-200, 2002.

64. Chelvanayagam S, Norton C: Practical management of faecal incontinence, In: Norton C, Chelvanayagam S, editors: *Bowel continence nursing,* Beaconsfield, United Kingdom, 2004, Beaconsfield Publishers, pp 229-237.

65. Doherty W: Managing faecal incontinence or leakage: the Peristeen Anal Plug, *Br J Nurs* 13(21):1293-1297, 2004.

16 *Bowel and Bladder Management in Children*

ANNE K. JINBO & MARIALIANA STARK
(Reviewed by Jane R. Starn & Janet Camacho)

OBJECTIVES

1. Identify the factors commonly accepted as "readiness criteria" for toilet training and the implications for timing of toilet training efforts.
2. Define the following terms: fecal incontinence, encopresis, functional constipation, primary nocturnal enuresis.
3. Explain the difference between primary and secondary enuresis and encopresis and between retentive and nonretentive encopresis.
4. Describe the pathophysiology of encopresis and the related clinical presentation.
5. Outline key factors to be included in the assessment and management of the child who has retentive encopresis.
6. Explain how each of the following contribute to fecal incontinence: imperforate anus repair, Hirschsprung's repair, myelomeningocele.
7. Outline the assessment and management of the child with a neurogenic bowel.
8. Describe the three developmental tasks involved in the acquisition of voluntary bladder control.
9. Explain what is meant by the term "dysfunctional voiding" and how it contributes to incomplete bladder emptying.
10. Outline the key factors to be included in the assessment of a child with dysfunctional voiding or urinary incontinence.
11. Briefly describe current theories regarding the causes of primary nocturnal enuresis and the related management options.
12. Describe the pathophysiology of the Hinman syndrome and the key components of appropriate management.
13. Compare and contrast the management of neurogenic bladder in a child to management of the adult patient with reflex urinary incontinence.
14. Identify major psychosocial factors to be assessed and addressed in the management of any child with bowel or bladder dysfunction.

Children are subject to many of the same problems associated with bowel and bladder dysfunction as are experienced by adults; in addition, children are subject to many congenital and developmental disorders affecting the bowel and bladder. This chapter deals with elimination issues unique to children.

BOWEL MANAGEMENT

FETAL DEVELOPMENT OF THE GASTROINTESTINAL SYSTEM

Normal bowel function in the infant and child is dependent partly on normal fetal development of the gastrointestinal (GI) system. Although a detailed description of fetal GI tract development is beyond the scope of this text, a brief review of the critical aspects that are most likely to be involved in congenital anomalies is provided.

Development of the GI tract begins during the fourth week of fetal life, when the primitive gut arises from the dorsal part of the yolk sac. The primitive gut can be divided into three segments: the foregut, the midgut, and the hindgut. The foregut develops into the pharynx, lower respiratory system, esophagus, stomach, upper portion of the duodenum, liver, pancreas, and biliary system. The vascular supply for these bowel segments is provided by the forerunner to the celiac artery. The midgut evolves into the small bowel distal to the orifice of the bile duct, the cecum, the appendix, the ascending colon, and most of the transverse colon. The blood supply for the midgut is provided by the superior mesenteric artery, and these segments of bowel are attached to the posterior abdominal wall by the dorsal mesentery. The hindgut forms the left transverse colon, the descending colon, the sigmoid colon, the rectum, and the proximal portion of the anal canal. The inferior mesenteric artery provides the blood supply for the bowel segments arising from the hindgut.

The midgut undergoes an interesting sequence of events during its development, and any defect in the normal sequence can produce congenital complications involving the small bowel and proximal colon. As the midgut lengthens and enlarges, it becomes too large for the developing fetal abdomen; as a result, the midgut herniates into the umbilical cord. When the fetal abdomen enlarges sufficiently to accommodate the midgut, these segments of bowel "return" to the abdominal cavity; however, they rotate in a counterclockwise position during their return (Fig. 16-1). The small bowel segment of the midgut is the first to return, and it passes into the abdominal cavity in a position that is posterior to the superior mesenteric artery. The ascending and transverse colon segments then return and assume a position anterior to the superior mesenteric artery. The mesentery for the midgut attaches to the posterior abdominal wall close to the duodenum and ascending colon, which causes these segments of the bowel to assume a retroperitoneal position. Abnormalities in rotation may produce obstructive syndromes in the neonatal period.

Another aspect of fetal development that is critical to normal GI function after birth is the establishment of a patent lumen. Normal development of the GI "tube" involves endodermal proliferation, which temporarily occludes the lumen of the gut. However, this period of occlusion is normally followed by recanalization (Fig. 16-2). Failure to recanalize the lumen may result in atresia (complete obstruction of the lumen), stenosis, cysts, or intestinal duplication.[1,2]

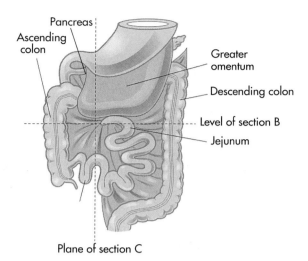

Fig. 16-1 Normal rotation of bowel in counterclockwise fashion during return to the abdominal cavity. (From Moore K, Persaud TVN: *The developing human,* ed 7, Philadelphia, 2003, WB Saunders.)

A final aspect of GI development that is critical to normal function is the separation between the GI and genitourinary systems. In very early stages of fetal development, the rudimentary reproductive, urinary, and intestinal ducts terminate in a common hollow cavity known as the "cloaca." At about week 4, the urorectal septum begins to form. This sheet of connective tissue divides the cloacal cavity into two separate compartments: the anterior compartment develops into the lower genitourinary tract, and the posterior compartment develops into the rectum and anal canal. Congenital anorectal defects such as imperforate anus occur when this developmental sequence is interrupted or altered.

FECAL ELIMINATION IN CHILDREN

Bowel function may be described in terms of stool frequency, stool consistency, and stool size (caliber). Unfortunately, it is difficult to define "normal" bowel habits in a healthy population because of the many variables that influence the frequency and consistency of fecal elimination. This variability is well documented among adult populations and is believed to be attributable in large part to differences

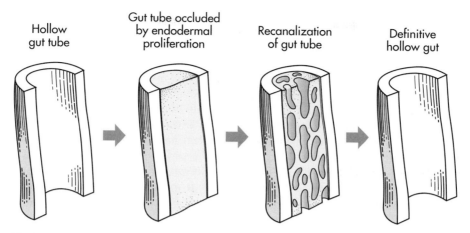

| Hollow gut tube | Gut tube occluded by endodermal proliferation | Recanalization of gut tube | Definitive hollow gut |

Fig. 16-2 Occlusion of bowel lumen followed by recanalization during fetal development. (Redrawn from Larsen WJ: *Human embryology,* Edinburgh, 1993, Churchill Livingstone.)

in dietary intake; for example, studies among adults in Western societies reveal a variability in bowel movement frequency ranging from three times daily to three times weekly. (Bowel movement frequency falls within this range for 94% to 99% of the study population.[2])

In infancy, normal stool frequency is much higher than among children and adults. For example, one study of newborn infants documented stool frequency ranging from one to nine stools daily during the first week of life.[2] Infants between 2 and 20 weeks of age typically have one to seven stools daily, with significant reported differences between breast-fed and formula-fed infants; breast-fed infants have fewer stools during the first week of life but a significantly higher number of stools thereafter as compared with formula-fed infants.[2] These differences in stool frequency gradually diminish after 8 weeks; by 16 weeks of age, when many infants have been introduced to solid foods, there is no difference in stool frequency between the two groups.[2]

Stool frequency among preschool children is reported to be comparable to stool frequency among adults, with significant variation reported among various populations. Individuals following high-fiber and vegetarian diets typically have a greater number of bowel movements than individuals following a meat-based, low-fiber diet. However, one interesting study compared stool frequency among subjects from Western countries and subjects from developing countries and found that stool frequency was lower in developing countries.[2]

There is limited information available regarding usual stool size and consistency in children because of the difficulty in obtaining precise information regarding stool characteristics from a large number of patients. (One factor contributing to this difficulty is the lack of clear and consistent definitions for terms used to describe stool consistency.) In infants, the daily stool volume has been reported to remain constant (at approximately 5 to 10 g/kg/day) until about the twentieth week of life, with variations between breast-fed and formula-fed infants as noted earlier. There is very limited information available regarding daily stool output (that is, stool weight) during childhood; it *is* known, however, that stool weight among "normal" subjects varies widely as a consequence of dietary variations. (The effect of diet on stool weight may be a result of changes in colonic bacterial flora, because bacteria are known to account for almost 50% of stool volume.[2])

ACQUISITION OF FECAL CONTINENCE

Total control over bowel elimination is generally achieved by 4 years of age,[3] and most children achieve bowel and bladder control during *waking* hours by age 3. To achieve continence, the child must have functioning sphincters, normal rectal sensation, and normal rectosigmoid motility. In addition, the child must demonstrate both physiologic and developmental "readiness." Brazelton identified both physiologic and psychologic criteria that must be met for a child to acquire continence and stated that readiness seems to peak for most children between 18 and 30 months of age. The two physiologic "readiness criteria" include *reflex sphincter control,* which can be demonstrated as early as 9 months of age, and *myelinization of the pyramidal tracts,* which is complete between 12 and 18 months of age. Azrin and Foxx recommended the addition of bladder control to the list of readiness criteria; they defined bladder control as the ability to empty the bladder completely with voiding and to stay dry for several hours. Psychologic and cognitive "readiness" is equally critical but less predictable in terms of time frames for accomplishment. Developmental criteria include motor skills such as walking to the bathroom, sitting on the toilet, clothing manipulation (such as pulling pants up and down), and flushing the toilet. Cognitive readiness, according to Azrin and Foxx, include the child's ability to communicate impending urination or defecation, either through facial expressions or posturing, and instructional readiness. Instructional readiness includes both receptive language (such as words to describe voiding or defecation) and the ability to follow one-step or two-step commands. Azrin and Foxx suggested that the most appropriate time frame for initiating toilet training for most children is between 24 and 30 months of age.[4] Brazelton and Azrin and Foxx provide guidelines for parents to use in toilet training their children. The approach advocated by Azrin and Foxx is particularly comprehensive and is associated with successful outcomes in their studies, although it may not be feasible for all parents.[5]

BOWEL DYSFUNCTION AND FECAL INCONTINENCE

Based on the previously cited time frames for "usual" acquisition of continence, one may consider a child who has not acquired bowel control by 4 years of age to be "fecally incontinent." Several terms are used to refer to bowel control problems among children, and these terms are defined as follows:

- *Fecal incontinence:* Fecal soiling associated with an organic or anatomic lesion, such as anal malformation, anorectal surgery or trauma, or neuromuscular disorder (such as myelomeningocele)
- *Fecal soiling:* Any amount of stool deposited in the underwear, regardless of the cause
- *Encopresis:* Fecal soiling usually associated with functional constipation; also used to refer to fecal incontinence not caused by an organic or anatomic lesion
- *Functional constipation:* Constipation not caused by organic or anatomic abnormalities *or* the requirement of medication to regulate bowel function after 4 years of age

Children with fecal incontinence fall into four main groups: children with functional fecal retention and overflow soiling (retentive encopresis), children with functional nonretentive fecal soiling (nonretentive encopresis), children with anorectal malformations, and children with neurologic lesions such as spina bifida (Fig. 16-3).

The pathophysiology of the dysfunction differs in each of these groups, and different management programs are required based on the underlying pathophysiology. Therefore, each of these groups is addressed separately in terms of management. However, accurate determination of the underlying problem is dependent on a thorough evaluation; thus, the key elements of assessment for any child with bowel dysfunction or fecal incontinence are presented first, followed by a discussion of specific problems.

History

Spending the time to obtain a thorough history is critical to gaining an understanding of the child's elimination disorder and its effect on the child and family. Key areas to be addressed during the patient and family interview include the medical history, developmental history, and behavioral assessment. Specific areas of inquiry for each of these areas are outlined in Box 16-1.

Fecal Incontinence

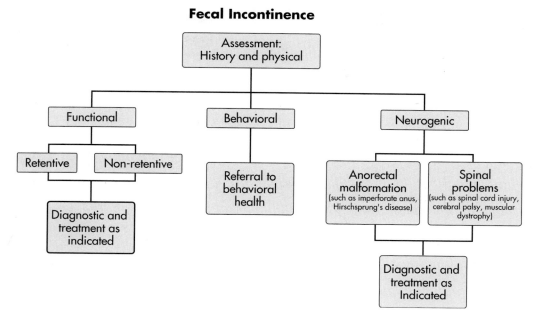

Fig. 16-3 Algorithm for assessment and management of fecal incontinence.

Physical Assessment

The focus of the physical assessment is on determining the presence and severity of fecal retention and ruling out potential organic causes of lower bowel dysfunction, such as disorders affecting the lumbosacral cord. Throughout the history and physical examination, the clinician should be alert to evidence of emotional problems requiring additional investigation.

To assess for fecal accumulation, the clinician inspects and palpates the abdomen and performs a rectal examination. Typically, hard fecal masses within the colon can be palpated through the abdominal surface; however, palpatory findings may be noncontributory if the child has retained stool throughout the colon but no hard masses. Therefore, a negative abdominal examination does not exclude the possibility of significant fecal retention throughout the colon.

The anorectal examination begins with inspection of the perianal skin for evidence of dermatitis,

fissures, or cellulitis; acute perianal cellulitis caused by group A streptococci has been documented among these children and requires aggressive treatment.[6] The anus is then inspected for placement and resting tone. An anteriorly displaced anus may lead to symptoms of constipation and straining at stool in some infants and children, although it is considered a variant of normal in most individuals. A patulous anus is indicative of denervation, typically caused by a spinal cord lesion. A digital rectal examination is then done to assess for retained stool and to evaluate sensory function and sphincter function. (It is important to defer this component of the physical examination until the clinician has established rapport with the child and to obtain the child's consent and cooperation before the examination is done.) The child is asked to tell the examiner when the examiner inserts the gloved lubricated finger into the rectum. On insertion, the examiner should evaluate resting resistance; normally, the sphincter is appreciated as providing passive resistance that is

BOX 16-1 History Taking Guidelines for Children with Encopresis

Past Medical History

- Medical treatment(s) or condition(s) that could lead to problems with constipation:
  - Anorectal anomalies such as imperforate anus or anorectal stenosis (treatment to date)
  - Hirschsprung's disease (aganglionic megacolon): age at diagnosis, management before and after diagnosis (usually managed by initial fecal diversion to "decompress" bowel, followed by resection or bypass of aganglionic segment or segments and anastomosis of proximal functioning bowel to anal canal)
  - Medications: anticholinergics, tricyclic antidepressants, sympathomimetics?
  - Chronic anal fissures or perineal dermatitis leading to painful defecation
  - Hypothyroidism (significant possibility only in child with delayed linear growth)*
- Onset of encopresis; history of constipation; family history of constipation
- Present stooling and leakage pattern (frequency, amount, consistency of voluntary bowel movements and incontinent episodes; thorough description of encopretic episodes)
- Past and current use of laxatives, enemas, and suppositories, and results obtained
- Dietary intake with special focus on intake of fiber and fluid and foods and fluids known to be constipating (such as large amounts of milk or milk products); decreased appetite
- History of urinary tract infections or daytime or nighttime wetting; abdominal pain

Developmental History

- Developmental stage at which problem with fecal elimination began
- Age at which child was fully trained (if child was ever fully trained) and any evidence of encopresis during training period
- Critical life events or transitions associated with onset of bowel dysfunction (such as entry into school); family or personal life stressors

- Time frame for achievement of other developmental milestones (such as walking): normal or delayed?
- Evidence of attention deficit problems (that is, difficulty staying on task) that could interfere with ability to establish a normal bowel pattern? Cognitive dysfunction or learning disability? (Note evidence that there is an increased incidence of learning disabilities among encopretic children.[†])
- Overall academic performance and classroom behavior
- Peer relationships: any identified problems?

Psychosocial Assessment

- Psychosocial conditions in child's environment that could be contributing to the problem with encopresis (such as marital issues causing tension, problems with siblings)
- Approach to discipline within family
- Indications of deprivation or abnormal patterns of nurturance
- Effect of encopresis on family: Disagreement or disruption within family related to the problem? Guilt and accusation related to the problem?
- Parents' beliefs and understanding re: problem and cause; child's understanding and beliefs re: the problem and cause (if child is able to discuss the problem)
- Past and present methods for handling the encopresis within the family, to include any punishment strategies (for example, has child been spanked or had privileges withdrawn?); consistency (versus variability) of response
- Child's usual temperament style and general behavior at home; any evidence of depression?
- Relationships with family members and friends; any social interactional difficulties?
- Any evidence of secondary gains resulting from the encopresis?

---

*Datum from Boon RF, Singh N: *Behav Modif* 15(3):355-371, 1991.
[†]Datum from Stern P, Lowitz G, Prince M, et al: *Neurotoxicology* 9(3):351-358, 1988.

circumferential and symmetric. The child should then be asked to "tighten the muscle as if trying to hold in gas or stool," an act that allows the examiner to assess voluntary sphincter contraction strength. The child can then be asked to "push down and out as if you are trying to push out stool or my finger;" this maneuver allows the clinician to assess for voluntary pelvic muscle relaxation. Abnormal findings include diminished resting tone, the inability to sense the examining finger, and the inability to voluntarily contract or relax the sphincter muscles; these findings are common among children with neurologic lesions such as spina bifida with myelomeningocele. (If there is a significant volume of retained stool in the rectal vault, the digital rectal examination should be repeated after removal of the retained stool; this requirement may delay the full examination until a follow-up visit.)

The lumbosacral area and lower extremities should be closely examined for further evidence of a neurologic lesion; for example, flat buttocks are seen in children with sacral agenesis, and a pilonidal dimple or a hairy patch is common in children with spina bifida occulta, which may be associated with a tethered spinal cord. The lower extremities should also be evaluated for sensation, symmetry, and motor function; children with neurologic lesions affecting the pelvic floor and sphincter muscles may also have sensorimotor dysfunction affecting the lower extremities.

Diagnostic Studies

Diagnostic studies are frequently indicated when initial evaluation reveals retained stool or evidence of neurologic deficits or when the child fails to respond to initial conservative therapy; these tests provide additional data regarding the structure and function of the colon, rectum, and pelvic floor. Tests that are commonly ordered include the following:[7]

Abdominal Flat Plate. The abdominal flat plate is a "plain" radiograph of the abdomen frequently beneficial in detecting retained stool throughout the colon that is not appreciated on abdominal palpation. The extent of the imaged stool found on the radiograph helps to direct appropriate treatment. In addition, a flat plate reassures the clinician and the family that the problem is not caused by some rare disorder that has been overlooked.[8] (This test can be particularly helpful for the patient in whom initial therapy fails.)

Barium Enema. A barium enema is a contrast study done to identify any evidence of specific disorders, such as Hirschsprung's disease, that would adversely affect fecal elimination. Barium enema is of particular benefit in identifying anatomic anomalies, such as malrotation or luminal lesions (polyps or tumors), that could contribute to constipation. Colonic and rectal motility can be indirectly assessed by fluoroscopy and analysis of the postevacuation film.

Colonic Transit Study with Markers. The colonic transit study is done to rule out a motility disorder as the cause of chronic constipation. The patient ingests a specified number of radiopaque pellets, and serial abdominal films are obtained to observe the progression of the markers through the colon. Segmental transit times for the right and left colon and the rectum are determined by plain abdominal radiographs performed on alternate days until at least 80% of the markers are excreted. (Physiologically normal adults pass 80% of the markers within 5 days and 100% within 7 days.) Retention of the markers in the right or transverse colon at 7 days is indicative of disordered colonic motility.

Anorectal Manometry. Anorectal manometry is one of the most commonly performed studies among children with encopresis. Pressure-sensitive probes or balloons are inserted into the rectum and anal canal at the levels of the internal sphincter and the external sphincter. The rectal balloon is then inflated to simulate rectal distension, and the response of the anal sphincters is evaluated. This test is extremely valuable in the detection of Hirschsprung's disease, in which the rectoanal inhibitory reflex (internal sphincter relaxation in response to rectal distension) is lost. In the child with retentive encopresis, common findings include diminished sensitivity to rectal distension and elevated anal sphincter pressures.

Radiographic Defecography. The radiographic defecography test is also known as an evaluation proctography and is useful in the evaluation of constipation caused by outlet obstruction. In adults, it is sometimes used to detect lesions such as rectocele or rectal intussusception; however, children are frequently less cooperative than adults, and this test is not widely used among the pediatric population.

Sphincter Electromyography. The sphincter electromyography test is done to identify patients whose chronic functional outlet obstruction is caused by failure to effectively relax the pelvic floor muscles during attempted defecation. Surface electrodes are applied to the perianal skin and are connected to a display monitor; the patient is then asked to tighten the muscles, relax the muscles, and "bear down" as if having a bowel movement. Failure to relax the muscles is evidenced by persistent or increased pelvic muscle electrical activity during the child's attempts to relax and to bear down. This group of patients generally responds well to biofeedback, in which patients relearn appropriate muscle control, including relaxation.

Rectal Compliance. The rectal compliance test is done to evaluate the rectum's ability to relax around a bolus of stool, thus providing temporary storage until defecation is convenient. To conduct the test, the clinician inserts an inflatable balloon into the rectum and a pressure probe between the rectal wall and the balloon. The balloon is then inflated to simulate rectal distension, and the rectal wall pressures are measured. Two patterns may be observed in children with fecal incontinence: (1) the child may exhibit abnormally high rectal wall pressures in response to limited rectal distension, that is, *diminished rectal compliance*; or (2) the child may exhibit abnormally low rectal wall pressures in response to rectal distension, that is, *increased rectal compliance*. Diminished compliance results in the inability to store stool and to delay defecation and is common among children with inflammatory processes such as Crohn's proctitis; these patients experience a constant defecatory urge at low rectal volumes. Increased compliance is commonly seen in children with chronic fecal retention resulting in persistent rectal distension; these children report diminished sensory awareness of rectal filling even at significant rectal volumes.

Colonic Manometry. The colonic manometry test is not commonly used but can be helpful in distinguishing between myopathic and neuropathic causes of functional fecal retention.

Laboratory Tests. Laboratory tests are indicated for selected children with encopresis based on data gathered in the history and physical examination. For example, thyroid function tests and measurements of electrolytes, calcium, and magnesium may be indicated to rule out or diagnose underlying pathologic conditions such as hypothyroidism. The only routine laboratory study is a urinalysis and possibly a urine culture and sensitivity for girls with encopresis, who are at increased risk for urinary tract infection.

MANAGEMENT OF BOWEL DYSFUNCTION AND FECAL INCONTINENCE

Fecal incontinence represents one of the most embarrassing and psychologically devastating problems of childhood. Fecal incontinence in children is generally caused by one of three pathologic conditions: encopresis, congenital conditions, or neuromuscular disorders. Each of these is addressed separately.

Encopresis

The prevalence of encopresis in the pediatric population averages about 2.8% among 4 year olds, 1.9% among 6 year olds, and 1.6% among 10 to 11 year olds.[9] Encopresis accounts for 3% to 5% of visits to a general pediatric outpatient clinic and up to 25% of visits to pediatric gastroenterologists.[10-12] Encopresis typically presents in children less than 7 years of age. Male gender seems to be a risk factor; studies indicate that the ratio between boys and girls is at least 3:1 and possibly as high as 6:1.[13,14] However, socioeconomic status, family size, ordinal position of the child within the family, and age of parents have not been found to correlate positively with incidence of encopresis. There *is* a correlation with enuresis, which may be attributable to the effects of retained stool and rectal distension on the adjacent bladder; 25% of children with encopresis also have enuresis.

Classifications. Encopresis is sometimes classified as primary or secondary and as retentive or nonretentive. *Primary encopresis* refers to the condition in a child who has reached 4 years of age and has never achieved sustained bowel control (that is, fecal continence lasting for at least 1 year), whereas *secondary encopresis* is used to indicate the condition in a child who has been successfully toilet trained and has maintained continence for at least 1 year and then "relapsed" in response to some secondary disorder.[15,16] Approximately 50% to 60% of all encopretic children have secondary encopresis. *Retentive encopresis* is the term used to refer to fecal incontinence clearly associated with constipation; these children retain stool and may even develop a megacolon. *Nonretentive encopresis* is defined as fecal incontinence in a child who has no evidence of constipation; it is usually additionally classified as primary nonretentive encopresis (incontinence in a child who has never acquired bowel control) and secondary nonretentive encopresis (incontinence in a child who successfully completes toilet training but later regresses).[8] It is generally believed that primary nonretentive encopresis may be caused either by an organic problem or by emotional stressors, whereas secondary nonretentive encopresis is almost always caused by psychologic issues.[8] Encopresis can also be classified as diurnal or nocturnal, but this classification is rarely used because nocturnal encopresis is quite uncommon.

According to the fourth edition of the *Diagnostic and Statistical Manual of Mental Disorders* (DSM-IV), the diagnostic criteria for encopresis include the following: repeated passage of feces into places not appropriate for that purpose (such as clothing, floor) whether involuntary or intentional; at least one such event a month for at least 3 months; chronologic age of at least 4 years and/or equivalent developmental age; and no physiologic or medical basis for the behavior except for mechanisms related to constipation (that is, not caused by a laxative or medical condition).[17]

Etiology. Although the cause of encopresis is poorly understood, Levine postulated that in many children encopresis represents a functional bowel disorder that can be at least partly explained from a developmental perspective; he hypothesized that as children pass through critical developmental stages, the environment, people in their lives, or critical life events may contribute to a functional bowel disorder. This hypothesis is supported by evidence that the history of many children with encopresis is positive for several of these "risk" factors.[13] Levine outlined the developmental stages and issues as follows:

Stage I: Early experience and predisposition (infancy and toddler years). Children with a tendency toward constipation during this period, because of genetic or dietary factors, are at greater risk for the development of encopresis when they are older. The major risk factor during this stage is functional constipation, which may develop as a result of immature bowel function, surgical correction of congenital anomalies (such as imperforate anus), parental overreaction to toileting, or aggressive bowel management. These factors may lead to voluntary withholding of stool, in which defecation is perceived as a negative experience.

Stage II: Training and autonomy (2 to 5 years of age). During this stage, the child is beginning to develop autonomy and independence, and potentiating factors for bowel dysfunction include psychosocial stressors (birth of sibling, mother's returning to work, parental discord) during toilet training, coercive or extremely permissive toilet training, fears of toileting (such as monsters that bite when one sits down on the toilet), and painful or difficult defecation.

Stage III: Extramural function (early school years). Extramural function refers to the time frame during which the child enters school. These children are faced with a new routine, which includes using the school bathroom or withholding stool until they return home. Dietary habits, such as excessive ingestion of milk and decreased intake of fruits, vegetables, and fiber, may contribute to constipation. Additional potential risk factors include frenetic life styles, psychosocial stressors that evolve with school relationships, and illness or injury that results in prolonged inactivity with a resulting change in bowel function.

Psychosocial stressors at any stage can cause enough distraction to prevent a child's full attention to the urge to defecate. Children with attention deficit disorder may be at greater risk because of their inability to sit still to finish a task. Physical or sexual abuse can also result in fecal soiling. The emotional distraction caused by the abuse is more often the cause for the fecal soiling than the actual physical abuse.

It is clear that the risk factors for each individual child are likely to be somewhat different; it is therefore critical to perform a comprehensive assessment as a basis for an individualized treatment plan.[13]

Clinical Presentation. There seem to be three major clinical patterns among children with encopresis. In more than 90% of cases, encopresis is the result of functional constipation. In this condition, retention of stool causes rectal distension, with resultant leakage of stool around the retained bolus. Because the rectum is chronically distended, the stretch receptors fail to signal the child that defecation is imminent. As a result, these children commonly have several fecal accidents per day. The stool size is usually small, and the consistency of the stool is generally loose. These children are sometimes misdiagnosed as having diarrhea based on parental reports of odorous, thin, ribbonlike, or diarrheal stools.

A much less common pattern of encopresis is the nonretentive pattern; children with this condition may experience stress-related diarrhea, which appears to be associated with the disorder known as irritable bowel syndrome among adults, or they may experience daily incontinence of stool that is of normal size and consistency. The third and least common pattern is manipulative soiling, in which the child uses incontinent episodes to manipulate the environment (for example, to avoid school or to passively display anger toward family members).

Almost all children with encopresis retain stool at least intermittently. Typically, the retention develops gradually over time. Some children with encopresis actually defecate daily but fail to empty the lower bowel effectively, and because of this failure to empty the bowel, stool gradually amasses in the rectum and colon. The child may be asymptomatic or may complain of recurrent abdominal pain. Retained stool may be palpable on abdominal examination (if the child has significant colonic retention) or may be evident only on rectal examination (if the retained stool is confined to the rectum).

As rectal and colonic distension progresses, sensory feedback from the bowel becomes impaired; that is, rectal distension no longer causes sensory awareness of the need to defecate. In addition, distension of the rectal wall overstretches the muscle fibers, which reduces contractile force. There is no awareness of the need to defecate and no propulsive force to eliminate the stool; as a result, stool continues to accumulate in the rectum, where continued water absorption creates a hard fecal mass. As the fecal mass becomes larger and harder, elimination becomes progressively more difficult and more painful; defecation may result in fissures or hemorrhoids. Painful defecation further contributes to the vicious cycle of stool retention.

Soiling occurs in the presence of retained stool because the retained stool causes sphincter dysfunction. The constant distension of the rectum causes persistent relaxation of the internal sphincter, mediated by the rectoanal inhibitory reflex. Relaxation of the internal sphincter permits liquid stool and mucus to seep around the impaction and into the anal canal. Continence past that point is dependent on external sphincter contraction; however, the child with chronic retention usually fails to sense rectal distension and fecal seepage into the anal canal and therefore does not voluntarily contract the external sphincter. Even if the child does recognize the leakage, he or she is able to contract the sphincter for only a short period of time. When the external sphincter returns to resting tone, the anal canal pressures are insufficient to prevent leakage, and soiling occurs. In addition, prolonged rectal distension and high intrarectal pressures can produce a "paradoxical" response of the sphincter; that is, increased rectal volume causes reduced sphincter muscle tone and increased risk of soiling, as compared with the normal response of increased sphincter tone.

Children with encopresis present with a wide range of associated symptoms. Children with recent onset of retention and incontinence typically complain of abdominal pain; in contrast, children with long-standing encopresis seldom complain of pain because they generally have developed tolerance to colonic distension. The presence of associated enuresis is also variable. In children who do present with enuresis, effective treatment of the stool retention may alleviate the child's problems with bladder control. Encopresis at night is relatively rare and seems to be associated with a poor prognosis.[13]

Assessment. The assessment of a child with encopresis requires a thorough history, a focused physical examination, and possibly radiographic studies or anorectal physiology testing.[15] Laboratory tests are generally not beneficial in the evaluation of children with encopresis. An abdominal radiograph may be useful when the history is vague or the child is not cooperative with the examination. Lumbosacral spine films or magnetic resonance imaging (MRI) may be needed if examination of the lower extremities indicates an abnormality or if any sacral abnormalities are noted. However, the history and physical examination are usually the only diagnostic tools necessary to identify retentive encopresis and to rule out organic factors. Few cases of retentive encopresis and even fewer cases of nonretentive encopresis have an organic origin.

Psychosocial Concerns. Encopresis has a major effect on life style and on self-esteem. The inability to control defecation is extremely humiliating to these children, who live in constant fear of discovery, exposure, ruthless teasing, and ridicule. In addition, these children are often punished and are told that their problem with incontinence is an attention-getting act or a result of their own laziness. They may be told that they are negligent when they fail to change foul-smelling undergarments after an accident. Parents fail to realize that the sense of smell in these children (as in all people) accommodates to their own odors and that the child is frequently genuinely unaware of the accident and the offensive odor. Even though these children live with daily emotional trauma, acting-out behavior is not common; instead, these children are likely to isolate themselves to varying degrees and to show excessive dependence.

Encopresis also has a tremendous influence on the other family members. Parents generally feel frustrated and possibly angry or guilty regarding their child's "failure to acquire continence." In addition, the fear of "accidents" may profoundly affect family activities; car trips, visits to friends, and even restaurants may be avoided because of the fear of embarrassment. Siblings may hesitate or refuse to invite friends over because of fecal odor or fear that the child could have an embarrassing accident. The stress generated by these limitations and adaptations may increase tension and conflict among family members and between various family members and the encopretic child. Thus, psychosocial factors should be an area of major concern when one is assessing and managing the child with encopresis.

Management. There is a limited body of evidence-based data that addresses the treatment of encopresis. To date, treatment has been experiential rather than evidence based and consists of education, dietary modifications (increased fiber and fluid intake), and the use of laxatives. A *Cochrane Database Systematic Review* in July 2001 found 16 randomized or quasirandomized trials of behavioral-cognitive treatment for defecation issues in children, involving a total of 843 children. The results indicated that behavioral intervention combined with laxative therapy improved fecal continence in children with encopresis.[9]

Biofeedback training may be used to assist with other behavioral measures. Biofeedback is based on reinforcement and is derived from psychologic learning theory. It uses instrument-assisted exercises to improve physiologic control. Biofeedback has been used with children with constipation and/or encopresis to improve rectal sensation, to strengthen and improve control of the external sphincter, and to coordinate muscle contraction and relaxation to achieve continence. (In more than half of the children with constipation/encopresis, the anal sphincter contracts instead of relaxing during defecation.[12]) The role of biofeedback in the treatment of fecal incontinence must currently be considered to be unproven; more studies are urgently needed.

Management of the child with encopresis is variable, depending on the specific form of the encopresis (retentive versus nonretentive) and on the unique characteristics of the individual patient and his or her family. Management of retentive encopresis and that of nonretentive encopresis are discussed separately.

Retentive Encopresis. Effective management of retentive encopresis requires a very comprehensive approach. Some clinicians recommend beginning treatment with intensive psychoeducation, to demystify the shame and blame around the stool accidents.[9,18] They emphasize the importance of reassuring the child and the parents that this is a common childhood problem and that it is no one's "fault."[9,13] The clinician should review the pathologic sequence of events leading to the current condition of a "stretched-out bowel," reduced sensory awareness of rectal filling, and reduced contractility of the colonic and rectal musculature. The overall principles of treatment are explained, and a specific treatment plan is developed with the child and parents. The importance of long-term follow-up care should also be addressed in this initial discussion regarding management.

The next phase of treatment is the cleaning-out phase, the objective of which is to eliminate all retained stool from the colon and rectum. This may be accomplished by enemas, suppositories, laxatives, or combination therapy. In selecting a cleansing protocol, it is important to assess for impaction, because the use of laxatives and suppositories may be contraindicated in these children. Laxatives cannot eliminate a true impaction, and the increased peristaltic activity can cause severe cramping pain, which may lead to an emergency room visit. Suppositories are contraindicated because they are unable to break up the impaction or to facilitate elimination of a large fecal mass; in fact, they generally become imbedded in and contribute to the fecal mass and fail to aid in the cleansing objective.[6]

Several protocols have been recommended for the cleanout phase of treatment. Levine recommended using as many as four 3-day cycles, as follows: day 1, two adult-sized Fleet enemas; day 2, bisacodyl suppository; day 3, bisacodyl tablet. He found that many children required four or even five cycles to obtain complete elimination of the retained stool.[13]

Another approach to cleanout is from the Developmental Medicine Center at Boston's Children's Hospital; these clinicians recommend an approach tailored to the age of the child, previous treatment, and history of trauma.[9] For children age 7 years or older who have no history of trauma, they utilize a 14-day cycle of alternating bisacodyl pills, bisacodyl suppository, and Fleet enema. For children less than 7 years of age and for children who cannot tolerate suppositories or enemas (because of previous trauma), they suggest polyethylene glycol without electrolytes, starting at 1 capful in 6 oz of fluid/day. The child with a long-standing impaction may require a higher dose or the addition of a stimulant such as senna or bisacodyl. The child and family need to be told to expect a large amount of stool output.

Other clinicians have tried variations of Levine's protocol; for example, Sprague-McRae reported success with the following adaptation: day 1, Fleet enema morning and evening; day 2, bisacodyl suppository morning and evening and Fleet enema in evening; day 3, bisacodyl tablet taken orally in evening. This team recommended a pediatric-sized Fleet enema for children between 4 and 7 years of age or less than 50 lb and an adult-sized Fleet enema for children more than 7 years of age or more than 50 lb.[19]

In 1994, Seth and Heyman reported successful cleansing without the use of enemas. Their approach was to use mineral oil at a dose of 15 to 30 mL/kg/day, not to exceed 240 mL/day; this was used only for children who were more than 1 year of age. These investigators documented initial cleansing within 3 or 4 days, with a 98% success rate and minimal side effects (one patient complained of abdominal cramps).[7] Administration of mineral oil is facilitated by keeping it cold and mixing it in a 1:1 ratio with a fat-based substance such as pudding, yogurt, or chocolate syrup.

Other clinicians have also reported beneficial results with mineral oil; for example, Abrahamian and Lloyd-Still found that 47% of their pediatric population became completely asymptomatic after treatment with laxatives and mineral oil, and an additional 36% reported effective control with laxatives after the original cleansing treatment.[5] Clinicians selecting mineral oil for initial cleansing are cautioned to avoid its use in very young children and in children with gastroesophageal reflux or vomiting because of the potential for and danger of aspiration.[7] In addition, it is generally recommended that the mineral oil be given 2 or 3 hours after meals or that a multivitamin tablet be given as part of the treatment because mineral oil inhibits absorption of fat-soluble vitamins.[5]

Children with severe impactions usually require hospitalization and oral or nasogastric administration of a polyethylene glycol-electrolyte solution; this approach may also be required for children who are unresponsive to outpatient management or who cannot cooperate with the cathartic procedure.[8,20]

After successful colonic cleansing, a program is initiated to establish regular evacuation of soft formed stool and to eliminate withholding of stool and the evacuation of large stools. Components of the bowel retraining maintenance phase include medications and behavioral interventions. Mineral oil is the most commonly recommended medication; the dose is titrated to produce soft formed stool, and it ranges from 2 Tbsp once daily to 6 Tbsp twice daily. Polyethylene glycol without electrolytes is frequently used for children who cannot tolerate the taste of mineral oil. Again, the dose is titrated to maintain soft formed stool, but it generally ranges from one-half to one capful/day.[9]

Additional medications that may be used include lactulose, malt soup extract (Maltsupex), Milk of Magnesia, Haley's M-O, senna (Fletcher's Castoria), and bisacodyl (Dulcolax). Suppositories and enemas may be used to stimulate defecation on an as-needed basis. Table 16-1 provides dosage guidelines for each of the commonly used softener or stimulant agents based on the child's age and size.

Medications are generally used for at least 3 months and may be used for as long as 6 months. The goal is to prevent recurrent stool retention and gradually to restore the colon and rectum to normal size and function. Parents generally need to be reassured that laxatives are safe and not habit forming and that their child will have the laxatives tapered off once normal bowel function has been reestablished. Parents are also taught how to titrate the doses of mineral oil and any other medications appropriately and how to intervene if the child fails to have a bowel movement for 2 consecutive days.

In addition to using stool softeners and stimulants to normalize fecal elimination, the child's diet should be modified to eliminate constipating foods and fluids (such as excessive intake of milk and other dairy products) and to increase the intake of fiber. (The transition to a high-fiber diet should be delayed until disimpaction has been completed.[21]) A dietary consultation may be helpful to the parents and child in determining ways to add fiber to the child's diet. The family should be provided with a list of fiber-containing foods (Table 16-2), and the child should be included in discussing ways by which to add fiber to the diet. It may be helpful to develop a sample meal plan so that the parents can see how to incorporate fiber-containing foods into daily menus. In determining the fiber-intake goal for a particular child, the clinician should be aware that the American Academy of Pediatrics has recommended 0.5 g of fiber/kg body weight up to a maximum of 35 g daily. Another formula for estimating fiber intake needs in children more than 2 years of age is as follows: "Child's age in years + 5 = Desirable grams of fiber per day" (for example, a 3-year-old child should receive 3 + 5 g, or 8 g, of fiber daily). The clinician also needs to remember that high-fiber foods are more filling and lower in calories than low-fiber foods; with a child's small stomach, there is the potential for inadequate ingestion of calories when a high-fiber diet is begun. In addition, high-fiber foods can impede the absorption of minerals such as calcium, iron, copper, magnesium, phosphorus, and zinc; therefore, the child's weight should be monitored, and it is usually helpful to recommend a multivitamin-mineral compound daily.

In addition to measures to establish soft formed stool, the management program must include a toileting routine. It is not sufficient to teach the child to respond promptly to the urge to defecate, because the urge to defecate may not develop for 6 to 9 months following the initiation of treatment. Thus, it is essential to establish a regular schedule for sitting on the toilet and attempting defecation; this promotes appropriate elimination of stool into the toilet and helps to stop soiling. Having the child sit on the toilet for 5 to 10 minutes after breakfast and dinner will take advantage of the natural increase in peristalsis following meals, which increases the chance of successful defecation. In addition to encouraging the child to adhere to an established

TABLE 16-1   Dosage Guidelines for Stool Softeners and Stimulants

TYPE OF AGENT	GUIDELINE
Stool Softeners	
Mineral oil (plain)*	Less than 1 year of age: not recommended Disimpaction: 15 to 30 mL/year of age, up to 240 mL daily Maintenance: 1 to 3 mL/kg/day
Lactulose or sorbitol	1 to 3 mL/kg/day in divided doses (Available as 70% solution)
Lavage	
Polyethylene glycol-electrolyte solution	Disimpaction: 25 mL/kg/hour (up to 1000 mL/hour) by nasogastric tube until clear; OR 20 mL/kg/hour for 4 hours/day Maintenance (older children): 5 to 10 mL/kg/day
Laxatives	
Barley malt extract (Maltsupex) liquid or powder	2 to 10 mL/240 mL of milk or juice (Suitable for infant drinking from bottle)
Magnesium hydroxide (Phillips' Milk of Magnesia or Haley's M-O)	1 to 3 mL/kg/day of 400 mg/5 mL (Available as liquid, 400 mg/5 mL and 800 mg/5 mL, and tablets)
Magnesium citrate	Less than 6 years: 1 to 3 mL/kg/day (single daily dose) 6 to 12 years: 100 to 150 mL/day (single or divided dose) More than 12 years: 150 to 300 mL/day (single or divided dose) Available as liquid: 16% magnesium
Senna preparation (Senokot)	Less than 2 years: consult manufacturer 2 to 6 years: 2.5 to 7.5 mL/day 6 to 12 years: 5 to 15 mL/day Available as Senokot syrup, 8.8 mg of sennosides/5 mL; also available as granules and tablets
Bisacodyl (Dulcolax)	Age 2 years or older: 1 to 3 tablets/dose Available in 5-mg tablets
Prokinetic Agent	
Cisapride	0.2 mg/kg/dose, three or four times/day Available as suspension, 1 mg/mL, and 5-, 10-, and 20-mg tablets
Rectal Suppositories	
Glycerin suppository	Use as needed to stimulate defecation
Bisacodyl (Dulcolax) suppository	2 years or older: $^{1}/_{2}$ to 1 suppository (Available in 10-mg suppositories)
Enemas	
Docusate sodium (Enemeez—MiniEnema)‡	One unit rectally—to be used as an enema and not as a suppository Available in bottles of 30 single-use 5-mL tubes
Mineral oil enema	2 to 11 years: 30–60 mL as single dose *Adolescents:* as retention enema, contents of one enema (range 60 to 150 mL)/day as single dose
Sodium phosphate (Fleet) enema	Less than 2 years: to be avoided 2 years or older: 6 mL/kg up to 135 mL

Information in table obtained from Baker S, et al. Medical position statement of North American Society for Pediatric Gastroenterology and Nutrition: constipation in infants and children— evaluation and treatment, *J Pediatr Gastroenterol Nutr* 29:612, 1999.

*If a mineral oil preparation is used, multivitamin supplementation is recommended because of the potential for reduced absorption of fat-soluble vitamins.

‡Information on Enemeez is not based on the Position Statement.

TABLE 16-2   High-Fiber Diet

GENERAL GUIDELINES		
Dietary fiber is beneficial in that it adds bulk to the stool, reduces stool transit time, reduces intestinal intraluminal pressures, and slows gastric emptying.		
Adequate fluid intake is essential when fiber is added to the diet.		
Fiber intake should be increased gradually to avoid unpleasant side effects.		
A good approach is to use the following chart to identify high-fiber foods and to replace low-fiber foods in the diet with high-fiber foods until the desired "fiber-intake goal" is reached.		

FOOD	SERVING SIZE	FIBER IN GRAMS
Breads		
Cracked wheat	1 slice	2.1
Raisin	1 slice	0.4
Rye	1 slice	1.2
White	1 slice	0.8
Whole wheat	1 slice	2.1
Hamburger roll or bun	1 at $3\frac{1}{2}$-in. diameter, $1\frac{1}{2}$-in. height	1.2
Bagel, 100% whole wheat	1	5.4
Bagel, oat bran	1	7.7
Bran muffins made with Kellogg's All-Bran or Bran Buds cereal	1	3.2
Bran muffin made with Kellogg's 40% Bran Flakes cereal	1	1.3
Pancakes	1 at 4-in. diameter	0.5
Taco shell (tortilla)	1	0
Cereals		
Kellogg's All-Bran	$\frac{1}{3}$ cup (1 oz)	9.0
Kellogg's Bran Buds	$\frac{1}{3}$ cup (1 oz)	8.0
Kellogg's Cracklin' Bran	$\frac{1}{3}$ cup (1 oz)	4.0
Kellogg's Most	3/4 cup (1 oz)	4.0
Bran flakes	1 cup	5.0 to 9.2
Fiber One	1 cup	27.5
Granola	1 cup	5.8 to 6.0
Grape Nuts	1/2 cup	5.4
Raisin Bran	1 cup	6 to 7.9
Oat bran, cooked	1 cup	6.4
Wheat germ toasted	1/2 cup	8.0
Macaroni, vegetable, tricolored	1 cup	5.8
Vegetables		
Avocado	Half	2.2
Asparagus (boiled, cut)	$\frac{1}{2}$ cup	1.1
Beans		
Azuki bean, cooked	$\frac{1}{2}$ cup	5.8
Black, cooked	$\frac{1}{2}$ cup	7.5
Garbanzo, canned	1 cup	9.1
Kidney, canned	$\frac{1}{2}$ cup	5.9
Mung, boiled	$\frac{1}{2}$ cup	5.8

Continued

TABLE 16-2   High-Fiber Diet—cont'd

FOOD	SERVING SIZE	FIBER IN GRAMS
Vegetables—cont'd		
Pinto, cooked	1/2 cup	7.3
Bean sprouts	1/2 cup	1.6
Broccoli, steamed or stir fried	1 cup	5.0
Brussel sprouts (boiled)	1 cup	7.2
Cabbage, shredded, boiled	1/2 cup	2.3
Carrots, drained, boiled	1/2 cup	2.3
Cauliflower, boiled	1/2 cup	1.1
Cucumber, raw	1 oz	0.1
Eggplant, peeled, drained	1/2 cup	2.5
Green beans, cut, boiled	1/2 cup	2.0
Green pepper	1 medium	0.8
Lentils, dry, boiled	1 cup	9.0
Lettuce	6 medium leaves	1.4
Mushrooms, raw	1/2 cup	0.9
Okra	1/2 cup	2.6
Peas, boiled, drained	1/2 cup	4.2
Radishes	10 medium	0.5
Spinach, boiled	1/2 cup	5.7
Squash, acorn, baked or mashed	1/2 cup	5.3
Tomato, raw	1 medium	2.0
Tomato, paste, canned	1/2 cup	5.4
Taro, sliced, cooked	1 cup	6.7
Turnips, boiled, mashed	1/2 cup	3.2
Fruits		
Apple with peel	1 medium	3.3
Apple, dried, rings	10 each	5.8
Applesauce, canned	1/2 cup	2.6
Apricots	2 medium	1.6
Apricots, dried halves	1/2 cup	5.0
Banana	1/2 small	1.6
Cantaloupe	1/4 whole	1.6
Cherries, sweet	10 large	1.2
Dates, dried	5	3.1
Figs, dried	5	8.7
Grapefruit, fresh	1/2 whole	0.6
Grapes, seedless	12	0.3
Guava	2	9.7
Lemon, fresh	1 slice	0.3
Mango	1 cup	5.0
Nectarines	1 medium	3.0
Oranges	1 small	2.4
Peach, fresh	1 medium	1.4
Peach, dried halves	10	12.2
Pear, dried, halves	10	13.1
Pineapple, fresh	1/2 cup	0.9

TABLE 16-2   **High-Fiber Diet—cont'd**

FOOD	SERVING SIZE	FIBER IN GRAMS
Fruits—cont'd		
Plums, fresh	2 medium	0.4
Pomegranate	1	5.5
Prunes, dried	10	7.8
Prunes, stewed	½ cup	7.0
Raisins	2 tablespoons	1.2
Strawberries	½ cup	1.7
Nuts and Seeds		
Almonds, dry roasted	½ cup	6.8
Coconut, fresh grated	1 cup	7.5
Coconut cream, canned	1 cup	6.5
Coconut cream, raw	1 cup	5.3
Coconut milk, fresh, frozen	1 cup	5.3
Coconut milk, raw	1 cup	5.3
Macadamia, chopped	½ cup	5.1
Mixed, dry roasted with peanuts	½ cup	6.2
Peanuts, boiled without shell	1 cup	5.5
Peanuts, dry roasted	½ cup	5.0
Pistachio, dry roasted	½ cup	5.0

From Seth R, Heyman M: *Gastroenterol Clin North Am* 23(4):621-636, 1994, and Hawaii Dietetic Association, 1997.

toileting routine, the entire family should be assisted to work on eliminating any negative issues regarding toileting that may have developed over time.

It is recommended that small rewards be used for positive reinforcement (such as stickers or special toys in the bathroom for preschoolers, stickers or hand-held computer games for school-age children, and magazines and the assurance of privacy for adolescents). The "reward" should not be costly, and special age-appropriate rewards should be earned only by more advanced achievement, such as a certain number of days without soiling. The goal is to help the child accept responsibility for his or her actions and needs but to avoid any sense of punishment for an accident.

In establishing the medication and toileting schedule for any individual child, it is important to be flexible and creative and to assist the child and family to incorporate the care routine into their daily schedule with minimal disruption. It is also important to monitor the child's response and to

taper the medications as the increased fiber and attention to toileting produce softer, more frequent stools. The goal is to wean the child from all medications once bowel function has normalized and the child has incorporated a high-fiber diet and routine toileting into his or her daily routine.

Nonretentive Encopresis. As noted earlier, nonretentive encopresis is most commonly caused by psychologic issues, although primary nonretentive encopresis may also be caused by organic problems. Therefore, it is essential to explore psychologic issues when assessing the child and establishing a management plan.

The assessment of a child with primary nonretentive encopresis may reveal an organic cause of the encopresis but more commonly will reveal a history of coercive toilet training and the failure to achieve complete fecal continence. The parents may have been punitive in their approach to toilet training, and the child may have begun to use soiling as a way of getting back at them. Alternatively, the parents may have been controlling and intrusive although not punitive; in this case, the child may have reacted with anger and resentment. If the assessment reveals either a punitive or controlling approach to toilet training and bowel management, the clinician should instruct the parents to stop trying to toilet train the child and to seek counseling and family therapy. The emphasis during counseling should be on development of positive parent-child relationships with appropriate use of positive reinforcement.

The history of a child with secondary nonretentive encopresis usually reveals psychosocial stressors in the home or the school environment that have caused the child to regress to an earlier developmental stage. Because the cause of the incontinence is psychologic, the focus during treatment is on encouraging the child to identify and talk about the stressful situation that precipitated the regression. The child is reassured that he or she is not at fault for soiling and that there has been no change in the parents' unconditional love. This reassurance can help to eliminate or reduce guilt and blame. In planning and implementing treatment for a child with secondary nonretentive encopresis, it is important to provide the child with time to develop some control over the psychologic crisis before introducing him or her to a bowel retraining program for correction of the fecal incontinence.

As noted earlier, the primary focus in treatment of the child with nonretentive encopresis is on resolution of the psychologic issues that triggered the bowel dysfunction. Secondary management usually involves implementation of a comprehensive bowel management program, which typically includes many of the elements already described under management of retentive encopresis: medications when indicated, establishment of a routine toileting program, encouragement to respond promptly to defecatory urges, periodic underwear checks, and positive reinforcement for appropriate toileting. The child or family may also be under the care of a psychologist or psychiatrist, or the clinician may observe signs and symptoms that prompt a follow-up psychiatric or psychologic consultation (such as conduct disorder, depression, or learning disabilities). Whenever the patient and family are under

psychiatric or psychologic care, it is critical for the continence nurse clinician to work in collaboration with the mental health professional. It may also be of tremendous benefit to enlist the cooperation of the staff at the child's school, preschool, or day-care setting.

Carefully monitored long-term follow-up care is critical for any child with encopresis. As explained, the initial goal is to establish regular voluntary elimination of soft formed stool and to eliminate withholding of stool and large fecal masses. Once an acceptable bowel elimination pattern has been in place for 4 to 6 months (such as two or three bowel movements per day), the child is gradually weaned off stool softeners. Data indicate that such a program results in complete and long-lasting remission in approximately 65% of the children, with an additional 30% reporting substantial improvement.[14] The children who continue to soil should have follow-up evaluation to determine the cause of the persistent problem; in some of these children, the problem may be paradoxical contraction of the external sphincter during attempted defecation.[14] Benninga and colleagues evaluated the effectiveness of biofeedback retraining in 29 patients with chronic constipation and encopresis ranging in age from 5 to 16 years. Sixteen of these children exhibited inappropriate contraction of their external sphincters, and eight evidenced diminished rectal sensation. Biofeedback training was effective in teaching 26 of the children how to relax the external anal sphincter and in normalizing rectal sensation in 18.[7] Therefore, biofeedback should be considered for children with intact nerve pathways but attenuated rectal sensation or compromised ability to correctly contract and relax the pelvic floor and sphincter muscles.

The ultimate goal in treating encopresis is to restore the child to normal bowel function and a normal life style and to prevent long-lasting psychologic and emotional problems that may develop secondary to chronic fecal incontinence. Parents frequently report an overall improvement in the child's demeanor, appetite, and level of activity after successful treatment. The success of the treatment program is highly dependent on the child's willingness to address his or her problem with encopresis and on the parents' willingness to assist the child to remain compliant with the treatment program. As outlined, the treatment program is usually multifaceted and long term and must be carried out by the family members themselves, who are frequently juggling multiple other responsibilities and complex schedules. It is therefore essential for the health care clinician to establish rapport with the child and family and to work collaboratively with them to establish a feasible treatment plan that incorporates the key elements of education, counseling, pharmacotherapy, and behavior modification.

Congenital Conditions Resulting in Fecal Incontinence

Several congenital disorders alter the normal neuromuscular function of the colon and rectum and can therefore lead to fecal incontinence. The most common of these are imperforate anus, Hirschsprung's disease, menigomyelocele, and neuromuscular disorders (such as cerebral palsy, muscular dystrophy, or hypotonia). Each of these disorders is briefly described, and then assessment and management of the child with neurogenic bowel dysfunction are addressed.

Imperforate Anus. The term *imperforate anus* is an umbrella term that encompasses a range of anomalies involving the anal canal and rectum. The common denominator in all of these anomalies is the absence of a visible anal opening. Some of these children are born with a fistula between the distal portion of the bowel and the perineum or urinary tract. The incidence rate is about 1 in 5000. The anomaly may occur in isolation or as a component of the VACTERL syndrome. (Infants born with the VACTERL syndrome exhibit vertebral, anorectal, cardiovascular, tracheoesophageal, renal, and limb anomalies.) Anorectal anomalies are typically classified as either "high" or "low" lesions, depending on whether the distal end of the bowel terminates above or below the puborectal component of the levator ani complex. Several classification systems have been developed to categorize the various anorectal anomalies more accurately. The one most widely used in the United States is the wingspread classification, which is outlined in Table 16-3.[22] In children with low defects, the distal end of the rectum and the anal canal traverse the levator mechanism and the striated muscle complex; however, the anal opening is situated anterior to the external sphincter. In some children, the anal opening is situated correctly at the external sphincter but is covered with skin. Ninety percent of children with

---

TABLE 16-3 Wingspread Classification for Anorectal Anomalies

FEMALE	MALE
High Lesions	***High Lesions***
Anorectal agenesis	Anorectal agenesis
With rectovaginal fistula	With rectoprostatic urethral fistula
Without fistula	Without fistula
Rectal atresia	Rectal atresia
Intermediate Lesions	***Intermediate Lesions***
Anal agenesis with rectovestibular fistula	Anal agenesis with rectobulbar urethral fistula
Anal agenesis with rectovaginal fistula	Anal agenesis without fistula
Anal agenesis without fistula	
Low Lesions	***Low Lesions***
Anovestibular fistula	Anocutaneous fistula
Anocutaneous fistula	Anal stenosis
Anal stenosis	
Cloacal Malformations	***Cloacal Malformations***
Rare Malformations	***Rare Malformations***

low defects have an identifiable perineal fistula.[1] Low defects can usually be treated effectively with simple dilatation or a minor perineal procedure.

With intermediate-level defects, the distal end of the rectum and the anal canal extend partially through the levator ani complex but then terminate, typically in a fistulous opening into the vagina (girls) or rectobulbar urethra (boys). Almost all these children present with fistulous openings into the perineum or urinary system.

In children with high-level defects, the distal end of the rectum terminates above the levator ani complex; these infants generally develop fistulous openings into the proximal end of the vagina in girls or into the prostatic urethra or the bladder in boys. (Alternatively, the rectum can end in a blind pouch with no fistulous tracts.[1]) Infants with high lesions often have associated anomalies involving the genitourinary tract, spine, and heart. High defects are more common in boys, although there are no other known genetic factors.

High lesions are characterized by an absence of the internal anal sphincter, although there may be a thickening of the distal circular muscle at the end of the bowel. The external sphincter is almost always present, at least in part. The levator ani and puborectalis muscles are usually present, although in patients with high lesions the puborectal muscle is small and is densely adherent to the urethra or vagina. These infants generally undergo diverting colostomy at birth and a reconstructive pull-through procedure between 3 and 9 months of age. This pull-through procedure involves mobilizing the distal end of the bowel, pulling it through the pelvic musculature, and creating an anal opening. The procedure currently favored is the Pena midsagittal anorectoplasty. Once the suture lines have healed and any necessary dilatations have been completed, the colostomy is closed.[2]

Complications occurring after the surgical pull-through procedure include stricture of the anocutaneous anastomosis, recurrent rectourinary fistula, mucosal prolapse, anterior anal malposition, constipation, and incontinence. Fecal incontinence is by far the most troublesome of the complications. The most important determinant of continence is the level of the initial lesion. All children with low

lesions achieve normal continence, but only a few children with high lesions achieve normal continence by the time of entry into school. Fortunately, most of these children continue to improve in terms of continence, and most are socially continent by the time they reach adolescence.

The level of the lesion can be partially inferred by the clinical presentation. In boys, if meconium appears anywhere in the perineum, either through an anocutaneous fistula or the median raphe of the scrotum, the lesion is low and can be treated by simple dilatation or perineal anoplasty. If meconium is eliminated in the urine but not directly onto the perineum, the lesion is almost certain to be high, and a diverting colostomy is probably indicated.[2] In girls, if the opening of the bowel cannot be seen, it is likely that there is a high rectovaginal fistula, which requires a temporary diverting colostomy and later reconstruction.

Hirschsprung's Disease. *Hirschsprung's disease* was first reported in 1886 by Hirschsprung, who believed that the condition was caused by colonic distension. It was not until the 1940s that the colonic distension was clearly understood to be secondary to the absence of ganglion cells in the distal portion of the colon and rectum. Currently, Hirschsprung's disease is a major cause of neonatal obstruction, and statistics indicate that 46% of all cases of Hirschsprung's disease are diagnosed in the neonatal period.[23]

Etiology. Hirschsprung's disease occurs as a result of arrested fetal development of the myenteric nervous system, although the specific causative factors are unknown. Normal development of the nervous system occurs in an orderly sequence; intermuscular neuroblasts migrate in a cephalocaudal direction, followed by intramural dispersion of neuroblasts to the superficial and deep submucosal nerve plexuses.[23] Hirschsprung's disease occurs as a result of an interruption in the cephalocaudal migration of nerve cells into the hindgut, which prevents the development of ganglion cells in Meissner's and Auerbach's plexuses. This neural "arrest" is believed to occur at about 12 weeks of gestation. The loss of ganglion cells produces an aperistaltic segment of bowel, which causes a secondary dilatation of the proximal bowel segment. The proximal border of the defective bowel is usually within the rectum or the sigmoid colon, although occasionally the entire colon is aganglionic.[1]

The incidence of Hirschsprung's disease is 1 in 5000; the male-to-female ratio is usually reported as 4:1, although in babies with long-segment disease the ratio is closer to 1:1. There is strong evidence for a genetic link, based on a significantly higher incidence among siblings of patients with Hirschsprung's disease.[23] There is no racial predilection.

Clinical presentation. The clinical presentation of Hirschsprung's disease is quite variable, depending on the length of the aganglionic segment and on the presence of complications such as enterocolitis. Babies with involvement of the entire rectum and sigmoid (and babies with total colon Hirschsprung's disease) are usually diagnosed very early in life, because they develop signs of intestinal obstruction as soon as feedings are begun (that is, failure to pass meconium, reluctance to feed, bilious vomiting, and abdominal distension). Plain abdominal films typically reveal multiple dilated loops of bowel with air-fluid levels, findings consistent with a distal bowel obstruction. Some infants develop enterocolitis and present with overwhelming sepsis (manifest by respiratory failure, hypovolemia, shock, coagulopathy with reduced platelet count, reduced urine output, and temperature instability). In these cases, prompt diagnosis and treatment are obviously essential for survival. A few of these infants actually develop intestinal perforation and peritonitis, although these complications are rare.[23]

Infants with short-segment disease (that is, disease confined to the rectum) may be incorrectly diagnosed and managed because their presentation is less dramatic and clear cut. These babies present with chronic constipation that may be managed initially with digital rectal dilatations and enemas. Some of these infants experience a temporary response to these measures, but most respond poorly and develop additional signs and symptoms of bowel dysfunction, such as failure to thrive, abdominal distension, and vomiting. The development of diarrhea in an infant with Hirschsprung's disease is an ominous sign because diarrhea is associated with enterocolitis, which has a high mortality during the first few months of life.

Interestingly, enterocolitis is rarely seen past the age of 2 years.

If the disease is not diagnosed during infancy, the child will continue to suffer from progressively more severe constipation; he or she may have ribbonlike stools with an offensive odor and massive abdominal distension with palpable fecal masses. Frequently, children with undiagnosed Hirschsprung's disease have a history that is positive for intermittent bouts of obstruction, fecal impaction, hypochromic anemia, hypoproteinemia, and failure to thrive.

Assessment. Diagnosis of Hirschsprung's disease is suggested by physical examination and radiographic studies and is confirmed by full-thickness biopsy of the bowel wall. A critical component of the physical examination for these children is the digital rectal exam, which is remarkable for the lack of fecal material in the anal canal and rectum and for the snugness of the rectal vault around the examining finger; in addition, withdrawal of the examining finger is typically followed by a forcible gush of flatus and offensive liquid stool. (This response to digital rectal examination is explained by the fact that, in the absence of ganglion cells, the internal anal sphincter fails to open in response to rectal distension; thus, fecal material and gas do not enter the anal canal normally. The examining finger serves to "open the door" for elimination of stool and gas.)

Diagnostic studies. Diagnostic studies commonly used in the workup for an infant with signs and symptoms of Hirschsprung's disease include flat-plate radiographs of the abdomen, contrast films of the colon and rectum, anorectal manometry, and full-thickness rectal biopsy. A plain radiograph of the abdomen with the patient in prone position shows significant gaseous distension that extends to the junction between ganglionic and aganglionic bowel. If a contrast study is done, it also reveals a distal collapsed bowel (the aganglionic bowel) and a proximal dilated bowel (the ganglionic bowel). A more definitive study is anorectal manometry, which reveals loss of the rectoanal inhibitory reflex, that is, loss of internal sphincter relaxation in response to rectal distension. A full-thickness biopsy reveals absence of ganglion cells and is considered to be the definitive study for the diagnosis of

Hirschsprung's disease; therefore, any child suspected of having Hirschsprung's disease by clinical and radiographic presentation should have a confirmatory biopsy done before any surgical intervention.

Treatment. Once the preliminary diagnosis of Hirschsprung's disease is made, the child is prepared for surgery. During the surgical procedure, serial biopsies are done, and the specimens are analyzed by frozen section to determine the level at which ganglion cells are present. A colostomy is then performed above the level of aganglionosis to decompress the bowel. If the entire colon is found to be aganglionic, an ileostomy is performed. Definitive surgery is postponed until the bowel is decompressed and an effective bowel preparation can be performed and typically until the infant is at least 6 months old. There are several surgical approaches to reestablishing continuity between the ganglionic section of the colon and the anal canal. In the Swenson procedure, the aganglionic colon is removed, and the normally innervated segment of colon is brought down and anastomosed to the anal canal just above the internal anal sphincter. The Duhamel procedure varies, in that the distal rectal stump is left in place and the ganglionic bowel is anastomosed in an end-to-end fashion posterior to the rectum. The Soave technique involves retention of the muscle layer of the aganglionic bowel; the mucosal layer is stripped away, and the ganglionic bowel is brought through the muscular sleeve and is anastomosed at the anorectal junction. Postoperative complications include recurrence of aganglionosis (possibly because of vascular compromise or a chronic inflammatory process leading to loss of ganglion cells), spasticity of the internal anal sphincter, fecal incontinence, and enterocolitis. Management of complications depends on the specific complication, its severity, and the morbidity associated with various management options. Recurrent aganglionosis may be managed medically if it is limited in severity or extent, whereas a spastic internal sphincter can be easily corrected with a posterior sphincterotomy. Enterocolitis is the most serious complication, accounting for 30% of deaths in young infants.[24] The management of fecal incontinence is discussed later in this chapter.

Spina Bifida. *Spina bifida* is an umbrella term that encompasses several congenital anomalies with a common element of a separated (nonfused) posterior vertebral arch. It is now recognized that these defects occur as a result of abnormal development of the neural tube and its surrounding structures.[25]

The incidence of neural tube defects is about 1 in 1000 in the United States, thus making this one of the leading causes of disability in children. There are some geographic variations in incidence, and studies indicate an increased risk among future pregnancies for couples who have one child with spina bifida.[25] The cause has not been clearly established; however, it is known that the defect occurs about the twenty-eighth day of embryologic development, and research indicates that one possible cause is a low level of folic acid during the preconception period.

There are three major forms of spina bifida, with varying degrees of neurologic involvement and bowel and bladder dysfunction. The most common is spina bifida occulta. In this form, patients have a bony defect in the spinal column, but no visible protrusion of the spinal cord or meninges into the defect. The defect may be manifest only by a dimple or hairy patch over the involved area of the spinal column; obvious neurologic deficits and bowel and bladder dysfunction are rare. In spina bifida with meningocele, one sees a visible bony defect and a visible herniation of the meninges and spinal fluid into a sac on the infant's back. The spinal cord itself is not involved in the herniation. If the surgical repair of the meningocele occurs without complication, the incidence of neurologic dysfunction (including bowel and bladder dysfunction) is rare. In spina bifida with myelomeningocele, the spinal cord, meninges, and spinal fluid herniate through the bony defect into a sac on the baby's back. The herniation of the cord causes significant sensory and motor loss below the level of the defect, and bowel and bladder dysfunction is almost universal.[26]

Management. Initial management of the infant with spina bifida complicated by meningocele or myelomeningocele involves closure of the sac and return of the meninges, spinal fluid, and cord to the spinal canal. If the child is born with an associated hydrocephalus, a shunt is placed as well. There is unfortunately no way to correct the nerve damage that has occurred prenatally; therefore, long-term management is focused on preservation of existing function, correction of orthopedic anomalies, management of hydrocephalus, preventive skin care, and bowel and bladder management. Management of the neurogenic bowel is discussed later in this chapter.

Neuromuscular Disorders. Many neuromuscular conditions can contribute to bowel and bladder dysfunction. These include brain lesions and spinal cord lesions that interfere with neuromuscular coordination and control, disorders affecting the myoneural junction, and diseases affecting the muscle itself. Table 16-4 outlines the most common of these lesions. The management of children with these conditions depends on the specific problem, its severity, and its effect on normal physiologic function. For most of these children, bowel management follows the general guidelines outlined in the section on management of neurogenic bowel dysfunction.

The initial emphasis in management of any child with a congenital anomaly is on correction of the anomaly to the extent possible, and long-term management is focused on normalizing function of the involved organs or systems. Children with anomalies involving the colon, rectum, and anus generally experience some residual sensory or motor compromise resulting from the defect itself or the fibrosis associated with surgical repair. Therefore, the management of children with congenital anomalies involving the colon, rectum, and anus can be discussed from the general perspective of neurogenic

bowel management; specific differences related to the underlying condition are addressed as appropriate.

Assessment of the Child with Neurogenic Bowel. The clinician must gain a complete understanding of the child's current bowel patterns before starting a bowel program and must closely monitor the child's response to treatment. Assessment must address developmental and psychosocial status in addition to past medical history, current bowel elimination patterns, and the bowel management program currently being used.[27] Specific factors to be addressed during the patient interview are outlined in Box 16-2.

Physical examination. The physical examination for any child with bowel dysfunction is outlined previously in this chapter. Specific areas to be examined in greater detail for the child with neurogenic bowel dysfunction include hygiene status, sensorimotor status, and anorectal function. In addition, it may be helpful to include a brief evaluation of sexual maturity, because children with myelomeningocele or a hormonal imbalance frequently experience precocious puberty as early as 8 years of age.

Hygiene status. The clinician should carefully evaluate the perineum for residual stool secondary to inadequate cleansing and for perianal skin breakdown or rashes secondary to poor hygiene. The child should be asked whether he or she can tell when an accident has occurred and, if so, how. The child who states that he or she is unaware should be taught to do routine checks so any accidents can be detected promptly and appropriate hygienic care initiated.

Sensorimotor status. The sensorimotor portion of the examination should receive particular focus in the child with a neurogenic bowel. When inspecting the anus for evidence of tone, the clinician should also be alert to the presence of hemorrhoids or anorectal prolapse; the latter is particularly common among children who have undergone anoplasty and those with a spinal disorder such as myelomeningocele. If a prolapse is present, the clinician should assess for bleeding and tenderness, because these findings may indicate the need for surgical correction.

A sensorimotor evaluation usually begins with testing of perianal skin sensation. The skin is

TABLE 16-4 **Neuromuscular Disorders that Cause Fecal Incontinence**

Brain	Cerebral palsy
	Degenerative central nervous system lesions
	Infections (meningitis)
Spinal cord	Spinal muscular atrophies
	Infantile poliomyelitis
	Spinal cord injuries
	Tumors or malformations
Neuromuscular disorders	Myasthenia gravis
	Botulism
Muscle diseases	Duchenne's muscular dystrophy
	Myotonic dystrophy

BOX 16-2 History Taking Guidelines for Child with Neurogenic Bowel

Current Bowel Patterns

- *Size and consistency of stools:* that is, "pellets," "balls," "logs," "ribbonlike" (obtain approximate length and diameter of stools if possible); liquid, mushy, soft, formed, hard, or variable consistency
- *Frequency and consistency of voluntary bowel movements (if applicable)*
- *Detailed description of stooling "accidents":* frequency (daily, multiple times weekly, etc.), any associated or precipitating events, volume of incontinent stools (smear, teaspoon, tablespoon, half cup, "diarrhea," etc.), number of underwear (or liners) soiled in 1 day, current management (Is child aware that an accident has occurred? Is child able to clean himself or herself up after an accident? Does school or day care staff assist with management?)
- *Sensory awareness of rectal filling and defecation:* Can child sense rectal distension? Is child able to differentiate among gas, liquid, and solid? Is sensory awareness consistent or variable, and, if variable, how often is child able to recognize rectal distension?* (It is helpful to ask the child to point to where he or she feels the urge to have a bowel movement; many children with diminished or absent rectal sensation point to the left abdomen, indicating that their sensory awareness is related to peristaltic activity as opposed to rectal distension.)
- *Current bowel management program:* Has a bowel program been established? If so, what does it involve-digital stimulation? suppositories? enemas? regular toileting? medications? (If medications taken, determine strength, dose, and frequency.) Is child independent in bowel program and medication administration, or is assistance needed-if assistance is needed, how much assistance and who is providing it at present? What is the frequency of the current program, that is, how often are medications taken? Are stimulants used to initiate defecation? Is routine toileting performed? Is the currently established bowel program effective? If not, what problems are associated with the current program?
- *Specific toileting behaviors:* What position does the child assume while toileting, that is, are his or her feet firmly positioned on the floor or in the air? Does the child have enough trunk stability to sit without having to support himself or herself? Is the child able to do a Valsalva maneuver effectively to "push the stool out"? (It may help to have the child demonstrate how he or she "pushes stool out.") If current bowel program includes routine toileting, how much encouragement does the child require to adhere to the program?
- *Dietary status:* Have any dietary modifications been made to address the problems with bowel function? If yes, what are they and what effect have they had? What types of high-fiber foods does the child eat and in what volume? What is the child's usual volume of liquid intake? Does the child have access to liquids in the school or day care setting? Is the child receiving any fiber supplementation, and, if so, what formula and in what volume? Is the child's dental status satisfactory, or are there dental problems contributing to inadequate fiber intake?
- *Goals and motivation:* What is the child's perception of the problem with fecal incontinence? What are the child's and parents' goals for management? How much assistance does the child require, and how much assistance and support are the parents able and willing to provide?

Medical History

The questions in this section are specific to the underlying cause of the neurogenic bowel dysfunction and are therefore grouped accordingly:

Imperforate Anus

- *Level of anomaly,* if known: Was defect a "high" or a "low" defect, and what prognosis was given at the time of repair? Were any tests done to evaluate the potential for continence?
- *Sacral anomalies:* Was sacrum intact, or were abnormalities noted? (This is significant because children with imperforate anus combined with sacral anomalies are at greater risk for incontinence.)
- *Urologic problems:* Were any urologic defects or problems noted? Were any tests completed to evaluate the urologic system?
- *Corrective surgeries:* Number of corrective surgeries performed and any available data re the specific procedures

BOX 16-2 History Taking Guidelines for Child with Neurogenic Bowel—cont'd

Medical History—cont'd

- *Medical-surgical* follow-up after repair: When was the last checkup by the surgeon? Are there problems with constipation and overflow stooling? Have any studies been done to rule out retained stool and dilatation of rectosigmoid colon?

Hirschsprung's Disease

- *Extent of colonic involvement and type of surgery done to correct the problem (if known):* Were any anal dilatations required postoperatively? If yes, when was the last procedure done? It is important to question the child or parents carefully re: the caliber of stools; ribbonlike or pencil-thin stools may be indicative of anal stenosis, which is a common complication after surgical repair of Hirschsprung's.
- *History of constipation after repair:* What are the current frequency and consistency of stools? Has there been any use of softeners, stimulants, enemas, or suppositories? (These children are at significant risk for constipation caused by anal stenosis, dilatations causing an aversion to defecation, incomplete removal of the aganglionic bowel, or recurrent aganglionosis.†)
- *History of enterocolitis* (fever, abdominal pain, and diarrhea): Treatment required.†

Myelomeningocele or Spinal Disorder

- *Level of lesion:* Children with lesions at or above the sacral cord usually present with a neurogenic bowel and bladder although some children have incomplete lesions with sparing of some of the sacral pathways (these children may retain some degree of bowel control).
- *Any additional neurologic or spinal cord problems,* such as tethered cord? If yes, is there any effect on bowel and bladder function?
- Mobility and independence in activities of daily living to include toileting: Is the child able to ambulate with or without assistive devices? Is the child able to self-toilet and to carry out his or her own bowel program? If not, how much assistance is required, and who is available to provide the assistance needed to implement the program? Are assistive devices needed to facilitate the patient's transfer to the toilet and ability to maintain balance while on the toilet?

- *Urologic status:* Current bladder management (that is, spontaneous voiding versus Credé's maneuver versus clean intermittent catheterization); history of chronic urinary tract infections and usual frequency of antibiotic therapy (there is a potential for antibiotic therapy to cause diarrhea and disrupt the bowel program)

Developmental Status

- *Time frame for achievement of developmental milestones:* The age at which toileting was introduced and the response to toileting. (The clinician should be aware that parents of children with congenital conditions sometimes tend to "excuse" the child from learning normal toileting behavior. The clinician should counsel the parents re the importance of normalizing their child's life as much as possible and should explain that the child should be exposed to normal toileting by 3 years of age unless the child is cognitively impaired.)
- *Current continence status:* Is the child continent of urine but incontinent of stool? If the child is managing the bladder with clean intermittent catheterization (CIC), at what frequency does the child catheterize? If child is in school, how much distance is there between the classrooms and the bathroom facilities? Do the bathroom facilities provide privacy? Does the child have accidents at school? If so, how often and how are these handled?
- *Current academic status:* Has the child been diagnosed with a specific disorder such as attention deficit disorder or mental retardation? Is the child in a regular classroom or a special education program? (If the child is in a special education program, ask about the services provided. Some special education programs provide toileting assistance.) How is the child's attendance record in school?

Psychosocial Status

- *Behavioral issues:* Is the child seeing a therapist for any behavioral or emotional problems?
- *Peer relationships:* What is the child's peer group like? Are the child's friends aware of the problem, and, if so, what is their response? Are the child's peers able to detect any odor or problem with stool elimination?

Continued

BOX 16-2 **History Taking Guidelines for Child with Neurogenic Bowel—cont'd**

Psychosocial Status—cont'd
- *Extracurricular activities:* Does the child participate in school or extracurricular events? Does the child attend sleepovers or camps? Does the child participate in sports? How is the problem with bowel function handled in these settings?

- *School and teacher support:* Are the school staff and the teacher aware of the child's medical needs and problems? Are they sensitive and supportive regarding the child's toileting needs?
- *Incentive program:* What type of incentive program is best suited for this child if a bowel program is implemented?

*Datum from MacLeod J: *Endoscopy Rev* 5 (Nov-Dec):45-56, 1988.
†Datum from Walker WA, Durie PR, Hamilton JR, et al: *Pediatric gastrointestinal disease,* vol 2, ed 2, St. Louis, 1996, Mosby, pp 2077-2091.

touched with a soft object (cotton-tipped applicator) and a hard object (tongue blade), and the patient is asked to report where he or she is touched and with what type of object. Sensory testing is particularly helpful in children with a history of imperforate anus or a spinal cord disorder because these children frequently have diminished sensation. Sensory function may be further evaluated by anorectal manometry, in which a balloon is inserted into the rectum and gradually inflated and the child is instructed to report the first sensation of rectal filling. Assessment of motor function includes reflex testing and assessment of volitional muscle contractions. The clinician assesses for the anal wink by stroking the perianal skin with a cotton-tipped applicator and observing for anal contraction. The clinician may also elect to evaluate for the presence or absence of the bulbocavernosus reflex (that is, anal sphincter contraction in response to gentle squeezing of the glans penis or gentle tapping of the clitoris); however, this test should be done only after a thorough explanation to the child and parents. A positive anal wink and bulbocavernosus reflex are indicative of intact motor neural pathways between the sacral cord and the pelvic floor. These reflexes are generally absent in children with neurogenic bowel disorders. The child's ability to voluntarily contract the external sphincter and pelvic floor muscles is evaluated during the digital rectal exam. The child who exhibits a significant reduction in anal tone and who lacks normal reflex contractions may be further evaluated with external anal sphincter electromyography. Children with neurogenic bowel disorders frequently exhibit diminished sensation,

absence of reflex sphincter activity, and the inability to contract the sphincter muscles on command. These findings have tremendous implications in terms of bowel management because the child with significant sensorimotor dysfunction will not be able to recognize rectal filling or to delay rectal evacuation; therefore, continence in these children is dependent on a bowel program that involves regularly stimulated defecation.

Ideally, the physical examination includes a careful digital rectal exam. The clinician should obtain the child's consent and cooperation and then should proceed with a digital examination as described previously in this chapter. (It is important to defer the physical examination until the clinician has established rapport with the child. It may be helpful for the clinician to confer with the primary physician about the results of his or her rectal examination if the child is reluctant to permit a rectal examination.) Critical components of the examination for a child with neurogenic bowel include the patient's ability to contract and relax the anal sphincter voluntarily, as well as the sphincteric response to insertion of the examining finger.

Diagnostic studies. Many children with neurogenic bowel require additional studies for complete evaluation of anorectal and sphincteric function. Studies commonly performed to identify possible etiologic factors for chronic constipation or fecal incontinence are described earlier in this chapter. Children with chronic constipation may require colonic transit studies or defecography to identify or rule out abnormal motility or outlet obstruction. The child with incontinence frequently benefits from anorectal manometry to evaluate sphincteric response to rectal distension.

Additional tests that may be indicated for children with neurologic lesions and evidence of neurologic decompensation include computerized tomography scans and MRI of the spinal cord. These studies are beneficial in identifying a tethered cord, which is a common cause of deterioration in bowel or bladder function among children with spinal cord anomalies.

Management of the Child with Neurogenic Bowel

General concepts. Effective management of any child with a chronic disorder requires establishment of rapport between the child and the clinician. This is particularly true for the clinician working with children who have disorders of elimination because the child needs to feel comfortable in talking about accidents and about his or her feelings regarding the problem with incontinence. Thus, a key aspect of nursing management for these children is the establishment of a positive working relationship.

A second key concept is the need for a team approach. Ideally, this team should include a mental health professional (a psychologist, psychiatrist, or counselor) in addition to the caregivers and health professionals. Counseling is frequently needed to assist the patient and caregivers to deal with feelings and frustrations regarding bowel dysfunction, to eliminate punitive management strategies and feelings of blame or guilt, and to incorporate positive behavior modification strategies into daily care. If the child is already working with a counselor, the continence clinician should establish contact with the counselor and should keep her or him apprised of the child's overall management plan and progress in achieving continence; this enables the therapist or counselor to provide reinforcement and support. If the child is not already working with a counselor and one is available through the continence center or the school program, a routine referral is usually beneficial. Many of these children are suffering silently and would benefit tremendously from counseling to help them deal with the problem of bowel dysfunction as well as any underlying disability.[28]

A third principle underlying any effective treatment program is the importance of education and involvement of the child and caregivers. The child and caregiver are ultimately responsible for implementing the treatment plan; therefore, they must be educated regarding the reason for the bowel dysfunction and the options for its management and must then be involved in decision making. Failure to do so is likely to result in a treatment plan that is theoretically and physiologically sound but not "user friendly" or "user supported"; such a plan is quite unlikely to be successful. For example, an early morning bowel program may not be practical if the child attends school and the caregiver works full time. Any program must take into account the life styles and schedules of the individuals involved. Similarly, preferences and preconceived ideas must be addressed. For example, the stimulus for defecation could be digital stimulation, a suppository, a minienema, or a volume enema; the preferences of the child and caregiver should be heavily weighted considerations in the decision regarding which stimulus to use for a given child. Children and caregivers should be questioned regarding previous use of medications and other bowel management strategies. They frequently have strong beliefs about the effectiveness of various agents or strategies based either on their prior experience or on things they have heard, and these ideas will heavily influence their perceptions regarding efficacy. Therefore, these perceptions should be considered when selecting strategies and agents for use in a bowel management program.

A fourth principle is the need for close follow-up care. Ideally, the child and caregiver are seen within 1 or 2 weeks after initiation of a bowel management program; however, such face-to-face follow-up care may not be feasible. In this situation, telephone follow-up should be utilized to assess progress in bowel management and to identify frustrations or problems associated with the recommended program. The clinician must stress to the child and family that each bowel management program is tailored to the individual child, that modifications are almost always required based on the child's response, and that follow-up care is critical to the success of the program. The clinician should also stress to the child and caregivers that fecal continence and improved bowel function do not occur instantaneously and that developing the optimal management plan (based on feedback and modifications) may take several weeks. It is frequently beneficial to send consultation and progress reports to the child's primary physician, to inform him or her of the recommendations made and the rationale, and to keep him or her apprised of the child's progress. This enables the primary physician to be supportive of the bowel management program when interacting with the child and caregivers.

The specific strategies utilized to normalize bowel function and establish continence for the child with a neurogenic bowel are dependent on the underlying disorder. Thus, the specifics of management are addressed according to the specific disease or condition.

Imperforate anus repair. The child who has had an imperforate anus may be incontinent as a result of impaired sensory and motor innervation or as a result of chronic constipation leading to overflow stooling. The specific contributions of each of these factors are determined by a thorough history and careful physical examination and by imaging studies to assess for retained stool and anorectal physiology testing to assess for sensorimotor function.

The child who has had an imperforate anus repair and who subsequently presents with incontinence but no symptoms of constipation should undergo imaging studies to assess placement of the neorectum and anal opening. If the imaging studies indicate appropriate placement, sensorimotor dysfunction is the most likely cause of the incontinence; treatment for these children usually involves a combination of dietary modifications, medications, enemas, and biofeedback. Heymen and colleagues reviewed biofeedback protocols used to treat these children and found that biofeedback was effective in improving pelvic muscle strength and improving sensory awareness of rectal distension. Specific protocols can be used to address an individual child's specific needs: enhanced awareness of rectal distension, or improved pelvic muscle contractility, or the ability to coordinate pelvic muscle contractions in response to rectal distension.[29]

Data regarding the use of biofeedback in treating children following imperforate anus repair are limited; however, Arnbjornsson and others concluded that children treated with biofeedback improved their squeeze pressures and use of their external anal sphincter, and they also exhibited decreased thresholds for sensory awareness of rectal distension. The addition of biofeedback to behavioral therapies produced clearly superior outcomes.[30] This author (AJ) has also found biofeedback helpful in treating these children and has identified a subgroup who have developed "nonrelaxing puborectalis syndrome," a paradoxical contraction of the external sphincter in response to a Valsalva maneuver and attempts to defecate. (The external sphincter contracts when it should relax, which prevents normal emptying of the rectal vault.) Biofeedback has been helpful in teaching these children to relax the external sphincter muscle, which then improves their ability to empty the rectal vault and reduces fecal accidents. Poenaru and colleagues also reported the beneficial effects of biofeedback in reeducating children with obstructed defecation caused by paradoxical contraction of the external sphincter.[31] Biofeedback is used in addition to dietary measures, medications, and judicious use of enemas and suppositories to maintain stool that is soft and formed.

Some of these children retain some sensory awareness of the "urge" to defecate, but they are unable to initiate a bowel movement; these children usually benefit from agents that stimulate rectal contraction and defecation (such as suppositories or minienemas). If diet regulation, medication, biofeedback, and stimulated defecation fail to provide positive outcomes, surgical intervention may be indicated, in the form of revision of the anus, an antegrade colonic enema (ACE) procedure, or creation of a colostomy.

For the child with a history of constipation and overflow stooling, the initial intervention is a cleanout protocol as discussed in the section on encopresis (see Table 16-1). After colonic cleansing, the child is placed on a program to prevent stool retention and promote regular bowel elimination. The key components of such a program are measures to keep the stool soft and formed (such as dietary modifications, medications, and use of suppositories or enemas when indicated) and behavior modification (such as regular toileting). If the child does not respond to these therapies, additional workup is indicated to assess for the possible development of a megarectosigmoid colon, which requires surgical intervention.

Hirschsprung's repair. Many children with fecal incontinence after Hirschsprung's repair present with obstructive symptoms. For these children, it is critical to determine and correct the specific cause of the obstruction. For example, anal stenosis or stricture can be relieved by dilatation or surgery. If there is no obstructing lesion but the child presents with chronic constipation, initial treatment involves cleanout followed by a program to maintain soft formed stool and regular elimination (that is, dietary modifications, medications, routine toileting, and enemas or suppositories when indicated). If the child fails to respond to these measures, further workup is indicated to assess for recurrent aganglionosis or a motility disorder; this workup typically includes colonic transit studies and full-thickness biopsy of the colon wall. Recurrent aganglionosis is treated surgically, whereas dysmotility is generally treated with medications. This author (AJ) has found that a few children with obstructed defecation after Hirschsprung's repair have a very spastic, high-tone external sphincter, and these children can improve their ability to relax the external sphincter through biofeedback. These children also require dietary measures, behavior modification, and judicious use of medications to keep their stools soft and to prevent recurrent constipation.

Myelomeningocele and other spinal cord disorders. The management of any individual child with a spinal cord lesion such as myelomeningocele is dependent on his or her level of sensorimotor function. Most of these children have profound sensorimotor loss; that is, most cannot sense rectal distension and cannot voluntarily contract the external sphincter to retain stool. Thus, most of these children are dependent on an effective stimulated defecation program to provide them with social continence.

Management of the child with sensorimotor impairment begins with establishment of normal bowel function. Many children are constipated and in an overflow-stooling pattern on initial presentation.

These children are placed on a cleanout regimen as previously described and then on a maintenance program to prevent recurrent constipation. The maintenance program includes dietary fiber or fiber supplements, fluids, and medications (stool softeners or softener/stimulant combinations) as needed. The child is also encouraged to sit on the toilet daily, and the parent is taught to ensure that the child is in a good position to eliminate stool (that is, upright position with feet flat on the floor). Frequently, the parent is asked to maintain a bowel record so the child's natural bowel elimination patterns can be determined and used as a basis for routine toileting attempts.

The child who retains some sensation of rectal distension and some ability to control his or her external sphincter may be able to regain continence through meticulous adherence to this behavior modification program. Biofeedback may also be helpful for this group of children, because it has been shown to be effective in reducing the threshold for sensory awareness of rectal distension and in improving the child's ability to contract the external sphincter effectively. However, it is generally recognized that effective use of biofeedback is dependent on preservation of an adequate number of nerve pathways and that the child with almost total sensorimotor loss is a poor candidate for biofeedback.

For the child with profound sensorimotor loss, it is usually necessary to initiate a stimulated defecation program, that is, a program to induce bowel elimination at routine intervals so that overflow stooling and fecal accidents are prevented. Such a program is used in combination with all the measures previously outlined to ensure colonic cleansing and to establish stool of proper consistency (soft and formed). A schedule for elimination is then established based on the child's usual patterns (as determined by a bowel chart). Finally, a stimulus that will induce defecation at the desired time is selected.

The most commonly used stimuli include digital stimulation, suppositories, minienemas, and volume enemas with a retention balloon. Digital stimulation is the least expensive of the options; however, it works only if the reflex arc is intact and is generally less effective for children with sacral lesions. Suppositories are available in several different formulations (see Chapter 15); they are widely available, inexpensive, and easy to use. As a result, they are frequently selected as a first choice, and they are effective for many children. Alternatively, minienemas may be used; these are gelatin ampules containing a liquid mixture of stool softeners and mild stimulant or irritant substances. The end of the ampule is formulated as an enema tip with a twistoff cap; the tip is inserted into the anal canal, and the fluid is slowly squeezed into the rectum. Minienemas are easy to use and well accepted by most children and caregivers; in addition, they are effective for the majority of users. However, they are considerably more expensive than suppositories, and this factor can be a significant deterrent to their use. An option that is generally limited to children in whom simpler strategies fail is a volume enema given with a retention balloon. This system is commercially available as a silicone-coated catheter with a 30- to 50-mL balloon and an enema bag. The Silastic formulation is particularly beneficial for children with spina bifida, who are at risk for development of latex allergy and who should therefore avoid exposure to latex whenever possible. (The clinician should be aware that the underlying catheter material is latex and the silicone coating does not provide complete protection; therefore, any child known to be allergic to latex should have a pure silicone catheter substituted.) The balloon is inserted into the rectum, inflated, and pulled against the anorectal junction to create a seal; the enema fluid is then administered. Once the enema fluid has been instilled, the child can transfer to the commode with the balloon still in place. After transfer, the child deflates the balloon and expels the colonic contents. For children with some intact sensory pathways, the balloon can also serve as a biofeedback device, increasing the child's awareness of rectal distension. (Alternatively, the enema fluid can be administered using the "cone tip" of a colostomy irrigation set.[6]) There are several factors to consider in implementing use of the volume enema with retention balloon. One is the age of the child. Blair and colleagues found that children less than 4 years of age have trouble following instructions and have less success with this approach.[32] Other problems include premature expulsion of the balloon and incomplete evacuation, despite high-volume enemas. This may be caused by a concomitant colonic dysmotility problem, possibly resulting from years of chronic constipation or laxative use. The child with colonic dysmotility may experience a slow return of the enema fluid that manifests clinically as a "diarrheal" pattern.[32]

In addition to the problems identified earlier, administration of these retrograde enemas is difficult, and this may limit the child's ability to achieve independence in care. One alternative to stimulated defecation programs is the MACE procedure (Malone antegrade colonic enema), which was introduced in the late 1980s.[33] This procedure involves removing and reimplanting the appendix in a nonrefluxing manner into the cecum; the other end of the appendix is brought out on the abdominal wall as a continent stoma.[34] This provides a catheterizable channel through which antegrade washouts are given to produce colonic emptying (Fig 16-4). One variation on this procedure is the insertion of a low-profile tube ("cecostomy button") into the stomal tract; the tube can be accessed daily for administration of the washout solution.[35,36]

In the last decade, there have been several modifications to the ACE procedure. One modification is the use of structures other than the appendix for creation of a catheterizable channel. When the appendix is not available or is unsuitable, a "neoappendix" can be created using the Monti technique. A segment of ileum or colon is detached from the GI tract with its blood supply preserved; this segment of bowel is reconfigured into a rectangle that is sutured into a tubular structure over a catheter. This tubular structure is then tunneled in an antirefluxing fashion into the bowel wall; it serves as a continent, catheterizable channel through which daily antegrade enemas can be administered. The location of the catheterizable channel has also changed; a number of surgeons have placed these ACE conduits (and stomas) in the splenic flexure, based on the fact that the solid stool that needs to be evacuated is found in the left colon. (Monti tubes

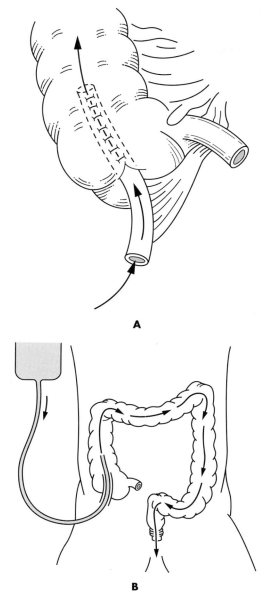

A

B

Fig. 16-4 Antegrade continence enema (ACE) procedure. **A,** Amputation of the appendix followed by reimplantation into the cecum and anastomosis of the opposite end to the abdominal wall to form a one-way opening into the cecum. **B,** Use of a stoma for antegrade colonic irrigations.

have also been placed at the splenic flexure.)[29] Finally, the surgical approach is changing; the ACE procedure is now being done laparoscopically.[37] The frequency of colonic washout varies, as do the type and volume of solution. The most commonly used solutions include normal saline, hypertonic phosphate, polyethylene glycol 3350 (Miralax), and tap water. Yerkes and colleagues studied the routine use of tap water as an irrigant, based on reports of hypernatremia following saline irrigations and electrolyte abnormalities with use of hypertonic phosphate solutions. They could not detect any significant hyponatremia or hypochloremia in any patient using tap water for continence irrigations. However, there is the potential for serious electrolyte imbalances, especially if large volumes of water are used; therefore, volumes should be monitored and electrolyte studies should be done periodically.[38] Kokoska and associates described their experience with irrigants; they reported positive outcomes with normal saline, polyethylene glycol 3350, and a 1:1 solution of glycerin and saline.[39] Because of the potential for electrolyte imbalance with all these solutions, they recommended serum electrolyte studies to assess a child's tolerance to a particular solution.[38,39] Graf and colleagues conducted a literature review on types and amounts of solution utilized for irrigation.[40] They found that the volume of irrigant varied from 80 to 1000 mL administered over a 5- to 60-minute time frame. In the majority of patients, colonic evacuation occurred within 1 hour of irrigant administration. The frequency of irrigations ranged from daily to weekly. These investigators concluded that the type of solution and volume and frequency of irrigation must be individualized for each patient.[40] The MACE procedure and its variants have now been performed for more than a decade. Reported complications include the following: stomal stenosis/necrosis, stomal leakage, difficulty catheterizing the stoma; pain with enema administration, wound infection, bowel obstruction from adhesions; appendiceal necrosis, hypertrophic granulation tissue at the stoma site, mucus discharge and dermatitis around the stoma, cecal volvulus, nausea and dizziness during phosphate enema usage, and hyperphosphatemia.[41] Children and parents need to be thoroughly informed regarding the procedure, long-term management requirements, and potential complications; the child and family must be motivated and willing to adhere to the enema regimen. Some centers believe that this procedure is more successful in children who are more than 5 years of age because they have a better understanding of the care and are more motivated.[40,41] In general, children and their families have been very satisfied with the MACE procedure. Foster reported that many children with neurogenic bowel, especially those with myelomeningocele, have benefited from this procedure and are willing to spend the time to complete a daily irrigation.[42]

Issues to consider in postoperative management include the potential for stomal stenosis, the importance of instruction in self-care with a focus on independence, and potential long-term complications. Stomal stenosis is prevented by daily stomal catheterization in the immediate postoperative period (until daily irrigations are begun). Instruction in self-care is begun as soon as the child is able to participate postoperatively. The clinician should direct teaching to the child and should consistently encourage the child and parent to minimize or eliminate parental involvement in the procedure. Potential long-term complications include irritant or infectious colitis and fluid-electrolyte imbalance. Children and caregivers should be taught to report abdominal pain, bloody or mucoid stools, fever, or signs of fluid electrolyte imbalance promptly to the physician. The clinician should also be aware that autonomic dysreflexia has been reported with high colonic retrograde enemas and is a theoretic possibility with antegrade irrigations.[42]

Children with neurogenic bowel dysfunction in whom conservative management and the ACE procedure fail still have the option of colostomy. Although this sounds like a radical intervention, the child and caregivers who have been dealing unsuccessfully with fecal incontinence and various bowel management regimens may actually find a colostomy to be a major relief. Colostomy provides control over fecal odor and fecal elimination and therefore gives the child a sense of security; a colostomy also eliminates problems with perianal skin irritation and the need to wear diapers.

DIARRHEA

As noted earlier, chronic constipation is a common contributor to incontinence in children. Diarrhea can also cause incontinence; it most frequently occurs as a response to an acute infectious process or as the result of a chronic condition or disease state.

Acute diarrhea is defined as an increase in the number of stools and an alteration in stool consistency, as compared with the patient's normal stooling pattern. It is usually caused by viral, bacterial, or protozoal agents. In children, rotavirus and Norwalk-like virus are responsible for up to 50% of acute diarrheal cases during winter months.[43] History will usually reveal a sudden onset of illness, and there may be other systemic symptoms, such as fever, cough, rash, or decreased activity level. With resolution of the infectious process, the diarrhea subsides, as do the incontinent episodes.

Chronic diarrhea is defined as an increase in the frequency, fluidity, or volume of stool, compared with the child's normal pattern, for longer than 14 to 21 days. Stool output in excess of 10 g/kg/day in infants and greater than 200 g/day in children is considered indicative of diarrhea.[43] Disease states that commonly lead to diarrhea include short gut syndrome, irritable bowel syndrome, Crohn's disease or ulcerative colitis, celiac disease, and cystic fibrosis. Children with peritoneal shunt infections commonly exhibit nausea, vomiting, and diarrhea as well as fever and abdominal pain. Children with congenital heart disease must be monitored closely during any episode of diarrhea, because it can be indicative of digoxin toxicity or worsening congestive heart failure (versus an episode of acute gastroenteritis). Oncology patients may develop chemotherapy-induced diarrhea. Children with cerebral palsy who have limited mobility are frequently plagued with impactions that exhibit as constant diarrhea (because the liquid stool seeps around the impacted stool in the presence of persistent internal sphincter relaxation); it is critical to carefully balance fiber, liquid, and stool softeners in these children and to assess for impaction before treating episodes of "diarrhea." Any child with diarrhea requires careful assessment, because diarrhea in children is typically symptomatic of another condition that needs to be addressed. Once the underlying problem is corrected, the diarrhea and incontinence typically resolve.

SUMMARY

Bowel management in the pediatric population is both challenging and rewarding. Fortunately, our society is moving toward a little more openness in discussion of elimination. There are more books for children and parents that explain problems with control of "poop" and "gas" and things that can be done to normalize and control their elimination patterns (Box 16-3). Once a rapport is established between the child and the clinician, children are usually very willing to work, and most respond well to positive reinforcement. A major challenge in working with these children is the need to obtain the ongoing support of the child's caregivers because many of these children have other medical priorities, and it can become overwhelming for a caregiver to

prioritize their many needs. This is a task that requires tremendous sensitivity and creativity on the part of the clinician as one addresses the child's and the caregivers' issues. Collaboration with the other professionals involved in the care of these children may be helpful in trying to obtain additional assistance in maintaining a bowel program for the child. Ultimately, the goals are not only to normalize bowel function and provide continence, but also to promote positive self-esteem; thus, the clinician must always remember that "... The young child is dependent on adults for many things, but the most important is a sense of being cared for ...."[44]

BLADDER MANAGEMENT

Urinary disorders are common among children, and children are vulnerable to some of the same urologic problems as those experienced by adults.

BOX 16-3   Resources

Websites

www.uoa.org (United Ostomy Association)
www.nafc.org (National Association for Continence)
www.aboutencopresis.com (Sponsored by Braintree Laboratories)
www.icpcs.org (International Center for Pediatric Colorectal Solutions)
www.iffgd.org (International Foundation for Gastrointestinal Disorders)
www.sbaa.org (Spina Bifida Association of America)
www.wocn.org (Wound Ostomy Continence Nurses Society)
www.suna.org (Society of Urologic Nurses and Associates)
www.simonfoundation.org (Simon Foundation)
www.ichelp.org (Interstitial Cystitis Association)

Educational Materials
Company Websites
www.mentorcorp.com
www.humanicare.com
www.us.coloplast.com
www.nafc.org
Books
Cho S: *The gas we pass,* Brooklyn, N.Y., 1994, Kane/Miller Book Publishers.
Gomi T: *Everyone poops,* Brooklyn, N.Y., 1993, Kane/Miller Book Publishers.
Hulme JA: *Bladder and bowel issues for kids,* Missoula, 2003, Phoenix Publishing.
Smith DP: *Improving your child's potty habits handbook,* Knoxville, 2003, PottyMD.
Smith DP: *Constipation handbook,* Knoxville, 2003, PottyMD.

However, problems with urinary function may manifest differently in children from the way they do in adults, with incontinence being the most common presentation. Urinary incontinence has been identified as the most common problem seen in pediatric urology practice.[45]

Children are at risk for urinary tract dysfunction for several reasons. The most obvious is the potential for congenital anomalies involving the kidneys, bladder, or urethra. However, a much more common factor is the ongoing development and maturation of the urinary tract and the neurologic pathways critical to volitional control of voiding. In addition to physical growth of the bladder-sphincter unit, continence requires a transition from the simple infant bladder, which empties by reflex, to the mature bladder, which is subject to complex neural control and inhibition. Another issue to be considered in the child with dysfunctional voiding or incontinence is the effect of cognitive development and the influence of toilet training. It is now known that toilet training can play a major role in the development of voiding dysfunction. This finding is particularly true when toilet training is begun before maturation of the critical anatomic structures and neurologic pathways.

It is thus clear that urinary incontinence and voiding dysfunction in the child may be a result of congenital anomalies, abnormal development or maturation of the neurologic pathways critical to volitional control of voiding, or developmental issues related to premature initiation of toilet training.

DEVELOPMENT OF THE GENITOURINARY SYSTEM

At birth, the kidneys occupy a large area of the posterior abdominal cavity. Although the kidneys continue to grow and develop during childhood, all the nephrons are actually present at birth. Urine formation and excretion begin by the third month of gestation and contribute to the volume of amniotic fluid.

In the infant, the bladder is an abdominal organ because of the cone-shaped pelvis. As the pelvis expands during childhood, the bladder becomes a pelvic organ and assumes the adult pyramidal shape. The urethra and bladder form a functional unit that work together to alternately store and eliminate urine. Coordination of bladder and urethral function occurs at three primary levels of the central nervous system: the cerebral cortex, the brainstem, and the sacral spinal cord. The relative influence of each of these control centers changes as the neurologic structures and pathways mature.

ACQUISITION OF CONTINENCE

In infants and young children, micturition is an involuntary act that is controlled by reflex activity coordinated at the level of the sacral cord and the pontine micturition center. During bladder filling, the tone of the sphincter muscles progressively increases to prevent leakage. When the bladder reaches its capacity, the micturition reflex is activated; that is, the detrusor muscle contracts and the sphincter muscles relax in reflex fashion to permit unobstructed voiding. Control of the periurethral striated muscles is fully integrated into the voiding reflex, even in infants.

During infancy and throughout the first year of life, voiding frequency remains constant at about 20 times per day. Over the first 3 years of life, the voiding frequency decreases to about 11 times per day, and the mean voiding volume increases fourfold. This increase seems to be primarily the result of an increase in bladder capacity, which is much greater than the increase in volume of urine.[46]

At about 2 or 3 years of age, the child becomes aware of the need to void and can learn to contract the pelvic muscles to briefly inhibit contraction of the detrusor muscle, thereby delaying urination. As the central nervous system continues to mature, the child learns to inhibit detrusor muscle activity, which enables him or her to achieve continence. At this point, micturition becomes voluntary.

Acquisition of bladder control is dependent on three separate events in development. The first is the development of the bladder into an adequate reservoir. For the first 12 years of life, the bladder capacity increases by about 1 ounce each year, which is expressed by the following formula: "Bladder capacity (in ounces) = Age in years + 2."[47] (Thus, a 6-year-old child should have a bladder capacity of 8 ounces, or 240 mL.)

The second event that is critical to continence is the establishment of voluntary control over the periurethral striated muscles and pelvic floor muscles. This usually occurs by 3 years of age. The third event is the most complex and involves the development of voluntary control over the micturition reflex. This occurs when the child gains the ability to voluntarily initiate or inhibit a detrusor contraction.

The acquisition of voluntary control over detrusor and sphincter activity requires a certain level of cognitive function. The development of voluntary control of voiding is a slow process and one that is subject to interference from factors such as pain, discomfort, or negative experiences associated with voiding. Such interferences may prompt the child to use emergency measures to prevent or postpone voiding for as long as possible; for example, the child may learn to use pelvic floor muscle contractions to inhibit bladder contractions, as opposed to normal central nervous system inhibition. Some children use these delay maneuvers only in certain circumstances, as when involved in playground activities; for other children, use of emergency inhibition measures becomes a habit leading to dysfunctional voiding and incomplete bladder emptying.

Development of central control over voiding is also subject to sociocultural influences. For example, in the farmlands of central China, rural Africa, and rural southern Europe, most children wear no underwear, and it is acceptable for them to void at any time outdoors, with girls squatting and boys standing. This is very different from Western societies, where there is a major focus on early acquisition of continence, and children are frequently shamed for bowel and bladder accidents.

It is evident that volitional control of voiding is dependent on intact nerve pathways as well as the processes of normal neurologic maturation and normal psychosocial development. Therefore, children with neural tube defects or other disruptions in the neuroanatomy of the lower urinary tract are at very high risk for voiding dysfunction and incontinence. The range of voiding dysfunction and incontinence among children with neurologic insults is quite variable, with the effect of any given lesion being dependent on its location and its severity.

With some neurologic insults, voiding dysfunction or incontinence may be the only symptom of the problem.

DYSFUNCTIONAL VOIDING

Dysfunctional voiding is the condition in which the child lacks awareness of progressive bladder filling and the impending need to void. At an unpredictable time, the child experiences an uninhibited detrusor contraction with sudden urinary urgency. The child typically responds by inappropriately contracting the sphincter muscles in an attempt to prevent urinary leakage. The child may also assume one of the dysfunctional voiding postures (that is, a boy may squeeze the penis, and a girl may press her fingers against the urethra or drop to a kneeling position, with her heel against her perineum). The child may or may not be successful in preventing leakage. If he or she is not able to inhibit the bladder contraction, incontinence will be the presenting symptom. Whether the child is able to prevent urinary leakage, he or she is at risk for incomplete bladder emptying secondary to inappropriate contraction of the pelvic muscles during detrusor contractions, which may result in urinary tract infection. The signs and symptoms of dysfunctional voiding are outlined in Box 16-4.[48]

ASSESSMENT OF THE CHILD WITH INCONTINENCE OR DYSFUNCTIONAL VOIDING

The assessment of any child with urinary incontinence or evidence of dysfunctional voiding begins with a detailed history and physical examination.

BOX 16-4 **Symptoms of Dysfunctional Voiding**

Urinary urgency
Incontinence
Lack of sensation of fullness
Dysfunctional voiding postures
Constipation
Abnormally frequent or infrequent voiding
Urinary tract infections

Box 16-5 outlines the assessment factors most critical to the management of a child with bladder dysfunction.[48] The voiding history is of particular importance and should include the child's present voiding patterns, the child's age when toilet training was started and when continence was achieved, the onset of the current problems and any associated events, and the child's and caregiver's perception of the problem and goals for treatment. Bowel habits need to be carefully explored, because chronic constipation can contribute significantly to bladder dysfunction, and neurologic lesions producing urinary incontinence are likely to produce fecal incontinence as well. The physical examination should focus on evidence of bladder distension, signs of spinal abnormalities, and evaluation of neurologic pathways affecting bowel and bladder function.[48] For a more in-depth discussion of assessment guidelines, refer to Chapter 12.

After a careful history and physical examination, the clinician determines the need for laboratory and radiologic studies. Routine tests usually include a urinalysis and urine culture; a blood urea nitrogen and creatinine assay may also be indicated to evaluate renal function. Urodynamic studies may be indicated to assess lower urinary tract function; however, these studies should be delayed until any infection has been eliminated and the urinary tract has been sterilized. Radiologic studies are ordered only if the findings on history and physical indicate the need, and they should be selected based on the provisional diagnosis (Table 16-5). For example, if there are physical findings consistent with occult spinal dysraphism, a plain film of the abdomen and pelvis can be obtained. The child with elevated blood urea nitrogen and creatinine levels will benefit from an ultrasonographic examination of the kidneys to evaluate upper urinary tract anatomy and function.

The voiding cystourethrogram should not be used as a screening test in children because it is often unpleasant, stressful, and traumatic for the child and is indicated only when anatomic causes of incontinence are suspected. Indications that a

---

BOX 16-5   **Guidelines for History and Physical Examination of Child with Urinary Incontinence or Dysfunctional Voiding**

History
- Circumstances and description of maternal pregnancy and delivery
- Child's acquisition of developmental milestones or any delays (to include details of bowel and bladder training)
- *Patient's perception of the problem* (description of voiding problem in the child's own words)
- Voiding habits: frequency, character of urinary stream, urinary symptoms, perceptions of complete versus incomplete emptying
- Number of voids/day or usual interval between voids
- Dry interval (time between voiding and incontinence or one episode of leakage to another) in child with incontinence
- Nocturia (number of episodes) or nocturnal enuresis
- Daily fluid intake (type and volume)
- Use of dysfunctional voiding postures (specific postures used, situations in which used)

- Urinary tract infections
- Family conflicts or evidence of family dysfunction; parental beliefs re: enuresis and response to enuretic episodes
- Family history of voiding dysfunction or incontinence (parents or siblings)
- Constipation or encopresis
- Any neurologic lesions or conditions
- History of surgery or hospitalization
- Previous treatment and response

Physical Examination
- Abdominal examination for evidence of bladder distension
- Inspection of back and buttocks for evidence of occult spinal dysraphism
- Inspection of genitalia and anus for any abnormalities
- Complete neurologic examination (perineal sensation, presence or absence of anal wink and bulbocavernosus reflex, anal tone)

TABLE 16-5   **Radiologic and Other Tests of Renal Function**

TEST	PROCEDURE	PURPOSE
Intravenous pyelography (IVP)	Intravenous injection of a contrast medium; medium secreted and concentrated in renal tubules; films made 5, 10, and 15 minutes after injection Disadvantages: produces poor renal outlines in newborns and young children; insensitive for the detection of acute, fecal inflammation; requires higher dosage of radiation; risk of reaction to contrast	Precise anatomic image of kidneys and can readily identify some urinary tract abnormalities (cysts, hydronephrosis); relatively sensitive for detection of cortical thinning or scarring
Voiding cystourethrogram (VCUG)	Contrast medium injected into bladder through urethral catheter until bladder is full; films taken before, during, and after voiding Disadvantages: relatively high effective radiation dose of 5.4 mSv; catheterization	Visualizes bladder outline and urethra; "gold standard" for the detection of reflux; permits grading of reflux according to standards; examines the urethra for stricture and the bladder for filling and emptying capacity
Renal cortical scintigraphy/ Radionuclide renal scanning	Radioisotopes injected intravenously and recorded with special camera and computer analysis Disadvantage: not useful in detecting obstruction	Measures renal function and renal blood flow by recording appearance and disappearance of radioactivity in each kidney; detects pyelonephritis and renal scarring even in early stages; useful in neonates; limited radiation; useful in patients with poor renal function; "gold standard" for diagnosis of pyelonephritis and renal cortical scarring
Ultrasonography	Transmission of ultrasonic waves through kidney areas to outline kidney mass; no radiation and noninvasive	Examination of the kidneys to identify hydronephrosis; examination of bladder to identify dilation of the distal ureters, hypertrophy of the bladder wall, and presence of ureterocele
Computed tomography	Narrow-beam x-rays and computer analysis provide precise reconstruction of area Disadvantages: expensive; high radiation dose	Provides both anatomic and functional information about kidney; especially valuable for distinguishing tumors and cysts; the definitive diagnostic test for acute pyelonephritis
Urine culture and sensitivity	Collection of sterile specimen that is plated to grow out organisms; any organisms then exposed to various antibiotics	To identify the concentration and type of bacteria in the urine; sensitivity testing determines the antimicrobial activity that various antibiotics exert against a specific bacterium

Continued

TABLE 16-5 Radiologic and Other Tests of Renal Function—cont'd

TEST	PROCEDURE	PURPOSE
Urodynamic testing	Uroflowmetry, measurement of postvoid residual urine, cystometrogram, and cystogram	Tests designed to measure the function of the bladder; not indicated in the routine evaluation of diurnal incontinence or voiding dysfunction in children; indicated for children with complex voiding dysfunction
Urinalysis (UA)	Method of collection an important aspect in interpreting UA results; bag results reliable only if negative; clean-catch method increases reliability; catheterization and suprapubic provide most accurate results	Laboratory evaluation of renal function; screen for presence of red blood cells, hemoglobin, leukocytes, nitrites, protein, and pH; to suggest the diagnosis of urinary tract infection, the three most useful components in evaluation: leukocyte esterase test, nitrite test, and microscopy

urinary tract disorder is the cause of the incontinence and that the cystourethrogram should be performed include severe urgency, urge incontinence, and urinary tract infection;[49] in contrast, a voiding cystourethrogram is not indicated for the patient with primary nocturnal enuresis (PNE) or as an initial assessment for the child with day and night wetting but no evidence of infection. If voiding cystourethrography is done, it should be done during urodynamic testing to minimize the number of urethral catheterizations.

Urodynamic studies are seldom needed in children with nonneurogenic voiding dysfunction and are indicated in these children only when the diagnosis is unclear and there is the potential for upper tract damage. In contrast, urodynamic evaluation is routinely indicated for children with spinal cord trauma or neural tube defects (myelomeningocele, lipomeningocele, or sacral agenesis), and yearly urodynamic evaluation is recommended for children with neurogenic bladder secondary to myelomeningocele. Urodynamic studies are also beneficial in the evaluation of bladder capacity and compliance in children with congenital anomalies affecting the lower urinary tract (such as posterior urethral valves, prune belly syndrome, and bladder exstrophy). Relative indications for urodynamic testing include suspected nonneurogenic neurogenic

bladder, cerebral palsy accompanied by persistent enuresis or voiding dysfunction, and persistent nocturnal and diurnal enuresis.[47]

After completion of the history, physical examination, and indicated laboratory and radiologic studies, the child's voiding problem can be classified as a functional disorder, a neurogenic disorder, or an anatomic disorder (Box 16-6). Management is then based on the specific classification and underlying cause. The discussion in this chapter is

BOX 16-6 Classification of Urinary Incontinence in Children

Functional Incontinence
Primary nocturnal enuresis
Nonneurogenic neurogenic voiding dysfunction
Nonneurogenic neurogenic bladder

Neurogenic Incontinence

Anatomic Incontinence
Urethral ectopia
Sphincter insufficiency
Exstrophy or epispadias
Short urethra
Trauma
Bladder outlet obstruction

on the functional and neurogenic classifications of urinary incontinence.

PRIMARY NOCTURNAL ENURESIS

It is important to define enuresis clearly and to differentiate between enuresis and incontinence. When enuresis occurs during the daytime or waking hours, it is called *diurnal enuresis,* a term that is synonymous with incontinence. When enuresis occurs during sleeping hours, it is known as *nocturnal enuresis,* which is a specific form of incontinence that is limited to sleeping hours in a child who is otherwise continent. Nocturnal enuresis is further classified as either primary or secondary; PNE is defined as bedwetting in children who have never been dry at night for a significant length of time. Secondary nocturnal enuresis occurs when a child who was dry at night for a period of at least 6 months begins to wet the bed again.

Epidemiology and Etiology

Except for allergic disorders, nocturnal enuresis is the most common chronic clinical problem encountered in pediatrics.[50] Nocturnal enuresis is more common in boys, whereas diurnal enuresis (daytime incontinence) is more common in girls.[51] Enuresis is more common among lower socioeconomic groups and in larger families. Genetic factors also seem to play a significant role in the development of enuresis. When both parents have a positive history of enuresis, 77% of the children develop enuresis, and when one parent has a history of enuresis, 44% of the children are affected with enuresis. The incidence among children with no parental history is only 15%. Research has provided additional evidence of a genetic cause in that a single region of chromosome 13 has been identified as a specific marker for PNE.[52]

The spontaneous cure rate for PNE is 15% per year after 5 years of age.[53] It is estimated that 1% of adults remain enuretic and that active treatment during early childhood will reduce the prevalence of enuresis in adulthood.[50]

Many explanations have been offered as to the cause of PNE, including emotional stress, physical problems such as pinworms and allergies, developmental delays, urinary tract disorders, psychologic

disturbances, antidiuretic hormone insufficiency, small bladder capacity, and "deep sleep."[51,54] Currently, PNE is generally considered to be caused by a maturational lag and is rarely associated with a significant psychopathologic condition.[55] Successful intervention is dependent on identification of the causative and contributing factors, which are generally not pathologic. Most children with enuresis (75% to 90%) fall into the PNE category.[56]

Assessment

The initial assessment of the child with enuresis should include a complete medical and social history, a physical examination, a urinalysis, and a urine culture. In the majority of cases, the history provides the most insight and guidance, because the physical examination, urinalysis, and urine culture are frequently negative.

Medical and Social History. The child with enuresis must frequently deal with multiple psychologic stressors, such as teasing, loss of sleep, and interference with peer activities such as sleepovers and camping trips. It is therefore critical to assess the effect of enuresis on the child's peer relationships and extracurricular activities. Another factor that significantly affects the child's response to the enuresis is the response of parents and other family members. The coping skills and management approach of parents and caregivers vary tremendously, and any negative or punitive response adds significantly to the child's stress. The clinician must therefore assess the parents' beliefs and feelings regarding the enuresis, their management techniques, and the overall family dynamics. Determining the parents' reasons for seeking treatment may provide useful information for the health care provider regarding parental attitudes and misperceptions.

The importance of parental attitudes and coping skills is reflected in a study in the United States that indicated that 16% of parents viewed bedwetting as a significant problem and one-third of them dealt with the issue by punishing the child.[57] It has also been documented that children in dysfunctional families who suffer from enuresis are at increased risk for emotional and physical abuse.[5] The management program for any individual child is always based to some extent on the family's beliefs about enuresis and the social structure of the home environment; however, inappropriate parental responses to the problem must always be viewed as a "red flag" and must be promptly addressed.

There are several other red flags to which the clinician should be alert when obtaining the child's history; these are signs and symptoms that may indicate a significant problem and that usually require consultation with or referral to a pediatrician, pediatric continence nurse specialist, or pediatric urologist. These include significant daytime incontinence, poor urinary stream, encopresis, and symptoms of urinary tract infection. Each of these findings point to a more complex problem requiring additional workup (Fig. 16-5).

Assessment of bowel function is an essential aspect of the history for any child with enuresis or voiding dysfunction. Constipation is common in children and is often overlooked in children with enuresis. As has been noted elsewhere in this text, constipation is a common contributing factor to

bladder instability, urinary tract infection, and encopresis.[58] Some studies have shown that effective treatment of constipation is effective in eliminating enuresis in a substantial number of children.[58]

The child with enuresis who also has daytime voiding dysfunction should undergo further evaluation, including a voiding record and assessment of functional bladder capacity. Children who present with frequent small-volume voids associated with urgency and posturing are likely to have underlying detrusor instability and small functional bladder capacity. These children need to be evaluated for any organic disorder; if none is found, they are frequently benefited by instruction in urge-inhibition strategies and a bladder retraining program as outlined later in this chapter and in Chapter 5.

In addition to the medical and social history, a brief developmental history should be obtained, and a description of any emotional or behavioral problems should be elicited. Current stressors in the child's life that could be contributing to the enuresis should be identified. If the child is known

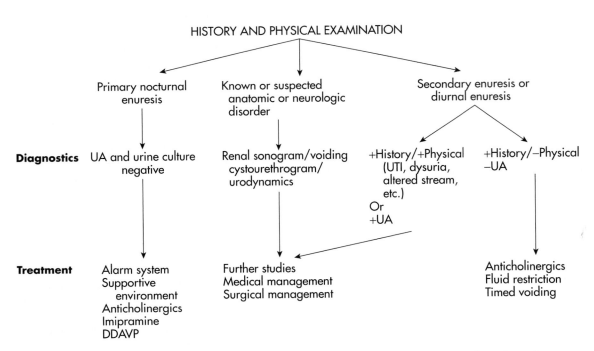

Fig. 16-5 Algorithm for assessment and management of a child with voiding dysfunction or urinary incontinence.

or suspected to have a serious psychopathologic condition, the treatment of enuresis should be postponed until the underlying issues have been addressed.

Physical Examination. The physical examination of a child with nocturnal enuresis should include an abdominal and genital examination, an observation of the voided stream (if the history is suggestive of any abnormality), and a brief neurologic examination to include the child's gait, muscle tone, peripheral reflexes, perineal sensation, and anal sphincter tone. The "red flags" for which the clinician should observe include the following: abdominal masses, such as evidence of bladder distension or retained stool; evidence of spinal anomalies, such as a pilonidal dimple or a hairy patch; abnormal neurologic findings, such as diminished reflexes, diminished sensation, or altered gait; and genital anomalies, such as epispadias, hypospadias, or urethral duplication. Most of these warning signs are obvious, but some are easily overlooked, such as subtle neurologic abnormalities.[59] Although it is important to be alert to subtle abnormalities in the physical examination, the physical exam for most children with PNE is normal.

Treatment. Four major factors should be taken into consideration when the clinician is developing a management plan for a child with enuresis: the effects of enuresis on the child, the age of the child, the response of the family and society to the child, and the psychosocial benefits of successful treatment.

Current treatment options for enuresis include behavioral interventions and pharmacotherapy. Hypnotherapy and acupuncture have also been used, but there is currently little research to support these treatment approaches. Although very few of these children or their parents require psychotherapy to address issues associated with enuresis, almost all of them benefit from motivational counseling.[60]

The reported success of each regimen must be attributed partly to the spontaneous "cure" of enuresis as the child outgrows the problem or to the increased attention directed toward the child. The evolution of multiple therapeutic options clearly indicates that no single treatment approach is ideal or even effective for all children. The treatment selected for any child with enuresis should reflect the child's developmental stage, and one example of a stage-appropriate intervention plan is outlined in Box 16-7. Most parents need assistance in understanding age-appropriate interventions and responses. Each of the strategies commonly used in the treatment of enuresis is briefly described.

Self-awakening. Teaching the child to awaken at night is the most straightforward approach to management of enuresis because it compensates both for increased urine production and for small bladder capacity. One technique for teaching self-awakening is to have the child rehearse a particular sequence of events every night before going to sleep.

BOX 16-7   Age-Appropriate Time Line of Interventions for Enuresis

3 to 5 Years of Age
- Educate parents regarding causes and incidence and correct any misconceptions.
- Teach good bedtime habits to the child: empty the bladder before sleep; limit fluids after dinner.
- Provide positive feedback for dry mornings.

6 to 7 Years of Age
- In addition to the above, begin a self-awakening program.
- Teach motivational techniques.

8 to 11 Years of Age
- In addition to the above, provide education and reassurance for both the child and the parents.
- Continue motivational techniques.
- Begin a program of bladder stretching.
- Instruct the patient to use an enuresis alarm.
- Instruct the patient to use desmopressin acetate for special events.

12 Years and Older
- In addition to the above, continue education and reassurance for parents and child.
- Instruct the patient to use an enuresis alarm.
- Begin a trial of desmopressin acetate for 2 to 6 months.
- Instruct the patient to use a combination of desmopressin acetate and enuresis alarm for 2 to 6 months.

The child is told to pretend that his or her bladder is full and it is the middle of the night. He or she awakens, gets out of bed, runs to the bathroom, and urinates. After the rehearsal, the child reminds himself or herself to get up during the night and to go to the bathroom to urinate if necessary. Another approach to self-awakening therapy is to use self-hypnosis with the hypnotic suggestion being that the child gets up to use the bathroom at night. One researcher has reported a 77% cure rate with the use of hypnosis in children more than 5 years old; however, the clinician must be aware that this was a small group of children and that these results would need to be replicated before one could assume widespread applicability.[61]

Behavioral measures to increase bladder capacity. The child with abnormally small bladder capacity can be taught to consciously attempt to "stretch his or her bladder" by consistently prolonging the time between voidings. (This is essentially the same program as urge inhibition and bladder retraining, which is used for adults with urge incontinence.) This approach is supported by studies suggesting that up to 85% of enuretic children have small bladder capacities and detrusor instability of nonorganic origin.[62] In addition, resolution of enuresis is consistently associated with increased bladder capacity and reduced diurnal voiding frequency, regardless of treatment method. Interestingly, children whose treatment included increased fluid intake showed greater improvement in bladder capacity and a greater reduction in enuretic episodes than children treated with fluid restriction.[63]

Motivational therapy. Motivational therapy involves a series of counseling sessions in which the child is encouraged to assume responsibility for his or her enuresis. A combination of approaches have been used, including reassurance, guilt removal, and emotional support by the health care provider and parents. Positive reinforcement and reward systems are used to enhance the child's self-esteem and to provide a positive incentive to remain dry at night. A common successful reward system is the use of stickers on a calendar. A predetermined reward is given to the child at the end of the week based on the number of dry nights achieved.

This method is successful in approximately 25% of children.[64]

Enuresis alarms. The theory behind enuresis alarms is to condition the child to associate bladder distension with awakening. The alarm system consists of a urine sensor that is attached to the child's underwear and a portable alarm box worn by the child either on his or her wrist or pajama top, depending on the model. Initially, the child awakens after or during voiding and takes responsibility for turning off the alarm and using the toilet. This process eventually conditions the child to awaken at the sensation of a full bladder rather than the sound of the alarm. Treatment may take as long as 3 to 4 months, and it is recommended that the child wear the alarm system until he or she has been dry for 3 weeks.

When used by children for 3 or 4 months in situations with parental support, the success rates are as high as 70% to 85%, with regression rates of 20% to 50%.[65] Because success depends on a cooperative and motivated child, alarm therapy is generally used for children 8 years of age and older. The adjunctive use of positive reinforcement, that is, provision of a reward after a predetermined number of dry nights, has been shown to add to the effectiveness of alarm therapy.

The cost of alarms is between $48 and $70. Many insurance companies will cover the cost if the prescription includes the term "medical device." For families who cannot afford the alarm system, a standard alarm clock that is set for 3 hours after the child goes to bed can be used as an alternative.

Pharmacotherapy. Thirty-two percent to 50% of physicians in the United States prescribe drug therapy for children with nocturnal enuresis; however, as early as 1972 it was recommended that drug therapy not be used as first-line therapy for enuresis because of the potential side effects and low overall efficacy. This recommendation still holds true today. Most clinicians recommend use of pharmacologic agents only for children in whom behavioral therapy has failed.

The two medications that are most commonly prescribed for enuresis are imipramine hydrochloride and desmopressin acetate (DDAVP). Imipramine is an effective agent in 60% of children so long as it is used continuously; however, it does not correct the underlying problem, and the enuresis usually returns if the medication is discontinued. The exact mechanism by which imipramine reduces enuresis is not known, but it clearly affects both the bladder and the urethra and is known to have weak anticholinergic activity as well as some alpha-adrenergic and beta-adrenergic effects; thus, it is likely to increase bladder storage capacity. The initial dose of imipramine is usually 25 mg for children 6 to 8 years of age taken 1 hour before bedtime. Children 8 to 12 years of age should receive 50 mg per night, and children older than 12 years of age are typically given 75 mg per night. In prescribing imipramine, the clinician should always strive to use the lowest effective dose. The drug should be administered for 2 or 3 months and then tapered off over 3 or 4 months. The two biggest drawbacks to the use of imipramine are the high relapse rate (more than 90%) when the medication is discontinued and the risk of toxicity.[66] Imipramine is potentially lethal even at low doses; therefore, serum levels must be monitored closely to prevent accidental overdosage.

The second medication that is commonly used in the treatment of enuresis is DDAVP, the synthetic analogue of the antidiuretic hormone vasopressin. This drug has been used in the treatment of nocturnal enuresis for more than 15 years. It reduces nocturnal urine production by increasing water reabsorption and urine concentration in the distal segments of the tubules. Originally, DDAVP was available only as a nasal spray, but now it is available in an oral preparation that is just as effective as the intranasal formulation. Some children respond to the 0.2-mg dose, but an increased response is usually seen with the 0.4- and 0.6-mg doses.[67] The starting dose for the intranasal preparation is 20 mcg or one spray into each nostril at bedtime. The dosage can be increased by 10 mcg weekly to a maximum dose of 40 mcg. Children with allergic rhinitis should take an antihistamine 1 hour before using the DDAVP nasal spray.

The duration of action for DDAVP is 10 to 12 hours. Adverse effects are rare but include epistaxis, nostril pain, nasal congestion, and headache. Most of the nasal effects are related to the use of nasal spray as a delivery vehicle; these effects should be eliminated with the use of oral preparations. The most serious side effects occur with either route of delivery and include water intoxication and seizures. It is therefore recommended that DDAVP not be administered to any child who is predisposed to the development of hyponatremia. Furthermore, children taking DDAVP should be instructed to restrict their fluid intake in the evening, and serum electrolytes should be evaluated after 1 week of treatment. Although there is the potential for adverse effects, most children have tolerated the DDAVP nasal spray without complications, and the oral preparation has been safely used for the treatment of enuresis in children 6 years of age and older for as long as 6 months.

DDAVP is considered a successful treatment for enuresis, but it does not provide long-term resolution of the underlying disorder. Relapse occurs in 90% of children when the drug is discontinued.[68] In addition, the cost of the drug (more than $100 per month) is prohibitive for many families. Finally, the one study comparing DDAVP with an enuresis alarm found superior results with the alarm.[69]

SUMMARY

Enuresis is self-limiting for many children; about 15% of untreated children experience spontaneous resolution each year. However, it is not self-limiting in all children. A Dutch study indicated that 0.5% of otherwise healthy adults 18 to 64 years of age still wet their beds regularly.[48] This means that about 10% of children with enuresis will remain enuretic throughout their lifetimes. Even for children who will undergo spontaneous resolution, treatment may be indicated and important. Studies indicate that children with enuresis and their parents do not regard enuresis as a trivial problem. It places a significant emotional burden on the affected child and a substantial financial burden on the parents. These findings support aggressive treatment initiated at the point that the enuresis becomes a problem for the child or parents. Low self-esteem is associated with enuresis and is known to be a risk factor for psychiatric disorders and problems with social adjustment; thus, the child should receive appropriate treatment as soon as he or she expresses the desire to "sleep dry."

NONNEUROGENIC FUNCTIONAL VOIDING DISORDERS

Complicated enuresis encompasses a wide range of functional voiding disorders in children who do not otherwise exhibit any evidence of neurologic impairment. Findings on history and physical examination that are indicative of complicated enuresis include significant daytime incontinence, a poor urinary stream, encopresis, and urinary tract infection. The assessment of these children should include a complete voiding and defecation history and an assessment of the child's functional bladder capacity (average voided volume) in addition to the data outlined in Box 16-5 and previously discussed in the section on PNE. Diagnostic studies indicated for these children include voiding cystourethrogram and renal and bladder sonogram. If the sonogram is nondiagnostic, the child should undergo intravenous pyelography with or without a renal scan. Children who have a history of urinary tract infection or sonographic evidence of bladder-wall thickening, ureteral dilatation, or hydronephrosis or a significantly elevated postvoid residual should be evaluated with a contrast voiding cystogram or videourodynamics study to detect any vesicoureteral reflux or bladder-sphincter dyssynergia.

Synthesis of the diagnostic data helps to classify the particular disorder, and such classification provides direction in terms of treatment. However, the clinician should be aware that the clinical patterns of small bladder capacity, detrusor hyperreflexia, lazy bladder, and Hinman syndrome may not be the distinct entities they seem to be when considered from a theoretic standpoint. In all probability, these "clinical classifications" actually represent different stages in the natural progression of nonneuropathic bladder dysfunction[70] (Box 16-8).

Small-Capacity Hypertonic Bladder

Children who develop recurrent urinary tract infections in the absence of any anatomic abnormality may experience symptoms of voiding dysfunction (such as frequency, urgency, urge incontinence, nocturia and enuresis, and dysuria) long after the

---

BOX 16-8 **Patterns of Voiding Dysfunction in Neurologically Intact Children**

· ·

Small bladder capacity
Detrusor hyperreflexia
Lazy bladder syndrome
Hinman syndrome

---

infection has been resolved. The abnormal voiding patterns that develop in these children actually contribute to their risk of recurrent infection.

The manner in which a urinary tract infection can induce dysfunctional voiding is as follows: when the bladder wall is inflamed, the sensory threshold is altered so the child senses bladder fullness at a significantly reduced volume. In addition, the detrusor muscle itself may become irritable, leading to detrusor instability (overactivity) and reduced compliance. The child may attempt to delay urination because of either pain or inappropriate setting; however, the inflamed detrusor muscle may fail to respond to the child's attempts to inhibit the detrusor contraction. The attempt to delay or interrupt voiding by contraction of the sphincter muscles creates a form of outflow obstruction (if the detrusor muscle is contracting at the same time). The resulting stop-and-go voiding pattern can lead to recurrent infection because bacteria can be carried from the meatus up into the bladder when voiding is interrupted in this manner.

Urodynamic studies in these children reveal a small-capacity bladder with elevated detrusor pressures during filling. As the bladder approaches capacity, the child experiences unstable (involuntary) contractions of high magnitude, resulting in severe urgency and urge incontinence (despite the child's efforts to maintain continence by voluntarily contracting the striated sphincter muscles). The outflow obstruction created by the child's efforts to maintain continence causes a sharp elevation in the intravesical pressures and may result in incomplete emptying. Sphincter electromyography is normal, but there may be complex repetitive discharges (pseudomyotonia) by the muscle during filling, which contributes further to the sense of urgency or to incontinence.

Detrusor Hyperreflexia

Detrusor hyperreflexia (neurogenic detrusor over-activity) refers to involuntary detrusor contractions of neurologic origin. Children with detrusor hyperreflexia have not yet acquired the ability to voluntarily inhibit the infantile voiding reflex. These children typically present with daytime symptoms of frequency, urgency, or sudden incontinence in addition to nocturnal enuresis. This clinical pattern does not seem to be caused by any urinary disorder or neurologic deficit; rather, it seems to occur as a result of a delay in central nervous system maturation. Children with chronic neurogenic detrusor overactivity may exhibit one or more subtle indicators of this delayed maturation: mirror movements (that is, similar motion in the contralateral hand when the individual is asked to pronate and supinate one hand rapidly), hyperactive deep tendon reflexes, ankle clonus, or posturing with a stress gait. Another subtle indicator sometimes seen in these children is left-handedness in a child whose family members are all right-handed, which may signify crossed dominance. However, the most significant finding is the use of specific behaviors to maintain continence, such as "Vincent's curtsy," in which the child drops into a curtsy pose to press the foot into the perineum. (The curtsy is a cover.) Alternatively, a boy may squeeze his penis.

Unstable (overactive) detrusor contractions are believed to result from an irritable focus within the bladder wall that triggers a detrusor contraction. When the bladder suddenly contracts and the child realizes that incontinence is imminent, he or she may attempt to prevent urinary leakage by contracting the pelvic floor and sphincter muscles. This maneuver, when successful, produces closure of the distal portion of the urethra first and the bladder neck second, which actually propels urine backward into the bladder. This obviously creates the risk of infection; therefore, all children who present with signs and symptoms of neurogenic detrusor overactivity should be screened for infection.

The sudden urgency triggered by the unstable detrusor contraction is usually followed by urinary leakage, unless the child is able to reach a bathroom quickly. However, there is the risk of incomplete emptying because the bladder muscle is contracting against a closed sphincter. Even if the child gets to the bathroom before leakage occurs, he or she may fail to adequately relax the pelvic muscles and striated sphincter, and so voiding occurs against some degree of outlet obstruction. Incomplete emptying then further exacerbates the problem with urinary frequency. In addition, the outlet obstruction produced by the partially contracted sphincter results in elevated voiding pressures, and the dysfunctional bladder muscle may contribute to elevated resting pressures. These elevated pressures impair the delivery of urine from the kidneys, which can eventually cause dilatation of the collecting system as well as recurrent urinary tract infection.[46]

Lazy Bladder Syndrome: The Infrequent Voider

The lazy bladder syndrome is the result of a long-standing habit of fractionated and incomplete voiding. Children with lazy bladder syndrome void primarily as a result of abdominal pressure because detrusor contractions are minimal or absent. These children typically present with large volumes of residual urine, and frequent infections are common. These children may go undiagnosed until the health care provider asks specific questions regarding voiding patterns, including frequency.

Infrequent voiders are usually older girls who are being seen as a result of recurrent urinary tract infections. The infections may or may not be symptomatic and may or may not be associated with episodic urinary leakage or nocturnal enuresis. When questioned, the child reports voiding as infrequently as twice daily (such as once in the morning and once at night). Most of these children had normal voiding patterns as infants, but after gaining bladder control they learned to delay voiding for extended periods of time. This pattern of infrequent voiding may result from an aversion to public bathrooms or from some aversion event or episode of dysuria occurring about the time of toilet training.

Although these children have extremely large bladders, they may experience episodes of urgency and urge incontinence when their bladders are filled to capacity, and they commonly strain during voiding. As noted, elevated postvoid residuals are common. These children may also be chronically constipated, and some may have a resultant encopresis. Urodynamic evaluation reveals a large-capacity, highly compliant bladder with variable contractility. Some children generate normal detrusor contractions, but in other children the detrusor contractions are either unsustained or absent. The voiding cystogram may demonstrate a failure to empty completely despite normal relaxation of the striated sphincter; this is consistent with the overall picture of myogenic failure resulting from chronic distension. Fortunately, vesicoureteral reflux is not generally seen. A sonogram may show mild thickening of the bladder wall, but trabeculation is generally absent or mild.

Nonneurogenic Neurogenic Bladder (Hinman Syndrome)

The nonneurogenic neurogenic bladder, also known as the Hinman syndrome, represents a cluster of clinical findings. The diagnosis is one of exclusion and is made when a child has all the clinical, radiographic, and urodynamic features of a neuropathic bladder but no evidence of a neurologic disorder. This condition is at the most severe end of the dysfunctional voiding spectrum.

Children with Hinman syndrome typically present with diurnal and nocturnal enuresis, urinary tract infection, constipation and encopresis, and morphologic changes in the lower urinary tract. Severe trabeculation (that is, a "Christmas tree bladder"), elevated volumes of residual urine, vesicoureteral reflux, and upper tract damage are often present. Functionally and radiographically, the bladders of these children strongly resemble true neurogenic bladders. However, in the majority of these children, a pediatric neurologic evaluation and an MRI scan of the spine fail to demonstrate any evidence of a neurologic lesion.

Dr. Hinman postulated that this syndrome develops as a result of unstable detrusor contractions and the responding contraction of the pelvic floor-striated sphincter muscle complex. This dyssynergic bladder-sphincter activity is believed to result in hypertrophy of the detrusor muscle and the trigone of the bladder, which causes increased ureteral resistance and eventual partial ureteral decompensation.

In addition, the dyssynergic bladder contractions result in elevated volumes of residual urine, which contribute to infection. Finally, the lack of coordination between the bladder and the pelvic floor, in addition to the detrusor overactivity, result in episodic urinary leakage.[71]

The key to diagnosis of the Hinman syndrome is the patient history. Both the child and the parents are interviewed to ascertain whether the voiding dysfunction began after a positive response to toilet training. Hinman believes that this disorder is a behaviorally based functional voiding disorder. He bases this belief on the finding that the disorder can be reversed by suggestion (hypnosis) and biofeedback, on the absence of any detectable neurologic or obstructive abnormality, and on the evidence of a "failure" personality and a domineering father among most of his patients. However, there is a subgroup of children who have demonstrable uropathy even before 2 years of age; among these children, the dysfunctional voiding pattern is apparently congenital. Older children presenting with evidence of Hinman syndrome must be carefully evaluated for psychologic factors contributing to the dysfunctional voiding pattern; if none are found, the child and parents can be reassured that the problem seems to be congenital.

Treatment is directed toward elimination of infection and correction of the dyssynergic bladder-sphincter activity. Specific measures include the administration of antibiotic and anticholinergic medications, the implementation of timed voiding, and bowel management measures to include disimpaction (if needed) followed by colonic cleansing and establishment of a routine bowel management program. It is crucial for the clinician to work with the parents and child to ensure that they have a clear understanding of the condition and of the management plan. The parents need to be encouraged to communicate confidence in their child's ability to overcome the bladder dysfunction, and they should be instructed to praise every measure of success in the program. These children generally need hypnosis or biofeedback to accomplish the necessary reeducation. A positive response to therapy is considered confirmation of the diagnosis.

NEUROGENIC BLADDER

It would be more accurate to describe the clinical picture classified as neurogenic bladder as "neuropathic vesicourethral dysfunction" because the entire lower urinary tract is involved in most children, and often the urethral dysfunction is more important than the bladder dysfunction.

Neurogenic bladder dysfunction can be caused by a lesion at any level in the nervous system, including the cerebral cortex, the spinal cord, and the peripheral nervous system. For example, up to 75% of children with cerebral palsy experience urinary incontinence. However, the most common cause of neurogenic bladder in children is abnormal development of the spinal column.[72] Children with myelomeningocele almost always have bladder dysfunction manifest as incontinence, and other spinal cord abnormalities, such as caudal regression syndrome, tethered cord, or tumors, can also cause incontinence. Sacral agenesis can result in neurogenic bladder, and this anomaly occurs in 1% of infants born to mothers with Type 2 diabetes. In addition, up to 5% of children with imperforate anus have a lumbosacral anomaly and neurogenic bladder. Although these disorders represent the most common causes of neurogenic bladder, any lesion affecting neurologic control of the bladder and sphincter can produce the dysfunctional voiding state known as neurogenic bladder.

The two most significant sequelae of neurogenic bladder dysfunction are upper tract deterioration and urinary incontinence.[73] The deterioration in renal function occurs as a result of the incoordination between detrusor muscle contraction and sphincter relaxation, a function normally coordinated at the level of the pons. This dyssynergia produces a functional obstruction at the level of the bladder outlet, which leads to high intravesical pressures, bladder muscle hypertrophy and trabeculation, vesicoureteral reflux, and upper tract deterioration. Another problem contributing to upper tract damage is recurrent infection, which is common because of incomplete bladder emptying and vesicoureteral reflux.

Many factors contribute to urinary incontinence in the child with a neurogenic bladder; these include detrusor overactivity, total or partial denervation of the sphincter, and poor bladder compliance occurring as a result of chronic urinary retention and outflow obstruction. Most commonly, the incontinence occurs from some combination of these factors.

It is not possible to predict the degree of bladder-sphincter dyssynergia or the behavior of the bladder based on the type of defect, level of lesion, or general clinical presentation of the infant or child; for example, children with myelomeningocele have widely varying patterns of voiding dysfunction, even when the level of the lesion is the same. Therefore, urodynamic testing and radiologic evaluation are considered essential components of assessment for any child with a neurologic lesion. Urodynamic evaluation is now recommended during the neonatal period at most pediatric centers in the United States. The rationale for this recommendation is that urodynamic evaluation provides essential information regarding the degree of dyssynergia and bladder-wall compliance and the risk for upper tract damage.[74]

In addition to initial assessment, it is critical to follow these children closely throughout infancy and childhood. It has been demonstrated that neurologic lesions can change throughout childhood, especially during early infancy and at puberty, when linear growth rates are the greatest. Children with completely intact nerve pathways or only partial denervation are especially vulnerable to progressive denervation and must be monitored carefully with periodic urodynamic and lower extremity evaluations to detect early signs of deterioration.

Children with low compliance and children with bladder-sphincter dyssynergia producing outflow obstruction are at great risk for upper tract damage and must be placed on intermittent catheterization and drug therapy early in life to lower the detrusor filling pressure and to prevent upper tract deterioration. Alternatively, infants may undergo temporary diversion at the level of the bladder (that is, vesicostomy).

Management

In managing the child with neurogenic bladder, the clinician must adhere to the following principles: preservation of renal function takes priority;

vesicourethral dysfunction is treated based on the nature of the objectively demonstrated abnormalities; both these principles must be realistically applied with consideration for the child's overall neurologic condition; and infection must be controlled. Because of advances in recent years (clean intermittent self-catheterization [CISC], medications, artificial sphincter, and augmentation cystoplasty), these principles and goals are achievable for most children.

A few children with incomplete spinal cord lesions can be managed by medication and voiding alone. For example, children who are continent but who experience urinary urgency may respond well to an anticholinergic agent, and children who have areflexic bladders and incomplete emptying with abdominal straining may benefit from an alpha-adrenergic antagonist to reduce urethral resistance.

CISC is currently the mainstay of treatment for children with neurogenic bladder because it bypasses the possibly dyssynergic sphincter, provides for complete bladder emptying, and supports continence so long as the functional bladder capacity is adequate. However, CISC is capable of protecting the kidneys only if the filling pressures within the bladder remain within acceptable levels.

For CISC to be considered effective, the program must be able to provide approximately 3 hours of continence between catheterizations with minimal reliance on pads to absorb leakage, and the child must be able to perform the procedure independently. Therefore, CISC may not be appropriate for children who lack the motivation or the manipulative skills necessary to perform the procedure accurately and consistently. CISC may also be ineffective or inappropriate in children who lack the necessary bladder capacity (either because of a small bladder or because of severe detrusor hyperreflexia unresponsive to medications) and children who have severe sphincter weakness resulting in continual leakage (Table 16-6).

If urinary storage is compromised by detrusor hyperreflexia, an antispasmodic medication is usually added to the treatment regimen. Oxybutynin is the most consistently effective agent, but propantheline or terodiline may be used if the child experiences adverse effects with the oxybutynin, and occasionally a combination of two agents is required. If medication fails to relieve the hyperreflexic contractions sufficiently

or if bladder compliance is low, an augmentation cystoplasty is indicated.

Clam ileocystoplasty is a common form of bladder augmentation, which is one of the major developments in the management of neuropathic bladder conditions. The bladder is almost completely bisected, and a section of ileum is then interposed as a "patch" to close the bladder while separating the two contractile halves of the bladder. This procedure increases bladder capacity by physically increasing the size of the reservoir and by eliminating detrusor muscle contractions.[74]

As noted, children with neuropathic bladder dysfunction are also at risk for stress incontinence because of partial or total denervation of the sphincter muscle. Children with minor degrees of genuine stress incontinence can usually be managed effectively with alpha-adrenergic agonists in conjunction with intermittent catheterization. Pseudoephedrine is the most frequently used agent, but imipramine and phenylpropanolamine can be used as alternatives. (The patient whose management is complicated by both detrusor hyperreflexia and stress incontinence can be given both pseudoephedrine and oxybutynin.) Children with severe stress incontinence in whom conservative therapy (CISC and pharmacologic therapy) fails usually require surgical intervention. Surgical procedures that have been used to treat stress incontinence include tubularization of the urethra and bladder neck, lengthening of the bladder neck, construction of urethral slings, and injection of bulking agents at the bladder neck. Unfortunately, these procedures have not demonstrated wide success among children; for example, the use of bulking agents is no longer routinely used because this procedure provides minimal long-term effects.[75]

Currently, the artificial urinary sphincter is considered the procedure of choice for boys. The "sphincter" is actually a soft urethral cuff that maintains urethral closure until the patient deflates the cuff via a pump device implanted in the scrotum; when the patient activates the pump, the fluid in the cuff is temporarily shunted to a reservoir in the lower abdomen. The child is taught to empty the bladder either by cuff deflation and CISC or by cuff deflation and abdominal compression.

TABLE 16-6   **Instruction in Clean Intermittent Self-Catheterization**

Assess readiness to learn	Is the child motivated and interested in learning CISC and becoming independent in care?
	Will the child be able to understand steps involved in performing CISC?
	Is the child able to perform simple sequencing or to follow three- to four-step commands?
	Is the child able to articulate questions or concerns that may arise?
	Does the child have sufficient trunk stability to sit on toilet or chair with hands free for CISC?
	Does the child have adequate fine motor coordination (can the child use a crayon/pencil for coloring or is the child able to string beads?)
	Is the child responsible enough to report problems such as difficulty with catheter insertion, bleeding, or signs of urinary tract infection?
Obtain supplies	Catheter (latex-free, plastic, polyvinyl, polyvinyl-hydrophilic, or closed system)
	Water-soluble lubricant
	Wipes or towel with soap and water
	Storage receptacle for catheter
	Mirror (if the child is able to use it with minimal confusion)
Instruct child in CISC	Explain the procedure, utilizing a diagram of the renal system.
	Position the child on the toilet (assess the child's ability to sit on the toilet).
	Wash hands.
	Identify the urethral opening:
	Girls: use a mirror or assist the child to learn to locate the urethra by touch.
	Boys: instruct the child to hold the penis straight up when inserting the catheter.
	Cleanse the perineum or glans.
	Lubricate the tip of the catheter.
	Insert the catheter gently; explain that resistance may be felt as the catheter passes through the sphincter and teach the child to use steady gentle pressure to advance the catheter until urine starts to flow; teach the child to advance the catheter another 1/2 to 1 inch to be sure the catheter is all the way in the bladder.
	Drain urine
	Gradually pull the catheter *out* to ensure complete emptying of the bladder (make sure the child understands to pull the catheter *out* to ensure emptying, rather than pushing the catheter *in*).
	Wash hands and the catheter after catheterization is completed.
Instruct child in catheter care	Wash the catheter with antiseptic soap and water (children with a significant history of recurrent UTIs may need to utilize a new catheter for each catheterization [this is a small group of patients]).
	With a smaller catheter, use a syringe to flush the catheter.
	Air dry the catheter and store in a container or plastic bag once dry.
Review complications	Bleeding may occur with trauma or UTIs; children with neuropathy should be reminded to insert the catheter with firm but *gentle* pressure and to avoid forcible insertion.
	Signs and symptoms of UTI include new or increased leakage between catheterizations, cloudy or foul-smelling urine, not feeling well.
	If the catheter is difficult to pass, helpful strategies include relaxation, reassessment, and repositioning of the catheter.

Continued

TABLE 16-6   Instruction in Clean Intermittent Self-Catheterization—cont'd

Review complications—cont'd	Leakage between catheterizations may indicate bladder spasticity and should be reported to the physician; medications may be required.
Teach the patient and parent "helpful hints"	If fluid intake increases, it may be necessary to increase the frequency of catheterization; however, this should be discussed with the physician.
	It may be helpful to reduce fluids before bedtime to reduce urine production during the night; in addition, it is important to catheterize just before going to bed.
	It is important always to take a "travel kit" when leaving home; the kit should include all supplies needed for catheterization away from home. The travel kit can be stored in the child's backpack, purse, or pocket.
	When traveling by air, the travel kit should be hand carried onto the plane.
	Perineal wipes are an acceptable substitute for soap and water when soap and water are not available.

CISC, clean intermittent self-catheterization; UTI, urinary tract infection.

(Abdominal compression is effective only if the urethral outlet is unobstructed; sphincterotomy may be performed if there is any element of outlet obstruction and the child prefers assisted voiding to CISC.) Complications associated with the artificial sphincter include erosion, infection, and mechanical malfunction.[76] If the male patient with major stress incontinence also exhibits low bladder wall compliance or detrusor hyperreflexia unresponsive to pharmacotherapy, augmentation cystoplasty is done in addition to placement of the artificial sphincter.

Girls with major stress incontinence are typically managed with bladder neck suspension, which is an effective (and less expensive) alternative to placement of an artificial urinary sphincter. The suspension increases urethral resistance and provides for improved storage, and CISC is used to empty the bladder effectively at regular intervals. Again, low bladder wall compliance or detrusor hyperreflexia unresponsive to pharmacotherapy is treated with augmentation cystoplasty in addition to bladder neck suspension.[74]

Another option for children with incontinence unresponsive to CISC and pharmacologic management is bladder augmentation combined with creation of a continent cutaneous stoma. Various techniques have been developed to create a continent catheterizable channel between the augmented bladder and the abdominal wall; for example, Mitrofanoff's appendicovesicostomy involves use of the appendix as the catheterizable channel into the augmented bladder. Continence can be further supported by surgically tightening or closing the bladder neck; however, it is first necessary to ensure that the patient is compliant with the CISC program. Common complications associated with bladder augmentation and a catheterizable conduit include stomal stenosis and bladder calculi.[77] For children whose bladder cannot be successfully augmented, a continent urinary diversion can be constructed using loops of bowel; examples of these procedures include the Benchekroun and Indiana reservoirs.

Although appliance-free continence is always the ideal outcome, such a goal may not be feasible for children with very compromised mobility or significant cognitive delay. In this situation, the goal becomes protection of the upper tracts and a manageable system for the caregiver. This may necessitate use of an indwelling catheter for girls or an external catheter for boys (with sphincterotomy, if necessary). Alternative management options would include a continent urinary diversion, which is managed by abdominal catheterization, or a standard urinary diversion, which is managed with an external pouching system. Again, the goal is to protect the upper tracts while establishing a management system that is appropriate for the individual child and caregiver.

PSYCHOSOCIAL ISSUES

This discussion of urinary and fecal incontinence in children has included a focus on the key developmental issues relevant to each particular condition. Normal psychosocial development is dependent on positive interactions between the growing child, the environment, and significant others. A child's perspective about his or her body is dependent on both the child's age and his or her life experiences. Incontinence may have different effects at different stages of a child's growth and development. A family's culture, social status, and economic status also influence the development of a child with chronic bowel and bladder problems.

Each stage of family development is characterized by a set of tasks, and each family develops their own unique coping style. Societal, cultural and geographic factors all influence family development and help to form the context for the family's beliefs, myths, taboos, role models, and patterns of adaptation. Families who have a child with an incontinence problem may experience emotional responses that parallel the emotions experienced by families of children with serious health problems; that is, the "grief response." Each family member must adapt, and the various family members are typically at different "stages" of adaptation at any given time. In addition, any crisis can result in an adaptation "setback," in which the various family members must deal with depression, anger, and similar emotions "all over again."

Functional families enhance their child's development; unfortunately, the opposite is true of families coping with chronic stressors in a dysfunctional manner.[78] There are noticeable differences in children and families who are able to cope with the problem successfully and to access the formal and informal resources in their communities. When families perceive their child's incontinence issue as totally negative and restricting, the child's functional status, school performance, and psychosocial competence are more likely to be impacted.

Although specific treatments, outcomes, and clinical services differ for children with fecal incontinence and those with urinary incontinence, these children and families share many common tasks and challenges: changes in daily routines such as management of frequent medical appointments, issues and challenges related to usual developmental transitions (starting school, development of autonomy in preadolescence, and initiation of sexual relationships), and adjustments related to the economic and psychosocial impact of the incontinence. Incontinence can profoundly affect the child's behavior, development, and interpersonal relationships; as noted, the specific impact varies and is affected by the child's developmental stage and the family's response. It is important to realize the potential impact of incontinence on the child's psychologic and social development and to address these issues in the overall management plan.

The primary care provider must obtain a history that identifies all of the issues related to the incontinence, including the parent's and child's perceptions and concerns regarding the problem and the treatment plan. This approach to assessment provides insight into the interactions between the child and parent. History taking that is comprehensive and sensitive to the parents' perceptions promotes the therapeutic process by conveying understanding and empathy to both the parents and the child.

There has been increasing effort by primary care providers to educate children about their condition; however, very few curricular materials take into account the various developmental stages of the children who need these materials. For example, most pamphlets are geared toward children in the 9- to 11-year-old range.[79] The clinician needs to select teaching materials and modify instructional approaches based on the child's developmental stage. As children progress from childhood to young adulthood, primary care providers should encourage them to take increasing responsibility for self-management as part of the usual process of developing independence and autonomy.

Children with incontinence issues may require a wide range of services from many different providers, including their primary care provider, behavioral health clinicians, public health nurses, and sometimes alternative sources of care. Their care may be spread over different sites, some of which may be located at a considerable distance from their home. Families may benefit from case management assistance. Nurses are ideal professionals for this care coordination because of their background in health, family, and child development issues.

School is the equivalent of the workplace for children. Primary care providers need to assist families with a school-aged child to ensure that the child is placed in a school that can meet his or her needs. Some children with incontinence issues require special education services because of the effects of the incontinence on their mental health or because of other comorbidities. However, most children with incontinence issues can participate in regular education with minor modifications. Plans need to be established for medication administration, management of incontinent episodes, and any other special care needs. Primary care providers are responsible for educating school personnel to minimize problems for the child and for the educators. Comprehensive prospective care of children with incontinence can eliminate or significantly reduce negative outcomes and assist the child with incontinence issues to reach his or her developmental potential.

Many children with chronic bowel and bladder problems face significant additional challenges as they are growing up. Some of these children are developmentally and/or physically challenged, and integrating them into public schools while meeting their complex needs is not always easy. Fortunately, in 1975, the United States Congress passed Public Law 94-142, the Education for All Handicapped Children Act, which established an educational bill of rights for children 5 to 18 years of age. This law ensures children access to a "free and appropriate public education," including "special education and related services provided at public expense, under public direction and supervision, without charge, which meet the standards of the state educational agency, and are provided in uniformity with the Individualized Educational Program (IEP)." This historic law was amended in 1986 by Public Law 99-457, which included the Handicapped Infants and Toddlers Program and extended services to children from birth to 21 years of age (in addition to other requirements). One requirement was for health care professionals to be involved in the development of an "Individualized Family Service Plan (IFSP)" for children from birth through 2 years, which is analogous to the IEP for older children.

In May 1997, Public Law 101-476, Individuals with Disabilities Education Act (IDEA), led to further expansion of services, to include mobility services, transition services, and services to support education of disabled children along with nondisabled children to the greatest extent possible (including one-on-one fulltime care by a registered nurse for children with complex medical needs).[43]

How do these laws affect care for these children? If a child needs to be catheterized during school hours or needs assistance with a bowel program, these aspects of their care are incorporated into the IFSP or IEP, and the services are provided in the school setting. If one goal of care is increased independence in activities of daily living, the IEP may incorporate interventions such as instruction in self-catheterization or self-toileting during school hours. It is not uncommon for teachers and school administrators to request education regarding the child's medical condition; nurses may need to provide this education in addition to developing a plan of care for bowel and bladder care.

The emotional and social needs of a child with bowel or bladder problems change as the child matures. Wearing diapers is not unusual for toddlers or preschoolers; however, as children make the transition into elementary school, a bowel and bladder program should be actively pursued to optimize their continence status. Teasing by peers can create many psychosocial problems. Gaining continence and being as normal as possible are goals for many of these children. Each child deserves a plan of care that will promote independence and provide continuity between home and school settings. In many instances, these children need additional support from therapists and counselors to help them deal with their emotions and social interactions, especially in the preteen and teenage years, when sexuality and body image are so important. Counseling services can be incorporated into the IFSP or IEP to ensure that the child's emotional needs are addressed as well as any behavioral issues that may arise. Support groups for these children are also helpful. The United Ostomy Association has teen, young adult, and parent groups that offer networking opportunities. In addition, annual rallies held in different locations across the nation help to bring these individuals together to share their experiences and to realize they are not alone. Participation in these programs also requires the adolescent to travel alone and to learn self-care. It is a time to test not only the teenager's (or young adult's) ability to care for himself or herself but also the willingness of parents to "let go" and encourage their son or daughter to seek independence.

To help overcome the stigma of incontinence, providers should encourage children and families with Internet access to use this avenue for seeking information and networking with others. Many individuals have benefited greatly from the information provided on various Websites.

SUMMARY

Urinary incontinence is a common condition among children and one that is potentially devastating, both in terms of renal function and in terms of psychosocial development. The evaluation of any child with voiding dysfunction or incontinence must therefore include screening for upper tract damage as well as careful assessment of the effect on life-style and self-esteem. For the child with simple PNE, treatment may be as simple as education and support for the patient and family or as aggressive as alarm therapy and pharmacotherapy. The level of intervention is determined by the child's age, the degree of effect on the patient and family, and response to prior treatment. For the child with dysfunctional voiding, the primary goal of intervention is to protect the upper urinary tracts; the secondary goal is restablishment or preservation of continence. These goals may be met through single or combination therapy; that is, behavior modification and biofeedback, pharmacotherapy, CISC, surgical intervention, or indwelling catheterization. The continence nurse plays a critical role in assuring comprehensive and holistic care for the child and family dealing with voiding dysfunction or incontinence.

SELF-ASSESSMENT EXERCISE

1. Explain why most experts recommend delaying toilet training until the child is at least 2 years of age, capable of communicating with parents, and interested in pleasing parents and caregivers.

2. Explain the differences between encopresis and fecal incontinence and implications for assessment and management.

3. Explain the sequence of events that typically results in retentive encopresis and the implications for management.

4. Identify at least one test that could be used to distinguish between a motility disorder and functional constipation.

5. Identify one cleansing protocol that relies at least partially on enemas and one that is dependent on laxatives and explain the importance of checking for impaction before selecting a cleansing regimen.

6. Explain how each of the following disorders contributes to fecal incontinence:
   (a) imperforate anus, (b) Hirschsprung's disease, and (c) myelomeningocele.

7. Identify key strategies for management of neurogenic bowel.

8. Define the term "dysfunctional voiding" and explain how it contributes to incomplete bladder emptying.

9. Outline management options for the child with dysfunctional voiding and incomplete bladder emptying.

10. List the current theories regarding the causes of PNE, indications for treatment, and treatment options.

11. List the primary goals of treatment for a child with neurogenic bladder and give the treatment options.

REFERENCES

1. Mazier W, Levien D, Luchtefeld M, Senagore A: *Surgery of the colon, rectum, and anus,* Philadelphia, 1995, WB Saunders, pp 6-8, 1128-1137.
2. Walker WA, Durie PR, Hamilton JR, et al: *Pediatric gastrointestinal disease,* vol 1, Philadelphia, 1990, BC Decker (St. Louis, Mosby), pp 90-108, 477-484.
3. O'Rorke C: Helping children overcome fecal incontinence, *Am J Nurs* 95:16A-B, 1995.
4. Christophersen E: Toileting problems in children, *Pediatr Ann* 5(20):240-244, 1991.

LIBRARY, UNIVERSITY OF CHESTER

5. Howe AC, Walker CE: Behavioral management of toilet training, enuresis, and encopresis, *Pediatr Clin North Am* 39:413-432, 1992.

6. Schmitt BD, Mauro R: 20 common errors in treating encopresis, *Contemp Pediatr,* 9(May):47-65, 1992.

7. Seth R, Heyman M: Management of constipation and encopresis in infants and children, *Gastroenterol Clin North Am* 23(4):621-636, 1994.

8. Boon RF, Singh N: A model for the treatment of encopresis, *Behav Modif* 15(3):355-371, 1991.

9. Schonwald A, Rappaport L: Encopresis: assessment and management, *Pediatr Rev* 25(8):278-283, 2004.

10. Levine MD: Children with encopresis: a descriptive analysis, *Pediatrics* 56:412, 1975.

11. Loening-Baucke V: Biofeedback treatment for chronic constipation and encopresis in childhood: long-term outcomes, *Pediatrics* 96:105, 1995.

12. DiLorenzo C, Benninga MA: Pathophysiology of pediatric fecal incontinence, *Gastroenterology* 126:S33-S40, 2004.

13. Levine M: Encopresis: its potential, evaluation, and alleviation, *Pediatr Clin North Am* 29(2):315-329, 1982.

14. Nolan T, Oberklaid F: New concepts in the management of encopresis, *Pediatr Rev* 14(11):447-451, 1993.

15. Stadtler A: Preventing encopresis, *Pediatr Nurs* 15(3): 282-284, 1989.

16. Stern P, Lowitz G, Prince M, et al: The incidence of cognitive dysfunction in an encopretic population in children, *Neurotoxicology* 9(3):351-358, 1988.

17. American Psychiatric Association: *Diagnostic and statistical manual of mental disorders,* ed 4 (DSM-IV), Arlinigton, VA 1997, American Psychiatric Association.

18. Rockney R: Encopresis. In: Levine MD, Carey W, Crocker AC, editors: *Developmental-behavioral pediatrics,* ed 3, Philadelphia, 1999, WB Saunders, pp 413-421.

19. Sprague-McRae JM: Encopresis: developmental, behavioral, and physiological considerations for treatment, *Nurse Pract* 15(6):8-24, 1990.

20. Ingebo K, Heyman M: Polyethylene glycol-electrolyte solution for intestinal clearance in children with refractory encopresis, *Am J Dis Child* 142:340-342, 1988.

21. Gunn V, Nechyba C: Constipation and encopresis. In: *The Harriet Lane handbook,* St. Louis, 2002, Elsevier, pp 63-265.

22. Smith E: The bath water needs changing, but don't throw out the baby: an overview of anorectal anomalies, *J Pediatr Surg* 22(4):335-348, 1987.

23. Rowe M, O'Neill J, Grosfeld J, et al: *Essentials of pediatric surgery,* St. Louis, 1995, Mosby, pp 586-593.

24. Roy C, Silverman A, Alagille D: *Pediatric clinical gastroenterology,* St. Louis, 1995, Mosby, pp 503-521.

25. Molnar G: *Pediatric rehabilitation,* Baltimore, 1985, Williams & Wilkins, pp 176-206.

26. Smith K: Myelomeningocele: managing bowel and bladder dysfunction in the school-aged child, *Progressions* 3(2):3-11, 1991.

27. MacLeod J: Fecal incontinence: a practical program of management, *Endosc Rev 5* (Nov-Dec):45-56, 1988.

28. Ludman L, Spitz L: Coping strategies of children with faecal incontinence, *J Pediatr Surg* 31(4):563-567, 1996.

29. Heymen S, Jones KR, Ringel Y, et al: Biofeedback treatment of fecal incontinence, *Dis Colon Rectum* 44(May):728-736, 2001.

30. Walker WA, Durie PR, Hamilton JR, et al: *Pediatric gastrointestinal disease,* vol 2, ed 2, St. Louis, 1996, Mosby, pp 2077-2091.

31. Poenaru D, Roblin N, Bird M, et al: The pediatric bowel management clinic: initial results of a multidisciplinary approach to functional constipation in children, *J Pediatr Surg* 32(6):843-848, 1997.

32. Blair GK, Djonlic K, Fraser GC, et al: The bowel management tube: an effective means for controlling fecal incontinence, *J Pediatr Surg* 27(10):1260-1272, 1992.

33. Malone P, Ransley P, Kiely E: Preliminary report: the antegrade continence enema, *Lancet* 336:1217-1218, 1990.

34. Churchill BM, Abramson RP, Wahl EF: Dysfunction of the lower urinary and distal gastrointestinal tracts in pediatric patients with known spinal cord problems, *Pediatr Clin North Am* 48(6):2-51, 2001.

35. Lee SL, DuBois JJ, Montes-Garces RG, et al: Surgical management of chronic unremitting constipation and fecal incontinence associated with megarectum: a preliminary report, *J Pediatr Surg* 37(1):76-79, 2002.

36. Duel BP, González R: The button cecostomy for management of fecal incontinence, *Pediatr Surg Int* 15:559-561, 1999.

37. Lynch AC, Beasley SW, Robertson RW, Morreau PN: Comparison of results of laparoscopic and open antegrade continence enema procedures, *Pediatr Surg Int* 15:343-346, 1999.

38. Yerkes EB, Rink RC, King S, et al: Tap water and the Malone antegrade continence enema: a safe combination? *J Urol* 166:1476-1478, 2001.

39. Kokoska ER, Keller MS, Weber T: Outcome of the antegrade colonic enema procedure in children with chronic constipation, *Am J Surg* 182:625-629, 2001.

40. Graf JL, Strear C, Bratton B, Housley HT, Jennings RW, Harrison MR, Albanese CT: The Antegrade Continence Enema Procedure: A Review of the Literature. *Journal of Pediatric Surgery* 33:1294-1296, 1998.

41. Erickson, BA, Austin C, Cooper CS, Boyt MA: Polyethylene glycol 3350 for constipation in children with dysfunctional elimination, *J Urol* 170:1518-1520, 2003.

42. Foster E: Surgical options for managing chronic fecal incontinence in children, *Progressions* 7(1):13-21, 1995.

43. Jackson PL, Vessey JA: *Primary care of the child with a chronic condition,* St. Louis, 2000, Mosby, pp 295-668.

44. Malloy T: *Montessori and your child,* New York, 1974, Schocken Books.

45. Hoebeke PB, Van Laecke E, Raes A, et al: Bladder function and non-neurogenic dysfunction in children: classification and terminology, *J Acta Urol Belg* 63(2):93-98, 1995.

46. Goellner MH, Ziegler EE, Fomon SJ: Urination during the first three years of life, *Nephron* 28(4):174-178, 1981.

47. Cendron M, Gormley A: Pediatric urodynamics: how, when, and for whom? *Contemp Urol* 9 (April):21-36, 1997.

48. Landa H: Pediatric incontinence, *Pediatr Urol Newslett* 1, 1996.

49. Himsl K, Hurwitz R: Pediatric urinary incontinence, *Urol Clin North Am* 18(2):283-293, 1991.

50. Hjalmas K: Pathophysiology and impact of nocturnal enuresis, *Acta Paediatr* 86:919-922, 1997.

51. Stark M: Assessment and management of children with nocturnal enuresis: guidelines for primary care, *Nurse Pract Forum* 5(3):170-176, 1994.

52. Eiberg H, Berendt I, Mohr J: Assignment of dominant inherited nocturnal enuresis to chromosome 13q, *Nat Genet* 10:354-356, 1995.

53. Wardy B, Uri A, Hellerstein S: Primary nocturnal enuresis: current concepts about an old problem, *Pediatr Ann* 20(5):246-255, 1991.

54. Norgaard J, Djuhuus J: The pathophysiology of enuresis in children and young adults, *Clin Pediatr* 32(special ed):5-9, 1993.

55. Chiozza ML: An update on clinical and therapeutic aspects of nocturnal enuresis, *Pediatr Med Chir* 19(5):385-390, 1997.

56. Garber K: Enuresis: an update on diagnosis and management, *J Pediatr Health Care* 10(5):202-208, 1996.

57. Haque M, Ellerstein NS, Gundy JH, et al: Parental perception of enuresis: a collaborative study, *Am J Dis Child* 135:809-811, 1981.

58. O'Regan S, Schick E, Hamburger B, et al: Constipation associated with vesicoureteral reflux, *Urology* 28:394-396, 1986.

59. Calamone AA: *Diagnosis and treatment of PNE*, monograph from proceedings of a closed symposium, Aventura, Fla., January 12, 1991, pp 14-17.

60. Miller K: Concomitant nonpharmacologic therapy in the treatment of primary nocturnal enuresis, *Clin Pediatr* 32(special ed):27-32, 1993.

61. Olness K: The use of self-hypnosis in the treatment of childhood nocturnal enuresis: a report of forty patients, *Clin Pediatr* 14:273-279, 1975.

62. Mahony DT, Laferte RO, Blair DJ: Studies of enuresis. IX. Evidence of mild form of compensated detrusor hyperreflexia in enuretic children, *J Urol* 126:520, 1981.

63. Starfield B: Enuresis: its pathogenesis and management, *Clin Pediatr* 11:343-350, 1972.

64. Schmitt BD: Nocturnal enuresis, *Pediatr Rev* 18(6):183-191, 1997.

65. Rappaport L: Prognostic factors for alarm treatment, *Scand J Urol Nephrol* 31(183):55-58, 1997.

66. Fritz GK, Rockney RM, Yeung AS: Plasma levels and efficacy of imipramine treatment for enuresis, *J Am Acad Child Adolesc Psychiatry* 33:60-64, 1994.

67. Mariani A: *Pediatric urology update 1998*, lecture presentation at Kaiser Permanente Hospital, Moanalua Valley, Oahu, Hawaii, July 15, 1998.

68. Rappaport L: Enuresis. In: Parker S, Zuckerman B, editors: *Behavioral and developmental pediatrics*, Boston, 1995, Little, Brown.

69. Moffatt MEK, Harlos S, Kirshen AJ, et al: Desmopressin acetate and nocturnal enuresis: how much do we know? *Pediatrics* 92:420-425, 1993.

70. Gool JD, van Vijverberg MAW, Jong TPVM: Functional daytime incontinence: clinical and urodynamic assessment, *Scand J Urol Nephrol Suppl* 141:58-69, 1992.

71. Hinman F Jr: Non-neurogenic bladder (Hinman syndrome). In: O'Donnell B, Koff SA, editors: *Pediatric urology*, ed 3, Stoneham, Mass., 1997, Butterworth-Heinemann, pp 245-248.

72. Bauer S: Pediatric urodynamics: lower tract. In: O'Donnell B, Koff SA, editors: *Pediatric urology*, ed 3, Stoneham, Mass., 1997, Butterworth-Heinemann, pp 125-138.

73. Robson W: Diurnal enuresis, *Pediatr Rev* 18(12):407-412, 1997.

74. Rickwood A: Management and outcomes in children with neuropathic bladder. In: O'Donnell B, Koff SA, editors: *Pediatric urology*, ed 3, Stoneham, Mass., 1997, Butterworth-Heinemann, pp 243-44.

75. Block CA, Cooper CS, Hawthrey CE: Long-term efficacy of periurethral collagen injection for the treatment of urinary incontinence secondary to myelomeningocele, *J Urol* 169:327-329, 2003.

76. Herndon CDA, Rink RC, Shaw MB, et al: The Indiana experience with artificial urinary sphincters in children and young adults, *J Urol* 169:650-654, 2003.

77. Surer I, Ferrer FA, Baker LA, Cearhart JP: Continent urinary diversion and the exstrophy-epispadias complex, *J Urol* 169:1102-1105, 2003.

78. Vessey JA, Rumsey M: Chronic conditions and child development. In: Allen PJ, Vessey JA, editors: *Primary care of the child with a chronic condition*, ed 4, St. Louis, 2004, Mosby, pp 23-43.

79. Perrin JM, Thyen U: Chronic illness. In: Allen PJ, Vessey JA, editors: *Primary care of the child with a chronic condition*, ed 4, St. Louis, 2004, Mosby, pp 335-345.

GLOSSARY

Abdominal Flat Plate Standard plain radiograph (roentgenogram, x-ray film) of abdomen commonly used to detect retained stool that is not palpable on abdominal examination.

Abdominal Leak Point Pressure Abdominal pressure at which urinary leakage is observed during straining, that is, the magnitude of abdominal force required to drive urine across the sphincter during bladder filling. In the normal individual, even maximum abdominal straining does not produce leakage.

Abdominal Straining Use of Valsalva's maneuver to increase intravesical pressure and to improve bladder emptying.

ACE Procedure Antegrade colonic enema: surgical creation of continent catheterizable channel between abdominal wall and cecum. This "one-way" stoma is used to perform regular colonic washouts to maintain continence.

Acontractile Detrusor Detrusor that cannot be demonstrated to contract during urodynamic studies.

Acute Incontinence Incontinence of recent and abrupt onset; may reflect new *onset* of urinary leakage or sudden *worsening* of preexisting minor incontinence.

Acute Urinary Retention Painful, palpable, or percussible bladder, when the patient is unable to pass any urine.

Adrenergic Mediating or mimicking the effects of sympathetic stimulation; stimulation of alpha-adrenergic receptors in the proximal portion of the urethra causes contraction of the smooth muscle and promotes urinary storage. Alpha-*adrenergic antagonists* are a class of drugs that relax the smooth muscle in the bladder neck and urethra; these drugs may *cause* or *contribute* to incontinence but can also be used to improve bladder emptying in patients with benign prostatic hypertrophy. Alpha-*adrenergic agonists* increase urethral resistance by increasing tone in the smooth muscle of the proximal portion of the urethra and bladder neck.

Anal Canal Passageway between rectum and outside of body; surrounded by internal and external anal sphincters and lined with multiple sensory receptors.

Anal Electromyography (EMG) Test used to assess the innervation of the external anal sphincter; may be done by glove electrodes (PNTML studies) or by needle electrodes placed into the external anal sphincter at several points and used to record the muscle response during voluntary anal sphincter contraction.

Anal Incontinence Involuntary passage of gas, liquid, or solid stool.

Anal Sphincter Repair Surgical correction of acute sphincter disruption secondary to trauma.

Anal Wink Test commonly used to evaluate the function of the sacral nerve roots. The perianal skin is lightly stroked while the examiner observes for anal contraction (a positive anal "wink").

Anatomic Bladder Capacity Volume of fluid that the bladder is capable of holding at the limit of its viscoelastic or accommodative properties; assessed while patient is anesthetized or sedated during cystoscopic examination.

Anorectal Angle Angle at junction of rectum and anal canal created by orientation and slinglike configuration of puborectalis muscle; believed to contribute to continence. Under resting conditions, angle is 90 degrees; during straining and defecation, angle straightens to 135 degrees.

Anorectal Manometry Study done to provide an objective measurement of anorectal sensation, pressures generated by the sphincter complex, and length of the anal canal; helps to quantify and localize any sphincter defects and to evaluate presence or absence of the rectoanal inhibitory reflex. Conducted by insertion of a small-diameter catheter with a balloon tip and pressure transducers through the anal canal into the rectum; intrarectal and intraanal pressures are measured at rest, during "squeeze," during Valsalva's maneuver, and in response to rectal filling.

Anorectal Physiology Testing General term for studies that provide a quantitative assessment of complex mechanisms involved in maintenance of continence; includes anorectal manometry, anal electromyography, defecography, and endoanal ultrasonography.

Anticholinergic Drugs that block the effects of cholinergic neurotransmitters; may cause urinary retention and constipation (adverse effects) but can be used therapeutically for patients with detrusor instability and urge incontinence and for patients with diarrhea related to increased motility.

Antidiarrheal Medications Agents such as anticholinergics and opiate derivatives that reduce intestinal motility.

Artifact Urodynamic data produced by inaccurate technique or physiologic events rather than pathologic condition. Examiner must be able to distinguish artifacts to interpret urodynamic data accurately.

Artificial Anal Sphincter Device composed of three components that are surgically implanted and used to restore continence for the patient with intractable fecal incontinence. The three components are a pressure-regulating balloon, an anorectal cuff, and a pump. (Device is currently considered experimental.)

Artificial Urinary Sphincter Three-component system that is surgically implanted and used to restore continence for the patient with intrinsic sphincter deficiency: soft inflatable cuff placed around the urethra or bladder neck, pressure-regulating balloon and reservoir placed in the abdominal cavity, and pump placed in the scrotum or labia. When cuff is inflated, it mechanically compresses the urethra to prevent leakage. Pump is used to deflate the cuff (by displacing the fluid into the reservoir) to permit voiding or catheterization.

Ascending Fibers Neuronal fibers unique to the distal portion of the colon that are probably involved in the coordination of reflex (colocolonic and colorectal) activity.

Atrophic Urethritis and Vaginitis Condition resulting from estrogen deficiency and characterized by thinning of the urethral and vaginal epithelium, sclerosis of the periurethral tissues, and persistent or recurrent subjective complaints of urinary frequency, urgency, and dysuria.

Augmentation Cystoplasty Surgical procedure designed to provide a low-pressure reservoir for the bladder. The dome of the bladder is split, the bladder is opened in a clam type of configuration, and a segment of isolated and detubularized bowel is anastomosed to the bladder.

Autoaugmentation of Bladder Surgical creation of a bladder wall diverticulum to increase bladder capacity and to interrupt detrusor contractility; designed to provide a low-pressure urinary reservoir.

Autonomic Dysreflexia Syndrome characterized by sweating, headache, and hypertension and caused by extreme stimulation of the autonomic nervous system; may occur in patients with spinal cord injuries above T6-T8 and precipitated most commonly by overdistension of the bladder, a hyperreflexic bladder contraction in the presence of detrusor-sphincter dyssynergia, or rectal distension.

Autonomic Neuropathy Damage to the autonomic nerves that innervate the bladder and gastrointestinal tract; associated with impaired detrusor contractility, intestinal hypomotility, and anorectal dysfunction.

Bacteriuria Presence of bacteria in the urine; may be further classified as *symptomatic* or *asymptomatic.*

Barium Enema Contrast study to identify anatomic abnormalities or luminal lesions; postevacuation film can be used to assess colonic motility indirectly.

Behavioral Therapy Any intervention in which the patient is taught to modify her or his usual behaviors to improve bladder and bowel control.

Benign Prostatic Hypertrophy Proliferation of cells within the prostate gland that produce glandular enlargement (benign prostatic enlargement); commonly associated with signs of "prostatism" (weak urinary stream with varying degrees of hesitancy, intermittency, urgency, frequency, nocturia, postvoid dribbling, or a feeling of incomplete emptying). Term "prostatism" is being replaced with "lower urinary tract symptoms" or "voiding symptoms."

Biofeedback Use of visual or auditory feedback to provide patient information regarding physiologic processes or functions, such as contraction or relaxation of the pelvic and abdominal muscles. May be subdivided into pressure (manometric) biofeedback and electromyographic (EMG) biofeedback. *Pressure biofeedback* is provided by pressure-sensitive probes or balloons placed into the patient's vagina or rectum; *EMG biofeedback* is most commonly provided by means of active surface electrodes applied to the perianal skin but may also be conducted by use of intraanal or intravaginal sensors (electrodes).

Bladder Organ for storage and elimination of urine; composed of the bladder *base,* which is fixed and nondistensible, and the bladder *body,* which distends easily to fill with urine.

Bladder Chart (Voiding Diary) Record kept by patient (or caregivers) that includes some or all of the following information: time and volume of normal voids, time and approximate amount of urinary leakage, type of activity associated with urine loss, number of pads or protective devices used in a 24-hour period, type and volume of fluid intake, time and amount of urine obtained by self-catheterization.

Bladder Management Program Strategies employed by individual (patient or caregiver) for the management of urinary elimination.

Bladder Outlet Obstruction Increased urethral resistance resulting in obstructed voiding; characterized by a poor or intermittent urinary stream and high detrusor pressures.

Bladder Retraining Behavioral strategy used for patients with urge incontinence. The patient is taught urge inhibition strategies and is then placed on a scheduled voiding program; the voiding interval is gradually lengthened to increase bladder capacity and establish a more normal voiding pattern.

Bowel Diary, or Bowel Chart Record kept by patient (or caregivers) that includes the frequency, volume, and consistency of both voluntary and involuntary stools and may also include data regarding food and fluid intake.

Bulbocavernosus Reflex Test used to evaluate the innervation of the striated muscles of the pelvic floor. The examiner gently squeezes the glans penis or the clitoris while observing for anal sphincter contraction. (Visible contraction is indicative of intact pathways.)

Bulk Laxatives Agents such as psyllium and carboxymethylcellulose that absorb fluid and thus help to normalize stool consistency; can be used to help correct either diarrhea or constipation.

BUN Serum study to determine blood urea nitrogen levels. Elevated levels are indicative of renal compromise.

Candida albicans Opportunistic yeast organism that readily invades damaged skin to produce a characteristic rash, that is, areas of confluent erythema with pinpoint satellite lesions visible at the periphery.

Cholinergic Mediating or mimicking the effects of parasympathetic stimulation (such as detrusor contraction). Cholinergic neural terminals release acetylcholine in response to parasympathetic stimulation.

Chronic Diarrhea Frequent elimination of mushy stool or episodic elimination of watery stool.

Chronic Intractable Incontinence Incontinence in individuals with cognitive or physical deficits that render them unable to participate in behavioral interventions and who are not candidates for surgical or pharmacologic correction of their incontinence.

Chronic Urinary Retention Nonpainful bladder, which remains palpable or percussible after the patient has passed urine.

Cleanser (Perineal) Liquid solutions or emulsions designed to remove effluent and bacteria; commonly contain water and a surfactant that helps to loosen soil from skin.

Clostridium Difficile Opportunistic pathogen that is a common cause of infectious diarrhea in patients who have received antibiotics; produces a mixed secretory-osmotic diarrhea.

Colon Large intestine, responsible for conversion of stool from liquid to solid and for storage and elimination of stool.

Colonic Motility Studies Study done to evaluate for colonic dysfunction in patient with refractory constipation; conducted by administration of oral contrast material, followed by serial radiographs to monitor progression through the colon.

Colostomy Fecal diversion (surgical creation of abdominal opening into colon to permit stool to exit onto the abdomen, where it is contained within a lightweight odorproof pouch); indicated for patient with intractable fecal incontinence.

Compliance (of Detrusor) Ability of the bladder wall to stretch to accommodate increasing volumes of urine without producing any significant increase in intravesical pressure; determined by dividing the change in bladder volume by the change in detrusor pressure. *Low bladder wall compliance* represents loss of the bladder wall's ability to stretch and store urine at low pressures.

Constipation Change in normal bowel habits characterized by a decrease in frequency of bowel movements, passage of hard, dry stools, or difficulty with stool elimination.

Continence Ability to control the elimination of stool and urine until a socially acceptable time and place for defecation and urination.

Continent Urinary Diversion Surgical procedure involving creation of a low-pressure reservoir using detubularized bowel or stomach and construction of a continent catheterizable channel between the reservoir and an abdominal stoma; may be used to arrest or prevent renal damage and to facilitate self-care in the patient with reflex urinary incontinence.

Creatinine (Serum) Serum analysis of creatinine levels; elevations indicative of renal damage.

Credé's Maneuver Use of manual pressure over the suprapubic area to increase intravesical pressure and improve bladder emptying.

Cystocele Herniation of the bladder into the vaginal vault; may be evident only during "bearing down" maneuvers.

Cystometric Bladder Capacity Volume of urine held by the bladder during urodynamic testing; generally recorded as either the volume at which the patient perceives a sense of bladder fullness or the volume when an overactive detrusor contraction causes premature voiding.

Cystometrogram Test conducted by insertion of a catheter with a pressure transducer into the bladder and the rectum to measure both bladder pressure and abdominal pressure. The bladder is then filled, and data are recorded regarding bladder capacity, sensory status, bladder pressures at baseline value and in response to filling, and presence or absence of involuntary bladder contractions (also known as "filling cystometrogram").

Defecating Proctography Test used to evaluate the function of the anorectal unit during defecation; conducted by filling the rectum with thick barium paste, positioning the patient on a radiolucent commode, and asking the patient to expel the paste during radiographic examination.

Defecation Forceful expulsion of stool from colon.

Delirium Acute confusional state that is reversible.

Dementia Irreversible alteration in mental status and cognition.

Detrusor Primary smooth muscle of bladder wall; plays an essential role in the storage and expulsion of urine.

Detrusor Hyperactivity with Impaired Contractility (DHIC) Condition sometimes seen in the elderly and characterized by bladder overactivity (unstable contractions occurring during the filling phase) in conjunction with impaired contractility and ineffective emptying.

Detrusor Hyperreflexia Term formerly used to refer to involuntary detrusor contractions associated with a neurologic disorder; new term is neurogenic detrusor overactivity.

Detrusor Instability (Overactivity) Involuntary detrusor contractions that cause urinary leakage (or reduced bladder capacity and urinary urgency) in patients who do not have neurologic disorders.

Detrusor Leak Point Pressure Detrusor pressure at which leakage occurs when the patient is at rest and is *not* straining; data can be obtained during cystometrogram or videourodynamic studies.

Detrusor Motor Area Collection of nuclei located in each frontal lobe that directly influence detrusor activity and are postulated to interact with other areas of the brain to provide the individual with "social continence" (that is, the ability to delay voiding until a socially appropriate time).

Detrusor Overactivity Umbrella term for involuntary detrusor contractions; most appropriately used when the specific cause for the involuntary contractions is unclear.

Detrusor Reflex Term used to refer to the complex series of events that result in detrusor contraction and bladder emptying; involves activation of proprioceptive stretch receptors in bladder wall in response to bladder filling, transmission of the sensory impulses to the brain, and neurally modulated sphincter relaxation and bladder contraction at a socially appropriate time and place.

Detrusor-sphincter Dyssynergia Loss of coordination between the striated sphincter and the detrusor muscle, that is, the sphincter does not consistently relax when the detrusor contracts (also known as "vesicosphincter dyssynergia"); produces functional obstruction of bladder outlet.

Detrusor Underactivity Detrusor contraction of insufficient strength and duration to empty the bladder effectively within a normal amount of time.

DIAPPERS Acronym for the most common reversible causes of incontinence: delirium, infection, atrophic urethritis and vaginitis, pharmaceuticals, psychologic conditions, excess urine production, restricted mobility, and stool impaction.

Diarrhea Increase in stool frequency, volume, or fluidity; in common use, an imprecise and subjective term. Objective definitions include "increase in stool weight to more than 200 or 250 g/day." May be classified as acute (lasting less than 4 weeks) or chronic (lasting more than 4 weeks) and as *secretory, osmotic, motility induced,* or *mixed.*

Digital Stimulation One option for stimulating defecation. Gloved lubricated finger is inserted into anal canal, and circular motions are used to stimulate relaxation of the internal anal sphincter and peristalsis in the left colon.

Disimpaction Removal of impacted fecal mass from rectum by digital breakup and removal with or without use of lubricating enemas.

Disordered Defecation Abnormal patterns of bowel elimination, such as diarrhea, constipation, or irritable bowel syndrome.

Double Voiding Double attempts to empty the bladder at each voiding; the patient is instructed to void, wait for a brief period of time, and then initiate a second detrusor contraction.

Dysfunctional Voiding Condition in which child lacks awareness of progressive bladder filling and impending need to void and therefore experiences uninhibited detrusor contractions with sudden urinary urgency. Typically, the child reacts by contracting the sphincter muscles or using perineal pressure in an attempt to prevent leakage. This behavior pattern places the child at risk for incomplete bladder emptying and urinary tract infection.

Dysfunctional Voiding Posture Position assumed by a child who is trying to inhibit a detrusor contraction; a boy may squeeze his penis, and a girl may press her fingers against the urethra or drop to a kneeling position with her heel against her perineum.

Ectopia Anatomic displacement, such as a ureteral orifice that empties into the vagina.

Electrical Stimulation Use of low-voltage electrical stimulation to improve the function of the urethral, levator, and detrusor muscles; based on findings that electrical stimulation causes contraction of the levator ani, periurethral striated muscles, and external anal sphincter and reflexly inhibits detrusor muscle contraction. (Used to treat both stress and urge incontinence.)

Elimination Diet Structured approach to elimination of foods and fluids that are poorly tolerated; involves elimination of common and known offenders (and additional restrictions if bowel dysfunction persists), with gradual reintroduction of foods one at a time once bowel function has normalized. Permits identification and restriction of poorly tolerated items.

Encirclement Procedures Surgical implantation of synthetic material or gracilis muscle to encircle and augment the anal sphincter. Gracilis muscle transfer is more commonly used. (Outcomes of gracilis muscle transfer may be enhanced by implantation of leads connected to a pulse generator that provides a continual stimulus to the muscle to contract. An external magnet is used to turn off the generator to permit defecation.) Gracilis wrap also known as *stimulated gracilis neosphincter procedure.*

Encopresis Fecal soiling in children usually associated with functional constipation; also used to refer to fecal incontinence in children that is not caused by an organic or anatomic lesion.

Endoanal Ultrasonography Alternative to needle electromyography for the assessment of pelvic floor function, specifically the sphincter complex; involves placement of sonographic probe in anal canal, which permits visualization of internal and external anal sphincters and identification of any disruption or thinning of sphincter complex. Particularly beneficial in evaluation of internal anal sphincter.

Enema Fluid administered intrarectally, usually intended to stimulate defecation.

Endopelvic Fascia Fibromuscular tissue (that is, connective tissue, smooth muscle, and vascular elements) that contributes to the support of the pelvic organs; condensations of the fascia are referred to as ligaments.

Enteric Nervous System Nerve plexuses located within the intestinal wall that play the primary role in mediation of peristaltic activity (also called the "intrinsic nervous system").

Enuresis Any involuntary loss of urine.

Enuresis Alarms One treatment option for children with nocturnal enuresis; goal is to condition child to associate bladder distension with awakening. Child wears urine sensor and portable alarm box that sounds an alarm when the sensor is activated; child is taught to get up, turn off alarm, and void.

Extrinsic Intestinal Innervation Type of innervation provided by autonomic nervous system. The sympathetic and parasympathetic fibers terminate on neurons of the intrinsic plexuses and serve to modulate colonic motility and secretion.

Estrogen Female hormone that normally accounts for 30% of female urethral resistance; estrogen deficiency is believed to be one etiologic factor for postmenopausal incontinence.

External Anal Sphincter Combination of smooth and striated muscle that encircles the internal anal sphincter and the distal portion of the anal canal;

provides both tonic (reflex) contraction and phasic (voluntary) contractions. Striated muscle is innervated by pudendal nerve; smooth muscle is innervated by enteric nervous system.

External (Condom) Catheters Condom-shaped devices that fit over the penis and connect to a drainage receptacle (leg bag or bedside bag); available in latex and nonlatex and in adhesive and nonadhesive forms.

Extraurethral Incontinence Leakage of urine from a source other than the urethra because of disruption of the anatomic integrity of the urinary system (such as a fistula or an ectopic ureter).

Established Incontinence Incontinence that cannot be easily reversed; usually caused by a pathologic condition within the urinary tract or neurologic system or by irreversible cognitive impairment.

Explosive Flow Pattern Exaggeration of the normal flow pattern, commonly seen in women (because of higher Qmax and Qave values and shorter flow times than those in men); considered variant of normal.

Fast-twitch Muscle Fibers (Type 2 Muscle Fibers) Comprise 30% of pelvic floor muscle fibers; physiologically designed to provide the rapid contraction needed to increase sphincter tone when there is a sudden increase in abdominal pressure.

Fecal Incontinence State in which an individual experiences a change in normal bowel habits characterized by involuntary passage of stool; may be further classified as passive incontinence (leakage that is not associated with urgency and of which the patient is unaware), urge incontinence (leakage associated with intense fecal urgency, the inability to delay defecation), or seepage and soiling (leakage of small amounts of stool between bowel movements in patient who is continent and able to delay defecation).

Fecal Soiling Any amount of stool deposited in the underwear, regardless of cause.

5-alpha Reductase Inhibitors Class of drugs that block the conversion of testosterone to dihydrotestosterone and thereby interfere with hormonal support for prostatic growth.

Flap Valve Theory of Fecal Continence Theory that increased intraabdominal pressure causes the anterior rectal wall to press down into the anal canal, thus occluding the anal canal and blocking the movement of stool.

Flutter Valve Theory of Fecal Continence Theory that intraabdominal pressure applied to a high-pressure area within the lower rectum causes the lower rectum to close and prevents passage of stool into the anal canal.

Folstein Mini-Mental Status Examination Validated screen commonly used to evaluate patients for cognitive decline.

Functional Bladder Capacity Amount of urine stored in the bladder before a sense of bladder fullness, urgency, or leakage prompts individual to urinate; determined by evaluation of the patient's bladder chart (either the range of voided volumes or the average voided volume). *International Continence Society recommends that this term be replaced with "average voided volume."*

Functional Constipation Constipation in children that is not attributable to organic or anatomic causes; also used to refer to the need for medication to regulate bowel function after 4 years of age.

Functional Incontinence Urinary incontinence caused by factors outside the urinary tract, such as immobility or cognitive impairment.

Functional Outlet Obstruction Obstructed voiding caused by failure of pelvic muscle and sphincter relaxation in the absence of any anatomic lesion.

Gastrocolic Reflex Increased colonic motor activity associated with eating; actually a misnomer, because the stimulus is not confined to the stomach and the increased motility is not confined to the colon.

Haustra (singular, Haustrum) Ringlike "pockets" characteristic of the colon; created by longitudinal muscle bands and circular muscle rings in colon wall.

Haustral Contractions Simultaneous contractions of the longitudinal muscle bands and a section of circular muscle in the colon; serve to increase exposure of the intestinal contents to the mucosal surface and gradually to move colonic contents distally.

Hinman Syndrome Functional disorder that closely mimics neurogenic (reflex) incontinence; characterized by unstable detrusor contractions and voluntary contraction of the striated sphincter in an attempt to maintain continence, which produces a functional obstruction of the bladder outlet (also known as "nonneurogenic bladder of childhood"). Clinical presentation includes diurnal and nocturnal enuresis, urinary tract infection, constipation and encopresis, and morphologic changes in lower urinary tract.

Hirschsprung's Disease Congenital anomaly characterized by absence of ganglion cells in the internal anal sphincter and distal portion of the rectum and involving variable lengths of the proximal portion of the colon; caused by an arrest in the cephalocaudal migration of neural cells during fetal development. Presents clinically as either intestinal obstruction or chronic refractory constipation, depending on the length of colon involved.

Hostile Bladder Function Term sometimes used to describe the potential for dysfunction in the lower urinary tract to cause distress in the upper tracts. Factors contributing to hostile bladder function include detrusor-sphincter dyssynergia, which produces urethral outlet obstruction, and low bladder wall compliance.

Impaired Detrusor Contractility (Detrusor Underactivity) Impaired contractile force of the detrusor, resulting in prolonged bladder emptying and/or a failure to achieve complete bladder emptying within a normal time span.

Imperforate Anus Umbrella term that encompasses a range of anomalies involving the anal canal and rectum and characterized by absence of a visible anal opening. May be further classified as "high" or "low" lesions, depending on whether the distal end of the bowel terminates above or below the puborectal component of the levator ani complex.

Incidence Number (or percentage) of individuals who develop a specific condition (such as incontinence) over a specific period of time.

Incontinence Impact Questionnaire Tool designed to measure the effect of urinary incontinence on an individual's quality of life.

Increased Daytime Frequency The complaint by the patient who considers that he or she voids too often by day.

Individualized Scheduled Toileting Program Program in which the patient is assisted or reminded to use the toilet "on schedule," with the specific times for toileting being determined by the patient's usual voiding patterns; used for selected patients with functional incontinence. Also known as "habit training" and "patterned urge response training."

Indwelling Catheter Catheter with retention balloon placed into bladder to provide continuous drainage; most commonly used for patients with reflex urinary incontinence or urinary retention who cannot be effectively managed by alternative programs. Indwelling catheters may be inserted via urethra or suprapubic incision.

Intermittent Catheterization Program of bladder management that involves regular evacuation of the bladder by means of in-and-out catheterization; may be used for patients with reflex urinary incontinence or patients with transient or chronic urinary retention.

Intermittent (Interrupted) Flow Pattern Flow pattern characterized by a saw-toothed configuration. Q_{max} is usually within normal limits, but Q_{ave} is typically low, and the voiding time is prolonged though the flow time may be short. Considered an abnormal pattern indicative of either impaired contractility or outlet obstruction. Pressure flow study is required to determine the particular problem.

Internal Anal Sphincter Continuation of the circular muscle layer of rectum; encircles anorectal junction and proximal 2 cm of anal canal. Controlled by autonomic nervous system.

International Prostate Symptom Score Tool designed to measure the symptoms associated with benign prostatic hyperplasia and their effect on quality of life.

Interstitial Cystitis Poorly understood chronic inflammatory condition of the bladder that commonly produces loss of compliance.

Intertrigo Mild inflammatory process that occurs on opposing skin surfaces as a result of friction and moisture; characterized by erythema, superficial linear erosions at the base of skin folds, or circular erosions between the buttocks.

Intrinsic Sphincter Deficiency Urinary leakage caused by a primary malfunction of the musculature within the urethra. *Note:* Urethral hypermobility and intrinsic sphincter deficiency may coexist.

Irritable Bowel Syndrome Chronic, recurrent functional defecation disorder characterized by abdominal pain, bloating and distension, and changes in stool frequency and consistency; may be further classified as constipation predominant, diarrhea predominant, or mixed.

Kegel's Exercises (Pelvic Floor Muscle Exercises) Exercise program involving repetitive contraction of the periurethral and pelvic floor striated muscles to increase muscle bulk and muscle strength.

Lactose Intolerance Condition characterized by lactase deficiency that results in reduced ability to metabolize lactose to absorbable monosaccharides; persistence of lactose within the lumen of the bowel induces osmotic diarrhea.

Lazy Bladder Syndrome Pattern of fractionated and incomplete voiding associated with minimal or absent detrusor contractions; characterized by infrequent voiding patterns, high postvoid residual volumes, and frequent infections. Cause believed to be chronic distension caused by infrequent voiding and resulting in myogenic failure.

Levator Ani Primary pelvic floor muscle; composed of multiple, named muscles that form a single functional unit.

Liquid Barrier Films (Skin Sealants) Mixture of polymers and solvents; when the solvents evaporate after application to the skin, the polymers dry to form an occlusive film. May be further divided into alcohol-based and alcohol-free liquid barriers.

Lower Urinary Tract Symptoms Term now used to describe the symptom complex formerly known as "prostatism" (that is, weak urinary stream with varying degrees of hesitancy, intermittency, urgency, frequency, nocturia, postvoid dribbling, or a feeling of incomplete emptying); shift in terminology caused by recognition that older women may present with the same symptoms.

Lower Urinary Tract Symptom Scores Tools designed to measure the effect of lower urinary tract symptoms on quality of life.

Magnetic Therapy (Extracorporeal Magnetic Innervation, or ExMI) Use of powerful magnetic field to induce electrical depolarization of the nerves and muscles of the pelvic floor, thus producing a strong contraction of the pelvic floor muscles; noninvasive therapy delivered by a "magnetic chair."

Manipulative Soiling Very uncommon form of incontinence, in which the child uses episodes of fecal incontinence to manipulate the environment or to passively display anger.

Marshall-Bonney Test Test used by some clinicians to differentiate between stress incontinence caused by urethral hypermobility and stress incontinence caused by intrinsic sphincter deficiency. The examiner places two fingers on either side of the urethra to support the bladder neck in normal anatomic position while the patient performs provocative maneuvers. (Lack of leakage indicates that the stress incontinence may be cured by surgical repositioning of the bladder neck.)

Material Safety Data Sheet Information sheet available from the manufacturer of skin care products that includes a complete listing of all ingredients as well as safety precautions.

Maximum Urethral Closure Pressure Difference between urethral pressure and bladder pressure, obtained through urethral pressure profile studies.

Maximum Urethral Pressure Gradient Difference between the maximum detrusor contraction pressure and the maximum urethral pressure measured at the point during bladder filling when urethral closure pressure is the greatest.

Megarectum Condition characterized by increased rectal compliance and reduced sensitivity to rectal distension. The overly distended rectum is unable to contract and empty effectively.

Melanosis Coli Black discoloration of mucosal lining of intestine associated with long-term use (at least 4 months) of some stimulant laxatives (such as senna, cascara, bisacodyl, phenolphthalein).

Microwave Thermotherapy Use of microwave heating with urethral cooling to induce ablation of the prostatic tissue while protecting the urethra and bladder neck. Studies indicate that the beneficial results are related more to improved detrusor function than to a significant reduction in prostatic volume.

Midurethral Sling Procedure Minimally invasive procedure designed to stabilize and support the urethra via placement of a tension-free sling at the midurethra, such as TVT and TOT procedures.

Minienema Gelatin ampules with enema tip that contain softener and stimulant agents used to stimulate defecation. Enema tip is twisted off, and medication is squeezed into rectum.

Mixed Diarrhea Diarrhea that is multifactorial in cause, such as diarrhea related to acquired immunodeficiency syndrome.

Mixed Incontinence Term used to refer to combination forms of incontinence, such as *mixed stress-urge incontinence.*

Moisturizer (Perineal) Topical creams used to restore water and lipids to the skin to improve its barrier function. Common ingredients include emollients to soften the skin, humectants to draw water into the stratum corneum, and occlusive agents to prevent evaporative water loss.

Moisture Barrier Product Formulations such as ointments, pastes, and creams that provide skin protection from irritants and moisture. Common ingredients include petrolatum, dimethicone, or zinc oxide, or a combination.

Motility-Related Diarrhea Diarrhea caused by disordered motility; for example, diminished motility results in bacterial overgrowth that can produce diarrhea, and increased motility compromises absorption and may result in osmotic diarrhea.

Motivational Therapy One treatment option for children with enuresis; involves series of counseling sessions in which the child is encouraged to assume responsibility for his or her own enuresis. Positive reinforcement and reward systems are used to enhance self-esteem and to provide a positive incentive to remain dry at night.

Motor Unit Anterior horn cell, its axon, and the several muscle fibers innervated by the horn cell.

Needle Bladder Neck Suspension Surgical procedures designed to correct urethral hypermobility by using sutures to suspend and support the anchoring tissues adjacent to the urethra and bladder neck; examples include the Stamey and the Raz procedures.

Neurogenic Bladder Bladder dysfunction caused by a lesion at any level in the nervous system; complex clinical picture with high incidence of upper tract deterioration and urinary incontinence.

Neurogenic Lower Urinary Tract Dysfunction Lower urinary tract dysfunction and incontinence caused by a disturbance in the neurologic structures and processes that control voiding.

Nocturia Interruption of sleep caused by the urge to urinate.

Nocturnal Enuresis Urinary loss that occurs only during sleep; may be further classified as *primary nocturnal enuresis* (that is, bedwetting in children who have never been dry at night for a significant length of time) or *secondary nocturnal enuresis* (recurrent bedwetting in a child who was dry at night for a period of at least 6 months).

Nonadrenergic, Noncholinergic (NANC) Receptors located throughout the detrusor wall that respond to adenosine triphosphate (ATP) rather than to adrenergic or cholinergic neurotransmitters; believed to play a modulatory role in detrusor function.

Nonneurogenic Functional Voiding Disorders Functional voiding disorders in children who do not otherwise exhibit any evidence of neurologic impairment; characterized by significant daytime incontinence, poor urinary stream, encopresis, and urinary tract infection.

Nonrelaxing Puborectalis Syndrome Condition characterized by paradoxical contraction of the external anal sphincter when the individual strains to defecate. Contraction of the sphincter and the puborectalis muscle prevents descent of the pelvic floor, straightening of the anorectal angle, and passage of stool into the anal canal (functional outlet obstruction). Also known as pelvic floor dyssynergia, anismus, spastic pelvic floor syndrome, rectoanal dyssynergia, or paradoxical external sphincter syndrome.

Nonretentive Encopresis Uncommon pattern of incontinence in children; characterized by stress-related diarrhea or by daily incontinence of stools that are of normal size and consistency. May be further classified as *primary nonretentive encopresis* (usually a psychologic problem caused by controlling or punitive toilet training) or *secondary nonretentive encopresis* (usually caused by psychosocial stressors that have caused the child to regress to an earlier developmental stage).

Normal Flow Pattern Pattern that resembles a bell curve that is slightly skewed to the left in men. Values are Q_{max} of 12 mL/second or more and Q_{ave} that is greater than 50% of the Q_{max}. In women, the Q_{max} and Q_{ave} values tend to be higher, and the flow and voiding times tend to be shorter.

Obstructive Defecation Disorders Condition characterized by difficult and incomplete evacuation of stool caused by obstruction of the anal canal. Obstruction may be functional or anatomic.

Osmotic (absorptive) Diarrhea Diarrhea caused by compromised absorption within the intestine. The reduced absorption increases fecal volume and also creates an osmotic force that attracts additional water into the lumen of the bowel (which further increases fecal volume).

Overactive Bladder Syndrome (also known as "Urge Syndrome" or "Urgency-Frequency Syndrome") Urgency, with or without urge incontinence, and usually with frequency and nocturia.

Overflow Incontinence Leakage associated with incomplete bladder emptying (that is, leakage that occurs when the bladder is full and the intravesical pressures are high). Leakage may or may not be associated with a detrusor contraction.

Overflow Stooling Pattern of fecal leakage seen in children with chronic stool retention and rectal distension characterized by frequent leakage of small amounts of stool.

Pad-weight Testing Test that objectively quantifies the volume of urinary leakage. The patient wears preweighed pads for specified periods of time or during specific provocative maneuvers, after which the pads are reweighed to determine the amount of urine lost.

Parasympathetic Nervous System "Maintenance" component of the autonomic nervous system. Stimulation of the parasympathetic pathways innervating the *bladder* promotes voiding by causing bladder contraction and indirectly reducing sphincter tone, and stimulation of the parasympathetic pathways innervating the *intestinal tract* increases motility and secretion.

Pelvic Floor Bony structures, endopelvic fascia, and muscles that support the pelvic organs and contribute to the sphincter mechanisms for both the urinary and intestinal tracts.

Pelvic Floor Relaxation Weakness of the pelvic floor support structures (that is, endopelvic fascia and muscles) that normally support the bladder neck and proximal portion of the urethra in the intra-abdominal position; the result is downward descent of the urethra and bladder neck during periods of increased intraabdominal pressure.

Pelvic Organ Prolapse Herniation of pelvic organs into and possibly through the vaginal vault caused by loss of normal structural supports.

Penile Clamp Plastic or metallic device lined with foam that is closed around the penis to prevent urinary leakage.

Penile Compression Cuff Soft band that is wrapped around the penis and secured with a Velcro fastener. The band incorporates a small bladder that is positioned along the ventral aspect of the penis and then inflated with air to partially compress the urethra.

Perianal Pouch Drainable "ostomy type" of pouch designed for application to perianal area and used for containment of stool.

Perineal Dermatitis Perineal skin damage resulting from exposure to stool, urine, or topical agents; may be further categorized as *irritant contact dermatitis* (inflammation caused by direct damage to the water-protein-lipid matrix of the skin) or *allergic contact dermatitis* (inflammation caused by a hypersensitivity reaction to an antigen).

Periurethral Bulking Procedures Surgical injection of biocompatible material into the urethral wall to increase urethral resistance; used for patients with intrinsic sphincter deficiency.

Periurethral Striated Muscle Mixture of slow-twitch and fast-twitch muscle fibers located adjacent to the membranous urethra in the male and adjacent to the rhabdosphincter in the female.

Pessary Intravaginal device designed to prevent pelvic organ prolapse or to support the bladder neck to reduce or eliminate urinary leakage.

Phasic Detrusor Instability Condition characterized by sensory urgency and hyperactive detrusor contractions and resulting in both sensory urgency and urinary leakage.

PNTML Studies Pudendal-nerve terminal motor latency studies; conducted on patients with suspected pudendal neuropathy to determine the time from electrical stimulation of the pudendal nerve until contraction of the muscle. Conducted using glove electrodes. The examiner inserts the gloved "electrode" finger into the anal canal, identifies the pudendal nerves, and stimulates the nerves with low-voltage electrical stimulation.

Pontine Micturition Center Two adjacent collections of nuclei located in the pons that provide two key functions in detrusor function: (1) mediation of the detrusor reflex and (2) coordination of bladder contraction and sphincter relaxation.

Postprostatectomy Incontinence Incontinence after prostatic surgery (usually radical prostatectomy) that may be caused by one or more of the following: sphincter dysfunction, detrusor instability, or reduced bladder compliance.

Postvoid Dribble Dribbling loss of urine that occurs after voiding, possibly because of retained urine in the distal portion of the urethra (male) or a urethral diverticulum or the vagina (female).

Postvoid Residual Urine Volume Amount of urine remaining in the bladder immediately after voiding; may be determined by catheterization or by bladder ultrasonography.

Powders Formulations that are designed to absorb moisture from the skin, thereby reducing frictional forces.

Power Pudding Bran mixture used to prevent constipation and normalize bowel function and consisting of $\frac{1}{2}$ cup of wheat bran flakes, $\frac{1}{2}$ cup of applesauce, $\frac{1}{2}$ cup of canned or stewed prunes, and $\frac{1}{2}$ cup of prune juice.

Pressure-flow Nomogram Chart developed to assist clinician in synthesizing and interpreting the data from a urodynamic pressure-flow study; for example, the International Continence Society (ICS) chart displays pressure flow values in three zones (unobstructed, equivocal, and obstructed).

Pressure-flow Study Physiologic study to evaluate bladder emptying; includes data regarding detrusor contractility and urinary flow rates. Conducted after cystometrogram. Filling catheter is removed, but pressure-sensitive catheter is left in place, and patient is asked to void on uroflow commode. Intravesical pressure is measured throughout voiding, and flow rate and flow pattern are determined by uroflowmetry.

Pressure Transmission Ratio Test performed to evaluate urethral resistance during provocative maneuvers such as coughing; performed by obtaining simultaneous measurements of intravesical and urethral pressures at rest and during a cough. (Pressure transmission ratio is calculated by dividing the change in urethral pressure during a cough by the change in *P*ves during a cough and multiplying the result by 100.)

Prevalence Total number of individuals with a specific condition (such as incontinence), as compared with the total population being studied, at a specific point in time.

Prolonged (Poor) Flow Pattern Flow pattern characterized by a low *Q*max and *Q*ave and a prolonged voiding time and flow time; indicative of compromised bladder emptying, caused by either bladder outlet obstruction or impaired contractility. Patient with poor flow pattern should have pressure-flow study to determine the specific problem.

Prompted Voiding Program in which the caregiver checks the patient on a regular basis, asks whether he or she is wet or dry, provides feedback regarding the accuracy of the patient's self-assessment, and offers assistance with toileting. Positive responses are praised, and incontinent episodes are managed without comment. Used for patients with functional incontinence related to compromised mobility or mild to moderate degrees of cognitive impairment.

Propagating Peristaltic Contractions Series of peristaltic contractions that serve to propel stool distally through the colon (also known as "mass movements").

Prostatism See *Lower urinary tract symptoms.*

Pruritus Ani Perianal inflammation and skin damage caused by intense itching and chronic scratching.

Pubococcygeus Muscle Component of levator ani muscle complex; consists of U-shaped muscle fibers that arise from the pubic bones, attach to the lateral walls of the rectum (and the vagina in the female), and extend around the posterior portion of the rectum. Also known as the "pubovisceral muscle."

Puborectalis Muscle U-shaped muscle (component of pelvic floor muscle complex) that originates along the posterior aspect of the symphysis pubis, passes posteriorly to form a sling around the anorectal junction, and returns to the posterior side of the symphysis pubis.

Pudendal Neuropathy Damage to the pudendal nerve resulting in a higher threshold for sensory awareness of rectal distension or a time delay in recognition of rectal filling.

Pabd Abdominal pressure as measured by rectal or vaginal pressure monitors during urodynamic testing.

Pdet Detrusor pressure, that is, the force created by the active and passive tension elements within the bladder wall; cannot be measured directly but can be calculated by subtracting abdominal pressure from intravesical pressure.

Pull-through Procedure for Imperforate Anus Reconstructive procedure in which the distal end of the bowel is mobilized and pulled through the pelvic musculature to terminate at a newly created anal opening.

Pves Intravesical pressure as measured by a pressure monitor inserted into the bladder; intravesical pressure represents the sum of the abdominal and detrusor forces acting on the contents of the bladder.

Q-Tip Test Test used by some practitioners to demonstrate urethral hypermobility objectively. A sterile lubricated Q-Tip is inserted into the urethra to the level of the bladder neck, and the patient is asked to strain down. (Upward movement of the Q-Tip reflects a downward movement of the bladder neck, which may be indicative of urethral hypermobility.)

Rectal Catheter Large-bore indwelling catheter placed into rectum and connected to bedside drainage bag for containment of large volume of liquid stool; associated with risk of anorectal necrosis and now considered inappropriate. (Alternatives are internal drainage systems and nasal trumpet inserted into rectum and connected to bedside bag.)

Rectal Compliance Ability of the rectal wall to distend with limited increase in rectal pressure, that is, to stretch and store stool at low pressures.

Rectal Compliance Study Study of rectal compliance; conducted by insertion of a balloon-tipped catheter with pressure transducers into the rectum and then progressive filling of the balloon while the corresponding changes in rectal pressure are recorded.

Rectal Prolapse Protrusion of the rectal mucosa into or through the anal canal.

Rectoanal Inhibitory Reflex Reflex relaxation of internal sphincter in response to rectal distension;

permits rectal contents to move into the proximal portion of the anal canal.

Rectocele Herniation of the anterior portion of the rectum into the vaginal vault; may be evident only during "bearing-down" maneuvers.

Rectum Last segment of large intestine; provides sensory awareness of impending defecation and temporary storage of stool.

Reflex Incontinence Involuntary loss of urine caused by an unstable contraction of the detrusor and occurring with diminished or absent sensory awareness of the urge to void.

Reflex Voiding Program Method of management for selected male patients with reflex urinary incontinence; the bladder empties by means of spontaneous contractions and leakage is contained by a condom catheter connected to a drainage bag.

Retentive Encopresis Incontinence associated with chronic constipation and overflow stooling; characterized by small loose incontinent stools several times daily.

Retropubic Suspension Surgical procedures designed to correct urethral hypermobility by elevating the urethrovesical junction; examples include the Marshall-Marchetti-Krantz and the Burch colposuspension procedures.

Rhabdosphincter Intrinisic striated muscle of the urethral sphincter; in boys and men, located in the membranous urethra, just below the apex of the prostate gland, and in girls and women, located in the middle third of the urethra.

Routine Scheduled Toileting Toileting program in which the patient is assisted to the bathroom on a fixed, predetermined schedule, most often based on the caregiver's convenience; commonly used in long-term care settings.

Sacral Neuromodulation Implantation of an electrode at the level of the S2 foramen to provide low-level electrical stimulation; believed to provide afferent input to sacral cord that inhibits the pathologic reflex interfering with voiding.

Saline Continence Study Study to quantify fecal incontinence; conducted by infusing saline into the rectum at a standardized rate and then documenting volume at which "first leak" occurs and total retained volume.

Sampling Reflex Sensory discrimination among gas, solid, and liquid that takes place when the internal anal sphincter relaxes and permits rectal contents to contact the numerous sensory receptors in the anal canal.

Secretory Diarrhea Diarrhea caused by significant increase in the volume of water and electrolytes secreted *into* the lumen of the gut; most commonly caused by infectious agents but can also be caused by noninfectious stimulants to secretion (such as unabsorbed bile acids).

Segmentation Contractions Contractions within the intestinal wall that create a back-and-forth mixing motion. These contractions expose the stool to the mucosal lining, which promotes absorption.

Self-awakening Programs to teach a child with primary nocturnal enuresis to awaken to the sensation of a full bladder; commonly involves teaching the child to rehearse the desired sequence of events (that is, waking to a full bladder, getting up and going to the bathroom, and returning to bed) and to remind himself or herself to get up to urinate during the night if necessary.

Sensory-Motor (Sensorimotor) Reeducation Programs to improve sensory awareness of rectal filling or sphincter control; requires intact cognitive function and intact neurologic pathways. Biofeedback commonly used but not always essential. Sensory retraining involves placement of an intrarectal balloon that is inflated to the point of first sensation and then gradually deflated as the patient learns to recognize lower levels of rectal distension. Sphincter reeducation may include pelvic muscle exercises (Kegel's exercises) or may involve education re pelvic muscle relaxation.

Sensory Urgency Condition in which unstable detrusor contractions (documented by urodynamic studies) are associated with a significant sense of urgency to urinate but no leakage.

SF-36 Standardized universal health assessment tool; stands for 36-item short form.

Simple Cystometrogram Procedure in which sterile water is introduced into the bladder via a catheter to evaluate bladder capacity, sensory awareness of bladder filling, and the bladder's response to filling and to provocative maneuvers.

Sling Procedures Surgical placement of strips of fascia or synthetic material underneath the urethra that are then anchored to retropubic or abdominal structures to elevate the urethra; designed to treat intrinsic sphincter deficiency by significantly increasing urethral resistance.

Slow-Twitch Muscle Fibers (Type I Muscle Fibers) Predominant muscle fiber in the pelvic floor; physiologically suited to provide sustained pelvic muscle tone over prolonged periods of time.

Sphincterotomy Surgical incision of the urethral sphincter to reduce urethral resistance; used in patients with reflex urinary incontinence and detrusor-sphincter dyssynergia who wish to manage their urinary incontinence with a reflex voiding program. Associated with a significant complication rate.

Sphincter Electromyography (EMG) Study that provides a graphic representation of the electrical activity recorded from pelvic floor muscles (using needle, wire, or surface electrodes); can be used to assess the integrity of neuromuscular innervation but cannot be used to evaluate muscle tone or strength. In the physiologically normal individual, the sphincter EMG reflects reduced voltage during a voluntary detrusor contraction (that is, appropriate sphincter relaxation).

Spina Bifida Umbrella term that encompasses several congenital anomalies that have in common separated (nonfused) posterior vertebral arches (a type of neural tube defect). May be further classified as *spina bifida occulta* (bony defect not accompanied by any protrusion of the spinal cord or meninges into the defect), *spina bifida with meningocele* (visible bony defect with herniation of the meninges and spinal fluid into a sac on the infant's back), and *spina bifida with myelomeningocele* (bony defect with herniation of the spinal cord, meninges, and spinal fluid into a sac on the infant's back). Myelomeningocele is associated with significant sensory and motor loss below the level of the defect, and bowel and bladder dysfunction is almost universal.

Stimulant Laxatives Agents that work by irritating the mucosal layer, decreasing segmentation contractions, increasing peristalsis, and decreasing colonic transit time, thus producing soft or liquid stools.

Stimulated Defecation Programs Programs that include both a routine schedule for fecal elimination *and* use of a peristaltic stimulant to initiate the defecation process; indicated for patients with sensory or cognitive deficits and patients with sphincter dysfunction.

Stool Softeners Agents that attract water to the fecal mass.

Stress Incontinence Involuntary loss of urine occurring when the intravesical pressure exceeds the maximum urethral pressure (typically during physical exertion such as coughing, sneezing, or sudden change of position). Leakage occurs in the absence of a detrusor contraction and is caused by sphincter dysfunction.

Suppository (Rectal) Solid form of medication shaped for intrarectal administration. Laxative suppositories are used to stimulate peristalsis in the left colon and rectum.

Sympathetic Nervous System "Fight-or-flight" component of the autonomic nervous system. Stimulation of the sympathetic fibers innervating the *bladder* promotes bladder filling by causing relaxation of the detrusor muscle and contraction of the musculature in the proximal portion of the urethra, and stimulation of the sympathetic fibers innervating the *intestine* causes reduced motility and reduced secretion.

Symptom Severity Index Tool to assess the severity of stress urinary incontinence and its psychosocial effect.

Timed Voiding Voiding on schedule; can be beneficial for patients who have reduced sensory awareness of bladder filling but who retain sufficient detrusor contractility to effectively empty the bladder.

Transepidermal Water Loss (TEWL) Rate at which water evaporates from the stratum corneum, which is an indicator for the integrity of the skin barrier.

Transient Incontinence Incontinence caused by reversible factors.

Transurethral Needle Ablation of the Prostate (TUNA) Use of low-level radiofrequency energy to create necrotic lesions within the prostatic tissue without damaging adjacent structures; produces only minimal reduction in volume of prostatic tissue but believed to destroy intraprostatic nerve fibers contributing to smooth muscle tone and urethral resistance. Similar procedure is *interstitial radiofrequency therapy*.

Transurethral Resection of Prostate (TURP) Surgical resection of the prostate by a urethral approach; commonly used for treatment of benign prostatic hyperplasia.

Transurethral Vaporization of the Prostate Surgical alternative to TURP in which electrodes are used to provide simultaneous vaporization and coagulation of prostatic tissue.

Tricyclic Antidepressants Pharmacologic agents with both anticholinergic and alpha-adrenergic agonist activity; used to increase urethral resistance and to reduce bladder contractility. (Used for children with nocturnal enuresis and adults with mixed stress-urge incontinence.)

Upper Urinary Tract Distress Threatened or impending impairment of renal function, as evidenced by febrile urinary tract infections, renal insufficiency, dilatation of the renal pelvis or ureter, or vesicoureteral reflux.

Urethra Collapsible tube extending from the bladder neck to the external meatus. In boys and men, the urethra is divided into four segments: the preprostatic urethra (also called the bladder neck), the prostatic urethra, the membranous urethra (which contains striated muscle fibers and is sometimes referred to as the external sphincter), and the distal (conduit) urethra.

Urethral Hypermobility Abnormal descent of the bladder neck and proximal portion of the urethra during activities that cause increased abdominal pressure. This abnormal descent is caused by pelvic floor weakness (pelvic floor relaxation).

Urethral Occlusion Devices Devices designed to prevent leakage as opposed to controlling it. Devices available for women include a urethral occlusion insert. Devices available for men include an occlusive penile cuff and a penile clamp.

Urethral Pressure Profile Test to measure urethral resistance, conducted by slowly pulling a pressure-sensitive catheter through the urethra while measuring urethral and intravesical pressures; provides a profile of urethral resistance at rest that is used to help diagnose intrinisic sphincter deficiency.

Urethral Resistance Algorithm Chart that uses a comparison of flow rates at maximum detrusor contraction pressure to determine bladder outlet obstruction.

Urethral Stent Stainless steel device placed at the level of the membranous urethra to reduce urethral resistance and to lower detrusor contraction pressure; used as an alternative to standard sphincterotomy for patients with reflex urinary incontinence who wish to manage with a reflex voiding program.

Urge Incontinence involuntary leakage of urine accompanied by or immediately preceded by urgency.

Urgency The complaint of a sudden compelling desire to pass urine that is difficult to defer.

Urge Inhibition Strategies Strategies used to inhibit the urge to void and delay voiding. Typical urge inhibition strategies include relaxation, distraction, and pelvic muscle contractions.

Urinalysis Analysis of urine to detect the presence of any abnormal substances (such as glucose, protein, red or white blood cells, bacteria, nitrites).

Urinary Frequency Voiding interval of less than 2 hours during waking hours.

Urinary Hesitancy Condition characterized by a prolonged time between initial attempts to start the urinary stream and time at which voiding actually begins.

Urinary Incontinence Symptom, sign, and condition as defined thus by the International Continence Society: "a condition in which involuntary loss of urine is a social or hygienic problem and is objectively demonstrable."

Urinary Retention Incomplete bladder emptying, typically defined by an abnormally high postvoid residual urine; sometimes further classified as *acute*, which is characterized by rapid onset and frequently involves a painful inability to void or to empty the bladder effectively, and *chronic*, which tends to be insidious and is sometimes unrecognized by the patient.

Urinary Stream Interruption Test Test used to evaluate pelvic muscle strength. The patient is asked to interrupt voiding, and the examiner determines (1) the patient's ability to interrupt the urinary stream voluntarily, and (2) the number of seconds required to do so. (Also used to help the patient identify the pelvic floor muscles.)

Urodynamics Group of tests designed to evaluate the transport, storage, and elimination functions of the middle and lower portions of the urinary tract; may be further classified as simple (tests that can be completed without an electronic monitor) and complex (tests that require the use of electronic monitoring equipment).

Uroflowmetry Screening study in which patient voids into a uroflow device that provides the following data: maximum flow rate (Qmax), average flow rate (Qave), voided volume, and flow time. Also provides graph of urine flow that permits clinician to determine flow pattern.

Urogenital Distress Inventory Tool designed to measure the effect of urinary incontinence on an individual's quality of life.

Vaginal Weight Cone Therapy Use of graduated intravaginal weights to assist the patient in strengthening the pelvic floor muscles. The weights provide sensory feedback to the patient and "remind" her to contract her pelvic floor muscles when she feels the weight beginning to slip out of position.

Videourodynamics Studies that combine pressure, flow, and sphincter electromyographic data with simultaneous lower urinary tract imaging (usually fluoroscopy); provides dynamic anatomic data as well as functional data. Considered the preferred study in patients with complex urinary incontinence, patients with hostile neuropathic bladder dysfunction, women with significant pelvic organ prolapse, or women with stress incontinence for whom surgical intervention is being contemplated as well as patients with recurrent urinary incontinence after a surgical procedure.

Visual Laser Ablation of Prostate Endoscopic laser ablation of the prostate; alternative to transurethral resection of prostate (TURP).

Voiding Cystourethrogram (VCUG) Physiologic tests of bladder function, that is, cystometrogram and pressure-flow study.

Voiding Dysfunction General term used to refer to any abnormality associated with bladder emptying.

Voiding Pressure Study (Pressure-Flow Study) Study that provides a graphic representation of urodynamic pressures (Pabd, Pves, and Pdet) and urinary flow; typically, the sphincter electromyogram is recorded as well. Test is conducted immediately after the filling cystometrogram (filling CMG) catheter is removed, and patient is assisted onto a uroflow device and asked to void (if multilumen catheter is used, catheter is left in place and patient is asked to void around it).

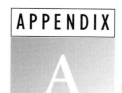

APPENDIX A

Self-Assessment Exercise Answers

CHAPTER I

1. Issues contributing to the variability in prevalence rates include differences in the definition of incontinence, differences in the population being sampled, and differences in study methodology. Studies that define incontinence very broadly (such as "any leakage of urine within the past year"), studies that sample higher-risk populations (such as patients seeing a urologist or gastroenterologist), and studies involving subjective report only (as opposed to objectively validated leakage) generate significantly higher prevalence rates. These findings point to the need to standardize the definitions of incontinence used for prevalence studies, the need to validate leakage objectively, and the importance of either conducting broad-based population studies or limiting any generalizations to the specific population sampled.

2. The groups at greatest risk for incontinence seem to be women and the elderly. For community-dwelling adults, average prevalence rates for urinary incontinence are about 27.6% among women and 10.5% among men; in studies addressing the severity of leakage among women, approximately 7% of community-dwelling women report leakage that is moderate to severe and "bothersome." For the institutionalized elderly, the prevalence rates are about 50%. Similarly, the prevalence of fecal incontinence among community-dwelling adults is approximately 2% to 5%, but the prevalence among institutionalized elderly persons approaches 50%.

3. (1) *Skin breakdown* may be attributable to the primary effects of prolonged contact between the skin and urine (such as contact dermatitis), the reduced tensile strength of macerated skin and the associated risk for friction injuries or spontaneous "cracks" in the skin, or the increased risk for pressure ulcer development (which may be the result primarily of the inactivity and immobility common among incontinent individuals).

    (2) *Injury caused by falls.* Nocturia and urgency are major risk factors for falls.

    (3) *Urinary tract infection* may be caused by the use of indwelling catheters, which leads to ascending bacteriuria, or to the use of absorptive products, which create a warm moist environment that is favorable to bacterial growth. In some patients, incontinence is caused by an underlying problem with urinary retention, which is associated with urinary stasis and infection.

4. *False.* Urinary incontinence is a very expensive problem, in terms of both direct and indirect costs. The last comprehensive analysis of costs related to incontinence management was based on 1995 data; at that time, annual costs in the United States were estimated to be $16.3 billion.

5. Overactive bladder/urge incontinence is associated with the greatest effect on quality of life; this can be explained by the effect of frequency, urgency, and uncontrolled large-volume urinary leakage on activities such as travel, social activities, and sleep. Fecal incontinence also has a devastating effect on quality of life, by severely limiting individuals' ability to work, go to school, or participate in social activities.

6. (a) *Stress incontinence.* Stress incontinence is defined as involuntary loss of urine during

physical exertion such as coughing, sneezing, or sudden exertion. Stress incontinence represents a problem with storage caused by sphincter dysfunction.

(b) *Overactive bladder/urge incontinence.* Urge incontinence is defined as the involuntary loss of urine accompanied by or immediately preceded by urgency. Urge incontinence is associated with overactive bladder syndrome and is suggestive of detrusor overactivity (that is, involuntary detrusor muscle contractions). It represents a problem with storage caused by bladder dysfunction.

(c) *Neurogenic lower tract dysfunction (reflex incontinence).* This condition involves loss of neurologic control of the lower urinary tract and is frequently associated with bladder-sphincter dyssynergia. Reflex incontinence represents a combined problem with storage and emptying and is caused by neurologic lesions above the level of the sacral spinal cord.

(d) *Chronic retention associated with urinary leakage.* Chronic retention involves incomplete emptying of the bladder, either because of weak detrusor contractions or resulting from bladder outlet obstruction; it may or may not be associated with urinary leakage. This type of incontinence represents a problem with emptying because of either bladder dysfunction or urethral obstruction.

(e) *Functional incontinence.* Functional incontinence is defined as urinary leakage caused by problems outside of the urinary tract. The most common etiologic factors are cognitive impairment and immobility. It is a problem with storage.

(f) *Extraurethral incontinence.* Extraurethral incontinence is leakage from a source other than the urethra, such as an ectopic ureter or a fistula. This is a problem with storage, although it is caused by factors other than the bladder or sphincter.

(g) *Nocturnal enuresis.* Nocturnal enuresis is leakage that occurs only during sleep. This type of incontinence is common among children. It is a problem with storage caused by factors other than the bladder or sphincter (such as deep sleep).

7. The trend in assessment is to begin with a careful history, physical exam, bladder chart, and basic laboratory studies and to limit complex urodynamic studies and imaging studies to patients with complex clinical presentations and specific indications of comorbidities, such as pelvic malignancy or renal compromise, and to patients scheduled for surgical intervention. The trend in patient management is to begin with the least invasive and least costly treatment (typically behavioral therapies), to use pharmacologic agents as adjunct therapy when indicated, and to reserve surgical intervention for patients in whom the more conservative therapies fail or who present with specific problems not amenable to behavioral therapies. In addition, continence care is becoming more multidisciplinary in focus, which represents an opportunity for the continence nurse.

8. Key responsibilities include the following: identification of risk factors; assessment to include relevant history, focused physical examination, assessment of bowel and bladder charts, bedside cystometry, and identification of common complications; establishment and implementation of an appropriate management plan to include dietary and fluid management, bowel training or stimulated defecation program, bladder retraining, prompted voiding, or scheduled voiding program, pelvic muscle reeducation without biofeedback, indwelling catheter management, intermittent catheterization program management, recommendations regarding skin care and containment products, and education and counseling; and identification of patients requiring referral for additional assessment or intervention.

CHAPTER **2**

1. Four goals of a comprehensive program for the individual with urinary incontinence are as follows:
- Reduction or elimination of urinary leakage
- Protection of upper urinary tracts against complications of voiding dysfunction
- Maintenance of perineal skin integrity
- Preservation of dignity

2. (c) The individual with bladder outlet obstruction resulting in high intravesical pressures and incomplete bladder emptying with high residual urine volumes is the individual at greatest risk for upper tract damage.

Reason: The urine transport system (that is, calyces, renal pelves, and ureters) is a low-pressure system. High intravesical pressures impede the delivery of urine to the bladder and place the patient at risk for recurrent urinary tract infections, hydroureteronephrosis, vesicoureteral reflux, and compromised renal function. In addition, high residual urine volumes are associated with an increased risk of urinary tract infection caused by the stasis of urine and resulting bacterial proliferation.

3. Antimuscarinic medications have a much greater effect on bladder contractility than on ureteral peristalsis because of the differences in regulation of the smooth muscle in the upper tracts as opposed to the lower tracts. In the upper tracts, the smooth muscles have tight connections that facilitate the rapid propagation of electrical impulses. These impulses are initiated in pacemaker cells in response to distension of the renal pelvis (with urine). Although the autonomic nervous system does innervate the upper urinary tracts, there are relatively few neuromuscular junctions in the upper tracts, and neural control is believed to play an indirect modulatory role only. In contrast, neuromuscular junctions are plentiful in the bladder, where the ratio of neuromuscular junctions to smooth muscle cells is almost 1:1; thus, neural control plays a *major* role in regulation of detrusor contractility, with parasympathetic stimulation promoting detrusor contraction and sympathetic stimulation promoting detrusor relaxation. Because neural stimulation contributes only weakly to ureteral peristalsis, anticholinergic medication has minimal effect, and because neural stimulation is the primary mechanism for innervation of the detrusor, it has a major effect.

4. The pelvic floor consists of the pelvic bones, pelvic fascia, and pelvic muscles. These structures provide support to the bladder and the urethra. The pelvic floor contributes to continence in two significant ways:

(1) The support structures help to maintain the bladder base and proximal portion of the urethra in an intraabdominal position, which ensures that any increase in intraabdominal pressure (as occurs with coughing, laughing, or lifting) is transmitted equally to the bladder and to the proximal portion of the urethra and the bladder base. This is important because urinary leakage will occur any time the intravesical pressure exceeds the intraurethral pressure.

If the bladder base and proximal portion of the urethra lose their intraabdominal position, sudden increases in intraabdominal pressure are transmitted to the bladder but not to the urethra, and there is increased risk of leakage.

(2) The muscular elements of the pelvic floor contribute to urethral closure. The periurethral striated muscle and the levator ani muscle are composed of both slow-twitch (Type 1) and fast-twitch (Type 2) muscle fibers. Contraction of the pelvic floor muscles engages the fast-twitch fibers, which provide a rapid increase in urethral closure pressure during periods of physical exertion. In addition, the slow-twitch fibers in these muscles provide for sustained contraction, which stimulates a spinal reflex that inhibits detrusor muscle contraction. The significance of the pelvic floor musculature to the maintenance (or restoration) of continence is evidenced by

the beneficial effects of pelvic muscle reeducation (Kegel's exercises) in patients with urinary leakage.

5. • *Anatomic integrity.* Urinary continence is dependent in part on the elimination of urine being delayed and controlled by a sphincter mechanism. Loss of anatomic integrity allows urine to bypass the sphincter mechanism, thus producing incontinence.

• *Neurologic control of the detrusor (bladder).* Voluntary initiation or delay of voiding is dependent on normal neurologic control of the bladder; that is, the neurologically intact person is able to recognize the sensations of bladder filling and is able to delay bladder emptying until a socially appropriate time. Many structures must function normally to provide this level of "social continence." Normal cerebrocortical function allows the individual to recognize the need to void and to inhibit lower centers to delay voiding until an appropriate time and place can be found, at which point the inhibitory signals are discontinued and voiding is allowed to proceed under the direction of the pons. The pons mediates the detrusor reflex and provides for coordinated voiding. When the bladder fills sufficiently to activate the stretch receptors in the bladder wall and inhibitory signals from the cortex are withdrawn, the pons mediates relaxation of the sphincter mechanism, followed by detrusor contraction. Communication between the central control centers (cortex and pons) and the bladder and sphincter is provided by the spinal cord, specifically the autonomic pathways and the sensorimotor pathways that control the pelvic muscles and rhabdosphincter.

Neurologic control of the detrusor can be compromised by any cerebrocortical lesion affecting the detrusor motor area or by any lesion affecting the pons or the spinal cord. If the lesion is above the level of the pons, the individual will lose social continence but will retain coordinated voiding; however, if the lesion is below the level of the pons (but above the parasympathetic outflow tract), the individual will lose both social continence and coordinated voiding. (In this situation, the detrusor will contract in response to parasympathetic stimulation, but the sphincter may remain partially or completely closed.)

• *Competence of the urethral sphincter mechanism.* A competent sphincter provides a "leakproof" seal during bladder filling and storage, even during sudden and precipitous rises in intraabdominal pressure. Normal sphincter function is dependent on normal urethral wall softness, adequate urethral mucus production, the integrity of the submucosal vascular cushion, contractility and innervation of the smooth and skeletal muscle fibers in the urethra and pelvic floor, and normal support for the bladder base and proximal portion of the urethra (so it is maintained in an intraabdominal position). Because many factors function jointly to maintain adequate urethral closure pressure, a deficiency in one component can sometimes be offset by competence of the remaining structures; however, significant deficiencies usually result in inadequate urethral resistance and urinary leakage.

6. *False.* In the past, it was believed that voiding was mediated primarily by the sacral "micturition center," with input and modulation from higher brain centers. It is now recognized that voiding in the neurologically intact individual is coordinated by the pons but modulated by the cortex and other centers in the brain.

7. The cortex provides for "social continence," whereas the pons is responsible for coordinated voiding.

The cortical centers include the detrusor motor area (a collection of nuclei found in each frontal lobe) and multiple other modulatory areas and structures that are believed to affect bladder control. The cortical centers provide for social continence primarily through inhibition of the pons, which allows the individual to delay voiding.

As the bladder distends, the stretch receptors in the bladder wall are activated, and this sensory input is interpreted by the cortex as the "urge to void." If the urge to void occurs at a socially inappropriate time and place, the cortex sends inhibitory messages to the pons. When a suitable time and place for voiding is located, the cortex releases its inhibitory control to permit voiding.

The pons responds to input from the cerebral cortex and sends appropriate messages to the bladder and sphincter; that is, when the cerebral cortex sends inhibitory messages to the pons, the pons in turn activates the sympathetic pathways to the bladder and sphincter, thus signaling the bladder to continue to stretch and store. When the cortex releases its inhibitory signals, the pons provides for coordinated voiding; that is, the pons activates somatic and parasympathetic pathways to initiate sphincter relaxation followed by detrusor contraction. Should cortical control be lost, the pons takes over and provides for coordinated voiding in response to bladder filling; this pattern is *normal* for the precontinent child but is abnormal thereafter.

8. (c) Alpha-adrenergic agonists may be helpful for patients with inadequate urethral resistance. This is explained by the finding that the receptors in the smooth muscle of the bladder neck and proximal portion of the urethra are primarily alpha-adrenergic, and stimulation of these receptors causes smooth muscle contraction and enhanced urethral closure.

9. The postmenopausal woman is at greater risk for urinary leakage because of the decline in estrogen levels. Maximum urethral closure pressure is lower in elderly women than in younger women, and estrogen deficiency is believed to play a major role. Estrogen is known to increase the sensitivity of the urethral smooth muscle to alpha-adrenergic stimulation, to support the integrity of the urethral epithelium and the submucosal vascular cushion, and to promote urethral mucus production. In addition, estrogen treatment has been found to reduce the irritative voiding symptoms associated with urge urinary incontinence.

10. Fast-twitch fibers provide for a rapid contraction, or "quick flick," which provides a brief but intense increase in urethral closure pressure and helps to maintain continence during sudden increases in abdominal and intravesical pressure (such as a sneeze). Slow-twitch fibers provide for a slow but sustained contraction. The slow-twitch fibers in the levator ani muscle provide prolonged support for the pelvic organs when the individual is in the upright (standing) position. Pelvic muscle reeducation programs must therefore address both the fast-twitch and the slow-twitch fibers.

11. Your response should include identification of the factors that signal the neurologic maturity necessary for acquisition of urinary continence and an explanation of the fact that neurologic maturation occurs at different ages in different children and any attempt to toilet train before the maturation of critical neurologic processes is inadvisable. The factors that signal sufficient neurologic maturity include acquisition of fecal continence, the ability to verbalize the urge to urinate, the ability to postpone urination briefly, and the ability to interrupt the urinary stream voluntarily.

12. Elderly persons are considered to be at greater risk for urinary incontinence because of the changes that normally occur in the central nervous system, urinary tract, and adjacent organs, that is, reduction in bladder capacity, nocturia, possible reduction in detrusor contractility, enlarged prostate and increased muscle tone in the prostatic urethra in men and reduced estrogen levels in women. In addition, elderly persons are at much greater risk for many pathologic conditions commonly associated with incontinence, such as cerebrovascular accident, Parkinson's disease, and Alzheimer's disease. Reduced mobility and side effects of medications are additional risk factors. However, incontinence should never be considered a normal part of

aging; it always represents an abnormal condition. The health care professional must remember that most elderly individuals retain continence, and those who develop problems with urinary leakage can frequently be assisted to *regain* continence.

CHAPTER **3**

1. Acute incontinence refers to the sudden onset of urinary leakage or sudden significant worsening of preexisting minor leakage. It is frequently caused by reversible factors, and in this case it is usually transient, but it may also be caused by an illness or injury that is not reversible, and in this case the "acute" incontinence will eventually become "chronic." In managing the patient with acute onset incontinence, the initial focus is on identification and correction of any reversible factors. Once all reversible factors have been corrected, the patient is reassessed, and a treatment plan is established for any residual incontinence.

   Transient incontinence refers to incontinence caused by reversible factors and is by definition correctable. Reversible (transient) factors may cause acute-onset incontinence or may cause exacerbation of established, "chronic" incontinence. The management of any patient with incontinence, whether acute or chronic, must therefore begin with identification and correction of transient (reversible) factors.

2. Reversible factors frequently play a role in the exacerbation of established, "chronic" forms of incontinence, and correction of these reversible factors can significantly reduce the frequency and severity of the incontinence. Therefore, the first step in management of any patient with incontinence is to correct the "transient" factors. The patient can then be reassessed to determine the pattern of any residual incontinence, and a long-term management plan can be established.

3. D = Delirium (reversible alteration in mental status), which causes or contributes to incontinence by compromising the individual's ability to sense and respond appropriately to the sensations of bladder fullness.

   D = Dehydration causes concentrated urine that may irritate the bladder and thereby contribute to irritative symptoms such as urgency, frequency, and dysuria.

   D = Dietary irritants have also been reported to cause "overactive bladder–type" symptoms (urgency, frequency, and possibly urinary incontinence); the most common offenders are caffeinated and carbonated beverages and alcohol, and some individuals are sensitive to acidic fruits and juices, milk, and highly spiced food.

   I = Infection (of the bladder), which increases bladder contractility and causes urinary frequency and urgency. In the older individual with compromised mobility, this change may precipitate incontinence (because he or she is unable to reach the toilet quickly enough to prevent leakage).

   A = Atrophic urethritis and vaginitis, which alters the integrity of the urethral, vaginal, and bladder tissues. This altered integrity increases the risk of stress incontinence (because of loss of urethral coaptation and thinning of the submucosal vascular cushion) and of urge incontinence (because of increased contractility of the bladder and increased sensory urgency).

   P = Pharmaceuticals. Some drugs alter muscle tone in the urethra, causing reduced urethral resistance and increased risk of stress incontinence; some drugs reduce bladder contractility, thus increasing the risk of urinary retention and overflow incontinence; many drugs alter mental acuity, sensory awareness, and mobility, thus compromising the individual's ability to interpret and respond to the sensation of bladder filling accurately.

   P = Psychologic problems. Psychologic problems, such as severe depression, interfere with the individual's interest in self-care and motivation to maintain continence.

   E = Excess urine production. Conditions such as hyperglycemia, diabetes insipidus, obstructive sleep apnea, or congestive heart failure can cause production of excessive volumes of urine, which may overwhelm the individual's continence mechanisms.

R = Restricted mobility, which interferes with the individual's ability to reach the toilet in time to prevent leakage.

S = Stool impaction. Stool impaction creates pressure against the urethra and produces an outflow obstruction; this obstruction may cause retention with overflow incontinence or may cause increased bladder contractility and urge-pattern incontinence.

4. The older individual is frequently borderline in terms of maintaining continence because of normal changes in the urinary tract that occur with aging. These "normal" changes include reduced ability to delay urination, increased frequency of bladder contractions, reduced strength of bladder contractions, increased postvoid residual volumes, and increased nighttime production of urine. In addition, many elders have reduced mobility. The decreased ability to delay voiding, reduced mobility, and increased frequency of bladder contractions place the individual at risk for incontinence; the addition of a transient factor that further increases bladder irritability and sensory urgency (such as urinary tract infection) frequently tips the balance and causes temporary incontinence. The younger individual has better ability to delay voiding, better mobility, and a more stable bladder muscle; urinary tract infection in this person typically produces frequency and urgency, but it does not cause incontinence.

5. *False.* Alpha-adrenergic agonists (such as ephedrine) do not increase the risk for stress incontinence. Alpha-adrenergic antagonists (such as doxazosin) increase the risk for stress incontinence because they cause relaxation of the smooth muscle in the bladder neck and proximal portion of the urethra. Alpha-adrenergic agonists actually increase smooth muscle tone and therefore help to prevent stress incontinence.

True. Angiotensin-converting enzyme (ACE) inhibitors may worsen stress incontinence because of the dry cough that is a common side effect. Such a dry cough increases the intraabdominal pressure and may result in urinary leakage in the patient with weak pelvic floor musculature.

False. Calcium-channel blockers do affect bladder function or continence. Calcium-channel blockers reduce smooth muscle tone and contractility and therefore have the potential to affect bladder contractility and urethral resistance. The dihydropyridine group of calcium-channel blockers is particularly likely to reduce bladder contractility, which may result in overflow incontinence. This class of calcium-channel blockers also increases nocturnal urine production, which can cause nocturia or enuresis. A common side effect of calcium-channel blockers is constipation, which in itself can contribute to frequency, urgency, leakage, and incomplete emptying.

True. Urinary retention is a potential side effect of medications or components of medications with anticholinergic properties. Anticholinergic medications block the effects of parasympathetic stimuli, which mediate bladder contraction. Urinary retention is therefore a common side effect of anticholinergic medications.

False. Workup for the patient with acute onset urinary incontinence should routinely include urinalysis because urinary tract infection is a common contributing factor, and many elderly individuals have no signs of infection or present only with new-onset incontinence and possibly some mild alteration in mental status. A culture of the urine should be sent if the urinalysis demonstrates evidence of infection such as leukocytes, nitrites, or bacteria.

6. The most typical presentation for the patient with benign prostatic hyperplasia is an overflow pattern of incontinence, resulting from mechanical obstruction to urinary flow. However, the patient may also present with urge-pattern incontinence attributable to the changes in the bladder muscle that occur with long-standing obstruction to flow. In this situation, the detrusor muscle hypertrophies in

an attempt to produce the contractile force needed to expel the urine past the obstructed urethra. Over time, the hypertrophic muscle decompensates and becomes inappropriately contractile; the increased contractility of the detrusor muscle may cause urge-pattern incontinence. However, this "detrusor overactivity" may also cause urgency and frequency but no leakage if the individual has good sphincter function and is able to reach the bathroom quickly.

7. As noted in the answer to question number 6, the detrusor muscle responds to long-standing outlet obstruction by becoming hypertrophic, which increases its contractile force; it also tends to decompensate and to become more contractile, which results in increasing numbers of involuntary contractions. For a period of time postoperatively, the detrusor continues to function as it did when there was obstruction to flow; that is, the detrusor contracts inappropriately and forcefully, producing acute incontinence.

8. Surgical procedures involving the pelvic organs may affect continence by altering the position of the bladder and urethra or by causing inadvertent damage to the nerve pathways mediating bladder contractility and sphincter function. The most common mechanism by which pelvic surgery alters continence is by its effect on nerve function. If the parasympathetic pathways are damaged, the patient typically experiences urinary retention with or without overflow incontinence. Conversely, damage to the nerves innervating the urethral sphincter mechanism tends to cause stress incontinence. Typically, the bladder sphincter dysfunction improves over time as the damaged pathways recover.

9. Reduced compliance results in high intravesical pressures during the filling phase. This elevation in intravesical pressure opposes delivery of urine from the kidneys (because the ureteral transport system is a low-pressure system), which causes hydronephrosis and progressive renal damage. In addition, the high intravesical pressures tend to damage the

ureterovesical junction. The damaged junctions may then permit reflux of urine, which further damages the kidneys.

10. Assessment of a patient with acute urinary incontinence includes the following: a detailed history of the presenting complaint; review of genitourinary, gastrointestinal, gynecologic/obstetric systems; past medical and surgical history; psychosocial assessment; correlation of symptoms with 3-day bladder diary (if feasible); a focused physical exam; and simple diagnostics (urinalysis and postvoid residual). Management includes reducing or eliminating any reversible causes (review DIAPPERS) followed by reassessment of continence status. Further treatment may be required if the incontinence persists and involves interventions specific to the type of chronic urinary incontinence (such as pelvic muscle exercises for stress incontinence symptoms).

CHAPTER 4

1. Urethral hypermobility (loss of anatomic support for the bladder base and urethra) is common among women as a result of factors such as vaginal delivery, hysteric- of pelvic floor support does not occur in men. Damage to the nerves and muscles of the sphincter mechanism may occur in either women or men; causative factors in women include obstetric trauma and trauma associated with pelvic surgery, and the primary causative factor in men is trauma caused by radical prostatectomy.

2. (a) *Bladder chart.* Provides data regarding frequency of leakage and triggering events

   (b) *Pad-weight testing.* Quantifies volume of urine lost during various activities/provocative maneuvers

   (c) *Pelvic exam.* This is a critical element of the evaluation for a woman with stress UI. The vaginal mucosa and urethra are inspected for evidence of estrogen deficiency (atrophic vaginitis/urethritis), and the clinician also looks for evidence of altered anatomic support for the bladder and urethra (e.g., evidence of cystocele, rectocele, or pelvic organ prolapse; urethral deviation as opposed to midline position of the urethra). Pelvic muscle function is evaluated, including contractile strength and endurance. The patient is asked to cough forcefully and the clinician observes for simultaneous leakage of urine (which is indicative of stress UI).

(d) *Anal wink and bulbocavernosus reflex.* Positive findings are indicative of intact nerve pathways between the sacral cord and the pelvis.

(e) *Cystometrogram/videourodynamics.* Provides for differentiation between leakage caused by sphincter dysfunction (SUI) and leakage caused by overactive bladder (UUI). Data provided may help to differentiate between SUI caused primarily by urethral hypermobility and SUI caused primarily by intrinsic urethral weakness (also known as intrinsic sphincter deficiency, or ISD). Videourodynamic studies provide fluoroscopic imaging with pressure flow studies, which permits clinician to correlate leakage with clearly visualized abnormalities (such as urethral hypermobility, pelvic organ prolapse, or open bladder neck/intrinsic urethral weakness). Videourodynamics are considered by some to be the "gold standard" for diagnosis of SUI.

(f) *Urethral pressure profile.* Provides data regarding maximum urethral pressure, maximum urethral closure pressure, and functional urethral length. This test has somewhat limited value because there are no clearly defined "normal" values; however, MUCP (maximum urethral closure pressure) <20 cm H_2O is generally considered indicative of intrinsic urethral weakness (ISD), and MUCP >30 cm H_2O is generally thought to "R/O" ISD. (Values between 20 and 30 cm of H_2O are considered indeterminate.)

(g) *Leak point pressure (LPP).* LPP reflects the amount of force required to force urine past the sphincter. Values < 60 cm H_2O are considered indicative of ISD, values between 60 and 90 cm H_2O are considered to be a "gray zone," and values >100 cm H_2O are generally considered to "R/O" ISD as the major cause of leakage. (Medicare requires LPP <100 cm H_2O for the diagnosis of ISD and coverage for urethral bulking procedures.)

(h) *Ultrasound.* Can be used to assess urethral mobility, pelvic organ prolapse, urethral vascularity, and pelvic muscle contractility

3. • *Patient selection criteria* for pelvic muscle exercise program include the following: intact anatomic support for urethra and bladder base; absence of significant pelvic organ prolapse; demonstrated ability to volitionally contract the pelvic floor muscles; and patient who is motivated and cognitively intact.

   • *Guidelines:* Clinician must first assist patient to accurately identify and isolate the pelvic floor muscles (either via digital exam or urine stream interruption test); must then establish an individualized exercise program based on the patient's initial strength and endurance; and gradually increase the goals as the patient gains both contractile strength and the ability to "hold" the contraction. Studies suggest that a strong focus on endurance is particularly beneficial for most patients. There are no clear guidelines on either the number of repetitions/day or the specific "approach"—most clinicians recommend 30–45 repetitions per day (3 sets of 15 exercises). Some clinicians separate "quick flick" exercises (for fast twitch fibers) and "contract and hold" exercises (for slow twitch fibers) but many use a combined approach (contract as hard as you can and hold for as long as you can). Regardless of approach, patients must be instructed to *relax* the muscle following each contraction (for 10 seconds or for a period of time equal to the contraction time). Once the patient demonstrates the ability to correctly contract the pelvic muscles, she is taught the "Knack" (purposeful contraction just prior to activities that cause increased abdominal pressure and urinary leakage.)

4. *Biofeedback* provides visual and/or auditory feedback regarding contraction of the desired muscle groups, which can help patients learn to isolate and contract the "target muscle group."

5. *Electrical stimulation* activates afferent pudendal fibers, which causes reflex activation of sympathetic and pudendal efferents; this results in contraction of the smooth and striated muscles in the pelvic floor and in reflex inhibition of the detrusor. More research is needed to clearly identify the benefits and role of e-stim in treatment of SUI; studies to date show comparable results for patients treated with pelvic muscle exercises/behavioral treatment and those treated with e-stim. Treatment typically involves 15–30 minute treatment sessions 1–3 times per week (@ 50–100 Hz). *Magnetic innervation* uses a powerful magnet to induce electrical depolarization of the nerves and muscles in the pelvic floor, resulting in a strong muscle contraction. One advantage to this therapy is its non-invasive nature; the patient sits, fully clothed, in the "magnetic chair." Preliminary studies show positive results but more data are needed.

6. *Indications for surgical intervention include:* initial therapy for patient with coexisting pelvic organ prolapse, loss of anatomic support and severe leakage, or marked ISD; initial therapy for patient with SUI caused by urethral hypermobility who prefers surgery to behavioral therapy; and second-line therapy for patient with SUI caused by urethral hypermobility who "fails" conservative therapy.
Options for patient with SUI caused by urethral hypermobility: (1) retropubic colpo- suspension (procedures that elevate and stabilize the tissues surrounding the bladder neck and proximal urethra in a retropubic and intraabdominal position, thus preventing urethral descent); these procedures do *not* provide urethral compression so are not good choices for patients with SUI caused by ISD. (2) mid-urethral tension-free sling procedures (minimally invasive procedures involving placement of a polypropylene mesh tape at the level of the mid-urethra; this stimulates collagen synthesis along the length of the tape, which secures and stabilizes the urethra at mid-point).
Options for patient with SUI caused primarily by ISD: (1) injection of a "bulking" agent into the urethral walls to increase urethral resistance (frequently requires multiple injections and repetitive treatments); (2) suburethral sling procedures (placement of a strip of fascia or synthetic material underneath the urethra); the ends of the strip are then anchored to retropubic or abdominal structures to elevate and slightly compress the urethra, thus increasing urethral resistance; and (3) placement of an artificial urinary sphincter.

7. Urodynamics are generally considered an essential element of the workup for a patient contemplating surgery because these tests can accurately differentiate SUI caused by urethral hypermobility from SUI caused by intrinsic sphincter deficiency. This is critical since the two conditions require different surgical procedures.

8. *Topical estrogen* reverses urogenital atrophy and helps to restore normal softness and coaptation to the urethral walls. Estrogen also helps to increase the sensitivity of the alpha adrenergic receptors in the bladder neck and proximal urethra to adrenergic stimulation.
Duloxetine (which is not yet approved by the FDA for treatment of SUI), is a balanced norepinephrine-serotonin reuptake inhibitor, and norepinephrine and serotonin are the two primary neurotransmitters for the smooth and striated muscles in the urethra. Thus this drug acts to increase sphincter tone and contractility and to increase urethral closure pressure. Very positive results in clinical trials but *not yet approved.*

9. *Pessaries* are intravaginal devices that support the urethrovesical junction in a more

anatomic position and also reduce pelvic organ prolapse.

Femsoft urethral plugs are disposable slender balloon-tipped devices that can be used to occlude the female urethra and to prevent leakage.

CHAPTER **5**

1. *Urge urinary incontinence* (urge UI) is defined as "the complaint of involuntary leakage accompanied by or immediately preceded by urgency." Urge UI may present clinically either as frequent episodes of low-volume leakage between voluntary voids or as major high-volume leakage associated with complete bladder emptying.

   Overactive bladder(OAB) syndrome is the term used to describe urinary urgency, *with or without urge UI,* and typically combined with urinary frequency and nocturia. The term "overactive bladder" is synonymous with the terms "urge syndrome" and "urgency-frequency syndrome."

   Detrusor hyperactivity with impaired contractility refers to a condition in which a patient with an overactive but poorly contractile bladder has a desire to void that is frequent and typically urgent, but because the bladder does not squeeze well, emptying during voiding is less than complete. It is most common in elders who have no evidence of bladder outlet obstruction.

2. Any five of the factors listed in Table 5-2 or Table 5-3

3. Increased urinary frequency, urgency, nocturia, and (sometimes) urge UI

4. (1) Initial evaluation including general history
   (2) Symptom review including simple frequency-volume chart
   (3) Assessment of both impact on quality of life and desire for treatment

5. • Identification of contributing factors
   • Assessment for conditions other than OAB that could produce the reported symptoms
   • Identification and characterization of symptoms
   • Identification of any transient factors contributing to OAB or impaired emptying

6. • Either sex: recurrent UI; UI associated with pain, hematuria, recurrent infection, voiding symptoms, radical pelvic surgery
   • Men: UI associated with prostate irradiation
   • Women: UI associated with pelvic radiation or suspected fistula; significant postvoid residual, pelvic mass, or significant pelvic organ prolapse

7. Life-style interventions: dietary and fluid control measures, weight control, smoking cessation, pelvic floor muscle training, urge suppression training, bladder retraining

8. Bladder training is a specific program designed to increase bladder capacity and to reduce urinary frequency; it is indicated for motivated and cognitively intact individuals with OAB symptoms or stress UI. It consists of comprehensive patient education with a focus on strategies for controlling urgency and delaying voiding, scheduled voiding programs with progressive extension of the voiding interval, and positive reinforcement.

9. Urgency suppression involves contraction of the pelvic floor muscles in an attempt to reduce the sensation of urgency and to inhibit the bladder overactivity that caused it. Key components include discontinuation of all movement and repeated pelvic floor muscle contractions. Sometimes specialized breathing techniques, mind distraction, and body relaxation techniques are included. Once the urge subsides, patients are instructed either to walk slowly to the bathroom and void or to wait until a predetermined time (if they are participating in bladder training).

10. Antimuscarinic medications decrease bladder contractility (reducing overactivity) during urine storage by blocking muscarinic receptors (cholinergic receptors) in the detrusor muscle.

11. • Implanted neuromodulation
    • Bladder augmentation

12. To date, clinical trials reveal that no single therapy provides easy, rapid, and dramatic cure for most individuals suffering with OAB. For patients who do not respond well enough to monotherapy, clinical trials do show better efficacy with a gradually stepped and combined therapeutic approach.

13. The actual approach depends on the individual clinical situation. For most patients, however, a treatment plan that utilizes the safest and least invasive therapies (often behavioral) first and adds or adjusts from there offers the best chance for meeting the patient's goals.

CHAPTER **6**

1. Functional incontinence can be defined as loss of urine and/or stool caused by factors outside the urinary and/or gastrointestinal tract that interfere with the ability to respond in a socially appropriate way to the urge to void or defecate.

2. (a) *Impaired cognition.* The individual loses the ability to interpret the sensation of bladder fullness accurately, to remember the socially appropriate response, to inhibit detrusor contractions until an appropriate time and place to void, to locate the toilet facilities, to prepare for toileting and/or perform personal hygiene. Additional mental impairments related to dementia that can affect continence include aphasia, agnosia, perceptual confusion, apraxia, and loss of executive function.

(b) *Poor motivation.* Functional incontinence can be caused in total or in part by poor motivation to be continent. A diagnosis of depression may result in impaired physical, mental, and social functioning, which can affect the desire and ability to be continent. In some situations, incontinence may be a conscious choice because the physical effort required to use the toilet is valued as being too burdensome such as in the presence of acute or chronic pain, weakness, and fatigue.

(c) *Immobility.* The individual is unable to reach the toilet facilities in a timely manner,

that is, before detrusor contractions overwhelm the continence mechanism. Functional incontinence results when timely access to a toilet, bedpan, urinal or commode is compromised by a loss of independent mobility. For example, incontinence can occur when a wheelchair-bound person or one dependent on a cane or walker cannot access a toilet because the only toilet facilities are inaccessible to a person requiring an assistive device (for example, the bathroom is located up a flight of stairs or is too small to accommodate a wheelchair or walker).

(d) *Impaired manual dexterity.* Compromised manual dexterity related to joint deformities and/or pain from arthritis can interfere with the ability to open bathroom doors, manage clothing, perform hygiene, or flush a toilet.

3. Functional incontinence in institutional settings is caused by a complex combination of factors, some of which are directly linked to the culture of the institution, as well as issues related to staffing, staff education and commitment to continence. Staff in institutions may not consistently respond to requests for toileting, properly execute a toileting program, or make necessary environmental changes that support continence.

4. Some changes in bladder function associated with aging also contribute to increased risk for incontinence. Older adults have a decrease in bladder size and increase in postvoid residual urine. This normal change of aging reduces functional bladder capacity and causes increased voiding frequency. In the presence of impaired mobility, increased voiding frequency can increase risk of incontinence because the older adult may not be able to reach the toilet in time consistently. Older adults can also experience increased urine production at night, that is, nocturnal polyuria. Frequent nighttime urination contributes to functional incontinence when an older adult has difficulty getting out of bed or takes excessive time to do so. Older adults can also experience increased frequency of uninhibited bladder contractions causing urgency and frequency, which can cause incontinence if impaired mobility and cognition interfere with toilet access.

5. A cognitive assessment helps to shed light on the functional cause of the incontinence and is the first step in planning appropriate interventions. A diagnosis of dementia does not mean that the incontinence cannot be treated. A treatment plan can be designed that capitalizes on cognitive ability and supports areas of deficit. For example, persons with agnosia may not be able to recognize the toilet but may be able to follow instructions on how to use the toilet. There may be significant memory problems, but reading signs that give directions on when to use the toilet may not be a problem. Even persons with significant cognitive deficits can benefit from a consistent toileting schedule.

6. The assessment for functional incontinence should include an evaluation of all factors that can influence timely access to a toilet or toilet substitute. When the clinician suspects functional incontinence, either alone or in combination with other types of incontinence, the evaluation should include a careful assessment of cognition, other mental impairments, motivation, fear, mobility and coordination, manual dexterity, the living environment, clothing, the use of containment products, devices or equipment that restrain independent movement, and the ability, motivation and education of caregivers to promote and support continence.

7. Environmental modifications that are relatively simple to implement but can make a significant impact on continence include the following:
   - Replacing chairs that make it difficult to rise to a standing position (such as recliners and chairs with deep cushions) with chairs with firm arms and cushions
   - Improving lighting in the bathroom
   - Replacing clothing with buttons, snaps or zippers with clothing with elastic waists
   - Removing obstructing objects from the pathway to the bathroom
   - Replacing the use of an adult brief containment product with a product that can be easily pulled up and down such as an incontinence undergarment

8.

	Indications	**Implementation**	**Limitations**
Routine scheduled toileting	Persons with significant cognitive impairment, who are unable to identify or communicate the need to void and/or defecate	The patient uses the toilet on predetermined routine such as every 2 hours or an institutional schedule such as: on awakening, before and after meals, and before bed.	Not highly effective but does decrease the number of incontinent episodes Caregiver dependent Continence relies on chance
Habit training	Persons with moderate cognitive impairment, who are cooperative with toileting, will void when toileted or reminded to toilet	A voiding pattern is discovered using a bladder record, and the person is reminded to use the toilet or is taken to the toilet before the identified voiding times.	Caregiver dependent Requires motivated caregivers who need extensive education concerning program Consistent compliance to the schedule essential for success; may not be realistic in many care environments

Continued

	Indications	**Implementation**	**Limitations**
Prompted voiding	Mild to moderate cognitive impairment, voids when toileted, does not recognize the urge to void or does not act on urge, but has enough cognitive ability that can be trained to recognize that urge and execute toileting behaviors	The caregiver will approach the incontinent person, question him or her about continence, and give positive reinforcement for desired behavior that includes recognizing wetness, urge, voiding on the toilet, and continence.	Caregiver dependent Requires motivated caregivers who need extensive education concerning program Very labor intensive, thus difficult to implement in institutional settings. Consistent compliance to the schedule essential for success; may not be realistic in many care environment

CHAPTER **7**

1. Reflex incontinence (reflex UI) refers to the involuntary loss of urine caused by a hyperreflexic (uncontrolled) contraction of the detrusor muscle in response to bladder filling or other stimuli. It typically occurs in the absence of any sensory urgency to void, and is caused by neurologic lesions affecting spinal cord segments C2 to S1. It is frequently accompanied by detrusor-sphincter dyssynergia (DSD).

2. Neurogenic detrusor overactivity is a form of detrusor instability that is caused by a neurologic disorder. There is loss of central nervous system control over bladder function, and the bladder contracts spontaneously (in reflex fashion) in response to bladder filling and to other stimuli. DSD (detrusor-sphincter dyssynergia) refers to loss of coordination between the bladder and the sphincter. Normally, the pontine micturition center coordinates sphincter relaxation and bladder contraction so voiding always occurs through an "open door." With loss of pontine control, the sphincter may contract constantly or at intervals throughout bladder contraction, thus producing bladder outlet obstruction.

3. This statement is explained by a brief review of normal voiding physiology and the pathways controlling bladder and sphincter function. Voluntary control of voiding and coordination between the bladder and the sphincter are mediated by the central nervous system, primarily the cortex and pons. (The cortex provides conscious awareness of the urge to void and the ability to delay voiding by inhibition of the pontine micturition center. The pons provides for coordination between bladder contraction and sphincter relaxation.) If the lesion is above the pons, voluntary control and the ability to inhibit the pons and delay voiding are lost, but coordinated voiding is maintained, and so this patient will exhibit the signs of urge incontinence. Patients with lesions between C2 and the pons typically do not survive because of damage to the vital centers. Patients with lesions below S1 typically develop overflow incontinence because the parasympathetic nerve pathway that mediates bladder contractions comes off the spinal cord at the sacral level (S2), and a lesion at this level destroys or damages the outflow tract that causes bladder contractions.

4. (1) *Urinary leakage.* Because of the loss of sensory awareness and voluntary control, most patients are unable to predict, delay, or voluntarily initiate voiding. This has

tremendous consequences in terms of quality of life and ability to resume usual activities. The assessment of a patient with reflex UI must include onset and duration of incontinence, patterns of leakage, present management, life style, and goals, and the management plan must include measures for prevention or effective containment of leakage.

(2) *Potential effect on upper tract function.* Most patients with reflex UI develop DSD, which causes bladder outlet obstruction; this predisposes the patient to incomplete bladder emptying and urinary tract infections (UTIs). Uncontrolled DSD and repetitive UTIs predispose to low bladder compliance, which impairs the delivery of urine from the kidneys. The presence of outflow obstruction, UTI, and reduced bladder wall compliance jointly produce a syndrome known as "hostile bladder function"—bladder dysfunction that threatens the upper tracts.

Long-standing failure to address DSD adequately and to ensure effective bladder emptying can result in renal insufficiency and renal failure. The assessment of any patient with reflex UI must include measures to rule out or quantify the degree of outflow obstruction, to measure postvoid residual, and to determine the detrusor forces during filling and emptying. The *primary* goal of any management plan must be preservation of renal function.

Thus, effective management of any patient with reflex UI must include measures to maintain low bladder pressures and effective bladder emptying, to prevent or promptly treat symptomatic UTIs, and to prevent or control leakage.

5. (a) The most appropriate management plan for this patient would probably be intermittent catheterization (IC). He has the mobility and the motivation, and IC would effectively empty the bladder without requiring high-pressure bladder contractions. IC would provide this patient with continence and with protection of the upper tracts.

(b) The most appropriate option for this patient would be an indwelling catheter, which would provide bladder drainage and preserve her current level of independence. Absorptive products are not a realistic option, because she would be unable to change them; in addition, her DSD presents a somewhat hostile bladder condition, and a reflex voiding program places this relatively young patient at risk for upper tract damage. The only other realistic option would be to consider a continent diversion with an abdominal stoma, which would facilitate catheterization for this chairbound patient; however, a continent diversion involves major surgery and the potential for other complications.

(c) Reflex voiding program with condom catheter containment would be the best option for this patient. He is not a candidate for spontaneous voiding at this time; he does not want to perform IC, and an indwelling catheter would increase his risk for UTIs and upper tract damage. His urodynamic studies indicate that a reflex voiding program should provide effective emptying and that his bladder is "nonhostile."

6. (a) This patient would benefit from alpha-adrenergic antagonists, because these drugs reduce urethral resistance and thus improve bladder emptying and reduce the detrusor forces required to empty the bladder. The patient would need to be counseled regarding the potential for orthostatic hypotension and the importance of dose titration and bedtime administration. The patient should also be counseled to avoid over-the-counter decongestants, because these drugs oppose the intended therapeutic effect of the alpha-adrenergic antagonist.

(b) This patient would benefit from anticholinergic medications, because these medications tend to reduce hyperreflexic detrusor contractions. The patient would need to be counseled regarding the potential for dry mouth, heat intolerance, constipation, and temporary blurred vision.

Patients with narrow-angle glaucoma must be evaluated by an ophthalmologist before beginning treatment with an anticholinergic agent.

7. (a) *False.* Prophylactic and suppressive antibiotic therapy regimens are recommended for the patient with reflex UI because of the risk for UTI and upper tract damage.

Antibiotic therapy is recommended only for individuals with symptomatic UTIs, because treatment of asymptomatic UTIs and suppressive therapy tend to produce resistant organisms and the risk for serious and "untreatable" UTIs.

(b) *True.* Autonomic dysreflexia is a potentially fatal complication for the patient with a cervical or upper thoracic cord injury and can be precipitated by bladder distension.

Noxious stimuli such as bladder distension are the most common "triggers" for the massive sympathetic discharge that is known as "autonomic dysreflexia." It produces dangerously high blood-pressure levels that cause stroke or death. Prompt treatment, that is, elimination of the noxious stimulus and administration of sublingual nifedipine or another antihypertensive agent, is essential.

(c) *True.* Patients with UTIs caused by urease-producing bacteria are at increased risk for formation of calculi.

Urease-producing bacteria, such as *Proteus*, increase the risk for stone formation because they split urea to form ammonia, which raises both the concentration of ammonia and the urinary pH; these increases promote the precipitation of ammonium phosphate and the formation of magnesium-ammonium phosphate stones.

8. In the management of the patient with reflex UI, the ultimate goal is always maintenance of renal function and preservation of life and general health. The patient with low compliance (that is, a high-pressure, low-volume bladder) is at great risk for progressive renal damage and premature death because low bladder compliance results in a "hostile bladder" that opposes delivery of urine from the kidneys.

Bladder augmentation and continent urinary diversion are two surgical approaches to creation of a low-pressure reservoir. Bladder augmentation involves enlargement of the bladder and interruption of the contractile muscle fibers. Continent urinary diversion involves creation of a low-pressure reservoir using small bowel or stomach segments. The reservoir is connected to the abdominal wall by a narrow catheterizable channel. These "low-pressure" reservoirs are drained at intervals by use of IC.

CHAPTER **8**

1. Urinary retention represents dysfunction in the voiding (emptying) component of the storage-voiding cycle. Emptying difficulties may greatly affect upper urinary tract function in the following ways:

- Retention results in high intravesical pressures that tend to collapse the ureters and to impede the delivery of urine from the kidneys to the bladder (whenever the intravesical pressures exceed the ureteral pressures, urine delivery is impaired.) This condition can result in hydronephrosis.
- Some patients with retention also experience reduced compliance or detrusor overactivity. Both these factors increase the risk for upper tract damage by increasing intravesical pressure during the storage phase of the storage-voiding cycle.
- If the patient has any vesicoureteral reflux, high intravesical pressures increase the volume and frequency of reflux, which increases the risk for upper tract damage.

2. The two primary processes resulting in retention are as follows:

(1) Bladder outlet obstruction caused by conditions such as prostatic hypertrophy or

creation of excessive urethral resistance during an antiincontinence procedure in a woman with stress incontinence

(2) Reduced bladder contractility caused by primary damage to the bladder muscle or by temporary or permanent interference with the nerve pathways that mediate detrusor contractility (such as postoperative retention caused by sympathetic stimulation and analgesic interference with bladder contractility, or loss of innervation from a spinal cord injury, multiple sclerosis, or diabetes)

If the retention is caused by obstruction, the focus of treatment is generally on elimination of the obstructing lesion. However, there is currently no effective mechanism for restoring detrusor muscle function or normal innervation; therefore, patients with impaired contractility are typically managed with supportive strategies such as behavioral methods to enhance bladder emptying, pharmacologic agents to reduce urethral resistance, or clean intermittent catheterization (CIC).

3. Acute retention is typically characterized by the sudden complete inability to void, and these patients are usually acutely symptomatic; they commonly present to the emergency department in extreme distress. In contrast, chronic retention usually occurs gradually and is characterized by progressive bladder distension and rising residuals accompanied by "overflow" voiding or leakage. The patient with chronic retention typically has "low grade" voiding complaints; he or she may complain of difficulty initiating the urinary stream, prolonged voiding times, weak stream, and postvoid dribble, or may be relatively unaware of the problem.

4. Strategies to reduce the risk of acute urinary retention in the postoperative patient include the following: avoidance excessive intravenous fluid administration; effective pain management; careful monitoring for evidence of retention, especially in patients who are heavily sedated or who have had spinal anesthesia; administration of alpha-adrenergic antagonists when indicated; and prompt in-and-out catheterization for the patient who is unable to void effectively (to prevent excessive bladder distension).

5. Lower urinary tract symptoms include indicators of impaired emptying (hesitancy, poor flow, straining to initiate the urinary stream, and intermittent or prolonged stream) and symptoms of impaired storage (frequency, urgency, and nocturia). In the past, these symptoms were collectively labeled "prostatism" because they were thought to be caused primarily by prostatic hypertrophy; it is now recognized that these symptoms are general indicators of lower urinary tract dysfunction, they occur in both men and women, and they may be produced by a wide variety of pathologic conditions. Thus, the constellation of symptoms is now known simply as LUTS (lower urinary tract symptoms).

6. Acute urinary retention typically involves total inability to void and is accompanied by increasingly severe abdominal pain, tenderness to palpation, and possibly related symptoms (nausea, tachycardia, diaphoresis). Chronic urinary retention usually involves progressive difficulty *emptying* the bladder; the patient typically presents with symptoms such as hesitancy, poor flow, straining to initiate the urinary stream, and intermittent or prolonged urination (but no pain or tenderness to palpation).

7. Urodynamic studies include pressure flow studies carried out during the voiding component of the micturition cycle; pressure-flow studies provide insight into both detrusor function and urethral function during voiding. Outlet obstruction is manifest by high detrusor contractile pressures coupled with low urinary flow rates, whereas impaired contractility is characterized by low detrusor contractile pressures accompanied by low urinary flow rates.

8. Static factors contributing to outlet obstruction include overall size of the prostate gland, and size of the median lobe; a significantly enlarged prostate gland contributes to outlet obstruction by causing urethral compression. Studies indicate that men with prostate glands larger than 30 mL are three times more likely to experience retention than men whose prostate glands are smaller than 30 mL. However, an enlarged median lobe can cause compression and retention even in the absence of significant overall prostate gland enlargement.

   Dynamic factors contributing to outlet obstruction include increased volume of smooth muscle and increased sympathetic tone within the prostatic urethra; these factors cause increased urethral resistance and thereby contribute to retention.

9. Surgical reduction of the prostate gland may not provide symptom relief for the patient with benign prostatic hyperplasia because there is very poor correlation among glandular size, degree of obstruction, and clinical symptoms. In addition, lower urinary tract symptoms may be caused by changes in the detrusor muscle itself that occur in response to prolonged obstruction; in this case, removal of the prostate would not necessarily relieve the symptoms.

   Finasteride is a 5-alpha-reductase inhibitor; it acts to inhibit the conversion of testosterone to dihydrotestosterone, which is a much more potent androgen. Finasteride interferes with androgenic stimulation of prostatic hyperplasia and has been shown gradually to reduce prostate size, specifically the size of the median lobe; it has also been shown to reduce the risk of acute urinary retention and surgical intervention. This drug seems to be most effective for men with large prostate glands; it works on the static component of urethral obstruction. Data from long-term studies indicate long-term efficacy and minimal side effects.

   Alpha-adrenergic antagonists oppose sympathetic stimulation at the level of the bladder neck and prostate smooth muscle.

The sympathetic nerve fibers mediate smooth muscle contraction and thereby produce increased urethral resistance. These drugs interfere with sympathetic stimulation, thus causing smooth muscle relaxation and reduced urethral resistance. (They work on the dynamic component of urethral obstruction.) Alpha-adrenergic antagonists have been shown to be effective in a wide variety of patients with urinary retention because of their ability to reduce urethral resistance. However, long-term data regarding their efficacy are not yet available, and these drugs cause a significant number of side effects.

10. • *Behavioral therapies.* Patient with chronic retention should be taught to space fluids regularly throughout the day and to avoid bolus fluid intake, to void on schedule, and to use "double-voiding" to improve bladder emptying. Patients with dyssynergia may benefit from biofeedback.
    • *CIC.* CIC is an effective tool for emptying the bladder and is generally considered the "treatment of choice" for patients with retention caused by reduced bladder contractility (assuming sufficient cognition, motivation, and manual dexterity).
    • *Indwelling catheterization.* Indwelling catheterization may be used on a short term basis to manage episodes of acute urinary retention, or it may be used to manage chronic retention in patients who are not candidates for CIC or other treatment strategies. (Indwelling catheterization is never considered first-line therapy for individuals with chronic retention; this approach should be limited to patients whose condition cannot be otherwise managed.)
    • *Alpha-adrenergic antagonists.* Alpha-adrenergic antagonists reduce urethral resistance and thus improve bladder emptying; they are particularly beneficial for patients with retention caused by excessive urethral resistance but may also be beneficial for patients with reduced contractility (because a poorly contractile

bladder empties more effectively when there is reduced outlet resistance).

- *Surgical removal of obstructing lesion or tissue.* This approach may be beneficial when the retention is caused by a specific obstructing lesion, such as a stricture or a urethral sling or an enlarged prostate. (Before undertaking surgical removal of the prostate, it may be helpful to perform urodynamic studies to quantify the factors contributing to the retention.)

11. • Assess patient's cognitive function, motivation, and ability to access the urethra before beginning the program.

- Teach the patient the principles and benefits of the program: use of a clean catheter to empty the bladder on a routine basis; reduced potential for serious long-term bladder and renal complications; reduced risk of incontinence; avoidance of an indwelling catheter.

- Use diagrams, models, and/or mirror to help the patient identify her urethral opening; begin teaching her to identify urethral meatus by touch. Assist the patient to insert a lubricated catheter into bladder and to drain urine; as the patient gains skill and confidence, shift your role to that of a supportive onlooker.

- Collaborate with the patient to establish an appropriate catheterization schedule based on her bladder capacity and fluid intake patterns; explain to her that the goal is to catheterize frequently enough to prevent leakage and significant distension. Use urodynamic data and bladder chart as tools to determine patient's bladder capacity; modify the catheterization schedule and fluid intake patterns until appropriate volumes are obtained during the majority of catheterizations.

- Work with the patient to ensure appropriate fluid intake, that is, adequate volumes fairly evenly spaced with reduction or elimination of caffeinated beverages and alcohol. (The alternative to evenly spaced fluids is further modification of the catheterization schedule

to provide more frequent catheterizations during periods of increased fluid intake.)

- Teach the patient proper care of the equipment.

- Teach the patient the early signs of infection (recurrent leakage) and the appropriate response (prompt notification of health care provider).

CHAPTER **9**

1. (**d**) Stress incontinence is the most common type of postprostatectomy incontinence (PPI) and is caused by damage to the sphincter mechanism; some of the voluntary musculature is removed along with the prostatic urethra, and there is also the potential for damage to the nerves or muscles of the remaining sphincter muscles.

   Urge incontinence (overactive bladder) may occur as well, either from persistence of high-pressure bladder contractions originally caused by the partial obstruction produced by the enlarged prostate or as a result of surgical damage to the nerves innervating the bladder.

2. (**c**) Data to date suggest that the factor most critical to maintenance of continence is the extent to which the maximum possible urethral length is preserved. Studies indicate that this approach reduces both the incidence of PPI and the prevalence of persistent PPI. In contrast, the impact of a nerve-sparing approach or preservation of the bladder neck is unclear; data from available studies are contradictory in terms of results. There *is* evidence that the incidence and prevalence of PPI are higher in men more than 65 years of age; however, current data do not clearly support any connection between age and persistent PPI.

3. • *Rhabdosphincter.* The rhabdosphincter is a striated urethral sphincter muscle that extends proximally from the point at which the ejaculatory and prostatic ducts open into the urethra, to a point 2.5 cm distal to the prostate gland. The prostatic portion of this muscle is removed during prostatectomy; however, the portion of the rhabdosphincter distal to the prostate gland is preserved and is critical to postoperative continence. Stress incontinence is more likely when there is damage to the sphincter itself or to the pudendal nerve, when scar tissue alters the mobility of the muscle, and/or when the urethra is shortened to a total length of less than 2.5 cm.

- *High-pressure bladder contractions.* Prostate tumors frequently cause some degree of bladder outlet obstruction; in response, the bladder becomes hypercontractile and mounts high-pressure contractions to overcome the resistance produced by the prostatic obstruction. When these high-pressure contractions persist after prostatectomy, they contribute to overactive bladder and urge incontinence. In addition, prolonged bladder outlet obstruction may cause hypertrophy and connective tissue infiltration of the bladder muscle, which results in poor detrusor compliance that further contributes to frequency and urgency postoperatively.

4. • *History.* Onset, duration, and frequency of incontinent episodes to include triggering factors and volume of leakage; any associated symptoms (urgency, frequency, dysuria, hesitancy, incomplete emptying, nocturia); impact on quality of life (current management, stress level, self-esteem, support system); medical-surgical history with focus on any presurgical incontinence, neurologic conditions, urethral stricture, or pelvic radiation; current medications; fiber and fluid intake (bladder irritants?); bowel function; cognitive and functional status.

- *Physical exam.* Neurologic exam (cognition, gait, balance, manual dexterity); abdominal exam to rule out evidence of bladder distension; anorectal exam (sensory status, sphincter tone and contractility, presence of fecal impaction).

- *Bladder diary* (time and amount of voided urine and episodes of leakage; fluid intake).

- *Cough test, urinalysis, and postvoid residual* (if any evidence of retention).

5. • *Fluid modifications:* Teach the patient to take in enough fluid to maintain dilute urine (at least 1.5 to 2 liters/day) and to limit intake of foods that may be bladder irritants (such as caffeinated beverages and foods containing caffeine).

- *Dietary modifications:* Teach the patient to consume sufficient fiber (along with fluid) to prevent constipation, because constipation increases urgency and frequency.

- *Pelvic muscle exercises:* Assist the patient to isolate the pelvic floor muscles and to learn to contract these muscles without contracting the accessory muscles (abdominal, buttock, and thigh muscles); then instruct the patient to contract these muscles for 10 seconds 15 to 20 times three times daily (the patient may have to "work up" to the 10-second "hold"); then teach the the patient to contract these muscles voluntarily immediately before activities that typically produce leakage.

6. • *Anticholinergic agents* (such as tolterodine): these agents reduce bladder contractility and help to alleviate symptoms of overactive bladder, such as urgency and frequency). These agents are indicated for patients with "urge-pattern" or "mixed" incontinence.

- *Serotonin-norepinephrine uptake inhibitor* (duloxetine): Serotonin and norephinephrine are the primary neurotransmitters for urethral sphincter contractility; therefore, a combined serotonin-norepinephrine uptake inhibitor has been evaluated for treatment of stress incontinence. Clinical trials have shown impressive improvement, and one drug (duloxetine) is expected to obtain Food and Drug Administration approval for use in the United States within the next year. This drug would be indicated for management of stress incontinence.

7. • *Urethral bulking procedures:* These procedures involve injection of a "bulking" material into the bladder neck and are considered a first-line surgical intervention. Advantages include the fact that the procedure can be done on an

outpatient basis and the low incidence of complications; disadvantages include the fact that repeated injections are frequently needed and the lack of durable results.

- *Suburethral sling procedure:* These procedures involve implantation of a strip of fascia or other material beneath the urethra to act as a "sling" that increases urethral resistance and holds the bladder in position during periods of increased intraabdominal pressures. These procedures are most likely to be used for patients in whom bulking procedures fail.
- *Artificial urinary sphincter:* This procedure involves implantation of a three-part device (a pump that is placed in the scrotum, an inflatable cuff that is wrapped around the urethra, and a reservoir that is implanted in the subcutaneous tissue); continence is maintained by the fluid-filled cuff, and the patient is taught to deflate the cuff to void (by pumping the fluid out of the cuff into the reservoir). This procedure is considered a last resort for men in whom other procedures have failed.

CHAPTER 10

1. Indwelling catheters are the primary risk factor for nosocomial urinary tract infections and are associated with multiple other complications including damage to the bladder neck and sphincter, bladder stones, urethrocutaneous fistulas, and bladder cancer. Use of indwelling catheters increases the cost of care as a result of these many complications. In addition, indwelling catheters can have a negative impact on the patient's quality of life.

2. • *An elderly woman in long-term care with frequent episodes of urinary incontinence (UI) related to midstage Alzheimer's disease:* No, an indwelling catheter is not indicated; she should be managed with a toileting program and absorptive products.
   • *A male patient being cared for at home by his frail wife, who is unable to take him to the toilet or to change absorptive products:* Possibly. An external catheter should be considered first, but an indwelling catheter *is* appropriate if it is the only way the patient can be effectively managed by the home caregiver.
   • *A paraplegic woman who is unable to position herself for self-catheterization and whose husband works from 7 AM to 5 PM:* Possibly an indwelling catheter would provide for elimination of urine and would prevent reflux and retention. She should be evaluated for a continent urinary diversion however.
   • *A patient with a pressure ulcer on the trunk and UI:* Yes, an indwelling catheter should be used until the ulcer is healed and then should be discontinued.

3. Latex catheters are soft, flexible, conformable, and low cost. However, they are inappropriate for patients with latex sensitivity, and they *may* cause increased urethral irritation as compared with silicone catheters (note conflicting data on this point). Silicone catheters have thinner walls and therefore a larger lumen, which promotes drainage. In addition, they are less likely to collapse with aspiration, they resist encrustation, and they *may* reduce urethral irritation. However, they are firmer and therefore much less comfortable than the latex catheters, and the balloons have a tendency to cuff and crease with deflation, which can result in painful removal. (The balloons also tend to "leak down" because they are more permeable; thus, the balloons should have fluid added as needed [PRN].) Silastic catheters are latex catheters coated with silicone; they provide the comfort and flexibility of latex *and* the durability and reduced encrustation associated with silicone. However, they are not appropriate for patients with latex sensitivity.

4. Studies to date have all focused on the impact of antimicrobial coatings on infection rates in acute care settings and short-term catheter use; studies have shown that silver coatings can reduce the incidence of infection for up to 20 days. Studies have not yet been done on patients with long-term catheters; however, empiric use of antimicrobial catheters is appropriate for these patients, especially those who are "high risk."

5. Use the smallest effective catheter size, such as 14 to 18 Fr for adults.
   Rationale: Smaller catheters minimize urethral distortion and preserve urethral elasticity; smaller catheters also reduce urethral friction, reduce discomfort, and maintain the function of the paraurethral glands (which helps to protect against ascending bacteria).
   5-mL balloon (for adults) inflated according to manufacturers' guidelines (usually 10 mL).
   Rationale: Proper inflation of a small balloon assures symmetric inflation and minimizes irritation at the bladder neck, which reduces bladder spasms, discomfort, and leakage. Small balloons also help prevent damage to the bladder neck (which protects against leakage long-term).

6. *False.* Large balloons *increase* the risk of leakage because of irritation to the bladder.

7. A morbidly obese woman in whom urethra cannot be visualized in supine position: Use the side-lying position with particular caution to prevent contamination.
   A male patient with an enlarged prostate: Use a Coudé-tipped catheter; apply large mound of lubricant to urethral opening (or instill 10 mL of lubricant into the urethra); use steady gentle pressure to advance the catheter.
   A female patient whose urethra has prolapsed into her vagina: Insert a sterile gloved finger into vagina; slide the catheter along top of finger and upward into urethra.

8. (a) The catheter should be secured to the lower abdomen.

9. • Keep loops of tubing straight; avoid kinks and avoid any dependent loops.
   • Keep the drainage bag below the level of the bladder at all times.
   • Keep the drainage bag off the floor.
   • Empty the drainage bag when half to two-thirds full to prevent traction on the bladder neck.
   • When emptying, do not allow the spout to contact the floor or the collection device.
   • Disinfect collection containers after each use; provide each patient with his or her own collection container.

10. • Maintain adequate fluid intake. *Yes.* It promotes antegrade flow of urine, which helps prevent retrograde migration of bacteria.
    • Keep urine alkaline if possible. *No.* Acidic urine is needed to inhibit bacterial growth.
    • Provide thorough meatal care with antibacterial soap and ointment twice daily and as needed. *No.* Studies have shown no benefit to the use of antibacterial soaps and ointments; current guidelines recommend *gentle* meatal cleansing with *minimal* manipulation of the catheter and avoidance of harsh antiseptics that could damage the urethral mucosa; petroleum-based creams and ointments should be avoided because they can degrade latex catheters.
    • Change indwelling catheters monthly change drainage bags every 2 weeks. *No.* Ideally, the schedule for catheter change should be individualized for the patient and should be determined based on type of catheter and tendency to obstruct. There is no evidence to support monthly catheter changes as beneficial. Disconnection of the system should be avoided, because maintenance of a closed system has been found to be a key element in prevention of catheter-associated urinary tract infection (CAUTI); therefore, the catheter and drainage bag should always be changed as a unit.

11. (1) Inadvertent removal by the patient
    (2) Leakage
    (3) Encrustation

12. Suggest to Janice that she connect her catheter to a sterile leg bag at the time of catheter insertion and that she use a length of tubing to connect the leg bag to her night drainage bag, *as opposed to disconnecting the catheter from the leg bag and then connecting it to the night drainage bag.* Maintaining a closed system is a key element in prevention of CAUTI.

13. (1) Catheter-meatal junction
    Implications: Cleanse the perineum before catheter insertion and use meticulous

sterile technique for insertion; avoid manipulation of the catheter (manipulation promotes bacterial migration); stabilize the catheter to prevent catheter manipulation; provide *gentle* meatal care.

(2) Catheter-drainage tube connection
Implications: Use and maintain a closed system; use the safe sampling port to obtain specimens; avoid routine irrigations; change the catheter and drainage bag at the same time.

(3) Drainage bag outlet device
Implications: Maintain the tubing and drainage bag below the level of the bladder; keep the tubing above the level of the drainage bag; do not allow the spout to touch the floor or collection container; provide each patient with his or her own collection container.

14. Biofilms are 1000 times more resistant to antibiotics than are free-floating bacteria. Catheters increase the risk for biofilm formation, owing to placement in a fluid environment and the fact that urine provides a layer of proteinaceous material that supports biofilm growth; hydrophobic catheters such as uncoated latex catheters and silicone catheters are particularly high risk.
Preventive measures:
- Use catheters with hydrogel (hydrophilic) coatings.
- Use catheters with antimicrobial coatings.
- Utilize all measures listed in the answer above to reduce the risk of CAUTI.

15. The patient is asymptomatic, so treatment is not needed. In addition, studies indicate that measures such as irrigations, topical antibacterials, and catheter changes are ineffective in eliminating bacteria, and treatment with antibiotics increases the risk for development of bacterial resistance and has no long-term benefit (the bacteria will recur).

16. Definition of term: Positive urine culture in patient with clinical signs and symptoms of bacterial invasion of the urinary tract, that is,

bladder spasms/leakage, suprapubic discomfort, burning sensation in bladder, cloudy malodorous urine, malaise, chills and fever, anorexia, flank pain, altered mental status (may be only indicator of UTI in an elderly patient)
Response:
- Remove the existing catheter; insert a new catheter and obtain culture and sensitivity testing from the new catheter (provides accurate culture and sensitivity results, hastens clinical improvement, and reduces relapse).
- Treat based on culture results.

17. The primary cause of leakage, other than luminal occlusion, is bladder spasms; bladder spasms can be caused by any of the following:
- *Fecal impaction:* Monitor bowel function and intervene to prevent constipation and impaction.
- *Unsecured catheters:* Check to be sure the catheter is properly secured at all times.
- *Large catheter or large balloon:* Use a 14- to 18-Fr catheter with a 5-mL balloon; do *not* insert a larger catheter or larger balloon in response to leakage (unless leakage is determined to result from a damaged bladder neck and urethra).
- *Concentrated urine:* Ensure adequate fluid intake.
- *Infection:* Obtain culture and sensitivity testing if all other causes of bladder spasms have been ruled out in a patient with leakage around a patent catheter.

18. (**b**) Infection with urease-producing bacteria

19. "Blockers" are patients who consistently and repeatedly develop catheter encrustation resulting in diminished urine flow.
Measures:
- Monitor catheter function and modify the catheter change schedule so the catheter is changed before it blocks.
- Increase the patient's fluid intake and maintain acidic urine.
- Consider routine instillations of acidic solution such as Renacidin (two sequential

instillations of less than 50 mL Renacidin two to three times/week; use gravity instillation to prevent damage to bladder mucosa).
20. *False.*
21. (**c**) Advance the catheter into the bladder slightly; attach the syringe to the balloon port and allow the fluid to return by gravity.
22. Advantages:
    - The patient can attempt a voiding trial without removing the catheter.
    - It eliminates risk of urethral trauma, urethritis, and urethral fistulas.
    - It provides easier management/access for the wheelchair-bound patient.
    - It minimizes interference with sexual activity.
    - It reduces the risk of infection.
    Disadvantages:
    - The patient may leak from urethra and may require surgical closure of the urethra.
    - It is associated with an increased risk for bladder stones.
    - Health care providers have less knowledge about care of suprapubic catheters.
23. - Autonomic dysreflexia
    - Bladder malignancy
24. - Remove the catheter before intercourse; replace after intercourse.
    - If catheter left in place:
      - Select a position that minimizes traction on the catheter and pressure on the bladder neck (such as a side-lying position).
      - Male patients: Fold the catheter back alongside the penis, secure with a condom, and use copious amounts of water-soluble lubricant.
      - Female patients: Tape the catheter to the abdomen or thigh so it is out of the way.
    - Empty the drainage bag and position it out of the way, OR remove the drainage bag and insert a catheter plug.
25. (**a**) Question him regarding any signs or symptoms of UTI or problems with constipation; reassure him that this is not harmful.

26. (**b**) 26-year-old male paraplegic with moderately severe bladder-sphincter dssynergia.
27. BioDerm External Collection System

CHAPTER 11

1. Intractable incontinence can be defined as incontinence with no potential for cure or improvement. These patients are usually unable to participate in behavioral programs secondary to cognitive, physical, or social barriers, and pharmacologic and surgical therapy is not recommended because they are not likely to be of benefit. These patients must therefore be managed with containment devices or absorbent products and skin care. The goals in managing these patients are maintenance of skin integrity and preservation of patient dignity.
2. (a) Fecal incontinence increases the risk for breakdown because stool contains residual enzymes that have been shown to produce epidermal damage. The combination of fecal and urinary incontinence can be particularly damaging because the alkaline environment created by the mixture potentiates the enzymes in the stool.
   (b) Underhydration or overhydration of the skin increases the risk for breakdown because physiologic levels of water content help to maintain the normal barrier function of the skin. When the skin is underhydrated, the cells shrink, and the change in configuration creates defects in the barrier. When the skin is overhydrated, it becomes more permeable and also more vulnerable to the effects of friction.
   (c) Elevated skin temperature may increase the risk for breakdown because it increases the permeability of the skin and creates an environment conducive to microbial overgrowth.
   (d) Alkaline pH is a risk factor for breakdown because the healthy stratum corneum has an acidic pH, which contributes to the barrier function of the skin. Alkaline pH is

associated with reduced barrier function and increased permeability.

(e) Cleansing procedures that damage skin lipids compromise the skin's ability to function as a barrier and render it more permeable and therefore more subject to microbial and irritant invasion.

3. (a) Irritant dermatitis is characterized by erythema and edema in the affected area, followed by development of vesicles and then by blistering and skin loss. Severe irritant dermatitis may resemble a chemical burn, with intense erythema, epidermal loss, and pain. Mild dermatitis may be associated with itching, but pain and burning become predominant as the dermatitis worsens. Management involves removal of the irritant and use of various barrier products (creams, ointments, pastes, or alcohol-free barrier films) to provide protection and to permit the skin to repair itself.

(b) Perineal yeast infection is characterized by an erythemic rash with pinpoint satellite lesions at the periphery. The rash may be confined to the perineum or may extend to the groin and inner thighs. A ruddy or purplish hyperpigmentation is common in long-term infections. Perineal yeast infections must be treated with an antifungal agent that is active against yeast organisms. The prescription drug of choice is nystatin; however, some over-the-counter antifungals are less costly and are frequently effective (such as miconazole or clotrimazole).

(c) Estrogen deficiency is common in the postmenopausal woman and is manifest by a pale, dry, and nonrugated vaginal mucosa and by complaints of itching, irritation, or uncomfortable "dryness." It is most effectively treated by estrogen applied topically.

4. Manufacturers are required to provide MSDS sheets for each of their products. These sheets contain a complete listing of ingredients as well as the results of dermal and ocular irritation tests and any ocular warnings. Products with ocular warnings may be more irritating and should be avoided for patients with sensitive or fragile skin.

5. (a) Cleansers are used to remove stool and urine from the skin while minimizing disruption of the skin barrier. They should be pH balanced and nonirritating and should leave minimal residue.

(b) Moisturizers are appropriately used to keep the skin supple and to maintain the skin's ability to function as a barrier.

(c) Moisture barriers create a barrier between the skin and exogenous irritants such as urine and stool. They may be formulated as creams, ointments, or pastes. Petroleum products, dimethicone, and zinc oxide are common ingredients. Pastes are dryer and more occlusive than creams and ointments and are usually used for patients who are at very high risk for skin damage or who have already sustained skin damage.

(d) Powders are formulated to absorb moisture and are typically used on opposing skin surfaces to minimize friction.

(e) Liquid film barriers are used to protect intact skin by providing a polymer film that forms a protective coating on the skin. Products that contain alcohol are contraindicated for skin that is damaged; alcohol-free barrier films may be used in these situations.

6. • Select a catheter with a nonkinking junction between the catheter tip and the drainage tubing.
   • Size the catheter appropriately.
   • Clean and dry the skin and clip or shave any loose hairs.
   • Consider a short-shaft external catheter, the Bioderm system, the AFEX system, or a urinary pouch for the male patient with a short or retracted penis.

7. • Urinary retention that cannot otherwise be managed
   • Management of terminally ill or severely ill patients
   • Management of patients with stage 3 or stage 4 pressure ulcers on the trunk or pelvis until the ulcer is healed

- Management of urinary incontinence in the homebound patient who is incapable of self-toileting and whose caregiver is unable to manage the patient with toileting or absorptive products. Catheters may also be used short term for monitoring fluid balance.

8. The catheter should be constructed of bonded latex or pure silicone and should be between 14 and 18 Fr in size; the balloon should be 5 mL and should be inflated with 10 mL.

9. Primary factors to be considered include the volume of urine loss and the patient's ambulatory status. Secondary factors include the patient's or caregiver's dexterity, the need to conceal the use of absorbent products, patient or caregiver preference in regard to various design features, and cost factors.

CHAPTER 12

1. Critical elements include a thorough problem-oriented history, a focused physical examination, a bladder chart, a urinalysis, and a postvoid residual (whenever there is any suspicion of retention). Additional studies and techniques may be indicated for selected patients who present with a complex clinical picture or signs of upper tract distress or who fail to respond to conservative management.

2. • Open-ended question regarding bladder control problem and effect on patient's or caregiver's life
   • Onset and duration of the urinary incontinence (UI)
   • Patterns of urinary elimination and bladder management strategies (such as use of containment devices, barrier products, or catheters)
   • Volume and type of fluid intake
   • Patterns of urinary leakage and any precipitating or associated events
   • Focused review of systems to include genitourinary, gastrointestinal, and neurologic systems, in addition to medical-surgical history and medication profile
   • Treatment goals

3. *False.* Although history has been shown to be a relatively reliable indicator for stress UI, patient descriptors of urge-pattern incontinence do not allow reliable prediction of detrusor overactivity, and the diagnosis of any type of UI requires a careful physical examination as well as a patient interview. However, Gray and colleagues found that the *combined presence* of urgency associated with leakage, diurnal frequency, and nocturia does appear to have predictive value for urge UI.

4. • General assessment of patient's functional status, that is, cognition, mobility, and dexterity
   • Assessment of genitalia and perineal skin. In women, assessment includes inspection of the vaginal mucosa to determine the presence of infectious or atrophic vaginitis, an assessment of pelvic muscle strength, and determination of pelvic floor integrity (any evidence of prolapse); rectal examination may be performed also to evaluate the strength of the anal sphincter and the presence or absence of fecal impaction. In men, the testes are palpated, and a digital rectal exam is performed to assess the size and contours of the prostate gland and the contractility of the anal sphincter.
   • Focused neurologic examination: This includes inspection of the back, buttocks, and lower extremities, perineal sensation, reflex motor activity (the bulbocavernosus reflex), and any additional indicators of neurologic deficits.

5. • *Digital examination:* One or two gloved lubricated fingers are inserted into the vagina, and the patient is instructed to tighten and lift. The examiner assesses the strength and duration of the contraction, the degree of finger displacement, and whether the contraction is circumferential.
   • *Urine stream interruption test:* The patient is instructed to begin voiding and is then instructed to interrupt the urinary stream. The observer determines the time required to interrupt the stream completely.

- *Pressure-sensitive biofeedback probe:* A pressure-sensitive probe is inserted into the vagina or rectum and is connected to a display monitor. The patient is asked to contract her pelvic muscles, and the observer notes the pressure generated by the contraction.

6. • Data generated by a voiding diary include diurnal voiding frequency, frequency of nocturia, and frequency of urinary leakage. Some diaries also provide information regarding voided volumes, approximate volumes of leakage, activities and events associated with leakage, and volume and type of fluid intake.
   • Guidelines for patient and caregiver instruction include the purpose and importance of the diary, the time for maintaining the diary (usually at least 3 days), guidelines for measuring voided volumes and for approximating fluid intake, and the importance of documenting events and activities associated with leakage.

7. (1) Postvoid residual urine volumes can be obtained by catheterization or by bladder ultrasonography.
   (2) "High" postvoid residual volumes are sometimes defined as less than 250 mL, but in other settings the definition of high PVR is greater than 25% of the total bladder volume.

8. Simple bedside cystometry involves placement of a catheter into the patient's bladder. The catheter is then attached to either a Toomey syringe or a manometer, and the bladder is slowly filled with sterile water or saline. The patient is instructed to report the following sensations: first sensation of filling, bladder fullness, urgency. The examiner observes for evidence of detrusor overactivity, that is, a precipitous but sustained rise in intravesical pressure accompanied by a reported urge to void and possibly leakage. Simple cystometry is valuable in the assessment of bladder sensation and the presence of detrusor overactivity in frail elderly individuals.

9. (a) *Uroflowmetry:* The patient is asked to void into a special device that provides a graphic printout of the flow pattern and data regarding the flow rate (that is, mL/second). Uroflowmetry is considered to be a screening test in that it detects problems with bladder emptying and serves to validate information gained later during the voiding pressure study. It provides no information regarding the bladder's ability to store urine. Four flow patterns may be seen: normal, which appears as a modified bell curve with no intermittency; explosive, which is an exaggeration of the normal curve and appears as an inverted U; poor, which is characterized by a low flow rate and prolonged time to emptying; and intermittent, which is characterized by a stop-and-start pattern, usually caused by the intermittent use of abdominal muscle contraction to augment bladder contraction. The poor and intermittent flow patterns are indicative of voiding dysfunction and the need for further workup. These patterns are usually caused by bladder outlet obstruction or by impaired detrusor contractility, and patients presenting with these patterns require a voiding pressure study for differentiation.

   (b) *Filling cystometrogram (CMG):* The patient is catheterized with at least a double-lumen (or two-catheter) system. (One lumen or catheter permits filling of the bladder, and the other contains a pressure-sensitive transducer that measures the intravesical pressure.) A pressure-sensitive catheter is also placed into the patient's vagina or rectum; this catheter measures abdominal pressures. The bladder is slowly filled with water or saline, and tracings that reflect the filling volume, the intravesical pressure, the abdominal pressure, and the detrusor pressure are obtained. The patient is instructed to report the first sensation of filling, the sensation of fullness, and the sensation of urgency. Data obtained from this study include the following:

- *Bladder sensation:* Hypersensitivity and hyposensitivity are identified. Hypersensitivity increases the risk for urgency, whereas hyposensitivity places the patient at risk for retention.
- *Detrusor response:* Detrusor overactivity is characterized by a sudden sharp rise in bladder pressure that produces urinary leakage or severe urgency and is followed by a drop in pressure to previous baseline indicating muscle relaxation.
- *Bladder capacity:* This is the volume of fluid held before study is terminated by patient's sense of urgency or by an unstable bladder contraction.
- *Bladder wall compliance:* Normally, the bladder wall stretches to accommodate increasing volumes of urine, and this accommodation is reflected by a minimal change in pressure as compared with volume. Normal compliance is considered to be at least 50 mL/cm H_2O. Low compliance is very significant in that high intravesical pressures impede the delivery of urine from the kidneys and place the patient at risk for upper tract distress.
- *Urethral sphincter competence:* The clinician determines urethral sphincter competence by performing an abdominal leak point pressure study during cystometrography. Any leakage is considered indicative of some degree of sphincter incompetence.

(c) *Sphincter electromyography:* The clinician performs sphincter electromyography by placing surface electrodes immediately adjacent to the anus or by inserting needle or wire electrodes into the pelvic floor muscles. The electrodes transmit electrical impulses generated at the level of the pelvic muscle membrane to a display screen. The electrical activity of the pelvic muscles, that is, appropriate versus inappropriate contraction, can then be observed during the filling and voiding phases of the micturition cycle. (For example, this study is helpful in the detection of detrusor-

sphincter dyssynergia.) It is important to realize that this test measures only electrical impulses and provides no information about muscle tone.

(d) *Abdominal leak point pressure:* Pressure-sensitive catheters are placed into the bladder as described earlier under "filling cystometrogram." The bladder is then partially filled, and the patient is instructed to perform a slow Valsalva maneuver. If leakage occurs, the examiner notes the pressure at which it occurred. As noted earlier, the competent sphincter will not leak, and any leakage is indicative of some degree of sphincter incompetence.

(e) *Voiding pressure study:* When the filling CMG is completed, the filling catheter is removed, and the patient is instructed to void into a uroflow device. This study provides data regarding the strength of the detrusor contraction, the urinary flow pattern, and any bladder outlet obstruction. The voiding pressure study is used to differentiate between retention caused by reduced detrusor contractility and retention caused by bladder outlet obstruction.

(f) *Videourodynamics:* Videourodynamics provide all the information provided by the studies listed earlier but also provide imaging data; that is, fluoroscopy is performed before and during bladder emptying to determine the presence or absence of reflux, any anatomic abnormalities, and the level and character of any outlet obstruction.

10. Patients should be evaluated with urodynamic studies whenever they present with a complex clinical picture or with symptoms of upper tract distress, whenever surgical intervention is contemplated, and whenever initial treatment has failed.

CHAPTER **13**

1. The enteric nervous system is contained within the bowel wall; it is made up of Auerbach's and

myenteric plexuses and the nerve fibers that arise from receptors in the colon wall. The intrinsic nervous system is the primary mediator for colonic motility, and the receptors of the intrinsic nervous system are most responsive to "local" stimuli, such as stretch or intraluminal irritants.

Extrinsic innervation serves to modulate the activity of the intestinal tract significantly and is provided by the branches of the autonomic nervous system. (The nerve fibers of the autonomic nervous system terminate on the ganglia of the intrinsic nervous system.) Parasympathetic stimulation increases intestinal motility, whereas sympathetic stimulation reduces intestinal motility. In managing the patient with a spinal cord injury resulting in loss of autonomic innervation, the clinician must use stimuli to which the intrinsic nervous system responds to stimulate defecation.

2. Normal sensory awareness includes both awareness of rectal distension and the ability to discriminate accurately among liquid, solids, and gases. Normally, rectal distension causes stimulation of sensory afferents in the rectal wall and pelvic floor, which transmit messages to the cord and then the cortex that result in conscious awareness of the need to defecate. This sensory awareness of rectal distension is critical, in that it alerts the individual to impending defecation and the need to contract the external sphincter. The second component of sensory awareness is the ability to identify rectal contents accurately. This identification occurs when rectal contents contact the sensory receptors in the proximal end of the anal canal. This component of sensory awareness permits the individual to expel gas safely in suitable locations, without fear of fecal leakage.

3. The internal anal sphincter surrounds the proximal end of the anal canal and is a condensation of circular muscle fibers. It is under autonomic control and is normally tonically contracted. It relaxes in response to rectal distension, a reflex known as the "rectoanal inhibitory reflex." The internal anal

sphincter is the primary continence mechanism at rest and does not provide continence during episodes of rectal distension.

The external anal sphincter surrounds the internal anal sphincter and the distal end of the anal canal. It is composed of both smooth and striated muscle and therefore has both reflex activity and the ability to respond to voluntary contraction. Normally, the external sphincter is tonically contracted at rest; with voluntary contraction, the anal canal pressure can be doubled, which provides for continence during periods of rectal distension. Normal anorectal function during defecation requires the individual to relax the external sphincter voluntarily. Individuals who lack the ability to relax the external sphincter voluntarily experience chronic difficulty with defecation (nonrelaxing puborectalis syndrome).

4. The pelvic floor muscles form a slinglike support around the anal canal. The puborectalis muscle passes from the symphysis pubis around the anorectal junction and then back to the symphysis pubis. This sling of support creates an angle between the rectum and the anal canal that is theorized to possibly play a role in continence. During rest (and continence) the angle is 90 degrees, but during defecation it straightens to 135 degrees.

5. Maximal contraction of the external anal sphincter can be maintained for no more than 3 minutes; beyond this time, continence is dependent on the rectum's ability to stretch and store stool at relatively low pressures. This ability to relax around a bolus of stool and to store the stool at low pressures is known as "compliance." The individual with normal compliance can store 250 to 510 mL of stool.

6. When there is sufficient distension to trigger a series of peristaltic contractions, stool is propelled into the rectum. Rectal distension causes activation of stretch receptors in the rectum and pelvic floor, which results in conscious awareness of rectal distension. Rectal distension also causes relaxation of the internal anal sphincter, which permits rectal contents to contact the sensitive anal mucosa.

This permits differentiation of rectal contents. In response to the conscious awareness of rectal distension, the individual voluntarily contracts the external anal sphincter, which maintains continence until the rectum relaxes around the bolus of stool. When the individual reaches a suitable time and place for defecation, he or she assumes a squat position, which straightens the anorectal angle and relaxes the external sphincter; these two actions permit stool to move into the anal canal. Voluntary straining causes descent of the pelvic floor and funneling of the anal canal; straining also increases intraabdominal and intrarectal pressures, which facilitates evacuation. Once evacuation has occurred, the anal canal pressure returns to normal, and the anal canal resumes its 90-degree angle to the rectum.

CHAPTER 14

1. Secretory diarrhea occurs as a result of increased secretion into the lumen of the bowel. It is caused by bacterial toxins or by other agents that stimulate excessive secretion, such as bile acids, fatty acids, prostaglandins, and substances produced by selected malignant tumors. The stool volume is typically greater than 1 liter per day, the pH is neutral, and the response to fasting is minimal (because the diarrhea is not caused by ingested substances). The stool osmolality gap is usually less than 40 mOsm/Kg because most of the osmotic content of the stool is provided by the electrolytes secreted into the lumen of the bowel.

   Osmotic diarrhea occurs as a result of diminished absorption and may also be caused by reduced bowel length, by atrophy of the villi, or by ingestion or production of substances that are osmotically active and serve to pull fluid into the bowel. Common etiologic factors for osmotic diarrhea include lactose intolerance, sorbitol, and saline-based laxatives. Stool volume is usually less than 1 liter per day, the pH is acidic, and fasting produces a significant reduction in stool volume. The stool osmolality gap is usually more than 50 mOsm/kg (because the diarrhea is caused by osmotically active agents that increase the osmotic content of the stool).

2. Diarrhea does not *cause* fecal incontinence, but it does increase the *risk* for fecal incontinence; this is because the anal sphincter mechanism is less competent for liquid stool, and large volume liquid stools can overwhelm the strongest sphincter.

3. • *Dietary modifications:* Two general types of dietary modifications may be beneficial for patients with diarrhea. One type is specific restrictions based on etiologic factors (such as lactose restriction for the patient who is lactose intolerant). The other type includes a variety of suggestions that are beneficial for most patients with diarrhea: restriction of gut "irritants" such as caffeine, spicy foods, and foods high in insoluble fiber; increased fluid intake to prevent dehydration; and increased intake of foods containing soluble fiber, such as oats, pectin, and germinated barley. (Soluble fiber helps to absorb water, thicken the stool, and promote the health and absorptive function of the colon.)

   • *Soluble fiber supplements:* Soluble fiber supplements (such as psyllium or guar gum) can be used to help thicken the stool. In addition, soluble fiber interacts with normal flora (probiotics) to produce compounds that help to maintain bowel health.

   • *Probiotics:* Probiotics are commercially available blends of normal intestinal flora that help to prevent diarrhea caused by antibiotics and also interact with soluble fiber to produce compounds that are beneficial to colonic health.

   • *Antidiarrheal medications:* Most antidiarrheal medications work by reducing motility; some improve absorption within the colon or bind to secretory agents. Antimotility agents are effective in reducing the volume and frequency of stools but should be used only after impaction and infectious diarrhea is ruled out. The most commonly used antimotility agent is loperamide, which also acts to improve sphincter tone.

4. Health care providers tend to define constipation as infrequent bowel movements, whereas patients use the term "constipation" to denote any difficulty with stool elimination (infrequent bowel movements, passage of hard stools, straining at stool, or a sense of incomplete evacuation). Thus, it is important to have the patient describe the specific symptoms they are labeling "constipation."

5. • *Normal-transit constipation:* This type of constipation is seen in patients who have essentially normal colon function and no obstruction to stool elimination; the symptoms most commonly reported by patients include hard stools or difficult evacuation, along with associated symptoms such as bloating or abdominal discomfort. Because colonic motility is normal in these patients, the constipation is thought to be caused by factors *extrinsic* to the bowel, such as inadequate fiber or fluid, inactivity, chronic failure to respond to the call to stool, or constipating medications.

   • *Slow-transit constipation:* This form of constipation is characterized by a marked reduction in the propagating contractions that normally propel stool through the colon and into the rectum; there are fewer propagating contractions in response to the normal stimuli of waking and eating, and the contractions that do occur are of significantly reduced amplitude, velocity, and duration. As a result, stool moves extremely slowly through the colon. These patients have very infrequent defecatory urges, severe bloating, and very large, very infrequent bowel movements.

   • *Obstructed defecation disorders:* Patients with obstructed defecation syndromes have difficulty initiating defecation and do not achieve complete rectal evacuation despite excessive and prolonged straining; they commonly report a "lumplike" sensation or a feeling of "blockage" in the anal area.

6. • *Fiber and fluid therapy:* Fiber and fluid therapy are generally considered first-line therapeutic approaches for individuals with

constipation, especially when the constipation involves hard dry stools. The goals are to ensure approximately 30 g fiber intake/day, along with adequate fluid (30 mL/kg body weight/day). For patients with normal-transit constipation, this intervention may be all that is needed to normalize bowel function. In contrast, patients with slow-transit constipation may actually experience *increased* bloating and discomfort; should this occur, the fiber should be discontinued.

   • *Laxatives:* Laxatives may be used to relieve acute constipation in individuals with normal-transit constipation; for patients with slow-transit constipation, laxatives frequently represent primary therapy. Laxatives can be categorized as bulk agents, osmotic agents, lubricants, or stimulants. For patients with slow-transit constipation, osmotic agents (saline-based laxatives, sorbitol, lactulose, or polyethylene glycol agents) are commonly required on a routine basis (and are now known to be safe for routine use); stimulant agents such as bisacodyl or senna are used as needed.

   • *Biofeedback:* Biofeedback is helpful in the management of patients with pelvic floor dyssynergia, a condition characterized by unconscious contraction of the pelvic floor muscles during attempted defecation. Biofeedback can be used to help the patient learn to coordinate abdominal muscle contraction and pelvic floor relaxation.

7. • *History:* Frequency of defecatory urges (and usual response); frequency of bowel movements; volume and consistency of stool; any aids to elimination; usual fiber and fluid intake; any feelings of incomplete evacuation; amount of straining required; any associated symptoms (bloating, cramping, etc.); medication profile (prescription and over the counter)

   • *Physical exam:* Screening for neurologic or thyroid disease; abdominal exam (any evidence of colonic distension); careful anorectal exam (evidence of rectocele, ability to effectively relax the sphincter in response to the command to "push my finger out," evidence of retained stool)

- *Motility testing:* for patients with suspected slow-transit constipation
- *Anorectal manometry, balloon expulsion test, defecography:* for patients with evidence of obstructed defecation

8. The pathology of irritable bowel syndrome (IBS) remains unclear; current theories include genetic predisposition, visceral hypersensitivity, and altered motility and transit. Dietary intolerance may also play a role, although there is no evidence to suggest that it is *causative.* There are no clear data regarding genetic influences; evidence to support the role of visceral hypersensitivity and altered motility include the following:

- *Visceral hypersensitivity:* Studies show that patients with IBS are hyperresponsive to visceral stimuli such as mechanical distension of the gut. (They report pain in response to gut distension.) The cause of this visceral hypersensitivity may be increased recruitment of silent receptors, increased responsiveness of the receptors, or changes in central nervous system modulation.
- *Altered motility and transit:* All patients with IBS present with alterations in motility; however, no single pattern is common to all individuals with IBS. Patients may present with diarrhea-predominant symptoms, constipation-predominant symptoms, or alteration between diarrhea and constipation. Those with diarrhea-predominant symptoms commonly exhibit increased small bowel motility, whereas those with constipation-predominant symptoms exhibit reduced motility.
- *Management:* Management of IBS is symptomatic and supportive and includes use of medications to control symptoms, behavioral therapy to address the psychosocial aspects of the condition, and education regarding the condition and its management, with reassurance that it is not life-threatening. Patients are encouraged to maintain a "diet, stool, and symptom" diary

and to modify their dietary intake based on their own intolerances. A highly restricted diet is rarely indicated.

9. • *26-year-old man with paraplegia secondary to spinal cord injury at L2:* This patient is at risk because a spinal cord injury disrupts the sensory and motor pathways that provide sensory awareness of rectal filling and voluntary control of the external sphincter. This means that this individual will not know when stool reaches the rectum and will not be able to delay defecation by contracting the external sphincter. He is also at risk for constipation because of reduced mobility. He will need to initiate measures to maintain a soft but *formed* stool and will need to regulate bowel elimination by a stimulated defecation program.

- *62-year-old woman whose medical history includes four vaginal deliveries (two forceps-assisted) and chronic constipation:* This patient is at risk because the vaginal deliveries, especially the forceps-assisted deliveries, may have caused sphincteric injuries that reduce her ability to contract the external sphincter effectively. In addition, the forceps-assisted deliveries and her chronic straining to eliminate constipated stool place her at risk for stretch injuries to the pudendal nerve. Pudendal nerve damage can compromise both sensory awareness of rectal filling and voluntary sphincter contraction. There is evidence to support vaginal delivery as the initial insult in a series of events that causes fecal incontinence in older women. (Events that are believed to contribute to the onset of fecal incontinence include the hormonal changes associated with menopause and the tissue changes associated with aging.)
- *18-year-old woman with IBD and proctitis:* Proctitis alters the rectum's ability to serve as a reservoir for stool. Continence in this situation can be maintained only for the length of time the external sphincter can be maximally contracted. Once the external sphincter relaxes, anal canal pressures fall and incontinence is extremely likely. (Leakage

occurs whenever rectal pressures exceed anal canal pressures.)

- *83-year-old man with advanced dementia and no history of bowel dysfunction:* This patient is at risk because the advanced dementia alters his ability to interpret the sensation of rectal filling accurately and to respond appropriately with external sphincter contraction or movement to a toileting facility.

CHAPTER 15

1. (a) *Interview:* Review of current problem: onset; duration; description of problem; current management; associated factors; frequency, consistency, and volume of voluntary bowel movements and incontinent episodes; sensory awareness of urge to defecate; ability to delay defecation; effect of problem on life style; life-style factors affecting bowel function (such as fiber and fluid intake, activity level, and all medications being taken). Focused medical-surgical history to include neurologic conditions, anorectal surgery or trauma, gastrointestinal disorders, obstetric history, diabetes, and history of abdominal or pelvic surgery; patient's and caregiver's goals for treatment

   (b) *Physical examination:*
   - General data: Mobility, dexterity, and cognitive status
   - Specific data: Abdominal inspection and palpation; inspection of perianal skin; inspection of anus at rest, with contraction, and with "bearing down" maneuver; test for anal wink; digital examination of rectum and anus to include assessment of patient's ability to contract and relax the sphincter muscle and an assessment of sphincter muscle function; palpation of rectal vault to determine presence or absence of retained stool or rectal lesions.

   (c) *Bowel chart:* Frequency, volume, and consistency of both voluntary and incontinent stools; may include data regarding dietary and fluid intake.

2. (a) *Anorectal manometry:* Provides objective measurements of anorectal sensation, pressures generated by the sphincter complex, and the functional length of the anal canal. A pressure-sensitive catheter with an attached balloon is inserted into the anal canal and rectum and connected to a computer that records transmitted pressures. The rectal balloon is gradually inflated, and the patient is asked to report "first sensation" and "full sensation." Pressures within the anal canal are measured at rest, during maximum voluntary contraction, and during a Valsalva maneuver. The length of the anal canal is determined by identification of the area of highest pressure (the anorectal junction) and measurement from that point to the anus.

   (b) *Endoanal ultrasound:* Endoanal ultrasonography involves placement of a sonographic probe in the anal canal; the sonographic probe provides visualization of the thickness and structural integrity of the internal and external anal sphincters and can identify any disruption, scarring, or thinning of the sphincter complex. Endoanal ultrasound is particularly beneficial in mapping the internal sphincter; mapping of the external sphincter can more effectively be accomplished with magnetic resonance imaging.

   (c) *Defecography:* Defecography reveals any problems with rectal emptying, such as rectocele or rectal prolapse or pelvic floor dyssynergia. A thick contrast paste is instilled into the rectum, and the patient is placed on a radiolucent commode chair while still films and fluoroscopy are obtained. This shows any problems that occur during evacuation.

3. Impaction causes continual rectal distension, which is a constant stimulus to internal sphincter relaxation. This explains the leakage of liquid stool that is frequently seen in patients with fecal impaction. Options for disimpaction include administration of softening and

lubricating solutions (such as mineral oil) per rectum, followed by manual breakup and removal, or administration of fecalytic solutions such as a 1:1 solution of milk and molasses. Once the rectal mass has been removed, colonic cleansing is accomplished by a combination of suppositories, enemas, and orally administered laxatives. (For example, bisacodyl could be given orally at night, followed by a hypertonic phosphate enema the following morning.)

4. Bulking agents act to retain fluid. In the patient with diarrhea, bulk agents have a "thickening" effect. The thickened stool is more easily retained by the anorectal sphincter mechanism than liquid stool. In the patient with constipation, the bulk agent attracts fluid, which softens the stool; in addition, the bulk and the fluid create a stool of larger diameter, which more effectively distends the colon to stimulate peristalsis.

5. The anorectal sphincter mechanism is most competent for formed stool. Liquid or mushy stool can leak through a compromised sphincter mechanism. Soft formed stool is also easy to eliminate without excessive straining. Small, dry stools require excessive intrarectal and intraabdominal pressures for elimination.

6. • Options for management of high-volume liquid stool include anorectal pouching systems, a nasal trumpet inserted into the rectum and connected to a bedside drainage unit, and use of balloon-tipped internal drainage systems specifically designed for management of high-volume liquid stool. Perianal pouches consist of a drainable pouch connected to an adhesive skin barrier constructed to conform to the perianal contours; these devices are frequently considered first-line management because they are noninvasive and inexpensive.
   • Nasopharyngeal airways have been used effectively for the containment of liquid stool; the flared end of the trumpet is inserted gently into the rectum and the "tube" end is connected to bedside drainage. Advantages include the ability to use this system when pouches are ineffective and the fact that it is inexpensive. Disadvantages include the fact that there are limited studies addressing use of the nasal trumpet in management of diarrheal stools. (However, those that have been done demonstrated both efficacy and safety.)
   • Low-pressure balloon-tipped systems are now available that have been designed specifically for management of large volume diarrhea stools; these commercial devices have demonstrated efficacy and safety and can be used for prolonged periods of time. The disadvantage is the fact that they are more expensive.

7. Elimination diets are helpful for patients who have chronic diarrhea caused by food intolerances. Such diets are used to identify the patient's specific dietary offenders. The patient is asked to maintain a record of all oral intake (including condiments and seasonings), fecal output, and intestinal symptoms for 1 week. The patient is then placed on an "elimination diet." Foods eliminated include any offenders identified by the diet and bowel chart and any *common* offenders (such as chocolate and dairy products). The patient is asked to follow this diet for 2 weeks; if the patient fails to improve, a more restricted diet is initiated. Once the patient demonstrates improvement, the "eliminated" foods are reintroduced one at a time at intervals of about 3 days. Such spacing permits verification of the specific offenders.

8. *76-year-old woman with a history of chronic constipation who presents with fecal impaction and leakage of liquid stool:*
   • *Disimpaction and colonic cleansing regimen* (such as bisacodyl tablets at night followed by hypertonic phosphate enema in the morning) till mushy stool is eliminated
   • *Measures to normalize stool consistency:* Adequate bulk (such as bran formula or "bulk laxative" begun at 1 to 2 tbsp/day and titrated based on patient response); adequate fluid intake (at least 30 mL/kg body weight/day); increased activity as tolerated

- *Patient education program:* Relationship of chronic constipation, fecal impaction, and fecal incontinence; establishment of regular schedule for attempted defecation and prompt attention and response to "urge to go;" as-needed (PRN) use of osmotic laxatives
- *46-year-old woman with complaints of fecal urgency and episodic fecal incontinence*
  - *Measures to thicken the stool* (bulk laxatives and dietary modifications)
  - *Surgical consultation* to evaluate appropriateness of sphincter repair
  - *Pelvic muscle exercises* (with or without biofeedback) to strengthen contractility and endurance of anorectal sphincter; instruction in "urge resistance" strategies to improve overall control and reduce anxiety
- *26-year-old man with a low-level spina bifida lesion*
  - *Measures to normalize stool consistency:* Bulk laxatives or bran formula; sufficient fluids to maintain soft formed stool
  - *Stimulated defecation program:* Program begun on an every other day basis; digital stimulation or suppositories or minienemas to stimulate defecation at desired times (stimulated defecation scheduled after meals); if he fails to respond to these measures, could use low-volume tap water enemas administered by a retention balloon, or could refer for antegrade colonic enema procedure (or colostomy)

CHAPTER 16

1. The ability to achieve bowel and bladder control is dependent on physiologic maturation of neurologic pathways critical to sphincter control, cognitive awareness of bladder and rectal distension, the ability to communicate the urge to urinate or defecate, the ability to follow one- or two-step commands, and the desire to achieve control and to mimic and please parents. Physiologic maturation of the nerve pathways is generally complete by 18 months of age. Achievement of the developmental criteria is much more variable. If the child exhibits developmental readiness at 2 years, it would be appropriate to begin toilet training because adequate neurologic maturity has been achieved by this point. However, parents must realize that developmental status is just as critical to effective training as neurologic maturity. If the child's communication skills and desire to please are limited at 2 years of age, it is better to wait until those skills are in place.

2. Fecal incontinence refers to fecal soiling caused by an organic or anatomic lesion, whereas encopresis refers to fecal soiling caused by functional constipation or a psychologic issue (functional constipation is stool retention produced by dysfunctional elimination patterns, that is, chronic delay in defecation and stool withholding). Although technically incontinence refers to a physiologic problem and encopresis refers to a behavioral or psychologic problem, in common use they may be used interchangeably or incorrectly. Thus, any child seen for encopresis should be carefully assessed for an organic or anatomic lesion contributing to dysfunctional defecation, and the child seen for fecal incontinence should be evaluated for a possible behavioral or psychologic component to the incontinence.

3. - The child begins to delay defecation for a variety of reasons, such as an episode of painful constipation, a change in daily routine, or school entry and discomfort defecating in a public bathroom. As stool is accumulated in the colon or rectum, the muscle fibers in the rectal and colonic walls become "stretched," which compromises contractility and the ability to eliminate the retained stool. In addition, the constant distension of the rectum alters sensory feedback so the child becomes less aware of the need to defecate. This reduction in sensory awareness and in colorectal contractility contributes further to stool retention, and the retained stool becomes harder and more difficult to eliminate. If the child does try to eliminate the fecal mass, he or she is likely to

598 *Appendix A*

experience pain and bleeding. This further reinforces the vicious cycle of stool retention. As the rectum or colon becomes progressively more distended with stool, the rectoanal inhibitory reflex stimulates constant relaxation of the internal sphincter, which permits liquid or mushy stool to leak around the fecal mass and to escape through the open internal sphincter. The lack of sensory awareness means that the child does not recognize the need to contract the external sphincter. Even if he or she did recognize the need and did contract the sphincter, leakage would occur when the sphincter muscle became fatigued and returned to resting tone (within 1 minute).

- Effective management requires education and counseling for the parent and child, an aggressive bowel cleansing regimen, and a comprehensive program to reestablish normal bowel habits (that is, softeners, stimulants, fiber, routine toileting, underwear checks, positive reinforcement, and psychologic care as indicated).

4. The most beneficial study is a colonic transit study with radiopaque markers. After administration of the markers, the child is followed with serial flat plates to determine areas of normal and abnormal motility. Barium enema with a postevacuation film or fluoroscopy can provide indirect evidence of motility.

5. • Several regimens use a combination of bisacodyl tablets and suppositories, and Fleet enemas; for example, one regimen calls for four 3-day cycles as follows: two Fleet enemas on day 1, bisacodyl suppository on day 2, and 1 bisacodyl tablet on day 3.
- Alternatively, some clinicians prefer mineral oil at a dose of 15 to 30 mL/kg daily, not to exceed 240 mL/day.
- It is critical to assess for impaction before starting a cleansing regimen because laxatives cannot eliminate a true impaction and are likely to induce severe cramping and even vomiting. Suppositories are also ineffective with impactions. The best approach to

elimination of a true impaction is a combination of digital breakup and enemas.

6. (a) Imperforate anus involves incomplete formation of the rectum, anorectal junction, and anal canal. There are varying levels of severity. Repair of imperforate anus involves mobilizing the distal end of the bowel, pulling it through the pelvic musculature, and creating an anal opening. The long-term prognosis for continence is variable and depends in great part on the severity of the original lesion; that is, "high" lesions, or those where the distal end of the rectum terminates above the levator complex, are likely to result in incontinence because the internal sphincter is absent and the external sphincter may be incomplete. Lower lesions, that is, those in which the anorectal junction and internal sphincter are intact, have a much better prognosis for continence.

(b) Hirschsprung's disease involves aganglionosis of the distal portion of the rectum and varying lengths of the proximal portion of the bowel. Repair involves resection of the aganglionic bowel with anastomosis of the normally innervated proximal portion of the bowel to the anal canal. Incontinence is a potential complication caused by a nonrelaxing internal anal sphincter and the potential for stricture at the anastomotic line, both of which can lead to chronic constipation and overflow stooling.

(c) Myelomeningocele is a neural tube defect involving herniation of the spinal cord through the bony defect, which results in profound sensory and motor denervation below the level of the lesion. Most children with myelomeningocele lack sensory awareness of rectal distension and also lack volitional control of the sphincter; therefore fecal incontinence is extremely common among this patient population.

7. Key interventions for the child with neurogenic bowel include the following:

- Cleansing regimens for children with retained stool
- Measures to normalize stool consistency, with the goal being soft formed stool
- Routine toileting and prompt response to defecatory urge for child who retains sensory awareness and sphincter control
- Biofeedback to improve sensory awareness and sphincter control in child with intact pathways but compromised function and child with nonrelaxing puborectalis syndrome
- Stimulated defecation program (digital stimulation, suppositories, minienemas, or volume enemas with retention balloon used to stimulate defecation on routine basis)
- Antegrade colonic enema procedure or colostomy for the child in whom the foregoing measures fail

8. Dysfunctional voiding is the term used to describe voiding that is obstructed by contraction of the pelvic floor and sphincter muscles. Typically, the pattern of dysfunctional voiding begins when the child responds to sudden urinary urgency (that is, an unstable detrusor contraction) by contracting the pelvic floor and sphincter muscles in an attempt to prevent leakage. The child may also use a squatting position or digital urethral pressure to prevent leakage. If this becomes a chronic voiding pattern, the detrusor muscle is always contracting against a "closed door," which leads to obstructed voiding and incomplete emptying.

9. Effective management involves elimination of any urinary tract infection (that is, antibiotic therapy), coupled with pelvic floor reeducation (such as biofeedback), timed voiding, and anticholinergic drugs if indicated to normalize the child's voiding patterns.

10.
- Current theories include a maturational lag, antidiuretic hormone insufficiency, small bladder capacity, "deep sleep," emotional stress, uropathologic disorders, and a genetic factor.
- Treatment is generally considered to be indicated whenever the enuresis is interfering with the child's life style, peer or family relationships, or self-esteem.
- Treatment is selected based on the child's age and response to previous treatments. Options include supportive education and counseling, instruction in self-awakening, behavioral measures to increase bladder capacity, motivational therapy, enuresis alarm therapy, and pharmacotherapy (with DDAVP or imipramine).

11.
- The goals of treatment are preservation of renal function, control of infection, and restoration of continence or effective management of leakage.
- Treatment options include clean intermittent self-catheterization, antispasmodic medications, bladder augmentation, alpha-adrenergic agonists or surgical procedures to control stress incontinence, and indwelling catheter or urinary diversion (as last resorts).

Urinary Incontinence: Pathophysiology and Treatment, including Self-Test

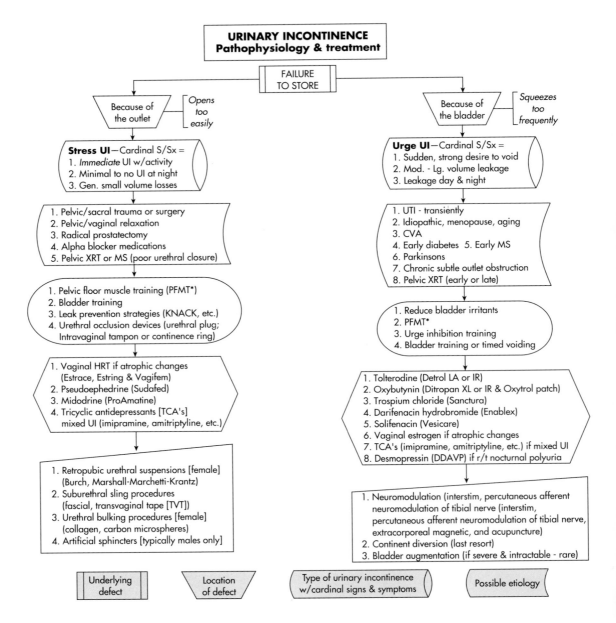

URINARY INCONTINENCE
Pathophysiology & treatment

FAILURE TO STORE

Because of the outlet — *Opens too easily*

Because of the bladder — *Squeezes too frequently*

Stress UI—Cardinal S/Sx =
1. *Immediate* UI w/activity
2. Minimal to no UI at night
3. Gen. small volume losses

Urge UI—Cardinal S/Sx =
1. Sudden, strong desire to void
2. Mod. - Lg. volume leakage
3. Leakage day & night

1. Pelvic/sacral trauma or surgery
2. Pelvic/vaginal relaxation
3. Radical prostatectomy
4. Alpha blocker medications
5. Pelvic XRT or MS (poor urethral closure)

1. UTI - transiently
2. Idiopathic, menopause, aging
3. CVA
4. Early diabetes 5. Early MS
6. Parkinsons
7. Chronic subtle outlet obstruction
8. Pelvic XRT (early or late)

1. Pelvic floor muscle training (PFMT*)
2. Bladder training
3. Leak prevention strategies (KNACK, etc.)
4. Urethral occlusion devices (urethral plug; Intravaginal tampon or continence ring)

1. Reduce bladder irritants
2. PFMT*
3. Urge inhibition training
4. Bladder training or timed voiding

1. Vaginal HRT if atrophic changes (Estrace, Estring & Vagifem)
2. Pseudoephedrine (Sudafed)
3. Midodrine (ProAmatine)
4. Tricyclic antidepressants [TCA's] mixed UI (imipramine, amitriptyline, etc.)

1. Tolterodine (Detrol LA or IR)
2. Oxybutynin (Ditropan XL or IR & Oxytrol patch)
3. Trospium chloride (Sanctura)
4. Darifenacin hydrobromide (Enablex)
5. Solifenacin (Vesicare)
6. Vaginal estrogen if atrophic changes
7. TCA's (imipramine, amitriptyline, etc.) if mixed UI
8. Desmopressin (DDAVP) if r/t nocturnal polyuria

1. Retropubic urethral suspensions [female] (Burch, Marshall-Marchetti-Krantz)
2. Suburethral sling procedures (fascial, transvaginal tape [TVT])
3. Urethral bulking procedures [female] (collagen, carbon microspheres)
4. Artificial sphincters [typically males only]

1. Neuromodulation (interstim, percutaneous afferent neuromodulation of tibial nerve (interstim, percutaneous afferent neuromodulation of tibial nerve, extracorporeal magnetic, and acupuncture)
2. Continent diversion (last resort)
3. Bladder augmentation (if severe & intractable - rare)

Underlying defect

Location of defect

Type of urinary incontinence w/cardinal signs & symptoms

Possible etiology

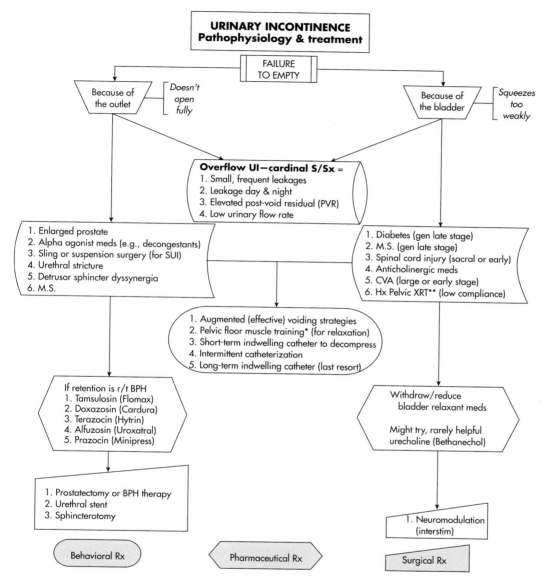

URINARY INCONTINENCE
Pathophysiology & treatment

FAILURE TO EMPTY

Because of the outlet — *Doesn't open fully*

Because of the bladder — *Squeezes too weakly*

Overflow UI—cardinal S/Sx =
1. Small, frequent leakages
2. Leakage day & night
3. Elevated post-void residual (PVR)
4. Low urinary flow rate

1. Enlarged prostate
2. Alpha agonist meds (e.g., decongestants)
3. Sling or suspension surgery (for SUI)
4. Urethral stricture
5. Detrusor sphincter dyssynergia
6. M.S.

1. Diabetes (gen late stage)
2. M.S. (gen late stage)
3. Spinal cord injury (sacral or early)
4. Anticholinergic meds
5. CVA (large or early stage)
6. Hx Pelvic XRT** (low compliance)

1. Augmented (effective) voiding strategies
2. Pelvic floor muscle training* (for relaxation)
3. Short-term indwelling catheter to decompress
4. Intermittent catheterization
5. Long-term indwelling catheter (last resort)

If retention is r/t BPH
1. Tamsulosin (Flomax)
2. Doxazosin (Cardura)
3. Terazocin (Hytrin)
4. Alfuzosin (Uroxatral)
5. Prazocin (Minipress)

Withdraw/reduce bladder relaxant meds

Might try, rarely helpful urecholine (Bethanechol)

1. Prostatectomy or BPH therapy
2. Urethral stent
3. Sphincterotomy

1. Neuromodulation (interstim)

Behavioral Rx

Pharmaceutical Rx

Surgical Rx

BPH, benign prostatic hyperplasia; CVA, cerebrovascular accident; HRT, hormone replacement therapy; Hx, history; MS, multiple sclerosis; PFMT, pelvic floor muscle training; r/t, related to; Rx, therapy; S/Sx, signs and symptoms; TCAs, tricyclic antidepressants; UI, urinary incontinence; UTI, urinary tract infection; XRT, radiation therapy.
*Pelvic floor muscle training consists of home exercises (Kegel), biofeedback, rectal electrical stimulation, and vaginal weights and cones.
Copyright 1996 by Marta Krissovich; updated 3/15/05.

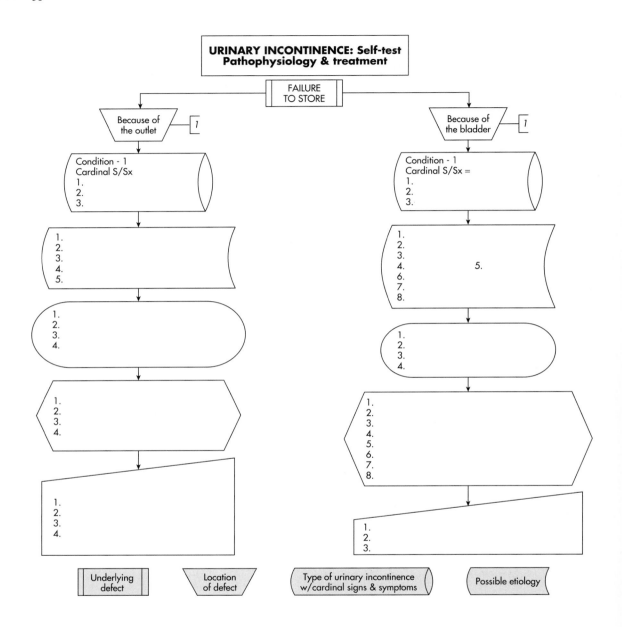

URINARY INCONTINENCE: Self-test
Pathophysiology & treatment

FAILURE TO STORE

Because of the outlet — 1

Condition - 1
Cardinal S/Sx
1.
2.
3.

1.
2.
3.
4.
5.

1.
2.
3.
4.

1.
2.
3.
4.

1.
2.
3.
4.

Because of the bladder — 1

Condition - 1
Cardinal S/Sx =
1.
2.
3.

1.
2.
3.
4.   5.
6.
7.
8.

1.
2.
3.
4.

1.
2.
3.
4.
5.
6.
7.
8.

1.
2.
3.

Underlying defect

Location of defect

Type of urinary incontinence w/cardinal signs & symptoms

Possible etiology

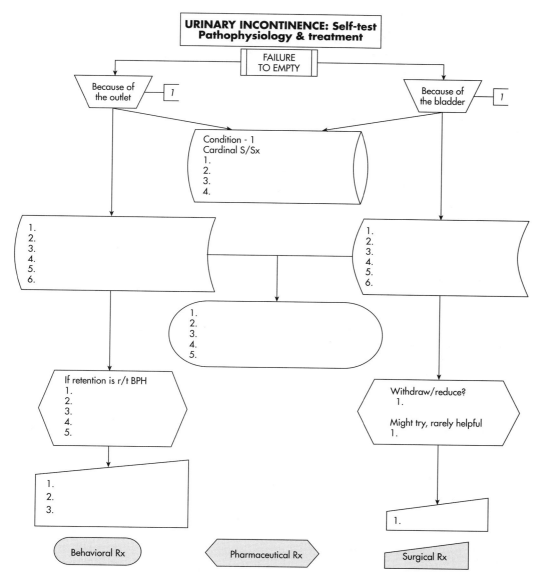

URINARY INCONTINENCE: Self-test
Pathophysiology & treatment

FAILURE TO EMPTY

Because of the outlet   1

Because of the bladder   1

Condition - 1
Cardinal S/Sx
1.
2.
3.
4.

If retention is r/t BPH
1.
2.
3.
4.
5.

Withdraw/reduce?
1.

Might try, rarely helpful
1.

Behavioral Rx

Pharmaceutical Rx

Surgical Rx

Copyright by Marta Krissovich, 1996; updated 3/15/05.

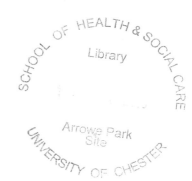
SCHOOL OF HEALTH & SOCIAL CARE
Library
Arrowe Park Site
UNIVERSITY OF CHESTER

Index